Textbook of
Communication
and
Education Technology
for Nurses

Textbook of Communication and Education Technology for Nurses

KP Neeraja
BSc BPR MSc (N) MA PhD
Professor in Nursing
Channapatna
Karnataka, India

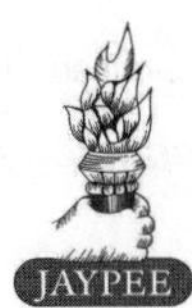

JAYPEE BROTHERS MEDICAL PUBLISHERS
The Health Sciences Publisher
New Delhi | London

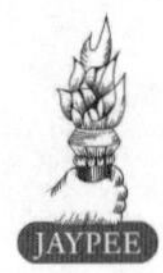

Jaypee Brothers Medical Publishers (P) Ltd.

Headquarters

EMCA House
23/23-B, Ansari Road, Daryaganj
New Delhi 110 002, India
Landline: +91-11-23272143,
+91-11-23272703+91-11-23282021,
+91-11-23245672
E-mail: jaypee@jaypeebrothers.com

Overseas Off ce

JP Medical Ltd.
83, Victoria Street, London
SW1H 0HW (UK)
Phone: +44-20 3170 8910
E-mail: info@jpmedpub.com

Corporate Office

Jaypee Brothers Medical Publishers (P) Ltd.
4838/24, Ansari Road, Daryaganj
New Delhi 110 002, India
Phone: +91-11-43574357
Fax: +91-11-43574314
E-mail: jaypee@jaypeebrothers.com

EU GPSR Authorised Representative

Logos Europe, 9 rue Nicolas Poussin
17000, La Rochelle, France
Phone: +33 (0) 6 67 93 73 78
E-mail: Contact@logoseurope.eu

Website: www.jaypeebrothers.com
Website: www.jaypeedigital.com

Inquiries for bulk sales may be solicited at: jaypee@jaypeebrothers.com

Textbook of Communication and Education Technology for Nurses

First Edition: 2011

Reprint: **2025**

ISBN 978-93-5025-350-2

Printed in India

Dedicated to

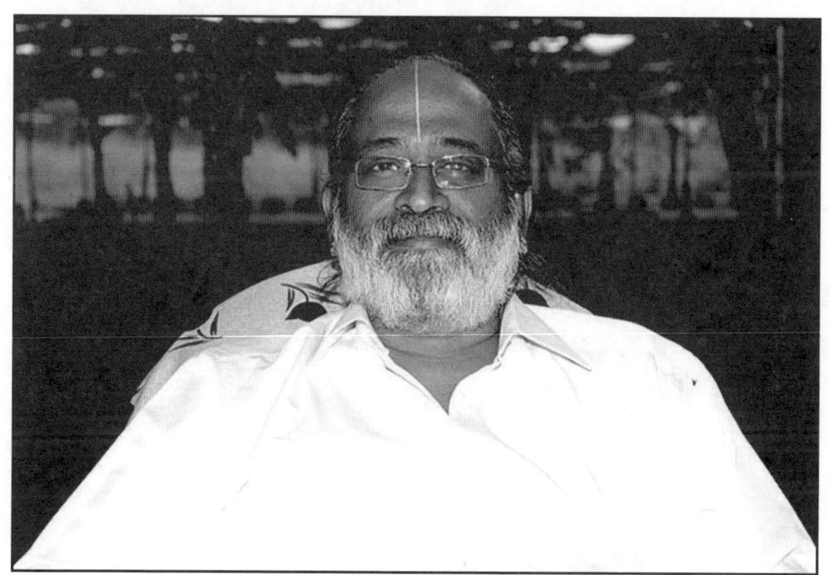

My Spiritual Father
Poojya Sri VV Sridhar Guruji

Foreword

With immense joy and honor, I am writing the foreword note for the present title the *Textbook of Communication and Education Technology for Nurses*. As a teacher of Dr KP Neeraja, I have seen her great contribution to the nursing profession by being an author of many textbooks in varied subjects. The knowledge, expertise, experience, dedication, determination, enthusiasm, and scholarship of Dr KP Neeraja's work can be seen in this textbook. This textbook has added another achievement in her life and a great treasure to the nursing knowledge. She is also a well-acknowledged author of many articles in the national and international journals.

Nursing is a scientifically rigorous discipline, which requires updated information on a regular basis to ensure best possible care provided to patients. The goal of nursing education is to develop scientifically sound nurses. To meet this goal, good nursing textbooks play a vital role. I am proud to announce that the timely publication of this book meets this gigantic task.

This textbook covers wide range of topics such as teaching methods, audio-visual aids, communication, health education, guidance, counseling and human relations. This book is useful not only for nurses but also for many other professionals such as doctors, psychologists, social workers, dentists, health educators, counselors, teachers, physical therapists, occupational therapists and many more professionals.

The great news for students about this book is, it covers the syllabus of Indian Nursing Council and various universities. It guides the nursing students to gain deeper theoretical knowledge and also the practical tips in teaching-learning process, audio-visual aids, communication, counseling, and guidance. The author has also provided questions of various universities questions at the end of the each chapter which will be helpful for the students for their exam preparation.

The faculty members of different disciplines will love to have this book on their reference shelf for day-to-day use in teaching the wide range of topics. I am sure it will become the Bible or Bhagavad Gita for the novice teacher as it walks through the teaching of subject matter in a simple way. The practical tips given in this book will help the inservice educator's to choose wide variety of topics to enhance the knowledge and skills of their learners.

The insight provided in this book meets the contemporary and future challenges that nursing students/ health team members and nurse/educators face, as care givers of the modern health care consumers. This book meets a compelling need to continue to prepare various health team members for leadership role in making health concerns a public priority.

I am confident that this book will receive a warm welcome by the nursing world and will go many more editions in future. I take this opportunity to congratulate Dr KP Neeraja and wish her all the best to write many more books of this kind and to be instrumental to the growth of nursing profession.

Mrs D Sujaya Lakshmi
MA (Anthro and Socio) MSc (N) MPhil (N)
Professor in Nursing

Preface

I obtained a great inspiration to write the *Textbook of Communication and Education Technology for Nurses* from my students and friends. During my interaction with them, they constantly encouraged and suggested me to bring out this new project. I am fortunate to have many well-wishers throughout the globe.

I took a few topics from my earlier books like Textbook of Nursing Education and Essentials of Mental Health and Psychiatric Nursing, Volume I and Textbook of Sociology for Nursing students.

The textbook comprises 15 chapters with schematic representations (wherever necessary). It covers mainly the syllabi of II BSc (N), PC BSc (N) and IV BSc (N), few topics will be helpful for MSc (N) too. At the end of each chapter, the various universities past years question papers like NTRUHS, RGUHS, MGRUHS, Kerala, Rajasthan and Punjab Universities of MSc(N), BSc(N), PC BSc (N) are given to facilitate quick attention of learners. It promotes a sensitive and holistic outlook in nursing education. I am confident that the book will meet adequately educator's as well as learner's needs. Maximum details given for each topic and language are made simpler and easier to meet the curricular requirements and quick understanding of topic. I am sure this book will serve as an ideal textbook for the professionals. I made earnest efforts to fulfill this need. Constructive criticism and suggestions are solicited to my e-mail ID: neerukp@yahoo.com

KP Neeraja

Acknowledgments

I would like to express a deep sense of gratitude to *"Almighty, the Creator"* who constantly provided support and blessed me in many ways in all my deeds in various forms.

With the deepest gratitude, I wish to thank my Spiritual Father *"Poojya Sri VV Sreedhar Guruji—Living Sai"* who gave consent immediately to my request, to dedicate this small token as "Puspham near to his Padam" . He blessed me to take up this project with lot of zeal in my mind and gave encouragement to pursue the work, I used to listen to his Gadyams continuously while working on the present work, which gave support in managing the stress associated with it and suggested the ways to overcome the problems.

I am very happy and indebted to my Teacher, *"Mrs D Sujaya Lakshmi"* who taught me "The Principles of Teaching" in 1986, agreed instantly to write a Foreword for my request.

I would also like to acknowledge and express my gratitude to *my students* (presently working in varied capacities as Teaching Faculty in Nursing Educational Institutions throughout the globe), *Seniors, Juniors, Friends, Teachers* and my son for their magnificent love, support and contributions in the creation of this book; without them I would not have completed the task fruitfully, they responded to my phone calls and assisted me in gathering materials with lot of interest.

My sincere thanks to Shri Jitendar P Vij, CEO, who responded and assured me by considering my request and made it possible to publish the book within a short span of time. I am very thankful to Mr Venu Gopal (Branch Manager) and Mr Ravi Kumar (Sales Manager) of Jaypee Brothers Medical Publishers (P) Ltd, Bengaluru who persistently provided support, motivated and given pressure that strived me to put hard efforts to achieve the task efficiently, cooperated with me and given valuable advice from the initiation to completion. I would like to appreciate and convey thanks to Ms Sunita Katla, PA to CEO, Mrs Samina Khan PA to Director-Publishing in head office for their patience, cooperation and strived sincerely along with me to publish the final draft of my book within limited time, these people are back force to complete this gigantic task competently.

Lastly, I would like to express my earnest gratitude to each member of my family who gave lot of mental support in accomplishing the task.

Contents

Philosophies of Education

PHILOSOPHY: AN INTRODUCTION

It is a scientific, systemic inquiry about the ultimate reality in the universe; it is the basis for understanding man. Etymologically, the term, 'Philosophy' has been derived from two Greek words: *"Philos"* means "love", *"Sophia"* means "wisdom". It is the loving and searching for wisdom and truth.

- 'Philosophy is the science of knowledge'—*Fitche*
- 'Philosophy is the science of all sciences'—*Coleridge*
- 'Philosophy is the mother of all arts'—*Cicero*

Philosophy refers to a certain way of thinking. It arises out of an attempt:

a. To arrive at the solution of a problem through the use of human reasoning and experience.
b. To find the deeper meanings of the problems.

Definitions

"Philosophy is a search for a comprehensive view of nature, an attempt at a universal explanation of nature of things"— *Henderson.*

"Philosophy is an unceasing effort to discern the general truth that lies behind the particular facts (i.e., the reality that lies behind the appearances)."

Meaning

- It is a search for a comprehensive view of nature, an attempt at a universal explanation of nature of things
- It is a living force, a way of life, an attitude towards life and a search for truth and reality. It is a speculation about the nature and value of things. It is a search for deeper and finer values of life
- Philosophy refers to, "Certain way of thinking, It arises out of an attempt – to arrive at the solution of a problem through the use of human reasoning and experience; to find the deeper meanings of the problems"
- Each individual should have a philosophy of life i.e., a set of standards, ideals which are based on the principles that he/she has chosen as being acceptable to him
- Philosophy is the study of the general principles and understanding all i.e., God, the world, and man himself, of origin, nature and the activities that come in the range of human experience. It is a comprehensive view of nature. Through philosophy man tries to understand himself and the world in which he lives. It answers the inevitable questions
- It is an inquiry into the wholesome of things
- It is what we believe and the principle which governs our life
- It is acting like a guide to have a concrete outlook on the world, life, human conduct and actions
- Philosophy is the earliest and the most original intellectual discipline
- Plato said, 'he who has a taste for every sort of knowledge and who is curious to learn and never satisfied may be termed as "philosopher"
- Questions of philosophical enquiry:
  - What is life?
  - What is man?
  - What is man's origin?
  - What is man's destiny or goal?

Philosophers try to answer these questions according to their own mature reflection and thinking.

These different answers lead to different philosophies, lives of great men prove that philosophy results in a certain way of life, beliefs, values and ideals formulated in terms of experiences and background of the person, who expresses them.

It is mostly an idea of what is possible and not a record of accomplished facts. Hence, it is hypothetical (it may or may not be proved true). There is no finality, it defines the difficulties and suggesting ways and means of dealing with them. Thus philosophy is described as a 'generalised thinking'.

Philosophy influences the daily life of every individual, it is particular way of looking at things, e.g. everybody will have their own philosophy of life i.e., some are pessimists, some are optimists, some are idealists, some are realists, some are materialists, some believe in destiny, some are atheists (do not believe in God) and so on.

Major Branches

- Metaphysics or discussion about the reality and the cosmos
- Epistemology or the theory of knowledge
- Ethics or the theory of morality
- Aesthetics or the discussion of beauty
- Logic or the study of ideal method of thought and reasoning

A well-marked attitude takes the shape of a particular school of philosophy or an 'ism'. There are different philosophical approaches, e.g. idealism, pragmatism, naturalism, realism, humanism etc.,

Relationship between Philosophy and Education

Philosophy, life and education are intimately linked with one another. Infact philosophy and education are like the two sides of the coin. While philosophy is the contemplative side, education represents the dynamic side (Table 1.1).

Thus philosophy is a major concern of education and there is, infact, an intimate relationship between philosophy and education. The truths and principles established by philosophy are applied in education. The arch of education will never attain complete clearness without philosophy. All the aspects of education are influenced by philosophy and there is a direct bearing between education and philosophy.

Philosophy Points out the way to be followed by Education

Education is the modification of child's behavior, whereas philosophy shows the way to be followed by educators in the modification of child's behavior. Education is a laboratory in which the philosophic theories and speculations are tested, thus education will be said as, 'applied philosophy'. Philosophy is wisdom, education transmits wisdom from one generation to the another.

Education is the best mean for the propagation of philosophy

A philosopher arrives at the truth after a great deal of contemplation on the real nature of the universe, man, his/her destiny and lays down aims, ideals and values and then he/she tries to live in accordance with them. He/she wants others to be converted his/her beliefs and live according to them, thus it can be achieved through education,

Table 1.1: Philosophy vs Education

Philosophy	Education
It sets the ideals, principles, goals, standards, values thus it is in reality and truth	Education works on values
It is the theory and speculative	It explains how to achieve the goals through man's educational efforts
It is the contemplative side	It is the practice
It deals with abstract ideas and ends the situations process	It is the active side (dynamic) It is the applied philosophy It deals with concrete and means
It is the art	It is the science
Philosophy formulates the method	It deals with the process of method

which is the best mean for the propagation of his/her philosophy. Education becomes more prominent than philosophy as action speaks louder than words or beliefs. Beliefs, philosophy are vital, thus it results in a prominent educational efforts.

All Great Philosophers are great educators

Philosophers reflected their views in their educational schemes. Most of the educational movements of the world own their origin to the philosophical schools of different philosophers. When a philosopher wishes to spread his/her ideals, beliefs, he/she formulates a scheme of education based on his/her philosophy, e.g. Socrates, Plato, Aristotle, etc. European philosophers like Locke, Rousseau, Spencer etc. were great educators. The great thinkers and philosophers of India are Goutham Buddha, Rabindranath Tagore and Mahatma Gandhi.

Philosophy determines the broad aspects of education

Philosophy provides aims of education, it determines the curriculum (course of study), methods of teaching, school discipline, role of teacher, school problems etc. philosophy will continuously influences and determines both the matter and the method of education. Thus philosophy contributes to the development of the educational theory and practice.

Influence of Philosophy on different aspects of Education

Philosophy and Aims of Education

Philosophy is the determining force in laying down the aims of education. Aims of education (moral, vocational, intellectual and spiritual) are based on views, ideals, beliefs, values, standards of philosopher. The philosopher struggles hard with the mysteries of life and arrives at his/her solution after mature reflection and thinking. He/she will suggest the ways and means of dealing with them through educational efforts. The educator selects the material for instruction, determines the methods of procedures for the attainment of goals. Thus the entire educational system proceeds with its foundation on sound philosophy, e.g. Idealism believes in self-enhancement and Naturalism prefers self-preservation.

Philosophy and Curriculum

Curriculum is the sum total of all the activities and experiences provided by the school to its pupil to achieve the aims of education. The philosophy determines the content and discipline that will promote curriculum. It is not fixed at all times, it changes in accordance with philosophy. Thus, curriculum differs with different schools of philosophy according to their own beliefs. Thus education needs leaders, who hold a sound comprehensive philosophy through which they can convince others and who can direct its consistent application to the formation to the function of appropriate curriculum.

The content of curriculum varies according to the philosophy it follows. For example:

Idealists emphasize higher values of life and prescribe the study of religion, ethics, logic, literature, arts and humanities.

Pragmatists advocate the study of functional subjects and social sciences, practical arithmetic, arts and crafts in their curriculum.

Naturalists are mainly concerned with Physical Sciences and direct experiences. The subjects are selected according to the aptitude and ability of the learner.

Philosophy and Textbooks

The textbooks must reflect the prevailing values of life fixed by philosophy, an appropriate textbook must be in accordance with norms of knowledge which the children are expected to know and accepted ideals of the society and the prevailing philosophy of education and the nation as a whole. Then only it will serve the desired purpose. The persons who select the textbooks must have standard of judgment, which should enable them to select the right type of books based on standard, supplied by philosophy. Through textbooks, the aims of education are realised. It will meet needs of ideals and principles.

Philosophy and Method of Teaching

Philosophy is a way of thinking and a way of working. Method is the process of establishing and maintaining contact between the pupil and the subject matter. Every system of education has its own method of teaching based on its own philosophical background. Method is the procedure through which aims of education are realised. Thus different schools of philosophy have laid down their own methods of teaching. For example:

- Idealism: advocates question, answer, lecture and discussion methods
- Naturalism: emphasises child-centred methods, like learning by doing and direct experience
- Pragmatism: recommends project methods, problem-solving method and socialized techniques

Philosophy and Discipline

Philosophy determines the nature and forms of discipline. Discipline is nothing but the conduct of the pupil. Internal discipline is concerned with inner code of conduct of the individuals sustain a nation. Philosophy and education are inseparably linked, they exist together, philosophy leads and education follows the path shown by philosophy. Discipline is mainly governed by the aim of education.

'Spare the rod and spoil the child' was the maxim for the guidance of teachers. In the past, perfect order and silence prevailed in the educational institutions, now we insist on self-government of students and free discipline.

Philosophy and the Teacher

Teacher is the backbone of the entire process of education. Philosophy of life should be in perfect consonance with the philosophy; the educational system is based on successful teachers. A teacher needs the study of philosophy as a person and as a teacher. A teacher is also having his/her own ideas and beliefs. Teacher influences the personality of the child and instills in him a new outlook and a new way of life. For example:

- Idealistic teacher is a person of high ideals, ethics and morals, he/she is role-model for the group of students
- Naturalism sees the teacher as the stage-setter and works behind the screen
- In pragmatism teacher is a friend and guide the pupil, facilitating the process of the growth of individual

Philosophy and Evaluation

Evaluation is the pivot of education system. It determines the extent to which aims and objectives are being attained, but also helps to bring about an improvement in the techniques and procedures of education. There is a close relationship between objectives, learning experiences and evaluation. It is therefore legitimate to ascertain how far our evaluation programme is in conformity with the philosophy that has determined the aims and objectives of education, its curriculum and its methodology. Evaluation takes into account the growth of the learner as a person with total personality development and in his/her total environment. Philosophical analysis, which is responsible for the movement of objectivity in the field of relationship between philosophy and environment.

General Impact of Modern Philosophies on Education

Common elements in all modern philosophies:

- Education has been psychologies, instructions are based on learner centred, individual differences have been recognized
- The principle of activity i.e., learning by doing is the common watchword
- Social discipline is a patent factor of educational development, the learner has to be trained for community life
- Democracy has been developed and it is the guiding factor of educational practices
- There is a scientific outlook on all matters of life
- The concept of discipline in education has undergone a radical change

Importance of Educational Philosophy to a Teacher

- To understand and accept the prevailing values of the society
- It results in intellectual development of the teacher
- It helps to improve the standard of his/her life
- It guides and improves the state properly
- It helps to bring about changes in various aspects of education
- It reforms the society

Principles of Education

The word 'principle' has two related meanings — A fundamental truth and a precept that serves to guide one's own actions (e.g. an educator).

Principles of education are generally accepted truths and precepts upon which educators has to base their decisions regarding educational outcomes and how best they can be achieved. These principles are the criteria by which an educator's efforts may be evaluated. They are also the 'guiding lights' for lesson planning and curriculum development.

1. Principle of Perception

Perception is a key issue in education, "The capacity to perceive, is the precondition to many forms of development" e.g. Cognitive, Affective, Musical, Kinaesthetic Perception etc.

The act of perceiving involves much more than just the functioning of our senses. Seeing, touching, hearing and feeling are simply the means of taking the information. For example:

- When I hear and see an ambulance. I perceive that someone is in need of and will receive medical attention or in emergency.
- I see markings on a piece of paper. I perceive words (provided I know the language) and I perceive meaning.

2. Principle of Integration

- To integrate means to bring together so as to form a whole
- There are various ways the principle of integration may be applied in education
- In order to learn, new information needs to be assimilated and this means integrating it with existing concepts, linking different concepts together to form conceptual wholes. This process is what allows one to form generalisations, draw conclusions, see new possibilities, make deductions, make judgments, compose and/or improvise music etc., indeed, it is fundamental to all but the most basic forms of mental activity
- Integration is central to interdisciplinary teaching, where knowledge and experience gained in different 'disciplines' is brought together around common themes, concepts and skills. One of the critical outcomes for education — An understanding of the world as a set of related systems, meaning that problem - solving contexts do not exist in isolation
- Integration also refers to "The bringing together of students from different ethnic and social backgrounds". But this is of little value if the content of education is drawn from one culture only. Education needs to be multicultural. Perhaps, it needs to be intercultural. As important to intercultural learning as is the understanding and appreciation of cultural differences is the recognition of similarities and common values.

3. Principle of Environmentalism

- Environmentalism essentially means concern and care for the environment. In contemporary usage, it generally refers to concern and care for the natural environment and to efforts to save the natural environment from the negative impacts of human development. Developing in students a commitment to environmental protection should be one of the primary concerns of education and of all educators (even music educators)
- But as a principle of education, environmentalism employs the broader definition of environment as the totality of external influences or factors affecting an individual. It is a recognition that what an individual becomes in life, is more dependent on external factors than on his/her genetic inheritance. There are several environments in which an individual finds him/herself, e.g. social, cultural, linguistic, physical, political, educational etc. The school and the various more specific environments that it comprises (e.g. classrooms) are controlled variables, meaning that the influence they exert on the learner can be controlled and made optimal for the purposes of education
- The quality of the learning environments that educators create is obviously one of the most crucial factors in the achievement of educational outcomes. The most successful learning environment is one that provides sensory experiences relevant to the learner, in terms of his/her social-cultural background, developmental levels, interests and psychological needs. It must also provide sensory experiences relevant to the current learning content (subject matter)
- A learning environment has several dimensions: visual, aural, tactile, social (interpersonal) and psychological. In all of these, the educator exercises a high degree of control.

4. Principle of Holism

- The principle of holism recognises that perception is a complex, multidimensional process that involves the whole self. It is not merely a process of taking in information. In order for incoming information to acquire meaning and to lead to purposeful action, it must be integrated or assimiliated into existing structures within the brain. Education is essentially about developing the concepts needed for the achievement of educational outcomes. A concept is an integrated whole that has cognitive and affective dimensions. Many concepts also are psychomotor or kinaesthetic, especially in music
- Concept development involves both divergent and convergent thought processes. Divergent thinking is where the mind, as the result of some stimulus (e.g. an idea, concept, problem, sensory experience etc.) makes links connections or associations with existing concepts or ideas already stored in the brain. Convergent thinking is where related concepts are integrated with the incoming information to form new and more complex concepts that may take the form of conclusions or generalisations

5. Principle of Developmentalism

To develop means "to advance, to expand or to grow into a more complex or complete form". The purpose of education is to develop individuals, ideally to the level of self-actualisation i.e. the fullest possible development of innate potential. In this regard, different forms of development are involved that correspond to different dimensions of being, i.e. cognitive, affective, spiritual, social, kinaesthetic, moral, aesthetic, creative, artistic etc.

For education to be properly developmental, it must proceed in accordance with ways in which human beings grow in all the ways identified above. Many forms of human development follow universal patterns that can be conceived in terms of stages and/or hierarchies.

6. Principle of Motivation

'Motivation' as per *Encarta World English Dictionary* has four meanings.

1. Giving of a reason to act: the act of giving somebody a reason or incentive to do something.
2. Enthusiasm: A feeling of interest or enthusiasm that makes somebody want to do something, or something that causes such a feeling.
3. Reason: A reason for doing something or behaving in some way.
4. Psychology: Forces determining behavior: the biological, emotional, cognitive, or social forces that activate and direct behavior.

Often a student's participation in the learning situation is motivated by the felt need to please others (teacher, parents, peers) or at least to meet their expectations. The orientation is outward and the motivation is said to be *extrinsic*. The need for acceptance (belongingness or love) has not been gratified sufficient that another need can become the impetus for action, e.g. the need for self-actualization. Motivation is *intrinsic* when it comes from within, not in response to external demands or prospects, but in response to individually felt needs and desires.

Extrinsic motivation is where participation in the learning activity is prompted by the prospect of either reward or punishment. It derives from factors outside or extrinsic to the learning situation, e.g. praise, marks, certificates, competition, special privileges etc. Extrinsic motivation can be either positive or negative. The latter can derive from the threat of punishment, sarcasm and ridicule.

Intrinsic motivation is inherent in the learning situation. The subject matter and/or activity arouses the student's interest and she/he participates willingly, not requiring extrinsic motivations such as rewards or punishments. When the outcomes of the learning situation are meaningful and relevant for the learner, extrinsic motivation is not likely to be necessary.

Abraham Maslow's conception of motivation involves a hierarchy of needs: for physiological well-being, for safety, for "belongingness" and love, for esteem, for self-actualization. Maslow suggests that once the needs at a lower level are gratified, the individual then becomes concerned with needs at the next higher level. When a need is gratified, it no longer acts as a motivator of behavior. The mature person, as Maslow sees him, is characterized above all by an ongoing process of "self-actualization." The mature person's behavior is no longer heavily dependent on what other people do to him/her or what they think or feel about him/her: He/she has been set free to explore the world and to discover new potentialities in himself/herself, which he/she can then try to define.

7. Principle of Inter-culturalism

The prefix 'inter' means "between; among; together; mutually or reciprocally" (*Webster American Dictionary*). Whatever root it is applied to, interaction is denoted, e.g. interdependent, interdisciplinary, international etc.

The concepts mutuality and reciprocity are particularly relevant when it comes to intercultural education. They are essentially synonyms and suggest that each of the cultures that are brought into interaction benefit and that the interaction is characterised by a shared sense of respect and openness.

Intercultural education is necessarily multicultural education. However, the reverse is not always true. One can learn about another culture without developing a respect for it and without discovering and appreciating common values, practices, customs and attitudes. In short, multicultural education does not necessarily stress interaction.

8. Principle of Outcomes based Education

Firstly, and most importantly, that education will always be based on outcomes. Most educators would argue that their work has always had this feature in that the achievement of outcomes (knowledge and skills) has always been the central concern of their efforts. The issue of specificity deserves some elaboration. The aims of a lesson (educational activity) should be presented as 'behavioral objectives' that state precisely what students are expected to do that gives evidence of and provide a means of assessing the learning that takes place. The 'doing' (behavior) needs to be identified in the setting out of the objective/outcome by an action verb. Verbs such as "Know, Understand and Appreciate etc." are not action verbs and should not be used therefore.

OUTCOMES: At the conclusion of the lesson the students will be able to:

1. Perform the Procedure systematically
2. Define the terms
3. Describe or explain in detail by understanding meaningfully.
4. Make at least three informative statements about the procedure

While being outcomes—Based is OBE's defining characteristic, other characteristics are generally acknowledged. These are:

* Increased learners' participation.
* The replacement of detailed and prescriptive syllabi with interdisciplinary 'themes'.
* A change in the role of teacher from dispenser of knowledge to facilitator of self-directed learning in an optimally interactive environment.
* Greater accommodation of individual differences in learning style and pace.
* Greater involvement of parents and public.

9. Principle of Multiple Intelligences

Related to the principle of holism is the recognition that the traditional idea of intelligence (as measured by IQ tests) is narrow and fails to account for the full range of human potential.

In 1983, Howard Gardner, professor of education at Harvard University, proposed his/her theory of multiple intelligences in which he/she identifies eight different intelligences:

* Linguistic intelligence ("word smart")
* Logical-mathematical intelligence ("number/reasoning smart")
* Spatial intelligence ("picture smart")
* Bodily-Kinesthetic intelligence ("body smart")
* Musical intelligence ("music smart")
* Interpersonal intelligence ("people smart")
* Intrapersonal intelligence ("self smart")
* Naturalist intelligence ("nature smart")

Gardner sees these intelligences as being autonomous faculties that can work individually or in concert with one another.

Functions of Education

A "purpose" is the "fundamental goal of the process—an end to be achieved. For example: Acquisition and transmission of Knowledge and information. " Functions are the "outcomes that may occur as a natural result of the process— by products or consequences of schooling", e.g. getting an award or degree after completion of duration of programme.

- Formation of healthy, social and formal relationships among and between students, teachers and others
- To predict future outcomes (decision-making).
- To seek out alternative solutions for solving the problem.
- To follow moral practices and ethical standards acceptable by society/culture.
- To develop communication and interaction skills, Understanding of human relations, ability to recognize and evaluate different points of view and ability to live a fulfilling life.
- To maintain self respect and give respect to others.
- Teach the cultural aspects of education.
- Capacity/ability to earn a living: career education by teaching job specific skills to have a livelihood.
- Capacity/ability to be a good citizen.
- Promotes sense of well being and creative thinking.
- Attains self esteem, self efficacy, self realization.
- Acquisition/clarification of personal values.
- Socializes people into key cultural values such as equality of opportunity, competition and religious morality.
- Emphasizes moral responsibilities in society that people should have towards each other.
- Higher talented people are given the most functionally important jobs for the society.
- Education produces the quantum of manpower that the economy needs at any time.
- Education equips manpower with skills.
- Adjust manpower to the changing needs of the society/economy.
- Revision of curricula in response to the dynamic rate of the economy.
- Qualities develop in individuals by education are: Honesty, respect, resourcefulness, truthfulness, handwork, leadership, faithfulness, initiative, creativity , punctuality, drive, foresight, regularity, Independence, reliability, care of public property, pomposity (tactical diplomacy).
- Functions towards individual—Education as integrated growth, trained for effective group life and social intercourse by a matured person. India is a land of diversities. There are diversities of religion, caste, languages, diet, dress, habits and physical environment. It is the function of education to bring unity in this vast diversity. Only then the best interest of the nation can be served and preserved.
- Dependence—Decreases as the child grows older and older, learns to obey and cooperate with others.
- Adaptability—Learner tries to adjust himself to his/her environment. He/she learns lot from his/her family and neighbourhood, It helps him greatly in adapting himself to situation and circumstances for the future. Thus his/her quality of adaptability provides the child with necessary power for developing habits and attitudes.
- Education as direction—Proper direction will enable children to have worthy interests in different phases of life. Direction is of two types—The environment which provides the child with a stimulus for his/her activity is external, while responses to that stimulus which process from his/her internal tendencies are internal.
- Education as preparation of individual for responsibilities and privileges of adult life children of today are adult of tomorrow. It is, therefore that preparation of individual child for responsibilities and privileges.
- Functions toward society—Education as a social function—Man is a social animal, he must live in and for society. In a social environment, a child's personality can develop best. The individual becomes what he/she actually is, mainly as a result of the interaction with his/her social environment. The mature members of the society pass on their own as well as their ancestors experiences, interest, findings, conclusions, traditions and attitudes to the younger and immature members of the society. All this has a great influence on the growth and development of the younger generation. In this way, the continuity of a society is maintained.
  - Education as continuous reorganization and integration of activities and experiences. We have to raise our people from local narrow prejudices of caste, community, region and provincialism to a broad national outlook. This is the domain of education.
  - Learner is active by nature. He/she cannot sit still. He/she must be busy in one activity or the other and this activity leads to his/her growth. It is, therefore, that growth never stops. It continues throughout life. If education is growth, as we have already noted, it must also never stop. It should also continue

throughout life. Thus in the growth and development of a learner, education plays the most vital part. It not only provides the learner with the rich resources of a good society but also induces him to make his/her own contribution on the maintenance and development of that society. Thus, by give and take process, the growth and development of the individual as well that of the society to which he/she belongs, is ensured.

– Conservative—Preserving all the old tradition, values, ideals, worthwhile customs and way of living
– Transmittive—Transmitting the culture heritage to the younger generation.
– Progressive—Reconstructing new experiences, unfolding new dimensions of knowledge, developing new capacities in the individual and furthering civilization and culture.
– Functions toward Nation—Inculcation of civic and social responsibility.
  The most important function of education in our national life is to make the rising generation, understand its rights and duties as individual citizens of a democratic country. It is because the very existence and progress of a nation depends on the proper education of the future generation. It is through education that social traditions, ideals and values are passed on to the future generation. These ideals and values strengthen democracy and reconstruct society.
– Training for leadership—Successful functioning of democracy needs efficient leadership in all spheres. of social, political, religious and educational activities therefore, the function of education is to develop qualities of leadership among the rising generation, for the service of the nation.

NURSING EDUCATION

Philosophy

It includes beliefs and values with regard to man in general and specifically man as the learner, teacher, nurse and the client and the beliefs about health, illness, society, nursing, and learning etc. Traditionally nursing education had adopted 'Children Philosophy' which was based on 'super-naturalism'. According to it, God is creator, redeemer and provider of man and the universe. The maxims of Christian philosophy are 'Love of God' and 'Love thy neighbour'. Every phase of nursing education has influenced by the philosophy upon which it is based.

Christian Philosophy considers man to be dualistic in nature i.e. man was created by God as a unit, (a composite made up of a body and a soul, possessing intellect and the likeness of God) and he/she was created for the purpose of serving him in heaven. Education based on this philosophy takes in all aspects of human life with the view in regulating and perfecting life in accordance with life of Christ, by which man may attain the eternal end for which he/she was created. It affects all aspects of the nursing student's life, i.e. spiritual, moral, intellectual, emotional, physical and social as they relate to the preparation of a Christian nurse motivated by supernatural motives. According to Christian philosophy, nursing is considered as, 'Profession of Charity'.

Spiritual Aspects

Religion should serve as the primary integrating factor in the development of the curriculum in a school of nursing. The principles of religion and morality are unchanging. By this stable truth, the nurse will be able to meet intelligently the changing conditions of modern social living. Religion provides the motives for the nurses to work effectively through religious principles.

Moral Aspects

Through understanding of moral principles governing man's conduct and action leading to the nurses to study 'ethics' (it is the philosophic science of human acts) from the point of the view of the order they should regard one another and man's ultimate destiny which they ought to help him to achieve and it also teaches the individual how to judge accurately the moral goodness or badness of any action. Nurse has to apply right conduct, in various situations of her/his daily life based on a sound moral character, adequate understanding and habitual application of proper moral standards. Nurse has to develop right conscience.

Intellectual Aspects

To provide a systematic development and training of the intellect, so that it may be enlightened, disciplined and disposed to function in accordance with the purpose for which it was created.

For the fulfillment of nursing functions, nursing education will give training in:
- Memory
- Direction of imagination
- Strengthening and expansion of the capacity for association
- Cultivation and training of the intellect
- Judge wisely
- Reason soundly
- Acquire prudence, wisdom and intellectual virtues
- Impart knowledge
- Provide opportunity for the student to analyse nursing care situations and problems, to apply various theoretical knowledge and skills in the field of clinical situation
- Development of communication skills, interpersonal relationship skills and interactional skills to express their thoughts.

Emotional Aspects

Nurse must be able to function as a mature, self-dependent and responsible individual and must be able to relate well to other people. It shows emotional maturity where by all her emotional needs were met.

The primary emotional needs are:
- Affection and love
- A feeling of belongingness
- Achievement or status i.e. prestige or self-esteem
- Approval from the group and from the authority figures

These needs must be met, if the student has to mature into a well integrated personality and who can use mature judgment and make the decisions in professional life.

Physical Aspects

To promote the harmonious development, physical needs also has to be met, to preserve her/his body and the essentials of her/his health. Nurse should have knowledge of how to guide others, who need assistance in learning, how to keep well or how to improve health.

Social Aspects

Nurse is a social being, who must work in society in relation to which, she has both privileges and obligations. Nursing is linked with social culture, in which nursing activities are carried out. The nursing student should be taught, to use her/his will power in gaining control of her/his own impulses. To acquire self-mastery and to be a virtuous member of a social group, nurse practices democratic principles.

Nursing is a service to individual, families and to the society. It is based upon art and science, which mold the attitudes, intellectual competence and teaching skills of the individual nurse, to help the people sick or well, to meet their health needs in medical direction.

Nursing is a social institution where:
- An organised group of people working together toward a common goal directly concerned with the welfare of the people
- A way of acting, specific to the group for the accomplishment of a common goal. The responsibility of nursing includes:
  - Prevention of illness
  - Promotion of health
  - Direct supportive and therapeutic care
  - Rehabilitation
  - Body-mind-spirit unity.

During the course of time, changes have taken place in the field of education, health care, sociocultural aspects, science and technology. There was need for change in the existing value systems and beliefs; changes had taken place in the field of nursing and nursing education also. It is not advisable to adhere to only one type of philosophy so, the nursing also is following the path of electism, i.e. to draw the best and useful aspects from various educational philosophies and make one's own philosophy.

Nursing is concerned with human welfare, it acknowledges the uniqueness of each individual. It considers health as a fundamental human right. Nursing is a service to individual, people or community without any distinction between caste, creed, sex or color, rich/poor, age or religion. Hence nursing is concerned with a philosophical outlook, i.e. 'the individual has intrinsic value and there is worth inherent in human life'.

Nursing requires critical thinking, logic and judgment; it is a problem-solving and decision-making process, nurse has to use a rational activity. Nurse is legally and morally accountable person.

The learning experiences should equip the learner with skills in problem-solving, decision-making and critical thinking.

Nursing actions are based on scientific principles, which are drawn from biopsychosocial sciences. Nursing curriculum should include Physical Sciences, Biological Sciences, Anatomy, Physiology, Microbiology and other relevant subjects.

Nurse will have active voice as a democratic citizen has some control over and responsibility for the political, legal, and social milieu related to health care matters, in which she/he lives.

Nurse is a socializing agent, consumer, advocate and protector. She/he has to play active role in bringing social change.

Nursing is a process to attain an end. It includes:
- Inherent purpose: The optimum level of well-ness of health of the individual
- Internal organisation: The series of actions to attain the aim of optimum level of wellness of health of the individual
- Infinite creativity: The dynamics of evolving unique, effective, efficient nursing activities for the achievement of the goal of optimum health

Nursing is a crucial component of multidisciplinary healthcare system, it reflects the independent, dependent and collaborative positions of the nurse involving respective functions. Nursing evolves as a holistic process with central and common philosophy, purposes, knowledge and functions. Nursing is a profession and nursing practice must reflect professionalism, professional adjustment and research.

Nursing roles in the order of priority are: Educative, Preventive, Promotive, Rehabilitative, Therapeutic and Supportive.

Democratic processes include in nursing role are: Authority by mutual consent, individual accountability, group activities, leadership and organizational set-up.

The requirements for professional nursing care includes: Clinical knowledge, judgment, technical competency, health knowledge, teaching skills, realisation of professional responsibilities. Philosophy will determine the selection of students, preparation of faculty, development of curriculum, attitudes towards client and community, personal life and professional growth of students and faculty.

It must be specific about the specialized functional roles and responsibilities within a profession and society. The purpose of nursing education is to prepare a person who can fulfill the role, functions and responsibilities of professional nurse within the society. The philosophy is developed by each faculty of individual school of nursing together with nurse leaders and nurse administrators. It should be clearly stated and directly related to the aims.

Concept and Meaning

"The unique function of the nurse is to assist the individual, sick or well, in the performance of those activities contributing to health or its recovery or to peaceful death thus he/she would perform unaided, if he/she had the necessary strength, will or knowledge and to do this in such a way as to help him to gain independence as rapidly as possible"— The concept of Nursing, Virginia Henderson (1958).

The essential components of professional nursing practice (according to American Nurses Association) include: care, cure and coordination. Nursing is based on scientific principles (systematized knowledge) and an art i.e., composed of skills that require expertisedness and proficiency for their execution.

Nursing is a dynamic, therapeutic and educative process in meeting the health needs of the society. Assisting the individual or family to achieve their potential for self-direction.

Education brings change in behavior of the individual in a desirable manner. It aims at all-round development of an individual to become mature, self-sufficient, intellectually, culturally refined, socially efficient and spiritually advanced.

Nursing education brings changes in the behavior of student nurse so as to prepare her/him to perform his/her roles effectively as an individual and as a good responsible citizen.

Strategies

Three phases are included in Nursing Education.

Pre-Nursing Education

The information about Nursing, to the prospective candidates, publicity and guidance about nursing education and its' prospectives, Orientation to nursing services, working conditions of nurses, career development, job avenues, opportunities and responsibilities of nurses etc. will be given. Booklets or brouchers can be developed like 'nursing as a career' 'profile of a nurse'. The prospective students can introspect, think, discuss and make a right decision. Careful and intelligent planning is required to develop personal and professional Career.

Nursing Education

Nurse educators has to select the candidate who is having interest for admission into nursing is the first step. They have to monitor continuously; implement the curriculum which consists of theoretical and practical hours of training in a critical manner, give equal weightage to develop the right attitudes, social and moral values, human relations, skills, ethics, civic sense, professional etiquette to have perfect background in nursing. Along with the technical skills, the personal qualities of the students also have to be promoted. Continuous evaluation of student's performance is essential. Educators have to take proper precautions to produce skilled and efficient nurses in order to provide qualitative health care services to the individual in specific and community in general.

Post-nursing Education

Nurse Educators has to develop teaching material and conduct research to improve the standards of nursing. Post-nursing education consists of orientation, supervision, inservice education, evaluation, research and registration.

After completion of the nursing training programme, the graduates or Diploma holders has to register their names along with education in professional organizations like State Nursing Council to be eligible to practice Nursing in the states and globally as registered Nurse, Midwife (Graduates and Diploma holders), Public Health Nurse (only for graduates); The membership will be renewed either annually or 2 - 5 years or life time membership (each council norms may varies).

The nurses after entering into job, still needs to be educated either in the form of in-service or continuing education, to update themselves to the modern technological advancement. The New graduates need to have a well-planned and organised orientation to the area of their posting. They must be oriented to the staff, equipment, working conditions and clients with whom they have to work. They need guidance and supervision in achieving professional standards. Nurses on the job must be evaluated periodically in terms of knowledge and performance and in-service education needs to be planned on the basis of their needs.

Steps for improving nursing education are: Development of educational material and Conducting Research and communicating its findings.

Historical Development of Nursing Education in India

- In 1871, Training for midwives were given for a period of six months with supervised nursing practice
- In 1918, first Lady Health Visitors course was started in Lady Reading Health School, Mumbai
- Later Diploma in General Nursing and Midwifery course was started with 3 years 9 months and later it was condensed to 3 years duration, again it was revised by INC now 3 years and 6 months
- In 1946, 4 years Basic nursing training programme started at RAK College, New Delhi and CMC Vellore
- In 1953, Post basic degree programme was started in Thiruvananthapuram
- In 1959, the first Master's programme in nursing was started at RAK College of Nursing, New Delhi
- In 1986, M Phil at RAK College of nursing, New Delhi was started
- In 1991, the first Doctoral programme in nursing was established in Institute of Nursing sciences, MV Shetty Memorial College, Mangalore.

Pattern of Nursing training programmes in India are:
- Vocational Nursing (at 10+2 level)
- Multi-purpose Health Assistants (after 10+2; 18 months duration)
- Diploma in General Nursing and Midwifery course (after 12 years of schooling, for 3 years and 6 Months)
- Basic BSc, Nursing (10+2 with sciences, 4 years duration)
- Post Basic BSc Nursing (after diploma nursing with 2 years of experience in clinical area and the course will be of 2 years duration)
- MSc (N) with any speciality (after BSc nursing with 1 year of experience either in teaching and in clinical area and the course will be of 2 years duration)
- M Phil in nursing (after MSc nursing the course will be of 1½ years–regular; 2 years–part-time)
- PhD in nursing (after MSc nursing 3 years duration—regular; after M.Phil nursing – 2 years duration)
- Short term courses—After diploma in Nursing (GNM). One year programs, like Neonatology, Oncology, Orthopedics, Cardiology and Neurology etc.
- IGNOU is conducting BSc(N) (Post basic and MSc (N) distance education programes.

Objectives of Nursing Education

- To prepare nurses who will provide expertized bed-side quality nursing care in the hospital
- Meets the needs of the individual, family in home in specific and educate the community in general. (Domicilliary Services – Home Health Services)
- To provide integration of health services and social aspects; theory and practice in generalized Public Health Nursing
- To provide an adequate, sound scientific foundation, intelligent nursing services to the needy population
- To understand the functioning of body and mind in health and disease
- To prepare nurses who will be able to work cooperatively with other health team members who will be engaged in health and welfare work
- To provide opportunities through curricular and extracurricular activities for the wholistic personality development of each individual student
- To ensure opportunities for initiative and resourcefulness, sense of responsibility for oneself and others with broad professional and cultural interest.

Purposes of Nursing Education

The basic purpose of nursing education is to prepare the nurses who, after completion of the educational programme, is able to plan for and provide comprehensive nursing care and health guidance to individuals and families according to their needs. The nurse must be prepared intellectually and morally enlightened and technically proficient. Nurse should be competent in teaching, oriented to community health and research-minded. Nurse must have the necessary knowledge, principles, skills and attitudes which are essential to professional nursing practices. Nursing students must develop competent health team members with sound judgment, intellectual and moral enlightenment, professional competence and expertise. The nurse educators should guide the learning activities of students by working as facilitators. The nursing educational training programme is to provide a broad based preparation with capacity building in students for doing the required nursing jobs with appropriate nursing interventions. The teachers should concentrate on the essential facts, skills and attitudes. The teachers should base their teaching on the nursing needs related to the real health problems of the community and in accordance with the job description.

FUNCTIONS OF NURSING EDUCATION

- The potential nurse with a fund of knowledge that she/he may draw upon during her/his career. The Knowledge of Psycho-social foundations, Biological Sciences help her/him to understand the biological foundation of illnesses as well as the psychological effects on those confronting a health care crisis, Such knowledge can help Nurse a more effective nurse
- Hands-on-practice—Nursing education typically asks student nurses to complete hands-on practice in a hospital during clinical training. During this time she will interact with actual patients under the watchful supervision of a licensed nurse with a background in nursing education. Hands-on experience can teach her

how best to practice such essential nursing skills, medication administration and patient charting. During this time she may turn to her/his supervisor and have the questions about patient care answered. This can help the nurse to enhance his/her skills in a low-stress environment.

- Different fields of nursing—An education in the field of nursing can provide a nurse with exposure to a variety of nursing specialties.
- Ongoing education—Nursing education involves yearly completion of a certain number of academic Theory as well as clinical hours. Completion of hours helps that, nurses have an up-to-date understanding of the latest advances in modern nursing theory, to undertake more tasks and to take more responsibility for their management of care of a client (individual or a community).
- Registration of nurses—The Graduates or the diploma holders has to register in state Nursing Councils to practice Nursing in respective country to protect the public - The public must be assured that nursing care, from the simplest to the most complex, is provided by properly qualified people who know what they are doing, know their limits and work within those limits and the legal protection of the nurse – if untoward situation arises protects the Nurses legally. As health professionals provide care in many fields and have many different skills, it is necessary that nurses work harmoniously together and collaborate with other health care providers for the good of the public. To that end it is important that each health professional knows as clearly as possible what may and may not be expected of each other.
- The role of the nurse in the future will encompass a wide range of activities from basic physical and mental care to complex technical procedures in the areas of health education, prevention of disease, treatment and rehabilitation in both the hospital and community.
- Nurses will need to continue to develop specialist skills in the face of advancing technology. The trend towards community care, the development of comprehensive planning organisations and the awakening of community consciousness of health needs will all act to emphasise the public health/community care.
- The nurse may become the primary contact worker or the nurse clinician and will need to be adequately prepared to bear broader health responsibilities.
- The generalist and specialist clinical functions have appropriately organised and supported by nurses carrying out management, teaching and research activities, because of the increasing dimensions in nursing in the future, it is believed that these supporting functions must now be expanded.
- Nurses should be encouraged to participate in the management of health care organisations and whenever nurses are involved in the outcome of decisions they should participate in the decision - making process.
- Scope of nursing practice—The promotion of holistic care, client focus, flexibility in practice, accountability, performance according to codes of ethics, conduct and competency standards, based upon appropriate educational foundations and on evidence of or research into practice.
- Most practitioners are engaged for most of their time in activities which can be described as core ie consistent with those depicted.
- Amplified or Expanded practice—"Within usual practice, some practitioners, stimulated by experience, increase knowledge and capacity for clinical judgement, perform activities or functions which have always been part of nursing practice, differently but more effectively".
- Extended practice—Nurse practitioners stimulated by the client's needs and guided by extensive experience and knowledge, will take on activities previously or currently performed by other health practitioners Amplify or extend role depends upon an expanded knowledge base evolved from experience and/or education
  - An expanded knowledge base evolved from experience and/or education.
  - A willingness to assume greater levels of responsibility.
  - Greater independence in practice.
  - An ability to critically reflect on practice.
- Practice in an emergency situation—Identifying the client's needs in an emergency situation, guided by extensive experience cond knowledge, the nurse will perform activities limited to this specific situation which would usually be performed by other health practitioners, to safely meet client needs in the specific emergency situation. The nurse's duty of care is contingent on his/her level of professional experience and education. The nurse in such a situation needs first to recognize that it is an emergency (and justify the definition of this situation as an emergency). If the treatment required would normally be provided by a medical practitioner or a well-equipped facility and if there is no danger to the patient in delaying treatment until these are available, there is no emergency and the nurse should accept the delay.

- The core scope of nursing practice is continuous with an encompassing area for amplification of practice. Amplification will be undertaken by some individuals, in some areas of their practice, through ongoing development of knowledge and skills. Along with experience, this increased level of performance will enable these nurses to undertake traditional nursing roles and functions differently and more effectively.
- The motive for the expansion of the scope of nursing practice is the delivery of more effective nursing care to clients. This extension is based on ongoing development of specific knowledge and skills.
- Nursing activities — that are congruent with the competencies of the nurse, where the client seeks assistance to meet activities of daily living because they are unable to assess and/or manage their own care.
- The client is the primary beneficiary of the nurse's actions, to provide contemporary nursing roles and functions aligned to consumer's needs.
- The practitioner can provide evidence that she/he has developed the knowledge, skills and attitude required for competent performance of the activity.
- The practice is based on prior educational achievement or validated outcomes of research.
- Delegation of Nursing Work—Nurses regularly delegate the responsibility for undertaking aspects of client's care to other people who may or may not be nurses, e.g. Nursing aids, Nursing assistants, the person to whom the activity is delegated has developed the knowledge, skills and attitudes required for competent performance of the activity.
  For example:
  - The client is stable
  - The person to whom the care is being delegated is competent to meet the complexity of the client needs
  - The impact on the client of the context and care giver within that context.
- Nursing is practiced in a variety of settings including homes, clinics, hospices, health centres, hospitals, workplaces and educational and research institutions.
- Recognize that nursing, in addition to clinical practice, may involve consultancy, administration, devising responses to changing health care needs. nursing is practiced in a variety of settings including homes, clinics, hospices, health centres, hospitals, workplaces and educational and research institutions.
- Recognize that nursing, in addition to clinical practice, may involve consultancy, administration, devising responses to changing health care needs.
- The roles of registered nurses in the education of patients and other nurses and as managers have been emphasised as needing further clarification and development.
- There is a need to recognize that the client's needs and of nursing services and that the client is knowledgeable about their own heath care needs and more demanding of quality services.
- To prepare competent and safe practitioners in a range of contexts. The use of core competencies is to frame nurse education, ensure there are consistent outcomes from education programmes for nurses at all levels, the current competencies are too global to effectively guide nurse education. The competency standards are only intended to inform curriculum development, not to produce a definitive curriculum. Nurse education may need to provide more development of undergraduate nurses in the areas of education and management.
- Nurses need to find new ways of ensuring that a continuum of care is provided.
- To prepare competent and safe practitioners in a range of contexts. The competency standards are only intended to inform curriculum development, not to produce a definitive curriculum.
- Education of nurses in the higher education sector should be continued in partnership with the health sector.
- Mechanisms for developing educational strategies to develop effective nursing leadership and management need to be established and supported.
- Managers need to be more flexible in their approach to work allocation.
- Nurses and society and the education sector need to appreciate the complexity of maintaining a skilled workforce, value that workforce and institute efforts to maintain viable numbers.
- To provide an adequate service based on a model of good practice.
- To convey a positive and contemporary image of its constituents and practice.
- Quality clinical placements are vital to the achievement of fitness to practise.
- Sufficient physical endurance, strength and mobility to perform required client care activities in a safe and effective manner for the entire length of the clinical experience, e.g. standing, walking, bending, squatting,

lifting or moving clients or objects weighing 25 to 50 pounds or more; Sufficient to perform manual psychomotor skills integral to patient care, e.g. Manipulate small equipment and containers (i.e., syringes, vials, ampules, and medication packages) to administer medication; Sufficient to independently assess patients and their environments, e.g. Collect data from recording equipment and measurement devices used in patient care, Detect a fire in a patient area and initiate emergency action and Draw up the correct quantity of medication into a syringe, Sufficient to physical monitoring and assessment, Sufficient to detect significant environment and client odors, e.g. Detect odors from client and environment; Sufficient to independently assess patients and to implement the nursing care plans that are developed from such assessment. For example: Detect changes in skin temperature, Detect unsafe temperature levels in heat-producing devices used in patient care, Detect anatomical abnormalities (i.e., subcutaneous crepitus, edema, or infiltrated intravenous fluid), Detect vibrations.

- Communication Ability: Sufficient ability to speak, comprehend, and write (print and cursive) in English and local language at a level that meets the need for accurate, clear, and effective communication eg: Give clear oral reports, Direct activities of others by providing clear written and oral instructions to others, Influence people's actions, Be able to communicate effectively on the telephone and Legibly convey information through writing.
- Sufficient to comprehend the written word, e.g. read graphs (i.e., vital signs sheets), Read and understand English print and cursive documents.
- Math Ability: Sufficient to do accurate computations, e.g. read measurement marks, Count rates, Read digital displays, Tell and measure time (i.e. count duration of contractions, etc.). For example: Accurately calculate medication dosages and intake and output.
- Critical thinking Ability: Sufficient to collect, analyze, integrate, and generalize information and knowledge to make clinical judgements and management decisions that promote positive patient outcomes. For example: Evaluate outcomes, Transfer of knowledge from one situation to another, Process information, Prioritize tasks, use long and short term memory, Problem solving.
- Emotional stability: Sufficient to assume responsibility/accountability for actions. For example: Establish therapeutic relationships and communicate in a supportive manner, Deal with the unexpected (i.e., client becoming critical, crisis), Handle strong emotions, Adapt to changing environment/stress, Focus attention on task and Monitor own emotions and be able to keep emotional control.
- Interpersonal Skills: Sufficient to interact with individuals, families and groups respecting social, cultural and spiritual diversity. For example: Negotiate interpersonal conflict, Establish positive rapport with clients, co-workers and faculty, Interact with others effectively.

Trends in Nursing Education

Records of civilization in ancient India exist from 2500 BC when the Indus valley civilization flourished. The sacred 'books of learning' the "Veda" were produced in the Vedic period from 1500 BC. The history of nursing in India goes back through the centuries to about 1500 BC. The beginnings in Nursing Education are shrouded in the mist of ancient myths (Wilkinson A. 1965).

The advent of Christianity and the teachings of Christ, which included the statements such as 'love thy neighbour as thy self', 'I was sick and ye visited me' enjoyed the care of the sick and the helpless. Charaka and Susruta leading authorities on the ancient Hindu system of Ayurveda (the science of life) though lived in the Christian era, they were not influenced by the Christianity. The following reference is found regarding the nurse in Charaka - Samhita:

Nurse: Knowledge of the manner in which drugs should be prepared and compounded for administration, intelligence, devotedness to the patient waited upon and purity (both of mind and body) are the four qualifications of the Nurse.

Subsequently, monastic orders further emphasized knowledge based health and nursing care. Nuns, monks had to acquire special knowledge and skills before being assigned to take care of the sick. The renounced Roman Matrons, Fabiola, Marceba and Paula stand out as early intellectuals associated with organisation of hospitals and nursing. Later, the many Christian religious orders emphasized the special knowledge needed by caregivers.

Modern Scientific Nursing: Nightingale's Model of Nursing Education

Florence Nightingale emphasized on cognitive knowledge and skills (1909). Preparation of nurses in Florence Nightingale's school of nursing at St. Thomas hospital included a years training with instruction by the Matron, the ward sister and the physician before assignment for 2-year hospital apprenticeship experience, during which students were granted stipends. These students were called 'ordinary probationers'. Those who did not receive stipend, but paid tuition for the first year were educated for higher positions and were called 'lady nurses'. Nightingale model of nursing education, the hospital based diploma school appears to have been the first model in almost all countries.

The most conspicuous and widespread modification of the Nightingale system had occurred in the United States and Canada and this is referred to as 'American system' or professional model in contrast to the British or Nightingale's apprenticeship model. A span of 60 odd years since nursing schools were first established in US divides itself into three periods of about 20 years each.

1. A pioneering period: 1873-1898

To provide decent conditions for both patients and nurses and to lay the foundations of an adequate nursing service.

2. Boom period in Nursing Education: 1893-1913

Every hospital wanted to have a school of its own. The number of schools of nursing increased tremendously. The young nursing profession organised its forces and tried its level best to control over expansion with the resulting slump in standards. Though laws were passed, variations existed in admission standards, in programs of instruction and also in the product of these schools.

Collaboration of nurse leaders in England and the US resulted in the funding of the *International Council of Nurses in 1899,* under the leadership of Ethal Fon Wick and Isabel Hampton. From its inception, the council worked toward professionalization of nursing in many countries and promoted national licensing, accreditation laws, and improvement in nursing education.

3. Period of standard setting and stock taking: 1913-1933

National League of Nursing Education under the leadership of Miss A Adelaide Nutting published standard curriculum for nursing schools in 1917. Nursing student's" preparation was service oriented rather than education oriented, as nurse educators did not hold advanced educational preparation. Gold Mark report identified many inadequacies in the education and concluded that advanced educational preparation was essential for teachers, administrators and public health nurses.

1940s–1960s: This period is considered as "Basic Science Era".

The Disease Body System Curriculum Model

The classic nursing curriculum model is the disease-based model, cross-gridded with body systems. In the curriculum the principles of nursing action lies in the disease itself:

- Disease or injury—etiology and nature
- Medical therapeutic management
- Nursing care.

Nursing care is deduced from knowledge of the disease and its medical treatment. In the traditional formulation of this curriculum model. Nursing trends to be highly programmed and prescriptive. For example: turn the patient Q2II, blood pressure Q4II etc. Nursing is dependent on the medical plan and medicine depended on the existence of the disease or injury.

Disease or injury/Medical plan/Nursing care.

Both Medicine and Nursing are derived through logical analysis of the preceding phenomena.

The method of the classic nursing curriculum is logistic with invariant relations among disease, medical therapy and nursing care. The curriculum focuses on the parts and is additive. Once the student learns all i.e., every disease then she/he is ready to graduate.

Another variant of the classic curriculum makes body systems than the disease entities. This alteration has the advantage of providing larger functional units: The body systems instead of the diseases. The components of the whole are how body systems rather than diseases and the curriculum is presented in logistic fashion.

In the 1940s, nurses concern for the whole person resulted in adding the psychosocial studies to the curriculum. This has supplanted the knowledge of the biologic systems which had previously dominated nursing education. With this change an emphasis on the interpersonal process in nursing intervention soon emerged. The focus in the 1940s led to the holistic approach in the 1950s in which the patient emerged as a logical focal point of the content presented in nursing schools and colleges. The person-centered approach conceptualized the patient as having common human needs and the goal of nursing was to meet these needs. Though systematic training in hospital schools had taken place, still traditional task oriented care was provided in hospital settings.

Brown (1948) a social anthropologist, reassessed nursing education at the request of national nursing council for war service, supported Winslow–Gold Mark report stressing on inadequacies in nursing education and stated that within 50 years, the education of nurses should occur in collegiate settings

1960s–1980s: Clinical Science Era

Impact of Abdellah on curriculum development:

Abdellah's work was the stimulus to two quiet different approaches to nursing – "A problematic approach and operational approach". The problematic approach led to two modes of care.

Those based on:

- Patient problems
- Nursing problems

The operational approach led to a typology of nursing acts and eventually to today's common focus on the nursing process – patient-centred approaches to nursing.

The Problem-based Curriculum Model

The selected problems may be patient problems or nursing problems. Often curriculum fail to differentiate between patient needs and patient problems. Such curricula often combine problematic and operational approaches, seeking solutions to patient problems and achievement of predetermined goals for patient needs. The principle of the curriculum is reflexive and rests on the interaction between man and his/her environment. A problematic mode allows for variance from patient to patient and from nursing act to nursing act. In the problematic method, each problem is considered to be unique and to have its own unique environment.

During the period nursing practice focused attention on individual / patient centred and family centered care. Social and behavioral sciences have occupied prominent role in curriculum research.

Nursing Education Programs

Masters', M.Phil and Doctoral programmes focussed on clinical specialization and on recent scientific advancements, issues or Problem oriented, Research advancements etc. Many nursing models emerge during this period, e.g. nurses role to promote behavioral stability of the patient (Johnson). Smith, Germaine and Gibbs (1971) identified specific nursing goals; prevention intervention model (Hodgman 1973) etc.

1980s–2000 AD: Political health - Scientific approach era

The model course around nursing acts. The curriculum is *operational* when focus is placed on selection among nursing acts. The curriculum is logistic when the acts are seen as an invariant sequence of steps to be followed with every patient, e.g. nursing process. In either case the focus is on what the nurse does, cognitive, psychomotor or affective behavior, basing on action principle stemming from the motivation to the act by the nurse agent. Nurse patient relationship promotes the sharing between nurse and the patient.

The movement of health for all and primary health care initiated people oriented, value based, holistic and humanistic approach to care.

Holistic Curriculum

Refers to the curriculum that takes a single subject matter in its entirely as the care of the educational programme. The most common subject matters are man and health.

1. Holistic curriculum asserts, the nursing is the profession that deals with the whole man in relation to his/her health.
2. Nursing is the profession, which deals with the 'whole of health' as it relates to man.

The curriculum focuses attention to the health and its relatedness to socioeconomic, cultural and political development, advancement in Bio-Medical Technology, Nuclear Medicine etc. Health can be perceived on a wellness-illness continuum. Birth to death life phase motion. Each course in such a curriculum is one reflection on the birth to death continuum, giving the student increased knowledge of the whole. Such a curriculum might organize its courses around life phases—infancy, childhood, adolescence, adulthood and old age.

People oriented/community oriented curriculum is geared to prepare nurse practitioners—community nurse practitioner, family nurse practitioner and in institutions—special units. Primary nursing is the answer to primary health care and primary nurse coming out of holistic curriculum would be able to participate in achieving health for all through primary health care organisation.

AIMS OF EDUCATION

Aim is a predetermined goal, which inspires the individual to attain it through appropriate activities. As education is a planned and purposeful activity, the aims are necessary in giving direction to the education (Fig. 1.1).

Factors determining Educational Aims

1. Philosophy of life: Education is the best means for propagation of philosophy. Philosophy and education are the two sides of a coin.
2. Elements of human nature, e.g. unfolding of the divine in man (Idealists).
3. Religious factors, e.g. buddha preached, ahimsa and truth are the two weapons which have to be prevailed in educational system.
4. Political Ideologies.
5. Socioeconomic factors and problems of the country.
6. Cultural factors—education has to preserve and transmit the cultural heritage and traditions from one generation to another.
7. Exploration of knowledge.

General Aims of Education

- Knowledge—it is essential for intellectual growth, good interpersonal relationship, healthy adjustment in life, modification of behavior, self-awareness and for social growth. Knowledge is power, attainment of knowledge is an important aim of education
- Complete living—education acquaints the person with activities of complete living, e.g. self-preservation, performance of social, political responsibilities and beneficial utilization of leisure time
- Harmonious personality development—harmonious cultivation of the physical, intellectual, emotional, mental, moral character and spiritual aspects of human development thus a well balanced personality development will take place with education
- Self-realization—education should help a person based on his/her potentialities what he/she is going to become
- Cultural development—every individual has to become cultured and civilized through education. Cultural development, if attained it gives refinement, aesthetic sense, concern and respect for others and their culture
- Vocational efficiency—education should prepare the child to earn his/her livelihood and make him self-sufficient and efficient economically and socially
- Citizenship—the child has to be educated to become a good citizen of his/her country. He/she should be beneficial to the society
- Leisure—leisure is a part of human life, where enjoyment and recreation occurs. It is needed to keep up rest and regain energy. Artistic, moral and esthetic developments can be inspired through the beneficial use of leisure time. Educate the child to utilize his/her leisure in creative and useful manner, based on ones' own interests, they can attain skills in the respective fields
- Development of leadership—Education should train the youth to assume leadership responsibilities in various fields like social, political, industrial and cultural fields

- Initiating the students to the art of living - education should enable a person to acquire the necessary interpersonal skills and adjustment abilities for successful and happy living together in society
- Education for increased productivity—education should help to satisfy this need through the production of manpower, i.e. people who are equipped with advanced scientific knowledge; complex, technical ability and efficient work experience
- Social and national integration–education should inculcate the feeling of oneness and belongingness
- Education for modernization–education should produce the people who are able to think and judge independently and effectively, intellectually efficient and technically competent persons must be prepared
- Education for cultivation of social, moral, spiritual values, and scientific advancement for national cohesion, socialism, secularism and democracy, fostering research in all areas of development, education for equality

Individual and Social Aims of Education (Ultimate Aim of Education)

Educational aims are correlative to the ideals of life. There are two ultimate aims of education—individual and social; of all other aims, these two are the most important because the remaining aims of education stress either the one or the other of these two. An individual is born with certain potentialities or natural endowments. It is the task of the education to develop them into a distinct individual personality. But personality development does not take place in a vacuum. It takes place in associating with others in co-operative living and in working together for the welfare of the group or society. We have to decide whether the individual and social aspects are totally contradictory to each other or is it possible to strike a balance between the two. In other words, it has to be decided whether the individual owes the existence to society or the society exists for the individual.

Educators who Emphasize Individual Aims of the Education

Rig Veda: Education is something which makes a man self-reliant and selfless.
M. Gandhi: By education, mean, an all round drawing out of the best in child and adult—body, mind and spirit.
Aristotle: Education is, the creation of a sound mind in a sound body.
Pestalozzi: Education is, the natural, harmonious and progressive development of man's innate powers.
Froebel: Education is the process through which the child makes internal and external.

Importance of Individual Aim

The Biologists Support to Individual

Aim of Education

Every individual is new and unique and different from others. He/she is a new experiment with life. We cannot change his/her nature just as we cannot change the color of his/her eyes. According to *Prof. Thompson* - "education is for the individual, its function is to enable the individual to survive and live out its complete life". Education is imparted to perceive the individual life. Community exists for the individual. Community being the means and individual being the end. Education should not set the means over the ends. Education is given for the sake of individual with a view to save him from destruction. Therefore, individual or not society should be the virtue of all educational efforts and activities.

The Naturalist's Support to the Aim

The naturalists like Rousseau and TP Nunn told that "the central aim of education is the autonomous (self) development of the individual". It is therefore that education should be according to nature which would make an individual what he/she ought to be. According to Rousseau, "everything is good as it comes from the hands of God, but everything degenerates in the hand of men". God makes all things good. Man meddles with them and they became evil.

The Psychologists Support to the Aim

The psychologists are of opinion that education is an individual process. No two children are identical in intellectual capacity and emotional disposition. It is therefore that a rigid and uniform curriculum for a large number of children is not justified. It should be replaced by a broad based and flexible curriculum. The work of education should be to find out the individual child's innate powers and possibilities and to provide the means by which he/she may enable to realize the highest of them. The teachers and books are the signboards to the road within.

The Spiritualists Support to Education

The spiritualists are of the view that every individual is a separate entity and responsible for his/her own actions. Since the spiritual development of man is individual the main function of education should lead the individual to self-realization and the realization of higher values in life. *Swamy Vivekananda* says, "Man is potentially divine. The goal is to manifest this potentiality within by controlling nature external and internal through education". *Lroothee* always said, "No one can be like another, but every one can be like the highest, how is that to be? Let every one be perfect in himself".

The Progressinists Support

According to this opinion, the progress and advancement of mankind is due to great individuals born in different periods of history. They include great scientists, inventors, explorers, religious leaders, social reformers and philosophers and the like. But for such individuals, the world would not have moved beyond what it was a few thousand years ago. It is only through the activities of such individuals that the world has become better and a happier place to live in. *Perry Nunn* says, "Nothing good enters the human. World expect in end through the free activities of the individual men and women and that educational practices must be shaped to accord with the truth". According to him, the purpose of educational efforts is to create conditions for the promotion of complete development of individuality.

Limitation of Individual Aims

- It makes an individual self-centred and indiscipline. He/she can be vain and only interested in his/her personal development and achievements. He/she is not interested in his/her fellow beings or society. The undisciplined person can be an undesirable individual in society. He/she will do anything perhaps, to gain his/her ends
- It ignores rich heritage: Great individuals have no doubt contributed much to the advancement and progress of mankind. But they could do so only after assimilating the rich heritage of thought and wisdom provided by society in the form of religion, tradition, arts and science

Social Aims of Education

As against the individual aim, there is the social aim of education. The individual is endowed with a social nature, he/she is social by instinct. An individual seems everywhere and always to be caught up in an intricate web of social relations. Without them the newborn baby would almost perish (The social process and the educational process are essentially one and the same). The individual cannot live alone by isolating from society.

The individual being a social animal will develop through special contact.

The social aim in its extreme form, regards the state as idealized super-human entity, over and above the individual. The state or society alone is the reality and the individual is only a throb in the social pulse. The state is the embodiment of reason, justice and morality. The individual is inferior to it in all respects. The supporters of the social aim of education do not conceive of an individual living and developing in isolation from society, in the words of *T. Raymont.* The isolated individual is a fragment of the imagination. According to *Ross*—individuality is of no value and personality a meaningless term apart from the social environment in which they are developed and made manifest.

According to *John Dewey,* social aim in education is stressed as education should make such individual to understand and appreciate the environment which he/she lives. He/she is ready to sacrifice his/her own desires if their satisfaction is harmful to others or if their gratification does not consist socially efficient and this social efficiency must be achieved by the positive use of individual powers and capacities in social occupations. A socially efficient individual is able to earn his/her livelihood. He/she also conforms to moral and social standards of conduct.

Gandhiji formulated the basic scheme with the objective of making people realize that education was not merely for the benefit of the individual, but for the needs of a predominantly rural and agrarian population.

State Socialism

The social aim of education in its extreme stage, neglects all the claims of an individual. Man is not born human, he/she becomes so. The state or society is superior to the individual in all respects. The individual citizen is totally subservient to the state, which is all powerful. The state has the right to mould and shape the individual so as to suit its own purposes or progress. The individual does not have the freedom to express his/her own views. The needs of society dictate the needs of education. The state uses the most convenient weapon for preparing individual to play different roles in society. He/she is to obey what the authorities dictate. His/her needs, usages and nature are completely ignored. The exponents of this school of thought believe in imparting education through social control and their watchwords in the educational process are discipline and obedience. The individual is to be given education not because he/she must develop his/her own individuality, but because he/she is required to serve the specific purpose, which the state has already determined. The state is supreme to dictate what shall be taught and how shall be taught. Discipline is its watchword, willing acceptance of authority is the method and obedience is the rule.

The social aim of education has been stressed upon by the following:

1. Education means the culture which every generation purposely gives to its successor in order to qualify, to keep and to improve the level attained — *Brown FJ.*
2. The teacher's aim is not to educate his/her students in the abstract, but for life in any existing society — *Bruebaker JS.*
3. Education is the process of reconstruction of experience, gives more socialized value through the medium of increased social efficiency—*Dewey.*
4. Education is an attempt in the part of the adult members of the human society to shape the development of the coming generation in accordance with its own ideals of life—*James Welton.*
5. True education involves three things:
   a. A sincere appreciation of one's country
   b. A readiness to recognize its weakness frankly and to wish for their tradition
   c. An earnest resolve to serve it to the best of one's ability, harmonizing and sub-ordinating individual interests to broader national interests.

The school has to build up this three-fold concept of patriotism. Thus the social aim of education finds expression in such concepts as education for social service, education for citizenship and education for social efficiency, e.g. ancient Sparta, ancient Greece, Italy (Fascist), and modern Germany.

Social Aim of Education in Democratic Countries

The social aim finds expression in such concepts as education for social efficiency. A society is considered to be efficient only, when it is physically strong, intellectually enlightened, economically self-sufficient and morally well disciplined. Such a society requires individuals who are physically fit, intellectually well - off, economically self-sufficient and morally high. It is only such individuals who can contribute really towards welfare of that society. In democratic countries the education aims at developing socially efficient individuals. Social efficiency implies social awareness, economic productivity and cultural and moral refinement. Social awareness will produce in the mind of the child, a sense of fairness in dealing with others, open mindedness to the ability to follow and lead as the situation warrants. Economic independence will help him to pull his/her own weight and he/she will not be a parasite or a drag on society, culture and moral refinement means that he/she will have a spirit of social service and self-sacrifice. He/she also conforms to a certain standard of conduct known as the 'moral conduct'. *John Dewey* says, "In the democratic and technological environment, the aim of education should be to enable the individual to control his/her environment and fulfill his/her possibilities". He/she further adds, "all education proceeds by the participation of the individual in the social consciousness of the race". This process begins unconsciously almost at birth and is continually shaping the individual's powers, saturating his/her consciousness, forming his/her habits training his/her ideas and arousing his/her feelings and emotions.

The individual is trained to be unselfish to part the needs and desires of others before his/her own. The experiences of the individual are communicated to others, so that they may benefit from them. There is no social satisfaction. The mind of the individual so socialized that he/she has an intelligent sympathy and good will for the whole social group. Accordingly school must teach the duties and responsibilities of individual citizens, they ought to train their students as a spirit of cheerful, willing or effective.

Synthesis between the Individual Aim and Social Aim

Apparently the two aims seem to contradictory and opposed to each other. The individual aim, if stressed greatly, will produce one, who are selfish, boastful and egoists. While extreme emphasis on social aim will create suppressed personalities and turn them into automation.

The two aims of education are complementary and not conflicting. We find neither the individual nor the society can exist without each other. The individual is the product of society; while the society in its own turn, finds its advancement in the development of the individual members.

John Adam says, "individuality requires a social medium to grow. Without social contacts we are not human. Individual development is not conceivable without being social. Human being has no meaning apart from society. Education has two-fold objects, 'the perfection of the individual and the good of the community'. Education is making good people as well as good citizen". *Humayun Kabir,* said "if one has to be creative member of the society, one must not only sustain one's own growth, but contribute something to the growth of the society".

According to *Ross,* "individuality is of no value and personality is a meaningless term apart from the social environment in which they are developed and manifested. Self-realization can be achieved only through social service and the social ideal of real value can come into being only through, free individuals who have developed valuable society and the individual. An individual can only develop in a progressive society and society can only make progress with developed individuals. The circle cannot be broken.

National Aims of Education

India has become a secular and democratic country, when India becomes free, there was a need for reorientation and restructuring of all our existing social, political and educational needs of the country. Aims of independent India were: preparation for democratic citizenship, increased productivity, national integration and achievement of goals. The total education system had to be reoriented and restructured to facilitate the achievement.

The Secondary Education Commission of 1952 *(Mudaliar Commission)* suggested the following aims of education in free India.

Democratic Citizenship

Education should prepare people for democratic citizenship. It means to train persons with capacity for clear thinking, receptivity to new ideas, clarity in speech as well as in writing and true patriotism.

Development of Personality

All round development of personality is an important aim of education. Education should develop the literary, artistic, aesthetic and cultural interests of students. For this purpose, subjects like art, music, dance, craft etc. should be included in the curriculum.

Development of Leadership

If democracy is to function successfully, there should be people to assume leadership in the social, political, industrial and cultural fields. Education should train the youth to assume such responsibilities.

Vocational Efficiency

For improving the poor economic situation of the country, the Commission emphasized the need for increasing productivity through vocational and technical efficiency. One of the aims of education is to develop vocational efficiency of the youth. Education will help to create a new attitude toward work and dignity of labour.

Initiating Students to the Art of Living

Through education, the child should learn the art of harmonious living. Education should enable a person to acquire the necessary interpersonal skills and adjustment abilities for successful and happy living together in society.

The *Kothari Education Commission* of 1964-66 proposed aims of education in India are:

Education for Increased Productivity

Increased productivity is an essential need of our country. Education should help to satisfy this need through the production of man power, i.e. people who are equipped with advanced scientific knowledge, complex technical ability and efficient work experience.

Social and National Integration

Education should include the feeling of oneness and belongingness. This is a very important aim of education in India which has the tendency to divide on the basis of language, culture, caste, religion and so on. This aim should be accomplished through some kind of public educational system and some form of obligatory national service.

Education for Modernization

The world is moving very fast with all kinds of scientific and technological advancements. India also should keep pace with the advancements of the modern world. Our education should aim at producing people who are able to think and judge independently and effectively. Intellectually efficient and technically competent persons must be prepared.

Education for Social, Moral and Spiritual Values

To integrate social, moral and spiritual values in the minds of children and young people. The curriculum should include instruction in these subjects by setting time for moral and spiritual instruction in all educational programmes. All religions should be given equal importance.

These are the educational aims for independent India suggested by the two commissions. Though we have come a long way in achieving these aims, still there is much more to be accomplished. Various commissions and committees appointed by the Government did periodic comprehensive appraisal of the existing educational scene in our country. Based on their reports, Government has drawn National Education Policies which specify the renewed aims and objectives of our education.

The National Education Policy of 1986 modified in 1992 have set the following educational aims in India are:

- All round material and spiritual development of all people
- Cultural orientation and development of interest in Indian culture
- Scientific advancement.
- National cohesion.
- Integration of body, mind and spirit.
- Furthering the goals of socialism, secularism and democracy.
- Man power development for different levels of economy.
- Fostering research in all areas of development.
- Education for equality.

Aims of Nursing Education

Nursing education is the professional education for the preparation of nurses, to enable them to render professional nursing care to people of all ages, in all phases of health and illness, in a variety of settings.

Factors Influencing Nursing Education

- Health needs of the people in the society
- Needs of the student
- Philosophy of nursing
- Current trends in general and professional education
- Advancement in Science and Technology.

Aims

- Man power development: Well-qualified, competent nurses are needed to meet the needs of people in the society. Nursing care is an important and integral aspect of health care. Nurse has to implement advanced scientific knowledge and professional skills in meeting the needs of people by adopting nursing process and its steps.

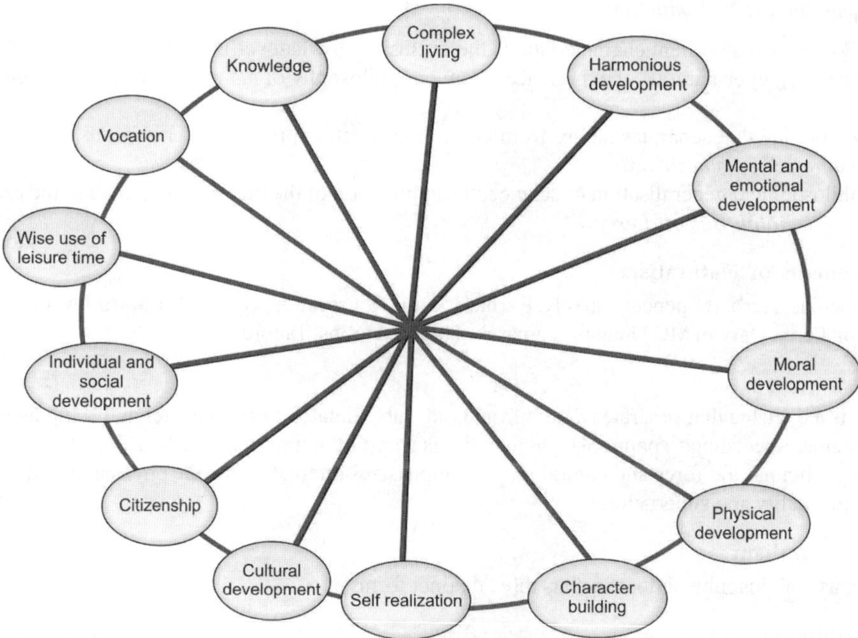

Fig. 1.1: Aims of education

- Nursing education should impart scientific and up-to-date knowledge in the area of Medical, Social, Behavioral and Biological Sciences.
- Inculcate the appropriate nursing skills and the right attitude to the students. Theoretical knowledge, and practical skills are essential for rendering intelligent and efficient nursing care.
- Nursing education should have sufficient theory content and practical experience.
- Nursing education should prepare nurses as good leaders to provide qualitative care. Nurses have to participate in decision-making and policy making in health care matters and allocation of resources for health development.
- Nurses have to implement health care programmes and health care services in community. They have to collaborate and coordinate health care functions. The nurse leaders are responsible for effective nursing education. Nursing education should aim to identify potential nursing leaders and facilitating for their development.
- To improve professional development of each nurse and their profession.
- For all round personality development of an individual nurse will develop and grow as a person of self-awareness, self-direction and self-motivation.
- Nursing should prepare nurses in participating scientific nursing research investigations, its results will be added up to the body of nursing knowledge.
- Nursing education should inculcate democratic values, e.g. respect to individuality, equality, toleration, cooperative living, faith in changes.

TRADITIONAL PHILOSOPHIES OF EDUCATION

NATURALISM

Introduction

It is a philosophical position adopted by naturalists, who approach philosophy from purely scientific point of view. They believe that nature alone represents the entire reality. There is nothing beyond/behind and other than nature.

Definitions

- "It is a system, whose salient characteristic is the exclusion of whatever is spiritual or indeed, whatever is transcendental (super-natural) of experiences from our philosophy of nature and man" – *George Hayward Joyce.*
- "It is the doctrine that separates nature from God, subordinates spirit to matter and sets up unchangeable laws as supreme" – *James Ward.*
- "It is a philosophical generalisation of science; the application of the theories of science to the problems of philosophy"– *Ralph Barton Perry.*

Chief Exponents of Naturalism

Bacon, Comenius, Herbert Spencer, Huxely, Bernard Shaw, Rousseau JJ, George Hayward Jayce, James Ward, Ralph Barton Perry, Darwin MC Dougall, Lamarck, Thomas Hobbs, Tagore.

Meaning

Naturalism is a doctrine that separates nature from God, subordinates spirit to matter and setup unchangeable laws as supreme. According to naturalists, human life is a part of nature, it is a self-sufficient entity having its own natural matter natural force and natural laws. It emphasizes on 'matter and the physical world'. It does not believe in spirituality and supernaturalism.

Forms of Naturalism

Naturalism, as a philosophical doctrine has three distinct forms:

Physical Naturalism

Nature is the reality, human life is wholly controlled and influenced by the eternal laws of nature, and it governs the human life, since it is moulded by natural laws. Reality does not exist within the individual. It is rather outside him, in the natural universe. Tagore calls, 'nature' as the 'manuscript of god' since human life is moulded and controlled by external nature, it should be in accordance with the natural laws.

Mechanical Naturalism

There is no spirit or soul, only matter is everything. Man is also matter, which is made up of atoms, empty space and motion. It regards man is merely a machine, governed by mechanical laws, he/she has no creative capacity, purpose or direction. This philosophy aims at training man as a good machine and keeping it in good working condition.

Thomas Hobbs, an Englishman described nature as an aggregate of things outside our mind which is moving in space.

Biological Naturalism

Based on Darwin, *Herbert Spencer's* view, by the process of growth and development man was energist identifying reality as a force of energy. Man's natural endowments (emotional and temperament) are the real springs of his/her behavior. If our behavior is according to our instincts, we feel happy, if not we feel unhappy and disappointed. Education should try to sublimate these natural impulses for socially desirable ends.

Development of Naturalism

Natural surroundings and freedom are the important factors for the growth and development of the child.

Thomas Hobbs, in 17th century described nature as an aggregate of things moving from one place to another.

JJ Rousseau in his/*her Emile* describes the education of a child is close to nature. Nature yields all kinds of good things, but the society of man grasps them and perverts them to evil ends. *Herbert Spencer* (19th century) used the word 'force' to describe 'reality'.

Naturalism and Education

Human nature develops according to the laws obeyed by heavenly bodies, as they move in their orbits. The duty of education is to learn, what these laws are and how to use those laws. Educational materials should be the facts and phenomenon of nature. Education makes the individual, a natural man.

Herbert Spencer's views, the educational objectives are: self preservation, securing the necessities of life, raising children, citizenship and education for leisure.

Naturalism gives maximum freedom and central position to the child. Watch words in naturalism are: 'Follow nature', 'Back to nature', 'Maximum happiness' and 'Utmost freedom to children', 'Instincts are basis of education', 'Senses are the gate ways of knowledge'. Naturalism believes that education should be according to the nature of the child, it advocates creation of conditions in which the natural development of the child can take place in a natural way. Textbooks, timetable, syllabus and even teachers are not so important for the learner, According to *Rousseau,* there are three sources of education, i.e. nature, men and things. The nature consists of natural development of organs and faculties, education from nature is to prepare a natural man.

Man is governed and directed by the laws of his/her own nature rather than those of social institutions. Thus naturalism is a revolt against the stereotyped system of education.

Naturalism and Education Process

- Education must confirm to the natural process of physical growth and mental development. Pupil will be given freedom to determine the form of the learning process, e.g. inductive methods of learning
- Education should be a pleasurable activity for children and it engages the spontaneous self-activity of the child
- Acquisition of knowledge is an important aspect of education related to body and mind. Punishment should be based on the consequences of wrong deeds, but with sympathy, its frequency will be reduced.

Naturalism and Aims of Education

- Self-realization.
- Self expression.
- Self preservation.
- Habit formation related to action and thought which are appropriate to the age.
- Cultivation of self-restraint and sense of value (*Herbert Spencer—biological school of naturalism*).
- Pleasure and pain are instincts of man are real guiding forces which are basis of the conduct of the child (*MC Daugall's view*).
- To make the child to adjust himself both physically and mentally to his/her environment and to the changing circumstances in life (*Lamarck's view*).
- Equip the individual to struggle for existence *(Darwin's view)* and ensure his/her survival (Herbert Spencer).
- Evolution of a better humanity through the transmission of not only physical traits, but also for the cultural ones.
- Education of the man as the 'back of God's creation'. Education should aim at the evolution of a better humanity through the transmission of not only physical traits, but also the cultural ones (*Bernard Shaw's view*).
- Education is universal spirit, according to the nature of the child (*Rousseau's view*).
- Development of individuality (*Sir Percy Nussy's view*).
- Struggle for existence and survival of the fittest (*Darwin's view*).
- Education should be according to the nature of the child's tenderness, capacities, instincts, likes and dislikes. It should aim at providing full opportunity for the development of natural endowments of the child.
- Perfect development of individuality will develop the child into a joyous, rational, balanced, useful and mature person.

Thus naturalism ignores the spiritual side of the child's personality by omitting the development of his/her will, conscience and morality.

Naturalism and Curriculum

- No fixed curriculum.
- Every child is given the right to determine his/her own curriculum.
- The child is expected to learn directly from nature through personal experiences.
- Naturalists give prominence to subjects like gardening, agriculture, nature study, art, crafts, botany, geology, geography and astronomy etc. as they are directly related to the nature of the child.
- The subjects should be correlated with the play activity of the child and with the life around him.

Naturalism and Methods of Teaching

- Naturalists are not in favour of direct training through teacher or textbooks.
- In the place of textbooks, they emphasize the value of 'concrete objects'.
- They advocate the direct experience of things and believe in the principle of 'learning by doing', e.g. observation and experimental methods.
- Direct methods are advised as to ensure the vocabulary of a student.
- In the training of science and mathematics "Heuristic method" is emphasized in the place of 'chalk and talk procedure'.
- Geography is through practical exercises, actual excursion and observation.
- Play - way method is used to develop spirit of joyful, spontaneous and creative activity.
- *Dalton plan* method is suggested, which gives freedom to the pupil to choose his/her own schedule of work. They learn through observation and experiment, self-government and self-effort.
- Naturalists emphasizes 'open air schools' self-government in schools and establishment of co-education in educational institutions.

Thus the centre of naturalism to the field of modern methodology of education is most outstanding and most abiding.

Naturalism and the Teacher

Teacher can neither interfere with the activities of children nor can impose his/her own ideas and ideals, will power upon them or a moulder of character formation. His/her place is 'behind the scene'. He/she is a 'spectator' or an 'observer' of the child's development. He/she cannot impose any activity, restrictions or limitations for the learner. He/she will allow the child, provided opportunity for free development of their own motives, growth and development in an atmosphere of non-intervention and freedom. He/she does not expect undue respect from his/her pupils nor does he/she pose as superior. He/she tries to understand the pupils and approves their behavior. Teacher cannot dictate to pupils, what they have to do.

According to naturalistic concept, a teacher is only a setter of the stage, a supplier of materials and opportunities. Teacher is a provider of an ideal environment and creator of conducive conditions to the natural development of the students.

Naturalism and Discipline

- Extreme discipline is not desirable, as it stands in the way of the child's natural development
- Free discipline may be applicable, as naturalists give utmost freedom to the child to do and learn whatever he/she likes, they do not advocate any sort of punishment for the child except that he/she is allowed to support the natural consequences of his/her actions.

For regulating the conduct of students, naturalists have evolved the concept of student self-government in tune with the demand of a democratic society.

Weaknesses of Naturalism in Education

- The simplicity of naturalistic educational practices may not be possible in urban areas.
- Higher order of discipline may not be possible as textbooks and teachers are not playing crucial role and leisure pace of learning through experience is taking place.
- The physical nature alone is not the power which can be used to control and direct education or any other human Endeavour. Nature alone cannot find peace or beauty, there is something higher, which can direct man's purposes, strivings towards positive ends.
- Lacks ideals, no place for spiritual values.
- No constructive suggestions to offer regarding a goal for educative effort thus it does not point to a higher end in the educational process.

Conclusion

Education is based on psychology of the child and in accordance with his/her nature. Naturalists keep the child in the forefront in the entire process of education. The teacher, school, curriculum, methods of training are not so important as the child, who has to be educated. Naturalists want the school, to provide conducive environment, which promotes the free development of the growing child.

Application of naturalism in Nursing Education

Nurse Educator can choose the teaching methods like projects method, demonstration, field trip etc. Teacher has to give liberty for the learner to select the problem and work on it; teacher can facilitate total personality development of the learner. Teacher will assist the student to utilize the leisure time in a productive manner in the form of extracurricular and co-curricular activities like NCC, NSS, sports, games, participating in competitions etc. Thus Educator facilitates learner's growth and development i.e., "sound mind in a sound body."

IDEALISM

Introduction and Meaning

The word, 'idealism' has been derived from 'ideal' or 'ideas'. Ideals or higher values are much more significant in human life than anything else. This philosophy seeks to explain man and universe in terms of spirit or mind. This philosophical thought, is originated by the great Greek philosophers, Socrates and Plato. They conceived ideas as the basis of their philosophy. Plato in his/her dialogues indicated the importance of mind and reason in the experience of man. Idealism idolizes 'mind and self'; it explains man and the universe in terms of 'spirit' or 'mind'. Man's spiritual nature is considered to be the very essence of his/her being.

Exponents of Idealism Philosophy

Plato, Socrates, Kant, Hegel, Berkley, Guru Nanak, Tagore, Mahatma Gandhi, Comenius, Kapila, Pestalozzi, Schopenhauer, Freebel, Dayanannda, Rusk.

Chief Assertions of Idealism

- Idealism believes in the 'universal mind' or 'God'. He/she is the creator and he/she creates entire world. It is the source of all human values. The goal of all human activities is the realization of 'universal mind' in his/her own self.
- It regards man as a 'spiritual being', superior to animals. Reality is found in the mind of man and in the external world.
- Main aim of human life is to achieve spiritual values i.e., truth, beauty and goodness. These values are absolute, undying and permanent, with these terms, man rises higher and higher in the moral plane, till he/she becomes one with the 'universal mind'. These are all attributes of God.
- God is the source of all knowledge and real knowledge is perceived in mind. According to idealists, knowledge gained through mind is more important, than knowledge gained through the senses.
- The world of ideas and values is more important than the world of matter. Idealism has full faith in eternal values which never change. They can neither be created nor destroyed.
- Man can express himself in language and communicate through various forms of art and culture. Man expresses his/her spiritual aspirations through morality and religion.
- Idealists maintain the distinctiveness and superiority of man's nature, not only from his/her spiritual capacities but also seen in his/her power and control over the environment.
- Man can change and manipulate the physical environment and shaping it according to his/her needs, he/she has also the power of controlling the spiritual and cultural environment and values, it can be represented by communication through art, culture, knowledge, morality and religion.
- Reality is spiritual. It exists in ideas, purposes, intangible values and internal truths.

Idealism in Education

Educational idealists believe that man is born with spiritual self. He/she can realize his/her spirituality and understand its true nature only through the agency of education. Education is expected to enlarge the boundaries of the spiritual realm. Ideals of race and its cultural pattern are preserved, transmitted and modified subsequently in the light of new situations.

Intellectual Training

The world is based on natural laws that are eternal and unchanging, logical consequence, physical laws are based on reason must be taught, as nature is simply the outer expression of an inner logical order.

Unique Nature of Man

In nature, man alone can understand logic order in existence through the power of his/her mind by reasoning and self-discipline. It is provided by the family and school, acquires an effort of mind and will. Social habits can be formulated with the process of rational development.

Idealism and Aims in Education

Idealism lays proper stress on the glory and grandeur of human life, which is the best creation of God. It has provided human life with high aims.

Exaltation of Human Personality

Education should lead to perfection in the individual. Human personality is of supreme value and constitutes the noblest work of God. The aim of education should be the exaltation of the self, which implies self-realization. It is the one i.e.specially associated with idealism, since man is a spiritual being, the divine in man should be unified and brought to his/her consciousness by means of education.

Self-realization

- Duties to self
  Cleanliness, neatness, moderation, satisfaction of all desires, self-control, self-sacrifice, punctuality, regularity, avoidance of obscenity, profanity and immoral language
- The function of education is to enable the individual to realize this unity within him and to establish a harmony between his/her nature and the ultimate nature of universe. Indian idealism practices liberation, mukti or nirvana as the ultimate aim of life.

Swami Vivekananda Explained the four-fold path

- Gnana (wisdom)
- Bhakti (devotion)
- Karma (action)
- Yajna (meditation)

  Idealist's aim at the full and complete training of man for manhood and not the development of some parts of man.

Acquisition and enrichment of Culture Environment

Man himself is the creator of cultural environment. It is a product of man's creative activity. Idealists therefore, emphasize that each child should enter into the cultural heritage of mankind which is free from the limitations of the material environment. Man has to preserve the culture, what he/she has inherited and also make to contribute the enrichment of that culture, so that the boundaries of spiritual realm will be enlarged. Education must help the individual in this contribution. Education should aim at providing the mean of acquainting the student with great achievements in art, literature, mathematics and sciences. Man should be able to invent, create, produce new and beautiful ideas and objects of community and society. Education should emphasize, encourage invention and creation as a part of culture.

Development of Moral Sense: Powers and Rationality

Intellectual development requires training in logical understanding and perception.

When the child develops moral sense, he/she is able to distinguish between right and wrong. Education should also develop the will power of the child, so that he/she may be able to follow the good and reject the evil. This power of truth, beauty and goodness which are the higher moral values.

Self-culture

The pupil has to learn:

- Polite behavior
- Good manners
- Self-control.

Industriousness
- Reliability
- Sincerity
- Perseverance.

Duties to Others
- The virtues of modest
- Respect for the opinions of others
- Cooperativeness
- Liberality and generosity
- Religious education.

Universal Education

Since all human beings are equally the children of God and are equal. In idealistic society, education should be universal without any distinction of caste, creed, color or social status.

Development of Inventive and Creative Powers

Man should not accept his/her physical environment as unchangeable. He/she should modify the environment according to his/her needs and mould it according to his/her own purposes through his/her inventive and creative skill. Education must foster those inventive power of man to ensure his/her mastery over the material given to him.

Idealism and Curriculum

In idealism, the curriculum will be selected based upon ideas and ideals. It aims to develop a true sense of appreciation of truth, goodness and beauty by which spiritual perfection will result. Spiritual act consists of moral, intellectual and esthetic events.

The three acts are inspired by the three corresponding desires of the spirit i.e., knowledge (gnana); feeling (bhakthi); and effort (karma); therefore the idealistic curriculum provides the training and cultivation of the intellectual, moral, esthetic acts for intellectual advancement of the child.

Language, Literature, Science, Social Studies and Mathematics are included in the curriculum. For aesthetic and moral development: Fine arts, Poetry, Ethics and Religion are provided.

Idealistic philosophy and education also insists on the creation of sound mind in a sound body. Therefore, physical exercises, hygiene, gymnastic and athletics are also included in the curriculum.

Thus the idealistic curriculum comprises of physical, intellectual and spiritual acts which will enable a man to develop completely.

Idealism and Methods of Teaching

- Self activity, project method, play way methods can be adopted to gain knowledge. (*Pestacozzi advocated*)
- *Froebel* developed 'kindergarten method'.
- Questioning, discussion, lecture method, single and group projects, imitation etc. also included as techniques of idealism.

Idealism and Discipline

- Strict discipline is essential for self-realization.
- Teacher's guidance is necessary at every step.
- As far as idealists are considered, freedom is not a means but it is an end.

Idealism and Teacher

- Idealist teacher has attained self-realization. He/she is a practical man based on ideal and virtuous life. He/she should live a life of contentment, contemplation, poverty and detachment. His/her personality is a source of inspiration for his/her students to follow and to learn the acts like a friend, a philosopher and guide.
- The teacher personifies reality for the students. The student understands and learns about the universe through his/her teacher.
- The teacher has to be a specialist in the knowledge in view of his/her students.

- Good teacher commands the respect of students by virtue of his/her own, high standards of behavior and conduct.
- Teacher initiates the pupil into the life of the intellect, but he/she provides standards related to attitudes, imitation. The social atmosphere of the school, pattern of speech, conduct and appearance encouraged in the school provide attitude for limitation by the student.

Weakness of Idealism in Education

- Scientific research study does not support the idealistic view of a spiritual universe.
- Ideals cannot be simplified.
- The social order today discourages imitation of ideas, ideals, behaviors and the standards that governed the lives of people of the older generation.
- The emphasis on good manners, polite behavior, docility, modesty sums out of tune with the present day world, where aggressiveness reiteration of demands, outspokenness and frankness are regarded as essential qualities in a competitive society.
- A polite, restrained manner may be mistaken for snobbery.
- Docility and modesty would be dubbed as evidence of diffidence.
- Overloaded information—selectivity in reading and learning has become a necessity.

Idealism and Nursing Education

To promote Moral, Spiritual, Emotional, Social, Psychological, Intellectual and Physical components among learners. Nurse Educator will introduce the principles of Idealism in teaching. In teaching method, like Questioning, Discussion, Project method, Play method, Lecture and Demonstration, Learning through immitation will be adapted based on the subject content, requirement of curriculum and felt needs of learners/organization. To enhance knowledge, feeling, efforts, decision making, e.g. able to differentiate right and wrong and select the right one; wisdom of the learner, the teacher will act as role model and guide and counselor.

REALISM

INTRODUCTION

Viewpoint

What is true and real in daily life is admissible; whose reality is not felt and unreal is inadmissible.
This doctrine is against spiritualism and opposes to idealism.

Meaning and Importance

- Realism is an outcome of scientific development
- By observation, experimentation and examination if it is found to be true, can be considered as real
- Realism is directly related to man and society
- Through realism, man is able to enjoy the comforts of society, after getting all the joys of life
- Realism provides education, which is useful for life where man can enjoy his/her activities and comforts in reality

Supporters of Realism

J Friedrich Herbart: He/she gave educational ideas on principles of realism and development of many-sided interests among the children. He/she explained, scientific effort has to be made by the teachers, which interest is for better welfare of the child and society. After identifying this analysis, interests among the children should be developed in the context of different circumstances of life.

Herbert Spencer: According to Herbert, education has to teach man to lead a complete life and live full happy life. The learner has to engage in the following acts in a desired manner.
- Self-preservation (care of health)
- Earning a living (preparation for vocation)
- Fulfilling responsibilities related to race preservation
- Fulfilling citizen responsibilities
- Utilization of leisure time

Franklin Bobit (American educationalist): Education should be provided according to the reality of life. Human responsibilities and obligations which are necessary to lead a happy life are:
- Acts concerned with language
- Acts concerned with hygiene
- Citizenship acts
- Ordinary social acts
- Leisure acts
- Acts of mental health
- Religious act
- Acts concerning race preservation
- Vocational behavior activities

Nature of Education

Scientific attitude based on realistic principle, where the learner can extends his/her knowledge, which he/she learnt through books can be developed.

Spiritual need has not considered as a real need of education.

Aims of Education
- Through education man leads a happy and comfortable life.
- It enables the man capable of earning by vocational form.
- To develop the memory of the child.
- To strengthen wisdom and power of decision-making.
- To create the capacity against struggles with adverse situations arising while earning a living.
- To meet the felt needs of individual (related to materialistic).
- To make the man as 'utilitarian' with the usage of mother tongue, experiments, demonstration and tours etc.
- Education will be provided according to the reality of life.
- To develop the child capacity for success in the struggles of future life.

Realism and Curriculum

Science, Mathematics, Hygiene, Vocational activities etc. have been given prominence in the curriculum.

Realism and Nursing Education

Nurse Educator will use project method, Demonstration, Field trip, Experimentation to promote observation, intellectual, Examination and analyzing skills among learners. Realistic approach, learning by doing observation etc. will be used.

PRAGMATISM

Introduction

It is derived from Greek word, 'pragmatism' which means 'practice or action; active and efficient'. A pragmatist lives in the world of facts rather than ideas or ideals. In American philosophy, 'pragmatism' means 'utility'. *William James* is the founder and father of this philosophy.

Chief Exponents of Pragmatism—William James, John Dewey, S. Kil Patrick, Margaret H and Mead

Meaning

Pragmatism is a matter of fact, treatment of things based solely on their practical utility. It is the element of utility that has the greatest appeal for a pragmatist. For him, utility is truth and truth is utility. Pragmatism believes in practical and utilitarian philosophy.

Pragmatism is a typical American philosophy. Americans experimented upon many new ideas and adopted those which proved useful for them in solving their day-to-day problems. Consequently they built up a 'Pragmatism of life', based on their own experiments and experiences. This is the pragmatic philosophy of life.

Man as a natural biological organism, schools become secular, scientific, practical, technical and scholarly pursuits became an extension of problem solving. The experiences which are helpful for the learner and help for direct training. It will be helpful for occupational activities.

Principles of Pragmatism

- Man creates his/her own values during the course of act. There are no fixed values for all times.
- Every truth is man-made product. There is nothing like absolute truth.
- Pragmatism laid special stress on the value of experimentation. It stands for testing every statement by finding out its practical implications. If these implications are desirable, the statement is accepted, otherwise it is rejected.
- True pragmatism is one, that helps in the solution of practical problems of life.
- Pragmatism should have meaning and utility in the solution of human problems (John Dewey).
- Pragmatism should be practical and useful in influencing the conduct of life and not a passive enquiry or contemplation.
- The growth of human personality takes place because of interaction with the environment. Man tries to adjust himself to his/her environment and this results in his/her growth. During the process of adjustment, man adopts himself to his/her environment but he/she also tries to mould the environment according to his/her needs, purposes and desires.
- Pragmatism has deep faith in democracy, it is a Government by the people, of the people and for the people. Through democracy only individual can realize the maximum development of his/her personality. This development is possible only in social context.
- Individual development also leads to the development of society.

Revolt against Traditionalism and Absolutism

Reality or truth works out in a practical situation whatever fulfils one's purpose and develops one's life is true.
- Movement in education is preoccupied with change
- Man shares his/her fundamental drives with other living creatures
- Moral values e.g. truth, goodness, beauty etc. have evolved through social processes
- Man has biologically unique features; the phenomenon of language gives him the power to reflect upon experiences to identify, criticize, evaluate and judge them
- Man and his/her universal are natural; man is an organism struggling to satisfy his/her need and to perpetuate himself in a natural world. The methods he/she has used in conserving life and satisfying his/her needs are scientific or empirical
- A new logic and concept of the nature of thought and enquiry.

Forms of Pragmatism

a. *Humanistic pragmatism:* Truth satisfies human nature and welfare as a whole. Whatever fulfils one's purpose, desires and develops one's life is true.
b. *Experimental pragmatism:* Which can be verified or whatever work is the true.
c. *Biological pragmatism:* It stresses the human ability of adaptation to the environment and that of adapting the environment to human needs.

Pragmatism in Education

It is a practical and utilitarian school of pragmatism; It believes in imparting education with reference to human needs. It enables the child to solve his/her daily problems and also to lead a better and happy life by creating new values.

Education therefore must have its intellectual, moral, esthetic, social and physical aspects. Pragmatism is the product of education, i.e. outcome of educational experiments.

Pragmatism of education is not an external application of readymade ideas to a system of practice. It is on the other hand, a formulation of the problems of right mental and moral attitudes which should help a person to meet the difficulties of contemporary social life—*Dewey.*

Pragmatism stands for progressive trends in education. According to pragmatism, activity lies at the centre of all educative process, which is progressive and flexible. It stands for freedom and worth of the individual.

Pragmatism works on the principle of democracy and education is a social necessity. Pragmatists believe that pragmatism is the product of educational practice and it has its effects on the various aspects of education. Educated person should be in command of skills and knowledge to meet and master the new problems that come in their lives.

Educational Applications

- The school becomes child centred, education will help the child to grow
- Education is centred in the experience of the children and this sense of need experienced by the children should be fulfilled
- In the school, the child learns the activities by practicing it, so the school has to provide conducive environment for the children. The child will learn most of the life things within the school. The teacher will act as a guide or counsellor. The pupil actively participates in the planning of activities with the teacher
- Cultivate creative interest among the child, intelligent cooperative effort is necessary
- Child centred education is to build a future centred society.

Pragmatism and Aims of Education

Creation of New Values

The pragmatist does not start with any fixed aims or scheme of values. The main task of the education is to put the education into a position of developing values for himself. The man has to create the values in the light of his/her own experience and felt needs. The child must learn, which values will fulfill and satisfy his/her needs and wants in the environment, he/she has to create such environment for the child.

Activity and Experience

For the creation of new values, activity and experience are essential. Education should therefore provide physical, intellectual, social, moral and esthetic acts as the media for the creation of values and for the development and selection of what the child wants to learn to satisfy his/her own needs for the present as well as for the future.

Personal and Social Adjustment

All the aspects are developed for meeting the individual and social needs of man, this will help him to cope with the varied problems and situations in life successfully. Direct the impulses, interests and abilities towards the satisfaction of the felt needs of the child in the environment.

Reconstruction of Experience

Pragmatists will provide a social setting for the development of cooperative and correlated learning in the school. Pragmatism emphasises adaptation to environment construction and reconstruction of experience and development of capacities to control the environment.

All-round Personality Development

The learner through pragmatism will develop physically, mentally, socially, morally and esthetically.

Pragmatism and Curriculum

Activity Curriculum

Pragmatists will not fix the curriculum in advance or in the beginning itself. Only an outline of the acts may be kept in view in the beginning and curriculum can be evolved according to the requirement of the situations. Thus, it will be a flexible and changing curriculum. While deciding it, the nature of the child and the multiple acts of life must be taken into consideration.

The curriculum should be based on child's occupations and activities, his/her own experiences learnt by doing the activities. The principle of integration and correlated activities should guide in curriculum construction.

Utilitarian Curriculum

It includes the subjects, which will impart knowledge and various types of skills, which the child needs in his/her present as well as future life. The curriculum is to be governed by the child's natural interests and felt needs during the successive stages of development. The experiences are provided which give knowledge and skills to the child. At the elementary stage reading, writing, arithmetic, nature study, drawing and handwork are provided.

At a later stage, practical subjects like Languages, Social studies, Physical Sciences, Mathematics and Hygiene are included in the curriculum. Agriculture for boys and Home Sciences for girls is prescribed. Training in some craft or vocation also advocated.

Principle of Integration
While deciding the subjects of curriculum, the principle of integration is kept in view. Instead of dividing knowledge into various subject fields, integrated knowledge around various problems of life is preferred. Pragmatism emphasises only the utilitarian aspect, so it will neglect useful subjects like art and poetry.

Pragmatism and Methods of Teaching

I. *Project method and practical oriented (learn—ing by doing):* According to pragmatists, the method of teaching are devised by the teacher in the light of real life situations. Education is not training or imparting knowledge, but to encourage training through self effort and creative activity. Knowledge is not only obtained from books, but also actually by doing the things.

II. *Provision of real life situation and touching and handling of objects, tools and making things:* Project methods are carried out in natural settings. The child is given a real and purposeful task to carry out. Thus the child gets knowledge and skills from the experience gained in accomplishment of that task.

Psychologically also these methods are effective because the child is always interested in doing things with his/her own hands.

The school, the curriculum and the subject matter all are considered from the child's point of view.

Six stages in this method:
- Providing a real situation
- Selection of the project
- Planning
- Execution of plan
- The evaluation
- Judgment of its utility

III. *Discussion, questioning and inquiry:* Methods also considered in philosophy of pragmatism.

Pragmatism and Discipline

- Purposeful and cooperative acts carried in a free and happy environment are conducive to good discipline Thus, they go a long way in the training of character and the establishment of self-discipline
- Self discipline is not exposed control by an external authority
- 'Pragmatism also emphasizes on social discipline through participation in cooperative acts in the school society
- Social discipline enables the child to have the virtues like toleration, mutual respect, sympathy, self-control, initiative, service of humanity and originality.

Pragmatism and the Teacher

- The teacher will create real life situation in which some problems may emerge and the child is interested in the solution of those problems
- The teacher will keep the pupil in the position of a discoverer and experimenter
- Teacher will not impose anything in the child. The child will decide his/her own goals, aims and purposes independently.

Strengths of Pragmatism in Education

- The student will learn the skills and meet his/her needs, prepared himself to live in society
- The student will try to meet the immediate felt needs
- The child learns the activities by doing. He/she will develop his/her qualities, abilities, thinking, reasoning, judgment based on either individual or social behavior
- Both teacher and student should explore in the adventure of seeking knowledge

- The pragmatic approach is based upon recognition of technological and industrialized felt needs
- Applicable in American settings.

Weaknesses of Pragmatism

- It does not give raise the question of the ultimate reality behind the things
- Artificiality in situation
- Problem solving activity may be pleasurable and challenging for the learners, but it may have little or no relationship with problems that occur in real life situations
- The teacher may be unable to cope with the demands of teaching
- Humanities, cultural acts have no place
- Teacher will act as information officer only. No faith in eternal truth, which is a stable body of knowledge
- Many gaps and deficiencies in the learning approach has been observed
- Denial of spiritual, cultural values are unpalatable
- Less practiced in Indian settings.

Conclusion

- Pragmatism emphasizes on child's individuality, his/her needs, interests and aptitudes. Principles of learning by doing, activity and experience, it stresses on integration of knowledge and relating the curriculum to real life situation, project method
- The teacher has to provide opportunities for act and to have the experience both in school and play ground
- The teacher is a friend and a helper
- The teacher should be alert, well informed and able to discuss the facts, subject matter with students

Pragmatism and Nursing Education

Nursing Educator will create a real life situation in which the learner will identify and select some problem based on his/her interest and specialization. He/she will does experimentation of discover by doing certain activities or research skills, work on that problem, integrate and correlation of activities and the facts analyses, concludes the findings, communicate its results. The teaching methods like project method, experimentation, demonstration, scientific enquiry etc. will be used. The learner will use self efforts, skill development, creative activities performs activity, observes and analyzes the situation. The learner will enhance intellectual, moral, esthetic, mental, social, moral, physical and clinical skills. Thus pragmatism has practical utility, provides cooperative and corelated learning experiences, construction and re-construction of experiences which will enhance clinical skills, experimentation skills among learners. Teachers will function as a guide, resource person and counselor.

MODERN CONTEMPORARY PHILOSOPHIES OF EDUCATION

Introduction

The world and its values are continuously changing, the educational system also changes from time to time. Each one philosophy has its own contributions and limitations; no one philosophy is complete in itself and can be applied successfully in all situations. Education has to be flexible and dynamic. It has to adopt, to the changing conditions and environment throughout the ages.

EXISTENTIALISM

Introduction

It is the youngest philosophy, described as modern 20th century philosophy, however a wide general recognition in educational field is not yet received.

Definition

A modern philosophy which is primarily built upon the work of the contemporary scholars of the 20th century.

Meaning

This philosophy views man as, participating in a world of things and events, human existence is the nature of man to exist, to stand out into reality, to participate in being, to be present to all.

Chief Exponents

Soren Kierkegaard (Danish philosopher); Jan Paul Satre (French writer); Karl Jaspers (German philosopher); Paul T; Reinhold Niebuhr.

According to Soren Kierkegaard (founder of existentialism), it is ultimate aim of man in life is 'to be that which is truly, man must accept the existence of God, is by faith, nor by reasoning'.

Later the thinkers did not consider God to be a necessity.

Jean Paul Satre, argued that human life has no purpose, existence is ultimate and that we must choose, by choosing, we become ourselves.

Assumptions

1. *The centre of existence is man rather than truth, laws, principles or essence:* The recognition of the individual existence, man makes himself through choices among many alternatives in the environment.

   Man is characterized by decisions, will and choice; certain uniqueness and mastery about the human person.
2. *The uniqueness and mystery of man:* The uniqueness of man comes from his/her emotions, feelings, perception and thinking. Man is the maker and master of culture. Man imposes a meaning on his/her universe.
3. *Man is not alone in the world:* Man is a social being, he/she is gregariousness in nature, and he/she cannot live in a state of anarchy. Life is seen as a gift and mystery. Man is free to choose commitments in life, he/she is the product of the choices. Man's existence is more important than his/her essence.
4. *Man cannot accept the ready-made concepts of existence forced upon him:* Man is free agent capable of shaping his/her own life and choosing his/her own destiny. We cannot treat people as machines.
5. *Self-knowledge:* Self - knowledge is the key to all truth and knowledge. 'know thyself' is the basic premise of this philosophy.
6. *Freedom and responsibility:* Based on freedom and responsibility, man can create his/her own values.
7. *Man is not complete:* Man has to meet the challenges in the changing society. He/she has to accomplish all tasks and activities.

Existentialism and Education

George Kneller has written 'existentialism and education'.

Educational Implications

- Becoming a human being, as one who lives and makes decisions about what he/she will do. Human existence and the value includes knowing oneself, social relationship and biological development etc.
- Trainers have to provide healthy atmosphere and environment for the children to find sense of securing encouragement, trustworthiness and acceptance.
- Children have to relieve from emotional stress, e.g. intense competition, harsh discipline, fear of failure.
- Each individual has to grow to understand his/her own needs and values and take charge of the experiences for changing them.
- Self-evaluation is the end of learning process. Education has to make the child to have free growing environment, fearless, understanding individuals.
- Classroom atmosphere has to prepare young people to become active, trust worthy and responsible.
- All school subjects should present situations for the development of human beings.
- The teacher should facilitate development of originality and creativity by providing necessary material and equipment.
- The teacher is in a position to foster individual growth tand he/she is the foreground and is the centre of attention.
- The teacher is very active and welcomes challenges to his/her ideas from the students.
- The democratic ideals must pervade the school environment in which the students has to grow.
- Concern and respect for the individual student should be the main concern of the school.
- Mechanization and impersonality are to be counteracted in schools.

Limitations in Existentialism
- Educational methods applied are said to be impractical.
- Time and effort consuming.
- The concepts like 'being' 'meaning' existence' 'person' are ambiguous and not clear.

Existentialism and Nursing Education
Nurse educator has to promote creativity among learners, teacher has to keep hard efforts to improve social aspect of health in learners. Teacher will provide conducive environment in teaching, learning situations which endorse the mental psychological and social aspects in development of learners.

PROGRESSIVISM

Introduction
It is an American philosophy, which is a revolt against the 'formal/conventional/traditional' system of education. It became popular, in 1929 the economic depression of USA adversely affected the educational system of the country.

Meaning
Education is centred around for the present life itself. The development of an individual and the society is only possible, when education facilitates the growth of every phase of the child.

Exponents
John Dewey; William James; G Thomas Lawrence; William Kilpatric. A large number of schools in Europe and USA were started this philosophy

Aims of Education
To develop the personality of an individual through providing a democratic environment in the educational institutions.

Progressivism and Curriculum
It should be based on the actual giving environment of the child. It must reflect his/her daily life.

Curriculum Includes
Political; Moral; Social; Vocational; Intellectual; Mathematics; General science, Languages; Integration of experiences.

Progressivism and Methods of Teaching
- Project method–active participation of the pupils in learning
- Socialized methods–to bring all the individuals into a group system of interaction
- Conferences
- Consultation
- Demonstrations and reform demonstrations.

Progressivism and the Teacher
The human elements, human beings are given more importance. The teacher has to meet the needs of learner as good human being.

The teacher, who is vital in education process and having richer, superior experience and can analyse the present situation. Teacher will act as a stage setter, guide and coordinator but he/she is not total authority, just he/she guides the situation.

Progressivism and the School
School is a cooperative enterprise, it provide conducive environment for democratic growth of the child.

Progressivism and Nursing Education

Nurse Educator will act as a guide, coordinator in teaching-learning activities. Provides democratic environment in Nursing Educational Institutions. The teaching methods like Project method, Demonstration method, Discussion, Conference, Consultation, Sociometry, Sociogram etc. will be used. Education is centered around the Social, Intellectual and skill development among learners.

BEHAVIORISM

Introduction

Person's behavior is the result of environmental conditioning. Man is a passive recipient, who reacts to external stimuli, he/she has no will or decision of his/her own or the capacity to take spontaneous action.

Principles

According to Skinner, each individual is having an 'ego', 'mind' centre of consciousness which enable him to choose any course of action, that he/she wanted to do. Individual's actions are predetermined by his/her heredity or immediate surroundings.

- Man is not separate from his/her surrounding environment
- Human behavior is controlled with creativity
- Reflexes and other patterns of behavior evolve and change as they increases the chances of survival of the species.

Techniques/Methods of Teaching

- Law of effect
- Reward
- Modeling
- Token economy
- Extinction
- Desensitization
- Flooding
- Response prevention and restraint
- Contingency management
- Negative practice
- Time-out
- Satiation
- Operant conditioning
- Reinforcement
- Shaping
- Programmed behavior
- Classical conditioning
- Reciprocal inhibition
- Cognitive learning
- Aversion
- Self-control technique
- Assertiveness training
- Contact
- Punishment
- Relaxation technique

Educational Applications

Systematic applications of principles of learning aims at changing maladaptive behavior with adaptive behavior.

Learning is governed by man's action and reaction to various media (oral, written, machine).

Learning occurs as a personal achievement through interaction between the learner and environment.

Advantages

- Man tries to understand, predict, influence and control human behavior with rapidity.
- Individualized instruction
- Auto instruction
- Self corrective
- Reinforcement provided by correct answers is a source of encouragement to the slow learners.

Limitations

- It requires technical proficiency
- Goals are not kept in mind, in controlling human behavior
- The concepts of freedom, capacity to choose, worthiness of individual will be completely lost.

Behaviorism and Nursing Education

Nurse Educator will utilize the skills and Behavior Modification techniques to promote the emotional health among learners. Systematic application of principles of learning will be adopted by teacher. The learners will easily adapts to any situations by utilizing the techniques and creates conducive environment to enhance their learning.

HUMANISM

Man is an end, not a means

Principles

The humanist emphasis is on literature.
He has to overcome the conflicts in his/her own time.

Directions

- Respect for language
- Ancient cultures
- Intellectuals for literary scholarship

Humanism Attitude is Reflected in Certain Value Systems

- Values are of the highest quality, benefit will occur
- Fall/decline in moral, esthetic standards, values results in violence and barbarism (undisciplined behavior, crude tastes and rude manners)
- Values are intellectual abstractions, eternal and unchanging
- Values are fundamental measures of human experience
- Human problems are problems of values
- Literature portrays man in historical circumstances and reflects moral decisions, civilized behavior
- Absolute and eternal values are inexpressible

The Role of Education in Humanism

- Children must be taught to respect language, a sense of language perfection
- Children must be trained in modern literary standards of academics

Curriculum

Music, Literature; central concern is respect for intellectual values and traditions.

Teacher

The teacher is expected to be well-read, well-trained in humanities subjects and superior attainment.

Humanism and Nursing Education

Nurse educator will keep sincere efforts for the promotion of linguistic development among learners. Nurses has to work in varied community settings, deal with people and their problems. The learners has to understand the language, which the patient is speaking, so only inclusion of languages in the curriculum has given weightage such that the learners will able to understand the client's problems; identify the needs, implements nursing process and meets the needs or clients in a systematic way by utilizing the theoritical knowledge and practical skills comprehensively. The teacher will act as a guide role-model and supporter for learners.

EXPERIMENTALISM

Experimentalists reject the laissez-faire individualism and permissiveness. They accept a naturalistic point of view, but they want the control and utilization of nature - not submission to nature. It accepts the perspective of evolution.

Ideas of Sociology Adapted by Experimentalists (according to John Dewey)

- Man is a social being and product of his/her environment

- Learning depends on environment
- Experimentalists ask people of the world, to appreciate and respect one another culture and to recognize that differences merely reflect environment circumstances
- Technology means progress in social development and social advance
- The goal of man is not only to survive but also to live a good life, economic well-being which is a motive for psychological and social behavior. The school is social institution, democratic philosophy of education has to be represented

Experimentalism and Nursing Education

Nurse educator will utilize scientific, systematic enquiry in meting the felt needs and demand needs of the client. They will promote skills among learners, e.g. scientific skills, interaction and interpersonal skills. In community health nursing practice, nurses will utilizes the resources in community and implement promotive, preventive, curative and educative activities will be implemented. Experimentalism philosophy, principles will be adapted both hospital and community clinical settings.

ECLECTICISM

Introduction

To familiarize with different philosophies, draw the best and essential points inspiration from all of them and make into one harmonious whole and build one's own philosophy of education. It is known as, the 'eclectic tendency' in education.

All the philosophies are oriented towards philosophy of life. it differs how one thinks about life; their own views related to life, different educationists formulated different philosophies. Some gave importance to spiritual and mental aspects of life, while others gave emphasis to the physical and social aspects. Man is a complex being with physical, mental, psychological, spiritual and social aspects of life. There should be a happy and harmonious life in various aspects related to life. A holistic philosophy of education which would help for the total development of the individual, is useful. No school of philosophy meets the entire requirements of varied situations in life. No system of education can be exclusively based on a particular school of philosophy. Infact, no educator is exclusively idealist, naturalist or pragmatist. For the modern educationists, it will be beneficial and effective, if they make a thorough study of these different schools of philosophy and then rearrange and relate the essential principles into one harmonious whole and thus build their own theory of the education with the best material. This would be basis for 'eclectic tendency' in education.

Definition

"The synthesis or harmonious blend of the diverse philosophies of education. It is the process of pulling out and putting together of the useful and essential aspects of various philosophies of education."

Meaning

- The fusion or synthesis of different philosophies of education
- The harmonization of principles underlying various tendencies and rationalization of educational practices - Munroe's view
- The process of putting together the common views of different philosophies into comprehensive whole

Need

- No philosophy is complete in itself. It cannot be applied successfully in all situations
- To find unity in diversity through eclectic approach
- To meet the changing needs and demands in the world and cultivate change in behavior, no need for the learners to stick to one dogma, ideology or philosophy
- Indian philosophers have always recognized the value of adjustment in the midst of conflicting ideologies. They always try to resolve the difficulties through peaceful and consistence means. So in Indian culture and civilization, we find deeprooted eclecticism and fusion

- There is a diversity of thinking in all aspects of human culture and civilization. The educator tries to discover some unity of thought in this diversity
- Uniform tendency or holistic approach is needed for Indian culture and its civilization
- The abilities and the talents of youth are properly channelized and utilized, the eclectic tendency is needed
- To promote good citizenship, equality of opportunity, universality in education, eclectic tendency is essential.

Areas of Agreement or the Eclectic Tendency at Work in Education

- Idealism stresses spirituality and absolute values; naturalism emphasizes the matter in man; pragmatism is regarded as a sort of compromise between spiritualism and materialism

The naturalistic philosophy moulds the individual in natural and physical environment; it follows natural environment and prepares the child to adapt himself to it. Idealism wishes the individual to fit him in the present day individualized and mechanized world, it goes to the extreme in the concept of changing the environment. To make the learner perfect with creative values and adjusting to the changing demands of eclectic tendency in society, education has started. The respect for the child as an individual and placing him at the centre of the educational process, which is a common feature in most modern philosophies of education.

Meeting Ground of all Philosophies

a. *Respect for child's personality:* Dignity and respect the child's personality. Child is the centre of educative process, the philosophies will mould the child according to their own view point.
b. *Powerful force of mind:* Mind is powerful force in the life of man.

   Idealists regard mind as a creator of its objects and a discoverer of its own laws. The mind and spirit together form reality–naturalists believe in the impact of environment on mind. The external world within the environment influences the mind and intellect. Pragmatists view the mind is a functional behavior.
c. *Free discipline:* Discipline is only a means and not end in itself. Self-government is acceptable of all, as a powerful means of inculcating discipline.
d. *Individual and social development:* Social efficiency and individual development are important aim of education.

   Health; Command of fundamental processes; Worthy home membership; Vocation; Citizenship; Worthy use of leisure; Ethical character; Enjoyment in freedom; Integrating personality.
e. *Curriculum:* Unity of mind and heart of people among divergent traditions of the country. Life centred curriculum for providing total experiences.

   Humanities, Language skills, Mathematics, Arts, Practical arts and Crafts, History, Geography, Sciences, Logic, Grammar, essential skills, desirable attitudes and social virtues are included in various curricula.

Methods of Teaching

- Play way method
- Learning by doing
- Direct experiences through projects and problem solving etc.

Teacher Training

Teachers, need to be prepared carefully for their role through courses of instruction and practical application.

   The educator seeks to find harmony among the various philosophical positions and a practical method for application of the finest principles needed in his/her educational work. Teacher puts altogether and creates an educational philosophy and practice of his/her own to suit the prevalent environment in which his/her institution exists.

Aims of Education

- Education should give a child, a command of the basic processes of learning.
- The child should become an efficient member of society.
- The development of moral character.
- Promotion of good health.
- Skillful training.

- To prepare the person to take his/her place in life.
- To be able to think, reason and to adapt himself to his/her environment.
- Interests and motivation of the child has to be improved.
- The child should be educated in favourable, congenial environment. Education has to promote or encourage the child to develop skills and knowledge.

Conclusion

We can easily find out, where a particular philosophy has succeeded and where it has failed and in this way, we can gain the good points of all of them. Infact, all these philosophy of education are complementary and not contradictory. if we take best from all the philosophies to have harmoniousness in nature idealism is fundamental while naturalism and pragmatism are contributory factors in the theory and practice of education. To establish new ideals and standards, there is a necessity to formulate a holistic philosophy, where all the best means of development of child will take place and narrow feelings, mutual ill wills can be overcome.

Electicism and Nursing Education

Holistic philosophy of education, where the knowledge of all philosophies will be used by Nurse Educator according to the learning situations and requirements of the learners, the course objectives will be attained by comprehensive, cooperative, coordinated effort, of all teachings factulty. Varied knowledge and skills will be incorporated in implementing Nursing activities. The total development of learners will be attained, they will become, skilful and efficient Nurses.

RECONSTRUCTIONALISM

Introduction

When political independence was achieved in India, the people realised that the educational system started by the British was against the nationalism, culture and traditions of the country. The criticism of the educational system was started even before independence, because it was according to the British policy and not in the interest of India. Its aim was simply to produce clerks who might help in running the British Government. At the same time its aim was to impose English culture, civilization on the Indians. In this educational system, Indian culture was deliberately neglected. Voice against this system has continuously been raised and it has been criticized persistently. In spite of the criticism, there education continues to run on the old lines. Several committees and commissions have been appointed to reform it, but no meaningful change has been brought so far. Education in our country is still impracticable and against Indian culture and traditions. Because of the impracticability of Indian education demands for its reform have been raised.

Meaning of Reconstruction

It may be understood in two forms. First, total change. Second, desirable change. Hereby educational reconstruction, we mean both the types of reforms. The present educational system undoubtedly does not represent Indian culture and traditions. So it should be changed totally or reformed gradually.

Total change is a difficult task and it requires deep thinking, money and research. Total change done in haste is harmful and it takes time and energy to bring it on right lines. So the method of bringing desirable reforms is better and convenient. So instead of changing the educational system totally, it should be reformed gradually. But whether it is a total change or gradual reform, our educational system must be based on Indian culture and traditions and at the same time it should be practicable also. By reform it is also meant that attitudes of all persons related to education, students teachers, administration etc should begin to change.

Main Elements of Reconstruction

1. *National culture and philosophy of life:* In educational reconstruction first of all we shall have to give freedom to our Indian philosophy and culture, the aim of which shall be to acquaint our students with our culture, customs, civilization, literature and history. For an all round development a person should be acquainted with his/her national culture and philosophy. So we shall have to familiarize our children with our culture and philosophy from very beginning in order. So we shall have to include these elements in our educational reconstruction.

2. *National education:* In our education we have to include national education policy. Our idea of national education should be so ambitious that it develops our national feelings and promotes our cultural development and all other types of advancement for the prosperity of the nation. This is real national education. The aim of national education should also be a development of mind and personality which may give rise to the feelings of self-control, self-regard, human love and sympathy in man.

   It should be the main aim of national education to acquaint man with his/her duties.

3. *Duty of government:* Educational reconstruction is a difficult task. For that help and interest of the government is necessary. Education takes the nation to the path of progress. So the Government has a great responsibility in this regard. The Government has to come forward in educational reconstruction and it has to provide money in its budget.

   After defence, education should be given utmost priority and it should be so organised that people extend their willing, cooperation. The Government has to pay attention on the entire education. Neglect of any respect will be harmful for the country. The Government has to pay equal attention on primary, secondary, higher, technical and vocational education. Only then it will be called as real national education.

4. *Duty of countryman:* Along with Government, the countrymen too have some duties in the educational reconstruction as citizens are indifferent, Government alone cannot do this work. They will also have to change their outlook and will have to adopt an attitude of respect and honour towards their culture, philosophy, and traditions. The leaders in the field of social, political, and educational activities will have to take the lead and participation in educational reconstruction.

Aims of Education

The primary aim of education is an all-round development of personality. It mainly includes physical, mental, moral and spiritual development. Along with it, reasoning, thinking, and intelligence should also be developed.

The aims of education is to develop faith in democratic principles.

To inculcate the feelings of social service in the student and create in him/her the capacity for adoption to environment and earning his/her living. Emotional integration with the people of other states should also be developed. People should also be taught the skill of utilizing their leisure in constructive activities. The things have to be paid attention in educational reconstruction. To create the ability to control factional tendencies such as communalism, casteism, regionalism, etc. for national integration. We should rise above narrow-mindedness, understanding and cooperation.

Curriculum

The curriculum will be based on the age, capacity, social status, environment and geographical conditions.

Free Education

Up to a stage, the education should be entirely free and this expenditure should be done by the state. It will be better, if education is free up to secondary stage. It is necessary to adopt democratic principles in curriculum and in the administration of educational institutions. General, technical, and vocational education should be provided and desirable changes should be made in primary, secondary and higher education.

Teaching Methods

In the teaching methods, the aim should not be only to pass examination but to develop necessary qualities and abilities also; so education should be activity centred. Teaching should be so organised that the student may become self-reliant.

Discipline

Education should be so organized and conducted that the problem of indiscipline may not arise at all, in the educational institution. For this, qualities like liberalism, tolerance and discretion may be developed in students.

Competent Teachers

Education cannot be beneficial in the absence of competent teachers. So proper arrangements for the training of teachers should be made. For this work, necessary changes are needed in the outlook of training institutions.

Examination

The prevailing examination system is defective, because it does not evaluated the ability of students properly. So such changes are to be made that the ability of students may be evaluate properly. The examination should be based on the work of the entire session. The defects of essay tests may be removed.

Guardians

The cooperation of teachers and guardians is needed in the reconstruction of education because the child passes his/her time in the company of both. So the education of guardians is also needed in this regard to fulfill their duties.

Healthy Environment

The work of educational reconstruction becomes easy if the schools are established in healthy environment.

Reconstructionalism and Nursing Education

Nursing curriculum includes National Education policy in General Education and Community Health Nursing; so that learners will be aware of the policy and its measures for implementations ablity of the students will be tested by practical examination by skill assessment. Teachers will function as supervisors and counselors. Demonstration project method, lecture method will be used to enhance the theoretical knowledge and practicals skills of learners.

QUESTIONS

- Agencies of Education (5 M, NTRUHS, June 2009 & 5M, MGRUHS, Aug, 2008)
- Agencies of education (5M, MGU, Oct, 2007)
- Aims of Nursing Education (5M, NIMS, Sept, 2010)
- Briefly explain philosophy and aims of education (10M, RGUHS, Sept, 2009)
- Bring out the relationship with Education and Philosophy(10M, RGUHS, Aug, 2010 & 15M, NIMS, Sept, 2010)
- Chief features of Existentialism (10M, RGUHS, Oct, 2008)
- Current trends in Nursing Education (5M, MGU, Dec, 2008)
- Define Education (2M, NIMS, May, 2007)
- Define Education. Explain the role of a teacher in nursing education. (2+10 = 12 M, NTRUHS, June 2009)
- Define Education. List various aims of Education, (3 + 5 + 8 M, Rajasthan UHS, Feb, 2008)
- Define Nursing Education (5M, RGUHS, April 2007)
- Describe Philosophy of Education (7M, Baba Farid UHS, 2010)
- Difference between Pragmatism–Naturalism (5M, MGU, Oct, 2007)
- Differentiate between Idealism - Pragmatism (5M, MGU, Feb, 2008)
- Discuss briefly aims and objectives of education. Explain the relation between Philosophy and education (15M, RGUHS, Oct, 2006)
- Discuss Education and Discuss its aims in context of Nursing Education (10M, Rajasthan UHS, March, 2010)
- Evaluation and accreditation of nursing education institutions (15M, RGUHS, Oct, 2009)
- Explain in detail about traditional Philosophers (7.5M, NIMS, Sept, 2010)
- Explain the relationship between philosophy and education (15M, RGUHS, M.Sc.(N), Oct, 2009)
- Explain Various Philosophies of Education, formulate a Philosophy for a 4 year B.Sc.(N) (6+8=14M, NTRUHS, June, 2009)
- Formulate a philosophy for M.Sc Nursing programme stating the importance of different philosophies (15M, RGUHS, Oct, 2009)
- Give the Meaning of " Philosophy of Nursing Education" (7M), Outline a Model of Philosophy for formulating a new School of Nursing (8M, MGRUHS, Nov, 2010)
- Give the Meaning of Philosophy of Nursing Education (7 M), Outline a Model of Philosophy for formulating a New College of Nursing (8M) Discuss the Organization Pattern of Education in India (15 M) (MGRUHS, Aug, 2008)

- Idealism (5M, MGU, Nov, 2009; 5M, NTRUHS, June, 2008)
- Identify and give examples of Philosophy seen in Nursing (5M, NTRUHS, June, 2007)
- List the various philosophies in Education , Explain the functions of Education, Discuss the maxims of teaching (3M+5M + 5M, NIMS, May, 2010)
- Name 4 Idealism Philosophers (2M, MGRUHS, Aug, 2008)
- Narrate Traditional Philosophies of Education (15M, NIMS, Sept, 2010)
- Philosophy of Nursing Education (5M, Baba Farid UHS, 2009; 5M, MGRUHS, Feb, 2009)
- Philosophy of Nursing Service (5M, NTRUHS, June, 2008)
- Pragmatism (5M, RGUHS, Aug, 2010; 5M, NTRUHS, June, 2007)
- Three aims of Nursing Education (3M, MGU, Dec, 2008)
- Trends and issues in Nursing Education(5M, MGU, Nov, 2009)
- What are the traditional philosophies? Explain any one suitable philosophy for nursing with examples (15M, NTRUHS, Feb, 2010)
- What do you understand by the term, "Philosophy" (2M), How are the Philosophy and Education are related to each other (8M), Discuss the Philosophy of Nursing Education (5M, MGRUHS, Nov, 2010)
- Write in detail the impact of modern technology in Nursing Education (15M, NIMS, Oct, 2008)
- Write in detail the role of a Nurse Educator in developing Nursing as a Profession (15M, NIMS, Oct, 2008)
- Write the Philosophy & Objectives of Nursing Education (5M, NIMS, Sep, 2010)

Indian Nursing Council

INTRODUCTION

Indian Nursing Council is involved in the operational management and regulation of services in the interest of society. This includes keeping up to date with tracking international developments, undertaking research in various relevant fields and adding new knowledge and insight to the practice of their profession.

INC is responsible for the corporate governance of Nurses and Nursing Professionals. This includes the issues of discipline, the promotion of health, proactively advising, alerting and offering comment to the Government on matters affecting the Nursing profession. However, the final democratic accountability and ultimate responsibility lays with the Government of India and Parliament.

Aims/Objectives

- To regulate the training policies and programs in the field of Nursing
- To bring about standardization of training courses
- To prescribe minimum standards of education and training of various Nursing programs
- To regulate these standards in all training institutions uniformly throughout the country
- To formulate the curriculum of varied courses and revise the curriculum whenever need arises
- To recognize Institutions/Organizations/Universities imparting Ph.D, M.Phil, Master's Degree, Bachelor's Degree, P.G. Diploma, Diploma, Certificate Courses in the field of Nursing
- To recognize Degree/Diploma/Certificate awarded by Foreign Universities/Institutions on reciprocal basis
- To promote research in Nursing
- To maintain Indian Nurses Register for registration of Nursing Personnel
- To Organize varied Training programs in coordination with National and International Voluntary organizations.

Functions

- An ongoing review of curriculum in response to national priorities
- An ongoing review of the education system with a focus on community based education
- Integrated education with a focus on problem-based learning to promote critical thinking
- Competency based education
- Protection of the rights and dignity of people
- To establish and monitor a uniform standard of nursing education for Nurses Midwife, Auxiliary Nurse-Midwives and Health Visitors by doing inspection of the institutions
- To recognize the qualifications under section 10(2)(4) of the INC Act, 1947 for the purpose of registration and employment in India and abroad
- To give approval for registration of Indian and Foreign Nurses possessing foreign qualification under section 11(2)(a) of the Indian Nursing Council Act, 1947
- To prescribe the syllabus and regulations for Nursing programs
- Power to withdraw the recognition of qualification under section 14 of the Act in case the institution fails to maintain its standards under Section 14(1)(b) that an institution recognized by a State Council for the training of Nurses, Midwives, Auxiliary Nurse Midwives or Health Visitors does not satisfy the requirements of the Council
- To advise the State Nursing Councils, Examining Boards, State Governments and Central Government in various important items regarding Nursing Education in the Country

Constitution of the Council

Section 3(1) of the Indian Nursing Council Act, 1947, provides for constitution and composition of the council consisting of the following (Fig. 2.1):

- One nurse enrolled in a state register elected by each State Council
- Two members elected from among themselves by the heads of institutions recognized by the INC for the purpose of this clause in which training is given:
  - For obtaining a University degree in Nursing
  - In respect of a post-certificate course in teaching of nursing and in nursing administration
- One member elected from among themselves by the heads of institutions in which health visitors are trained
- One member elected by the Medical Council of India
- One member elected by the Central Council of the Indian Medical Association
- One member elected by the council of the Trained Nurses Association of India
- One midwife or auxiliary nurse-midwife enrolled in a State Register, elected by each of the State Councils in the four groups of State mentioned below, each group of States being taken in rotation in the following order namely:
  - Kerala, Madhya Pradesh, Uttar Pradesh and Haryana
  - Andhra Pradesh, Bihar, Maharashtra and Rajasthan
  - Karnataka, Punjab and West Bengal
  - Assam, Gujarat, Tamil Nadu and Orissa
- The Director General of Health Services, ex-officio
- The Chief Principal Matron, Medical Directorate, Army Headquarters, ex-officio
- The Chief Nursing Superintendent, Office of the Director General of Health Services, ex-officio
- The Director of Maternity and Child Welfare, Indian Red Cross Society, ex-officio
- The Chief Administrative Medical Officer (by whatever name called) of each State other than a Union Territory, ex-officio
- The Superintendent of Nursing Services (by whatever name called) ex-officio from each of the States in the two groups mentioned below, each group of States being taken in rotation in the following order, namely:
  - Andhra Pradesh, Assam, Maharashtra, Madhya Pradesh, Tamil Nadu, Uttar Pradesh, West Bengal and Haryana
  - Bihar, Gujarat, Kerala, Karnataka, Orissa, Punjab and Rajasthan
- Four members nominated by the Central Government, of whom at least two shall be nurses, midwives or health visitors enrolled in a State register and one shall be an experienced educationalist
- Three members elected by parliament, two by the House of the People from among its members and the other by the Council of States from among its members.

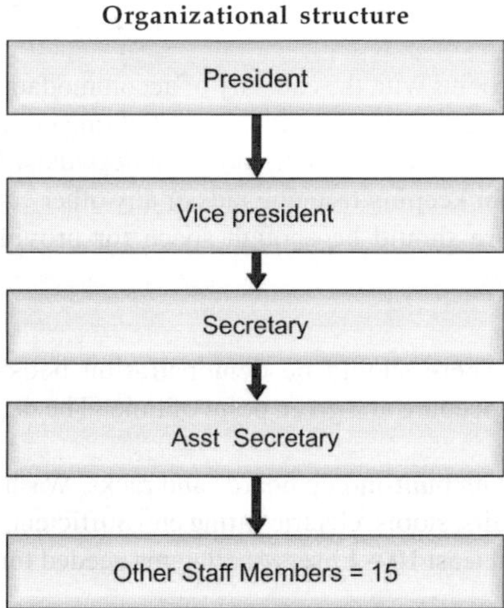

INC Committees

1. Executive Committee of the Council: To deliberate on the issues related to maintenance of standards of Nursing programs.
2. The Nursing Education Committee: To deliberate on the issues concerned mainly with Nursing education and policy matters concerning the nursing education.
3. Equivalence Committee: To deliberate on the issues of recognition of foreign qualifications.

Norms/Guidelines/Establishment of Nursing Education Institutions

The authority which desires to open a school/college of Nursing has to furnish the following documentary proof to the INC and comply with the following:

- Any organization under the Central Government, State Government, Local body or a Private or Public Trust, Mission, Voluntary registered under society Registration Act or a Company registered under company's act wishes to open a School/College of Nursing, should obtain the No Objection/Essentiality Certificate from the State Government
- The INC on receipt of the proposal from the institution to start the nursing program (School/College), will undertake the first inspection to assess suitability with regard to physical infrastructure, clinical facility and teaching faculty in order to give permission to start the program
- After the receipt of the permission to start the nursing program from the INC, the institution shall obtain the approval from the State Nursing Council and Examination Board/University
- Institution will admit the students only after taking approval of State Nursing Council and Examination Board/University
- The INC will conduct inspection and permission will be given year by year till the first batch completes.

Physical Facilities

Building

The College/School of Nursing should have a separate building. The college/school of Nursing should be near to its parent hospital having space for expansion in an institutional area. Minimum Land area recommended by INC for a school/college of Nursing is four acres of land owned and possessed by the applicant to set up the proposed nursing school/college(annual intake of 20 students). For every additional 10 seats, an additional constructed area of 2000 square feet should be increased. Constructed area can be increased in a phased manner between first and second year. For a College/School with an annual admission capacity of 60 students, the constructed area of the school/college should be 23720 square feet.

Adequate hostel/residential accommodation for students and staff should be available in addition to the above mentioned built up area of the Nursing College/School respectively.

The Minimum physical facilities which are required in the school/college are listed.

Class Rooms

There should be at least four class rooms with the capacity of accommodating the number of students admitted in each class. The rooms should be well ventilated with proper lighting system. There should be built in Black/Green/White Boards. There should be space to accommodate a desk/dais. A big table and a chair, podium for the teacher and racks /cup boards for keeping teaching aids or any other equipment needed for the conduct of classes also should be there. There should be enough space for providing proper and adequate seating facilities for the students in the class.

Laboratories

a Nursing practice laboratory: There should be demonstration beds in proportion to the number of students practicing a Nursing Procedure at a given point of time (The desired ratio being 1 bed: 6 practicing students.

It should be fully equipped with built-in-cup boards and racks. Wash-basins with running water supply, adequate furniture like table, chairs, stools, electric fitting etc. Sufficient, adequate inventory articles should be there sufficient number i.e., at least 10 – 12 sets of all items needed for the practice of Nursing procedure by the students.

b. Community practice laboratory: It should have all required articles needed for practicing nursing procedures in a community set-up.

c. Nutrition laboratory: It should have facilities for imparting basic knowledge about food and to practice the cooking for the healthy as well as for the sick. The furnishing equipments should include work-tables, cooking stoves or gas connection/fittings, wash-basins with running water—supply, cutlery, trays, plates, diabetic scales, cooking utensils, racks/shelves, refrigerator, pressure cooker, mixie and cup boards for storage of food items.

The details of the constructed area is given in below for admission capacity of 60 students:

Teaching Block

Sl No.	Teaching Block	Area (Sq Feet)
1	Lecture Hall	4 @ 1080 = 4320
2	Nursing Foundation Lab	1500
	CHN	900
	Nutrition	900
	OBG and Paediatrics lab	900
3	Pre-clinical science lab	900
4	Computer lab	1500
5	Multipurpose Hall	3000
6	Common Room (male & Female)	2000
7	Staff Room	1000
8	Principal Room	300
9	Vice Principal Room	200
10	Library	2400
11	A.V. Aids Room	600
12	One Room for each Head of Departments	800
13	Faculty Room	2400
14	Provisions for Toilets	1000
	Total	**23720 Sq Ft**

Hostel Block

Sl No.	Hostel Block	Area (Sq Ft)
1	Single/Double Room	24000
2	Sanitary	One toilet and one bathroom (for 5 students) – 500
3	Visitor Room	500
4	Reading Room	250
5	Store	500
6	Recreation Room	500
7	Dining Hall	3000
8	Kitchen and Store	1500
	Total	**30750 Sq ft**

Grand Total: 23720 + 30750 = 54470 Sq Ft.

School and College of Nursing can share laboratories, if they are in same campus under same trust, that is the institution is one but offering different nursing programs. However they should have equipments and articles proportionate to the strength of admission and the class rooms should be available as per the requirement stipulated by INC of each program.

Clinical Facilities

School/College of Nursing should have a 120-150 bedded Parent/Affiliated Hospital for 40 annual intake in each year.
- Distribution of beds in different areas
  - Medical 30
  - Surgical 30
  - OBG 30
  - Pediatrics 20
  - Ortho 10
- Bed occupancy of the Hospital should be minimum 75%
- The size of the hospital/nursing home for affiliation should not be less than 50 beds
- Other specialities/facilities for clinical experience required are as follows:
  - Major OT
  - Minor OT
  - Dental
  - Eye/ENT
  - Neonatology with Nursery
  - Communicable disease
  - Community Health Nursing
  - Cardiology
  - Oncology
  - Neurology/Neurosurgery
  - Nephrology etc.
  - ICU/ICCU
- Affiliation of psychiatric hospital should be of minimum 30-50 beds
- The Nursing staffing norms in the affiliated hospital should be as per the INC norms
- The affiliated hospital should give student status to the candidates of the nursing program
- Affiliated hospitals should be in the radius of 15-30 kms
- 1:3 student patient ratio to be maintained

If the institution is having both GNM and B.Sc (N) program, it would require 240 bedded parent/affiliated hospital for 40 annual intake in each program to maintain 1:3 student patient ratio.

Collegiate Program

Qualifications and experience of teachers of College of Nursing are as in table below.

Sl N	Post, Qualification and Experience
1	Professor-cum-Principal Masters Degree in Nursing 10 years of experience and minimum of 5 years of teaching experience Desirable: Independent published work of high standard/Doctorate Degree/M.Phil
2	Professor-cum-Vice Principal Masters Degree in Nursing 10 years of experience and minimum of 5 years of teaching experience Desirable: Independent published work of high standard/Doctorate Degree/M.Phil
3	Reader/Associate Professor Masters Degree in Nursing 7 years of experience and minimum of 3 years teaching experience Desirable: Independent published work of high standard/Doctorate Degree/M.Phil
4	Lecturer Masters degree in Nursing 3 years experience
5	Tutor/Clinical Instructor M.Sc (N) or B.Sc(N) with 1 year experience or Basic B.Sc(N) with post basic diploma in clinical speciality

M.Sc (N) Program

If parent hospital is super speciality hospital like cardiothoracic hospital/cancer, M.Sc(N) program can be started with annual intake of 10 M.Sc(N) in cardiothoracic/cancer. The nursing faculty recruited should be as given below:

Professor cum Coordinator	1
Reader/Associate Professor	2
Lecturer	1

The above faculty shall perform dual role

B.Sc(N) and M.Sc(N) program

Annual intake of 60 students for B.Sc(N) and 25 students for M.Sc(N) program

Teaching faculty	B.Sc (N)	M.Sc (N)
Professor-cum-Principal	1	
Professor-cum-Vice Principal	1	
Reader/Associate Professor	1	2
Lecturer	2	3
Tutor/Clinical Instructor	19	
Total	24	5

One in each speciality and all the M.Sc (N) qualified teaching faculty will participate in both programs. Teacher student ratio = 1:10

GNM and B.Sc (N) with 60 annual intake in each program

Professor-cum-Principal	1
Professor-cum-Vice Principal	1
Reader/Associate professor	1
Lecturer	4
Tutor/Clinical Instructor	35
Total	42

Two M.Sc (N) qualified teaching faculty to start college of nursing, for proposed less than or equal to 60 students and 4 M.Sc (N) qualified teaching faculty for proposed 61-100 students, and by 4th year they should have 5, 7 M.Sc (N) qualified teaching faculty respectively. Preferably with one in each speciality i.e., Med-Surgical Nursing, Paediatrics Nursing, OBG Nursing, Community health Nursing and Psychiatric Nursing.

Note

- No part time nursing faculty will be counted for calculating total number of faculty required for a college
- Irrespective of number of admissions, all faculty positions (Professor to lecturer) must be filled
- For M.Sc (N) program appropriate number of M.Sc faculty in each speciality has to be appointed subject to the condition that total number of teaching faculty ceiling is maintained.

Basic B.Sc (N)

Teaching Faculty	Annual Capacity	
Annual intake	40-60	61-100
Professor-cum-Principal	1	1
Professor-cum-Vice Principal	1	1
Reader/Associate Professor	1	1
Lecturer	2	4
Tutor/Clinical Instructor	19	33
Total	24	40

Teacher student ratio = 1:10

Part time teachers/External teachers

Sl No.	Faculty
1	Microbiology
2	Bio-chemistry
3	Sociology
4	Bio-physics
5	Psychology
6	Nutrition
7	English
8	Computer
9	Hindi / Any other language
10	Any other Clinical Disciplines
11	Physical Education

(The above teachers should have post-graduate qualification with teaching experience in respective area)

- All nursing teachers must possess a basic university or equivalent qualification as laid down in the schedules of the INC Act, 1947. They shall be registered under the State Nursing Registration Act
- Nursing faculty in Nursing college except tutor/instructors must possess the requisite recognized post graduate qualification in nursing subjects
- Holders of equivalent post graduate qualifications, which may be approved by the INC from time to time, may be considered to have the requisite recognized post graduate qualification in the subject concerned
- All teachers of nursing other than Principal and Vice Principal should spend at least 4 hours in the clinical area for clinical teaching and/or supervision of care every day.

School of Nursing

Qualifications of Teaching Faculty

Principal	M.Sc (N) with 3 years of teaching experience or B.Sc (N) Basic/Post Basic with 5 years of teaching experience
Vice Principal	M.Sc (N) or B.Sc (N) Basic/Post Basic with 3 years of teaching experience
Tutor	M.Sc (N) or B.Sc (N) Basic/Post Basic or Diploma in Nursing Education and Administration with 2 years of professional experience

For School of Nursing with 60 students (i.e., an annual intake of 20 students):

Teaching Faculty	No. required
Principal	1
Vice Principal	1
Tutor	4
Additional Tutor for interns	1
Total	7

Note: Teacher Student ratio should be 1:10 for the sanctioned strength.

Reason for revising the syllabus

- Too old syllabus
- Too much advancement and its impact—Educational technology
- National Health Policy/Population Policy/Priorities of the Government
- Latest Techniques of Communication
- Advances in Medical Sciences
- Modern trends in Evaluation
- Level and aspirations of new entrants to Nursing
- Demands of the consumer for quality care
- Equalization of Educational programs globally.

Curriculum Guide

- Helps the institutions to plan the programs effectively
- Experiment with new material and methods of teaching
- Discourage following traditional methods blindly
- Motivate to go above mediocrity and aim at the best
- Encourage all teachers to aim at quality.

ACCREDITATION OF NURSING EDUCATIONAL INSTITUTIONS IN INDIA

Accreditation for universities in India is required by law, unless the university was created. "It is emphasized that fake institutions have no legal entity to call themselves as University/Vishwavidyalaya and to award 'degree' which are not treated as valid for academic/employment purposes. Quality Assurance and Accreditation of Nursing is standardization of Nursing schools and colleges. Indian Nursing Council (INC) and State Nursing Councils, Government and Universities and Board are the accreditating agencies for Nursing educational institutions.

Definitions

- "The act of granting credit or recognition (especially with respect to educational institution that maintains suitable standards), A commission is responsible for the accreditation of Nursing Educational Institutions"
- "The act of accrediting or the state of being accredited, especially the granting of approval to an institution of learning by an official review board after the school has met specific requirements".
- "A process whereby a professional association grants recognition to a school or health care institution for demonstrated ability to meet the predetermined criteria for established standard by the Councils"

Objectives

To improve quality of Nursing education in the country

Specific objectives

- To review the strategies used for quality improvement in nursing education in the country
- To agree upon guidelines on quality assurance and accreditation of institutions
- To provide recommendations on the roles and function of nursing educational institutions, nursing councils or regulatory bodies and national authorities on the quality of education

Functions

- To ascribe or attribute to; credit with
- To supply with credentials or authority; authorize
- To attest to and approve as meeting a prescribed standard
- To recognize (an institution of learning) as maintaining those standards requisite for its graduates to gain admission to other reputable institutions of higher learning or to achieve credentials for professional practice
- To believe
- To give official recognition to sanction; to authorize
- To certify or guarantee as meeting required standards
- To furnish or send (an envoy etc.,) with official credentials

The health workforce plays an important role in strengthening of the health system. However, this workforce must be adequate in number, competent and motivated. Nursing Educational institutions , Nursing councils and authoritative bodies can play a significant role in producing qualified graduates, Post Graduates and Diploma Holders. An adequate, competent and motivated health workforce can save lives and is an important building block for health system strengthening. In addition to quality assurance, institutions should be accredited by nursing councils or national regulatory bodies to ensure quality. The authorities concerned should develop guidelines for the schools to follow and should accredit the schools. The results of the accreditation are usually made available to the public.

The accreditation process should take into account curriculum models, instructional methods and staffing policy of public health institutions; educational resources for the student population and for the delivery of the curriculum, including library, lecture halls, laboratories, computers and provision for field practice; description of methods used for assessment of their students and a mechanism for program evaluation.

Expected outcomes

- The development of guidelines on quality assurance and accreditation of institutions
- The councils have guidelines in establishment of quality assurance and accreditation systems in their own organizations

Quality can be defined in various ways based on interpretation

- Technical interpretation: a specific characteristic of an object, its properties
- Philosophical interpretation: the essence of an object
- Practical interpretation: achievement or excellence
- Metaphysical interpretation: the meaning of excellence itself
- Scientific interpretation: something to be desired.

Quality is subjective and is based on an individual's background, perspectives and standards. It is everyone's wish or desire to have quality or to be of quality. The pursuit of quality is a continuous cycle which involves the development of standards, quality audit, quality assessment, quality assurance, quality improvement and accreditation.

In the era of quality orientation, human rights and a consumer-driven society, the quest is for the best quality of education. Educational Institutions are expected to provide quality education and perform their roles effectively in producing qualified graduates who will meet the needs and expectations of society. Each institution is required to develop its own mechanism to ensure quality; this is sometimes called quality assurance. The national authoritative body or INC ensures quality by setting the standards of education, approving the curriculum and recognizing and accrediting the school. The quality of nursing education could be evaluated by councils to have many indicators such as standard curriculum, number of qualified teachers, number of students passing the university or board examination, number of students receiving a nursing license upon graduation, number of students getting jobs upon graduation, number of research grants and number of publications in peer review journals. The Indian Nursing Council prescribes the syllabus for all training programs, including unit plan and hours of each subject, scheme of examination and admission criteria. This ensures that the education offered in all nursing institutions is uniform. Minimum standards are also set for the physical facility, teaching facility and clinical facility to start a nursing program. The Indian Nursing Council conducts yearly or periodic inspections of the institutions in order to ensure that the set standards are being implemented.

Quality Cycle

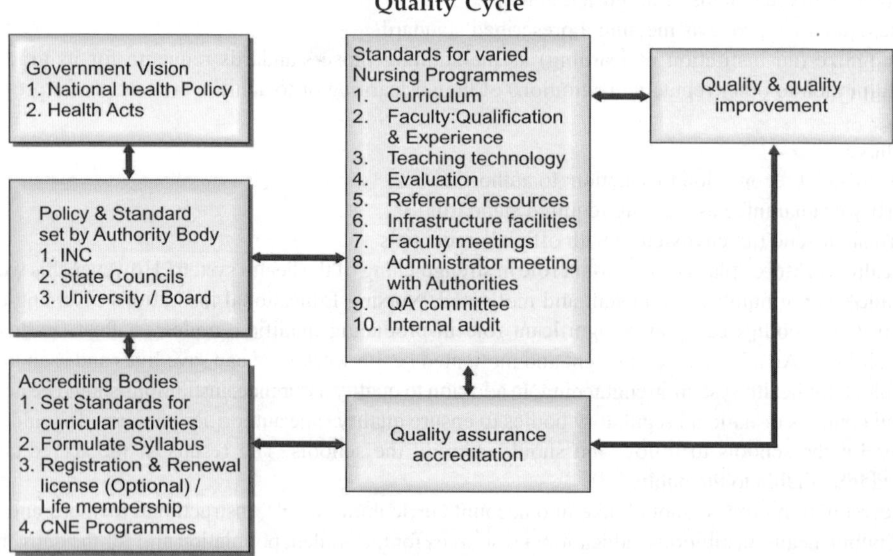

Source: Modified from – QA & Accreditation of Nursing & Midwifery Institution report of regional WHO workshop, 2009.

Strategies or methods used for quality improvement in educational institutions.
- Standards for curriculum and educational institution
- Upgrading of student admission criteria
- Recruitment of students by Merit
- Curriculum revision
- Upgrading of level of nursing education, i.e. from Diploma to PhD program
- External committee to review the test or sit in on the final examination
- Formal study for higher degree of teachers
- Refresher courses for teachers for updating their knowledge as per technological advancement, e.g. CNE, Faculty Development Programs, Staff Development Education Programs
- Nursing Council offering comprehensive examination to all institutions at National level.

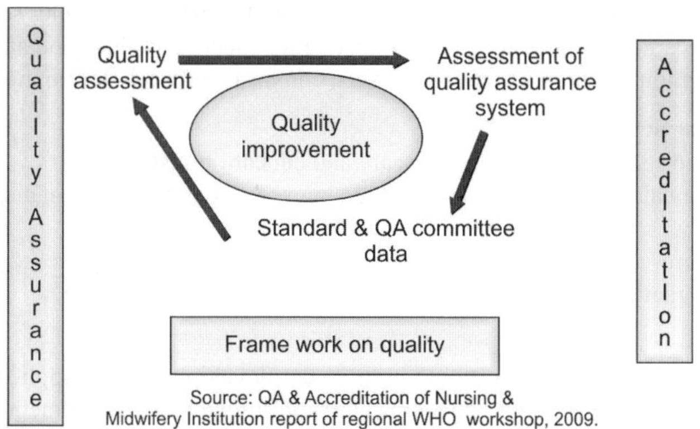

Source: QA & Accreditation of Nursing &
Midwifery Institution report of regional WHO workshop, 2009.

Nursing councils in India set standards of curriculum and educational institutions and accredit nursing educational institutions.

Quality Assurance

The goal of education is to prepare people to function properly in society according to societal needs. Quality assurance (QA) is one of the mechanisms developed by educational institutions to ensure that graduates attain adequate standards of education and training.

1. Internal QA—refers to the audit and assessment done by a team from within the organization.
2. External QA—refers to the audit and assessment done by a team from outside the organization, with the purpose of making the evaluation more objective. There should be tools for audit and assessment. The audit examines whether the school has performed the activities described in the checklist. The auditor simply checks "yes" or "no" column. The assessment aims to judge the level of quality. On the assessment form, criteria and a score for achievement are given for each item. The assessor selects the column that reflects the level of achievement. The total score indicates the readiness or level of quality. The institution must review the results and improve the quality in areas that are not yet at the highest level, while maintaining the quality of those that already meet the standards. Indian Nursing Council may integrate some new components in current accreditation guidelines, may encourage some nursing schools to establish a QA system.

Affiliation of Nursing Educational Institutions

Definitions

"To receive into close connection or association (with a larger body, group, organization, etc.); adopt as a member, branch"

"To adopt or accept as a member, subordinate associate, or branch".

"To associate (oneself) as a subordinate, subsidiary, employee, or member".

"To become closely connected or associated".

"Adoption; association or reception as a member in or of the same family or society".

Nursing Educational Institutions has to be affiliated with Government, University (for Colleges) Boards (Schools) and to the councils (State and National i.e., INC), to meet the requirements of educational programs and standardized as per National and International standards. First inspection is conducted on receipt of the proposal received from the Institute to start any Nursing program prescribed by INC. Then followed by every year the institution will be recognized or affiliated by the respective University, Three years once council's inspection will be conducted to maintain the uniform standards.

NURSING PROGRAMS

Philosophy of PhD Nursing in India by INC

To Prepare Nurses to function in super speciality areas who are required in tertiary care institutions, entrusting limited Public Health functions to Nurses after providing adequate training and increase the ratio of degree holding vis-a-vis diploma holding nurses. There is an acute shortage of Nursing faculty in under graduate and

Post Nursing program in India. Doctoral education is essential to prepare Nursing scholars to improve the quality of Nursing Education and practice in India. Doctoral education builds upon and extends competence acquired at the under graduate and post graduate levels, emphasizes theory development and research skills.

The Functions of Nurse Scholars
- To assume leadership roles in complex health care and education systems
- To develop a theoretical and empirical base for Nursing practice in both current and emerging health care systems,
- To conduct Nursing research and participate in developing health care policies
- To evidence based practice for clinical effectiveness.

Purpose

To prepare Nurse scholars who will contribute both to the development and application of knowledge in Nursing for enhancing quality of Nursing Education, Nursing Research, Nursing Practice and dissemination of Nursing knowledge

Objectives
- Conduct Research relevant to Nursing
- Develop Nursing Theories and Nursing Sciences
- To synthesize knowledge from Nursing and other allied Sciences
- To develop and test theory that affects health status
- To demonstrate the leadership skills in Nursing Practice, Nursing Education and Nursing Research
- To disseminate the results of theory development and Research.

M.Sc. Nursing Program

Philosophy

The Master of Science in Nursing Program is offered by institutions of higher education and is built upon Bachelor's curriculum in Nursing, recognized by INC. The program prepares Nurses for leadership position in Nursing and Health Fields who can function as specialist Nurse Practitioners, Consultants, Educationists, Administrators and Investigators in a wide variety of Professional setting in meeting the National priorities and the changing needs of the society. The program prepares Nursing graduates who are professionally equipped, creative, self directed and socially motivated to effectively deal with day to day problems within the existing constraints and act as an agent of social change. The program encourages the accountability and commitment to lifelong learning which fosters improvement of quality care.

Objectives

The Graduates of Master of Science in Nursing Program demonstrates:
- Increased cognitive, affective and psychomotor competencies and the ability to utilize the potentialities for efficient nursing performance
- Expertise in the utilization of concepts and theories for the assessment, planning and intervention in meeting the self care needs of an individual for the attainment of his/her fullest potential in her/his field of speciality
- Ability to practice independently as a Nurse specialist
- Ability to function effectively as educators and administrators
- Ability to interpret health related research and develop initial competencies in conducting research
- Ability to plan and initiate change in the health care system in practice and in the delivery of health care
- Leadership qualities for the advancement of the practice of Professional Nursing
- Ability to establish collaborative relationship with members of other disciplines for maintaining and improving health care
- Interest in lifelong learning for personal and professional advancement

On Completion of the two year M.Sc Nursing program, the graduate will be able to:
- Utilize/apply the concepts, theories and principles of nursing science
- Demonstrate advance competence in practice of nursing
- Practice as a nurse specialist

- Demonstrate leadership qualities and function effectively as nurse educator and manager
- Demonstrate skill in conducting nursing research, interpreting and utilizing the findings from health related research
- Demonstrate the ability to plan and effect change in nursing practice and in the health care delivery system
- Establish collaborative relationship with members of other disciplines
- Demonstrate interest in continued learning for personal and professional advancement
  Super Speciality Hospital are eligible to start M.Sc.(N) provided they have respective speciality beds.

Eligibility

A candidate seeking admissions shall have:
- Passed B.Sc Nursing (Basic) or Post basic B.Sc Nursing or Post Certificate B.Sc Nursing
- Minimum of 1 year of experience after obtaining B.Sc Nursing (Basic), in a hospital or in Nursing educational institution or in community health setting. For candidate with Post Basic B.Sc in Nursing degree no such experience is needed after graduation
- Registered in State Nursing Council as a Registered Nurse & Registered Midwife

Criteria for selection of candidates

The selection shall be based on merit judged on the basis of aggregate of marks obtained in the University examination from first year to final year B.Sc (Basic) Nursing or Post Basic B.Sc in Nursing and marks obtained in the selection test.

Duration

The course of study shall be for two academic years.

Course of study

In the MSc, 1st year, the following four subjects shall be common to all candidates irrespective of the subject specialty chosen:
- Advanced Concepts of Health and Nursing
- Biological and Psychosocial Foundations of Nursing
- Education and Nursing Education
- Biostatistics, Research Methodology and Nursing Research
  These four subjects will be called as common subjects.

Nursing Specialty shall be the subject specialty chosen by the candidate. In the M.Sc, 2nd year, the subject 'Administration and Nursing Administration' shall be common to all candidates irrespective of the subject specialty chosen. Nursing specialty – II shall be the branch of specialty chosen by the candidate.

Distribution of Theory and Practical teaching hours

Sl N	Subject	Theory Hrs	Practical Hrs	Total Hrs
First Year				
1	Advanced Concepts of Health and Nursing	150	90	240
2	Biological and Psychosocial Foundations of Nursing Sec-A: genetics, Embryology and Patho-Physiology Sec-B: Psychosocial Foundation of Nursing and Epidemiology	120	—	120
3	Education & Nursing Education	200	100	300
4	Biostatistics & Research Methodology and Nursing Research	150	50	200
5	Nursing Specialty I	100	275	375
Second Year				
1	Administration and Nursing Administration	200	100	300
2	Nursing Specialty II	100	275	375
	Dissertation		250	250
	Total	**1020**	**1140**	**2160**

Attendance

- A candidate pursuing M.Sc Nursing course shall study in the concerned department of the institution for the entire period as a full time student. No candidate should join any other course of study or appear for any other examination conducted by any other university in India or abroad during the period of registration.
- Every student shall attend symposia, seminars, conferences, journal review meetings and lectures during each year as prescribed by the department/college/university and not absent without valid reasons.
- Candidate who has put in a minimum of 80% of attendance in the theory and practical assignments separately shall be permitted to appear for M.Sc Nursing examination, provided she/he has completed the course and has shown satisfactory progress mentioned in the logbook.
- Any student who fails to complete the course in the manner stated above shall not be permitted to appear for the University examinations.
- The Principal should notify in the college notice board attendance details at the end of each term without fail under intimation to the university.

Internal Assessment Marks

There shall be continuous internal assessment. The marks for internal assessment set apart for theory and practical in each subject. These shall be a minimum of two tests and two assignments in each subject, the average of which shall form the marks for internal assessment. The Principal should notify on the notice board the internal assessment marks of the students at the end of each term without fail under intimation to the university. The Principal of the colleges shall send the internal assessment marks of the candidates both in theory and practicals to the university. A student must secure at least 50% of total marks for internal assessment in a particular subject in order to be eligible to appear in University examination in that subject.

Distribution of Internal Assessment Marks for various subjects

First Year		
Sl N	**Subject**	**Internal Assessment Marks**
1	Advanced Concepts of Health and Nursing	20
2	Biological and Psycho-Social Foundation of Nursing Sec-A: genetics, Embryology and Patho-Physiology Sec-B: Psycho-Social Foundation of Nursing and Epidemiology	 10 10
3	Education and Nursing Education Sec-A: Education Sec-B: Nursing Education	 10 10
4	Bio-statistics, Research Methodology and Nursing Research Sec-A:Bio-statistics Sec-B:research methodology and Nursing Research	 10 10
5	Nursing Specialty I Theory Practical	 20 20
	Total	**120**
Second Year		
1	Administration and Nursing Administration	20
2	Nursing Specialty II Theory – One Paper Practical – I	 20 20
	Total	**60**

Monitoring Progress of Studies

Every candidate shall maintain a logbook and record of her/his participation in the training program conducted by the department such as journal reviews, seminars, etc. The faculty members and peers will assess the presentations using relevant checklists given M.Sc Nursing logbook. The presentations made by the candidate should be mentioned in the logbook. The logbook shall be scrutinized and certified by the HOD and Head of the Institution and presented in the University practical examination.

M.Sc Nursing log book

The university has prescribed log book, it may be got printed by all the Nursing colleges having M.Sc Nursing course. The format given in the logbook shall be followed by all the PG students.

Dissertation

Each candidate pursuing M.Sc Nursing course is required to carry out work on selected research project under the guidance of a recognized post graduate teacher. The results of such work shall be submitted in the form of dissertation. The dissertation is aimed to train a graduate student in research methods and techniques. It includes identification of problem, formulation of a hypothesis, search and review of literature, getting acquainted with recent advances, designing of a research study, collection of data, critical analysis, interpretation of results and drawing conclusions.

Every candidate shall submit to the Registrar (Academic) of the University in the prescribed proforma, a synopsis containing particulars of proposed dissertation work within six months from the date of commencement of the course on or before the date notified by the university. The synopsis shall be sent through the proper channel.

The dissertation should be written under the following headings:

i. Introduction
ii. Aims or objectives of study
iii. Review of literature
iv. Material and methods
v. Results
vi. Discussion
vii. Conclusion
viii. Summary
ix. References
x. Tables
xi. Annexure

A declaration by the candidate for having done the work should also be included, and certified by the guide, HOD and Head of the Institution. Four copies of dissertation shall be submitted to the Registrar (Evaluation) through proper channel, along with a soft copy (CD), three months before the final examination. Acceptance of the dissertation is a pre-requisite for a candidate to appear for final examination (University norms may be varied).

Examination Pattern-First Year

Theory Paper	Subject	Duration (Hrs)	University Exam Marks
1	Advanced Concepts of Health and Nursing	3	80
2	Biological and Psycho-Social Foundation of Nursing Sec-A: genetics, Embryology and Patho-Physiology Sec-B: Psycho-Social Foundation of Nursing and Epidemiology	3	40 40
3	Education and Nursing Education Sec-A: Education Sec-B: Nursing Education	3	40 40
4	Biostatistics, Research Methodology and Nursing Research Sec-A: Biostatistics Sec-B: Research Methodology and Nursing Research	3	40 40
5	Nursing Specialty I	3	80
	Sub Total Theory		**400**
	Nursing Specialty I Practical		80
	Total		**480**

Criteria for pass

To be declared as pass in the M.Sc I year, a candidate has to pass in all the prescribed subjects for the I year. A candidate shall secure in each of the common subjects not less than 50% marks prescribed for University examination (40 out of 80) in theory papers (exclusive of internal assessment marks). A candidate shall secure not less than 50% of marks prescribed for University examination separately in theory (40 out of 80) and practical examination (40 out of 80), exclusive of internal assessment marks.

Carryover

A candidate who has passed in any of the three subjects, but has failed in any two subjects, is permitted to proceed to the II year. However, such a candidate shall have to pass all the failed subjects before becoming eligible to appear for II year M.Sc (N) University examination.

II year examination

The University examination consists of dissertation, written papers (theory), practical examination and viva-voce examination.

Practical: There shall be no practical examination in Nursing Administration. There shall one practical examination for Nursing II in the subject specialty chosen.

Viva-voce: 60 marks, the distribution of marks shall be—Component 1:50 marks and Component 2:10 marks.

Component 1: 50 marks, all examiners will conduct viva-voce jointly on candidate's comprehension, analytical approach, expression, interpretation of data, communication skills and knowledge of all components of course contents of nursing specialty subjects chosen by the candidate. It includes presentation and discussion on dissertation also.

Component 2: Pedagogy (Teaching skill) 10 marks, a topic will be given to the candidate at the beginning of practical examination. She/he is asked to make a presentation on the topic for 8-10 minutes.

Examination Pattern-Second Year

Theory Paper	Subject	Duration (Hrs)	University Exam Marks
1	Administration & Nursing Administration	3	80
2	Nursing Specialty II	3	80
	Sub Total Theory – 2 papers		160
	Practical – I		80
	Viva-voce		60
	Total		**300**

Criteria for pass

To be declared pass in the M.Sc II year a candidate has to pass in all the prescribed subjects for the II year fulfilling the Common and Specialty subject criteria, and secure total aggregate of marks of 150/300 in the University examination.

- Common Subject: A candidate shall secure in the common subject not less than 50% marks prescribed for the University examination (40 out of 80) in theory paper, exclusive of internal assessment marks
- Nursing Specialty Subject: A candidate shall secure not less than 50% of marks prescribed for University examination, separately in theory (40/80) and practical including viva-voce 70/140) examination. The internal assessment marks shall not be added to any component.

Declaration of Class

- A candidate having appeared in all the subjects in the same examination and passes that examination in the first attempt and secures 75% of marks or more of grand total marks prescribed* will be declared to have passed the examination with distinction
- A candidate having appeared in all the subjects in the same examination and passes that examination in the first attempt and secures 65% of marks or more but less than 75% of grand total marks prescribed* will be declared to have passed the examination in First Class

Eligibility for degree

A candidate shall have passed in all subjects of M.Sc I year and II year to be eligible for the award of degree.

---

*The grand total marks prescribed for I year is 600 marks (Internal Assessment marks (120) + University examination marks 480) and for II year it is 360 marks (Internal Assessment marks (60) + University examination marks 300)

B.Sc. Nursing Program

Philosophy

Education is a lifelong process and a graduate Nurse emerging out of the Universities should be tuned to learning throughout life. The graduate must bloom into a cultivated, creative, self directed, knowledgeable person whose education has encouraged a continuous process of development as a person, professional, citizen and an agent of social change. Health is a state of well-being that enables a person to lead psychologically, socially and economically productive life. Health as a right for all people, individual, families and communities have responsibility towards maintaining their health. Nursing contributes to the health services in vital and significant way in the health care delivery system. It recognizes the National Health goals and is committed to participate in the implementation of National Health Policies and programs. It aims at identifying health needs of the people, planning and providing quality care in collaboration with other professionals and community groups. Scope of nursing practice encompasses provision of promotive, preventive, curative and rehabilitative aspects of care to people across their life span in wide variety of health care settings. Practice of nursing is based upon application of basic concepts and principles derived from the Physical, Biological and Behavioural Sciences, Medicine and Nursing. Nursing is based on values of caring and aims to help individuals to attain independence in self care. It necessitates development of compassion and understanding of human behaviour among its practitioners to provide care with respect, dignity and protect the rights of individuals and groups. Undergraduate Nursing program is broad based education within an academic framework specifically directed to the development of critical thinking skills, competencies and standards required for practice of professional Nursing and Midwifery as envisaged in National Health Policy 2002. The teachers have the responsibility to be role models and create learning environment that enables students to acquire inquiry driven, self directed learning and foster an attitude of lifelong learning.

Undergraduate Nursing education program prepares its graduates to become exemplary citizen by adhering to code of ethics and professional conduct at all times in fulfilling personal, social and professional obligations so as to respond to national aspirations.

Aims

- Prepare graduates to assume responsibilities as professional, competent nurses and midwives in providing promotive, preventive, curative and rehabilitative services
- Prepare nurses who can make independent decisions in nursing situations, protect the rights and facilitate individuals and groups in pursuit of health, function in the hospital, community nursing services and conduct research studies in the areas of nursing practice. They are also expected to assume the role of teacher, supervisor and manager in a clinical/public health setting.

Objectives

On completion of the four year B.Sc. Nursing Program, the graduate will be able to:

- Apply knowledge from Physical, Biological and Behavioural Sciences, Medicine including alternative systems and Nursing in providing nursing care to individuals, families and communities
- Demonstrate understanding of life style and other factors, which affect health of individuals and groups
- Provide nursing care based on steps of nursing process in collaboration with the individuals and groups
- Demonstrate critical thinking and skills in making decisions in all situations in order to provide quality care
- Utilize the latest trends and technology in providing health care
- Provide promotive, preventive and restorative health services in line with the national health policies and programs
- Practice within the frame work of code of ethics and professional conduct and acceptable standards of practice within the legal boundaries
- Communicate effectively with individuals and groups, and health team members in order to promote effective interpersonal relationships and team work
- Demonstrate skills in teaching to individuals and groups in clinical and community settings
- Participate effectively as members of health team in health care delivery system
- Demonstrate leadership and managerial skills in clinical and community settings

- Conducted need based research studies in various settings and utilize the research findings to improve the quality of care
- Demonstrate awareness, interest and contribute towards advancement of self and of the profession
  Duration of the course shall be four (4) years including internship
  Medium of instruction and examination is English

Admission Eligibility

A candidate seeking admission should have:

- Passed the two year Pre-University examination or equivalent as recognized by the University with science subject, Viz., Physics, Chemistry and Biology
- Students of vocational courses: 10+2 vocational course of State Government with cognate subject namely domestic nursing and Physics, Chemistry and Biology as optional subjects
- Obtained at least 45% of the total marks in science subjects of the qualifying examination; if belonging to a SC or ST, should have obtained not less than 40% of the total marks in science subjects of the qualifying examination
- Completed 17 years of age at the time of admission or will complete this age on or before 31st December of the year of admission
  Working days in the academic year not less than 260 working days including University examinations.
  Attendance required for admission to examinations: 80 % of attendance in both theory and practical separately in each subject before admission to the examination.

Internal Assessment

- A minimum of three written examinations and practical assessments shall be conducted in each subject and the average marks of the three examinations shall be taken as the final internal assessment marks
- A candidate failed in any subject should be provided an opportunity to improve internal assessment by conducting a minimum of two assessments both in theory and practicals separately and the higher of the present and previous final internal assessment marks shall be considered for the University examinations
- If a failed candidate does not appear for any internal assessment examinations in the failed subject(s) the internal marks awarded for the previous examinations shall be carried over for subsequent appearance(s)
- The internal assessment marks should be submitted to the Principal by the respective HOD/teacher concerned atleast three weeks before the commencement of the Theory Examinations and he/she shall forward a copy of the same to the Registrar or an officer authorized by him/her to receive the same, atleast two weeks before the commencement of the Theory Examinations

Re-admission after discontinuation/Break of study

Every student shall attend her/his theory, practical and clinical classes on all working days unless she/he is granted leave of absence by the Principal. If a student absents continuously for a period of 91 days or more and seeks permission to attend the course within one year after discontinuation, her/his application shall be forwarded to the registrar with the recommendations of the Principal. If the Vice-Chancellor is satisfied with the reasons he may grant leave of absence attaching such conditions as he may deem necessary. Candidates who are absent for continuous period of one year or more without permission shall be deemed to have forfeited the admission into the course and her/his studentship shall stand cancelled without any further notice.

Course of study

The course of study and the scheme of examination for 4 YDC B.Sc., Nursing Degree shall be as follows:

Course duration	:	4 years
Weeks available/year	:	52 weeks
Vacation	:	08 weeks
Gazette holidays	:	03 weeks
Examination (incl preparatory)	:	04 weeks
Available weeks	:	37 weeks
Hours/week	:	40
Practical	:	30 hours/week

Theory	:	10 hours/week
Internship practical	:	48 hours/weeks
Hours available/academic year	:	1480 (37 weeks X 40 hours)

Course of Instructions

First Year

Sl No.	Subject	Theory (hrs) (Class and Lab)	Practical (hrs) (Clinical)	(In hrs)
1	English *	60		
2	Anatomy	60		
3	Physiology	60		
4	Nutrition	60		
5	Biochemistry	30		
6	Nursing Foundations	265 + 200	450	
7	Psychology	60		
8	Microbiology	60		
9	Introduction to computers	45		
10	Hindi/regional language *	30		
11	Library work/Self study			50
12	Co-curricular activities			50
	Total Hours (1480)	930	450	100

Second Year

Sl No.	Subject	Theory (hrs) (Class and Lab)	Practical (hrs) (Clinic)	(In hrs)
1	Sociology	60		
2	Pharmacology	45		
3	Pathology	30		
4	Genetics	15		
5	Medical-Surgical Nursing (Adult incl Geriatrics) – I	210	720	
6	Community Health Nursing – I	90	135	
7	Communication & Educational Technology	60 + 30		
8	Library work/Self study			50
9	Co-curricular activities			35
	Total Hours (1480)	540	855	85

Third Year

Sl No.	Subject	Theory (hrs) (Class and Lab)	Practical (hrs) (Clinical)	(In hrs)
1	Medical-Surgical Nursing (Adult incl Geriatrics) – II	120	270	
2	Child Health Nursing	90	270	
3	Mental Health Nursing	90	270	
4	Midwifery & Obstetrical Nursing	90	180	
5	Library work/Self study			50
6	Co-curricular activities			50
	Total Hours (1480)	390	990	100

Fourth Year

Sl No.	Subject	Theory (hrs) (Class and Lab)	Practical (hrs) (Clinical)	(In hrs)
1	Midwifery and Obstetrical Nursing		180	
2	Community Health Nursing – II	90	135	
3	Nursing Research and Statistics	45	*	
4	Management of Nursing Services and Education	60 + 30		
	Total Hours (540)	225	315	

Internship (Integrated Practice)

Sl No.	Subject	Theory (hrs) (Class and Lab)	Practical (hrs) (Clinical)	(In hrs)
1	Midwifery and Obstetrical Nursing		240	5
2	Community Health Nursing – II		195	4
3	Medical-Surgical Nursing (Adult and Geriatrics)		430	9
4	Child Health		145	3
5	Mental health		95	2
6	Research Project		45	1
	Total Hours (1690)		1150	24

Note:
- Internship means 8 hours of integrated clinical duties in which 2 weeks of evening and night shift duties are included
- Internship should be carried out as 8 hours /day @ 48 hours/week
- Students during internship will be supervised by nursing teachers
- Fourth year final examination to be held only after completing internship

Scheme of Examination

First Year

Theory	Subject		Assessment		
		Hours	Internal	External	Total
1	Anatomy and Physiology	3	25	75	100
2	Nutrition and Biochemistry	3	25	75	100
3	Nursing Foundations	3	25	75	100
4	Psychology	3	25	75	100
5	Microbiology	3	25	75	100
6	English	3	25	75	100
7	Introduction to Computers		25	75	100
	Practical & Viva Voce				
1	Nursing Foundations		100	100	200

Second Year

Theory	Subject		Assessment		
		Hours	Internal	External	Total
8	Sociology	3	25	75	100
9	Medical-Surgical Nursing-I	3	25	75	100
10	Pharmacology, Pathology, Genetics	3	25	75	100
11	Community Health Nursing-I	3	25	75	100

12	Communication and Education Technology	3	25	75	100
	Practical and Viva Voce				
2	Medical-Surgical Nursing-I		100	100	200

Third Year

Theory	Subject	Assessment			
		Hours	Internal	External	Total
13	Medical-Surg Nursing-II	3	25	75	100
14	Child Health Nursing	3	25	75	100
15	Mental Health Nursing	3	25	75	100
	Practical and Viva Voce				
3	Medical-Surg Nursing-II		50	50	100
4	Child Health Nursing		50	50	100
5	Mental Health Nursing		50	50	100

Fourth Year

Theory	Subject	Assessment			
		Hours	Internal	External	Total
16	Midwifery and Obstetrical Nursing	3	25	75	100
17	Community Health Nursing-II	3	25	75	100
18	Nursing Research and Statistics	3	25	75	100
19	Management of Nursing Services and Education	3	25	75	100
	Practical and Viva Voce				
6	Midwifery and Obstetrical Nursing	3	50	50	100
7	Community Health Nursing	3	50	50	100

Post Basic Diploma Programs (Short term courses)—Competencies/Purposes

Post Basic Diploma in Oncology Nursing

To train nurses to:
1. Provide quality care to patients with an actual or potential diagnosis of cancer.
2. Manage and supervise patient care in clinical and community settings.
3. Teach nurses, allied health professionals, patients and communities in areas related to oncology nursing.
4. Conduct research in areas of oncology nursing.

Post Basic Diploma in Nurse Practitioner in Midwifery

To train nurses to:
1. Provide quality care to mother and neonate.
2. Manage and supervise care of mother and neonate at all the three levels of care.
3. Teach nurses, allied health professionals, patients and communities in areas related to mother and neonate care.
4. Conduct research in areas of mother and neonate care.

Post Basic Diploma in Neonatal Nursing

The purpose of the course is to train nurses to:
1. Provide quality care to neonates.
2. Manage and supervise care of neonates at all the three levels of care.
3. Teach nurses, allied health professionals, patients and communities in areas related to neonatal nursing.
4. Conduct research in areas of neonatal nursing.

Post Basic Diploma in Psychiatric/Mental Health Nursing

The students after completion of the course will be able to:
1. Provide quality nursing care to individuals suffering from mental and emotional disorders.
2. Manage and supervise care of mentally ill patients in clinical and community settings.
3. Teach nurses, allied health professionals, family members and communities in areas related to psychiatric nursing.
4. Keep pace with the developments in other related discipline for effective management of psychiatric patients.
5. Conduct research in areas of psychiatric nursing.

Post Basic Diploma in Emergency and Disaster Nursing

The purpose of the course is to train nurses to:
1. Provide quality care in emergency and disaster situations.
2. Manage and supervise patient care in pre hospital and hospital settings.
3. Teach nurses, allied health professionals, patients and communities in areas related to emergency and disaster nursing.
4. Conduct research in areas of emergency and disaster nursing.

Post Basic Diploma in Critical care Nursing

The purpose of the course is to train nurses to:
1. Provide quality care to critically ill patients.
2. Manage and supervise care of critically ill patients.
3. Teach nurses, allied health professionals and family members in areas related to critical care nursing.
4. Conduct research in areas of critical care nursing.

Post Basic Diploma in Cardio - Thoracic Nursing

The purpose of the course is to train nurses to:
1. Provide quality care to patients with cardio thoracic disorders.
2. Manage & supervise care of patients with cardio thoracic disorders.
3. Teach nurses, allied health professionals and family members in areas related to cardio thoracic nursing.
4. Conduct research in areas of cardio thoracic nursing.

Post Basic Diploma in Orthopaedic and Rehabilitation Nursing

The purpose of the course is to train nurses to:
1. Provide quality care to patients with Orthopedic and Neuromuscular disorders.
2. Manage and supervise care of patients with Orthopedic and Neuromuscular disorders.
3. Participate in rehabilitation of patients with Orthopedic and Neuro-muscular disorders.
4. Teach nurses, allied health professionals, parents and communities in areas related to Orthopedic and Rehabilitation nursing.
5. Conduct research in areas of Orthopaedic and Rehabilitation Nursing.

Post Basic Diploma in Neuro Science Nursing

The purpose of the course is to train nurses to:
1. Provide quality care to neuro patients.
2. Manage and supervise care of neuro patients.
3. Teach nurses, allied health professionals, patients and communities in areas related to neuro patients.
4. Conduct research in areas of neuro science nursing.

Post Basic Diploma in Operation Room Nursing

The purpose of the course is to train nurses to:
1. Provide quality care to patients in OR
2. Manage and supervise patient care of patients in OR
3. Teach nurses, allied health professionals and family members in areas related to OR nursing
4. Conduct research in areas of OR nursing.

Diploma in General Nursing and Midwifery Program

Philosophy

Modern Nursing is a dynamic, therapeutic and educative process in meeting the health needs of the individuals, the family and the community. Nursing is one of the health professions which functions in conjunction with other health care agencies in assisting the individuals, families and communities to achieve and to maintain desirable standards of health.

Since nurses provided and will undoubtedly continue to provide a large part of health care, their training should equip them with professional expertise to meet the changing demands of society and their expanding role therein. To achieve this, emphasis must be laid to impart the knowledge and skills most relevant to the health care needs of the community and the country as a whole. This must also be accompanied by a corresponding change in professional attitudes.

The International Council of Nurses states that the unique function of the nurse is to assist the individual, sick or well, in the performance of those activities contributing to health or its recovery (or to peaceful death) that she/he would perform unaided if she/he had the necessary strength, will or knowledge. And to do this in such a way as to help her/him gain independence as rapidly as possible. Indian Nursing Council recognized that basic nursing education is a formally recognized programm of study providing a broad and sound foundation in the behavioural, life and nursing sciences for the general practice of nursing, for a leadership role and for the post basic education in specialties for advance nursing practice. The Council believes that this basic course in nursing should prepare nurses for occupying first level positions in nursing in all kinds of health care settings. The Council recognizes that nursing is a profession which is influenced by advances in science and technology. It believes that skills in all aspects of communication are also essential for learning and for the practice of nursing.

The Council also recognizes that the nature of nursing is such that a substantial portion of learning of the students is acquired in the clinical field of practice. It further recognizes that interdependence of or nursing and allied professions and occupations in promoting, maintaining and restoring health and prevention of diseases.

The Council believes that it has a responsibility in helping the students to develop pride in their profession besides keeping them abreast with current knowledge and professional trends for a successful career ahead.

Aims

The Diploma course in General Nursing and Midwifery is geared to the health needs of the individual, family, community and the country at large. The aims of the course are:

- To prepare nurses with a sound educational program in nursing to enable them to function as efficient members of the health team, beginning with the competencies for first level positions in all kinds of health care settings
- To help the nurses to develop an ability to cooperate and coordinate with members of the health team in the prevention of disease, promotion of health and rehabilitation of the sick
- To help nurses in their personal and professional development, so that they are able to make maximum contribution to the society as useful and productive individuals, citizens as well as efficient nurses
- To serve as a base for further professional education and specialization in nursing
- To prepare nurses to keep pace with latest professional and technological developments and use these for providing nursing care services

Objectives

The nurse on completion of this course will be able to:

- Demonstrate competency in providing health care to individual, sick or well, using nursing process:
  - Assess the nursing need of clients from birth to death
  - Plan and carry out appropriate action to meet nursing needs
  - Provide effective nursing care for maintaining best possible level of health in all aspects
  - Promote self care in people under their care
  - Apply problem solving techniques in nursing practice

- Evaluate effectiveness of nursing care
- Apply problem solving techniques in nursing practice
- Evaluate effectiveness of nursing care.
- Apply knowledge from the Humanities, Biological and Behavioral sciences in functioning as a nurse
- Function effectively with members of the health team and community applying the knowledge of human relations and communication skills in his/her work
- Participate as member of the health team in delivery of curative preventive, promotive and rehabilitative health care services
- Mobilize community resources and their involvement in working with the communities
- Demonstrate use of ethical values in their personal and professional life
- Demonstrate interest in activities of professional organizations
- Recognize the needs for continuing education for professional development
- Demonstrate basic skills in teaching patients and giving nursing care to them
- Demonstrate basic skills in administration and leadership while working with other members of health team and community
- Assist in research activities.

Admission Policies

Admission policies are based on the kind of program being offered by the school and the kind of candidates who, it is felt, will be most likely to pursue the course of studies successfully and profitably. These policies need to be carefully formulated and made known to those concerned with recruitment and selection so that the students finally admitted will meet the requirements of the program. Dropouts are inevitable but their number can be minimized by the formulation of policies consistent with objectives of the program and by adherence to these policies as far as prevailing conditions will permit.

Academic Qualifications

- 10 +2 passed/Pre-degree course/HSC /VHSC or its equivalent qualifications
- Students from science discipline with aggregate of 45% marks in Physics, Chemistry and Biology are preferable

Personal and Social Fitness

- Age limit 17-35 years
- Only medically fit students should be admitted

Others

- Transfer is allowed from one school to another only with sufficient reasons with permission from concerned authorities. Student shall not be allowed migration from one state to another state
- There should be provision for health services for the students such as:
  - An annual medical examination
  - Vaccination against Tetanus, Hepatitis B, any other communicable diseases as considered necessary
  - Free medical care during illness
  - A complete health record should be kept in respect of each student. The question if continuing the training of a student, with long term chronic illness, will be decided by the individual school

Year-wise distribution of weeks, days and hours of the course

Maximum hours/weeks/students shall be 36 to 40 including classroom instructions and clinical field practice.

1 year	46 weeks	1656 hrs
2 year	46 weeks	1656 hrs
3 year	46 weeks	1656 hrs

Note: Out of 52 weeks in one academic year, total of 6 weeks are deducted i.e. 4 weeks vacation, one week preparatory leave and one week for examination, Sundays and Gazetted holidays are to be considered as holidays.

Course instruction and Supervised Practice

First Year

	Subjects	Theoretical Hours	Supervised Practice
1	Biological Sciences Anatomy and Physiology Microbiology	 90 30	—
2	Behavioural Sciences Psychology Sociology	 40 20	—
3	Fundamentals of Nursing Fundamentals of Nursing First Aid Personal Hygiene	 175 20 20	612 hrs (17 weeks)
4	Community Health Nursing Community Health Nursing-I Environmental Hygiene Health Education and Communication Skills Nutrition	 80 20 20 30	
5	English	30	—
	Total (I year)	**575**	**612**

Second Year

	Subjects	Theoretical Hours	Supervised Practice
1	Medical-Surgical Nursing-I (incl Pharmacology)	140	828 hrs (23 weeks)
2	Medical-Surgical Nursing-II (Specialities)	120	
3	Mental Health and Psychiatric Nursing	70	216 hrs (6 weeks)
4	Community Health Nursing	—	84 hrs (2 weeks)
4	Computer Education	30	
	Total	**360**	**1116 (31 weeks)**

Third Year

	Subjects	Theoretical Hours	Supervised Practice
1	Midwifery & Gynaecology	120	756 hrs (21 weeks)
2	Community Health Nursing-II	100	216 hrs (6 weeks)
3	Paediatric Nursing	70	288 hrs (8 weeks)
	Total	**290**	**1260 hrs (35 weeks)**

Internship Period

	Subjects	Hours
1	Educational Methods & media for Teaching and Practice of Nursing	45
2	Introduction to research	40
3	Professional Trends & Adjustment	40
4	Administration and Ward Management	45
5	Health Economics	20
	Total	**190**

Breakup of Clinical Experience

Medical-Surg Nursing I & II	252 hrs	6 weeks
Paediatric Nursing	126 hrs	3 weeks
Psychiatric Nursing	126 hrs	3 weeks
Community Health Nursing	168 hrs	4 weeks

Midwifery	168 hrs	4 weeks
Student's area of interest	84 hrs	2 weeks
Total	924 hrs	22 weeks

2 weeks of night clinical experience has to be given during this period with night supervisor.

Total clinical experience in GNM Program

Subject	Supervised practice – hrs	Weeks
Nursing Science	612	17
Medical-Surg I & II	1080	29
Community Health Nursing	744	20
Psychiatry Nursing	342	9
Paediatrics	414	11
Midwifery & Gynaecology	924	25
Area of interest	84	2
Night duty	—	2
Total	4200	115

No night duty experience in 1st year, only 8 weeks of night duty experience throughout the training period. Total working hours 8 hrs clincials, 1 hr class or 1 day theory and 5 days clinical in a week.

Records to be maintained by the students in the clinical area.

First Year

Nursing care plan	4 in Medical/Surgical wards
Daily diary	
Health talk	1 each in urban and rural community field
Family study including Family care plan	1 each in urban and rural community field
Health assessment of an individual in the family	1 each in urban and rural community field
Community profile	1 each in urban and rural community field

Second Year

Medical Ward	
Nursing care plan	2
Case study	1
Case presentation	1
Drug study	1
Surgical Ward	
Nursing care plan	2
Case study	1
Case presentation	1
Drug study	1
Psychiatry Ward	
Nursing care plan	2
Case study	1
Case presentation	1
Drug study	1
Process recording	2
Mental status examination	4

Third Year

Paediatric Ward	
Nursing care plan	2
Case study	1
Case presentation	1
Drug study	1
Observation report	2 on new born
Maternity Ward and Gynaecology Ward	
Nursing care plan	2 + 1
Case study	1 + 1
Case presentation	1 + 1
Drug study	1 + 1
Daily diary	Urban and rural community field
Health talk	2 each
Family Health Nursing Care Plan	2 each
Group Project	1 each

Scheme of Examination

Sl N.	1 year	Total marks	Internal assessment	Council/Board's Examination	Duration of Exam (Hours)
1	Bio Sciences	100	25	75	3
2	Behavioural Sciences	100	25	75	3
3	Fundamentals of Nursing	100	25	75	3
4	Community Health Nursing-I	100	25	75	3
	Practical I Fundamentals of Nursing	100	50	50	

Sl N.	2nd year	Total marks	Internal assessment	Council/Board's Examination	Duration of Exam (Hours)
1	Medical-Surgical Nursing I (Including Pharmacology)	100	25	75	3
2	Medical-Surgical II (Specialities)	100	25	75	
3	Mental Health & Psychiatric Nursing	100	25	75	3
	Practical I Medical-Surgical Nursing	100	50	50	
	Practical II Psychiatric Nursing	100 (only School exam., No Council Exam)			

Psychiatric exam for Psychiatric Nursing has to be conducted at the place of Clinical experience at the end of clinical instructions by School itself and internal assessment marks shall be sent to the Council/Examination Board.

Sl N	3rd year	Total marks	Internal assessment	Council/Board's Examination	Duration of Exam (Hours)
1	Midwifery and Gynaecology	100	25	75	3
2	Paediatric Nursing	100	25	75	3
3	Community Health Nursing II	100	25	75	3
	Practicals				
1	Midwifery & Gynaecology	100	50	50	
2	Paediatric Nursing	100	50	50	
3	Community Health Nursing II	100	50	50	

Job Responsibilities of Professionals in College of Nursing

Principal

Educational qualification and experience

Masters Degree in Nursing—Total 10 years of experience with minimum of 5 years teaching. Registered in State Nursing Council.

Job summary

Principal is the administrative head in the College. He/she should hold qualification as laid down by INC. In Government settings, Principal will be directly responsible to the Director of Medical Education/Director of Health and Family Welfare services, In private settings under Management authorities., principal is responsible for implementation of Curriculum and revision of curriculum for various courses and Planning and Organization, implementation of Curricular, Co-curricular and Extracurricular activities and Research activities in College of Nursing. The Principal should be the controlling authority for the budget of the institution and also be the drawing and disbursing officer. The Principal and Vice-Principal should be gazette officers in Government schools and of equal status though non-gazette in non-government schools.

Shares teaching activities, provides guidance and Counselling services to the teaching faculty, Non-Teaching Programs and students., Organizes workshops, seminars, conferences, CNE and In service Educational Programs (Faculty Development and Staff Developmental Programs), assists the National Council (INC) and State Nursing Council, Government and Universities as adhoc inspector or resource person in formulating educational policies, materials and assisting in maintaining the standards in Nursing Educational Institutions, Assists the University in conducting examinations, workshops, Curricular revision and Educational policies.

Administration

- Develops Philosophy and Educational Policies, Objectives for educational program
- Identifies, evaluates and secures resources
- Planning ,Organizing, Staffing, Directing, Coordinating, Cooperating, Reporting and budgeting of all college activities
- Advertising and calling for the candidates for Nursing Program
- Scrutinizing applications—Preparing merit list and calling them for interview
- Conducting interview through the committee and selecting candidates and informing them
- Planning for orientation program for new students and staff
- Delegation of teaching work load and departments to each faculty along with teaching materials
- Identifies the present needs of learners related to educational program
- Selects and organizes learning experiences
- Coordinates University, Government/Management, allied officiating agencies for implementation of college activities
- Formulates the plan of action
- Acts as a Democratic, Autocratic, Lasize-faire leader based on the situation
- Principal in Private college settings will discuss with management and solves the issues related to fixation of salaries, increments, facilities for students and any inter departmental issues
- Communicating with other departments, agencies or individuals in connection with the program
- Maintaining students records, admission register, results, registers of teachers and students etc.
- Countersigning records of each department, library and hostel after annual verification by the concerned in charge of the department and the warden in case of the hostel
- Providing the supply of audio-visual aids, teaching materials as requested by the concerned department in charge
- Placing indents with the government for stationery, uniform for certain category of class IV servants in Government Schools and in Private schools coordinating with Management and Government authorities for coordinating schools' activities
- Purchasing furniture, equipments, books and journals as per requirement of the office, hostel and Nursing department

- Authorizing repairs of vehicles and purchase of oil, petrol and minor parts of replacement
- Sending proposals yearly for new items costly equipments etc., to the authorities
- Maintaining income and expenditure registers
- Seeing that monthly pay bills are sent in time, so also T A bills or any other type of bills
- Assisting the auditors in submitting tax reports & Budget
- Monitoring that office-timings and other rules of service are observed
- Writing annually the confidential report of staff and teachers
- Holding meetings with teachers, staff of office, hostel staff, students and their committee
- Representing the School and the profession on various organizations and varied Resource committees.

Organizing

- Determines the position, scope and responsibility of both teaching and non-teaching staff
- Analyses the job to be done in terms of needs of education program
- Prepares the job description, indicate the line of authority, responsibility in relationship and channels of communication by means of organization chart and other methods
- Considers preparation, ability and interest personally in equating responsibility
- Delegates authority commensurate with responsibility
- Maintains a plan of work load among staff members
- Provides an organizational framework for effective staff functioning such as organizing meeting of the staff.

Directing

- Fill the vacancies with qualified personnel, suitable professionals and recommends the candidates for promotion based on qualification and experience of the individual staff.
- Subscribes and encourages developmental aspects with reference to welfare of staff and students.
- Directs activities of staff working under them.
- Conducts adequate Staff Developmental Programs—Orientation programs, Faculty Development programs to enrich their knowledge.
- Guides and encourages staff members in their job activities.
- Consistently makes administrative decision based on established policies.
- Facilitates participation in community, professional and institutional activities by providing time, opportunity for support for such participation.
- Involve actively in designing educationally sound program.
- Develops positive attitude among staff and learners.
- Utilizes the resources in the development of total program and appreciates their contribution.
- Provides freedom for staff to develop active training course content within the framework of curriculum.
- Promotes staff participation in research.
- Procures and maintains physical facilities as per standards.
- Encourages the staff to actively contribute to the welfare of student activities.

Coordinating

- Maintains and utilizes effective Communication strategies
- Coordinates activities relating to the programs, e.g. conducts and follow up by regular meetings, Initiating the ways of cooperation
- Interprets nursing education to other related disciplines and to the public

Controlling

- Provides for continuous follow-up and revision of education program.
- Maintains recognition of the educational program by utilizing accrediting bodies.
- Maintains adequately and up to date records.
- Prepares periodic reports which revise the progress and problems of the entire program.
- Prepares, secures approval and administrates the budget.

Instruction

- Conducts Faculty Development progrmmes, Faculty meetings to assess the extent of completion of syllabus for specific batch of students, and assess if any need for further improvements.
- Contacting agencies, institutions, for arranging field visits, clinical experiences etc. such that students will get the best possible or maximum experience within the scheduled time.
- Initiating changes in curriculum keeping within the guidelines of the syllabus.
- Cooperating with the state council/board to conduct examinations by providing all facilities.
- Guiding students in filling examination forms, registration fees and seeing that they are submitted to the council in time.
- Teaching the subjects.
- Guides the faculty in preparation of Master Rotation Plan and Clinical Rotation Plan.
- Preparing and displaying weekly/monthly class, schedule, clinical experience of rotation plan etc. in consultation with tutors.
- Maintaining records of examination results.
- Communicating to the council about any relevant information regarding students.
- Encouraging teachers to experiment with newer methods of teaching and to find out newer clinical areas which would provide the best possible exposure of students, to that clinical area.
- Encourage and supporting co-curricular and extracurricular activities.
- Issuing transcripts to students.
- Assists the faculty in completion of difficult subjects.
- Plans for participating in educational programs for further development.
- Recognizes the needs for continuing education for staff and provides stimulation of opportunities for such development.
- Participates as a teacher in the educational program and deals with complicated topics.

Guiding

- Encourages students in their studies, research projects and writing up of the publication.
- Provides and maintains a program for recruitment, selection and promotion of students.
- Provides for systematic guidance program for staff members and students.

Counselling

- Counsel students and teachers in solving their personal and professional problems.
- Promotes group morale and Group Etiquette.

Miscellaneous

- Encouraging faculty members to take up further studies, attend Seminars, Workshops and participate in professional activities
- Participating in activities of the professional organization
- Encouraging students to actively participate in SNA activities and to join TNAI as a life member
- Arranging graduation and lamp lighting ceremonies with the assistance of teaching faculty
- Meeting visitors and discussing issues, pertaining to the school program
- Meeting parents or guardians of the students as and when necessary
- Preparing for the cooperation with inspectors from the state level bodies or national council.

Professor

Educational qualification and experience:

- Masters Degree in Nursing
- Total 10 years of experience with minimum of 5 years of teaching
- Registration in State Nursing Council.

Job summary

The professor is overall in charge and responsible for the departmental activities, and assists the Principal or the head of the Institution in administration, shares teaching activities, provides guidance and Counseling services to the teaching faculty, Non Teaching Programs and students, Organizes workshops, seminars, conferences, CNE and In service Educational Programs (Faculty Development and Staff Developmental Programs), assists the National Council (INC) and State Nursing Council, Government and Universities as adhoc inspector or resource person in formulating educational policies, materials and assisting in maintaining the standards in Nursing Educational Institutions. Assists the University in conducting examinations, workshops, Curricular revision, Educational policies.

Administration
- Assists the administrator in formulating Philosophy, Policies and educational objectives of educational programs.
- Utilizes opportunities through group action to initiate improvement of the educational program.
- Explains educational philosophy and policies to Teaching Faculty.
- Directs the activities of staff working in the department.
- Assists the administrator in implementation of Curricular, Co-curricular and Extracurricular activities.
- Based on the situations exhibits varied leadership roles.

Teaching
- Identifies the needs of the learners in terms of objectives of the program by utilizing records of previous experience, personal interviews, Performance appraisals and observations.
- Assists learners in identifying their needs.
- Selects and organizes learning experiences in accordance with educational objectives.
- Participates in curriculum development, implementation and evaluation of the Courses.
- Plans the educational activities and departmental activities, Job responsibilities of teaching staff.
- Ascertains, selects and organizes facilities, equipment and materials necessary for learning.
- Organizes Curricular, Co-curricular and Extracurricular activities in the institution.

Helping the learners to acquire desirable attitudes, knowledge and skills
- Creates conducive teaching and learning environment.
- Assists learners in utilizing problem solving techniques.
- Uses varied and appropriate teaching methods effectively.
- Uses incidental and planned opportunities for teaching.
- Encourages learners to assume increasing responsibility for self development.

Evaluating learner's progress
- Recognizes individual differences in appraising the learners progress.
- Uses appropriate devices for evaluation.
- Measures and describes quality of performance objectivity.
- Helps learners for self evaluation.
- Participates in staff evaluation of learners progress.

Recording and reporting
- Maintains and uses adequate and accurate records
- Prepares and channels clear and concise reports
- Shares information about learners needs and achievements with others concerned with instruction and guidance
- Participates in the formulation and maintenance of comprehensive record system.

Guidance
- Conducts guidance programs in the educational institution
- Give guidance within own field of competence
- Helps the learner with special problems to seek and use additional help as indicated.

Counseling
- Helps the learner to grow in self understanding.
- Promotes continuous growth and development towards maturity.

- Continues to develop competence in problem solving process.
- Cooperates in and/or initiates group activities in development and evaluation of studies.
- Utilizes findings of research.
- Makes data available concerning learners and concerning methods of teaching and evaluation.

Research
- Guides the students and faculty in their Research activities.
- Helps the students to conduct Research studies and communicates the Research findings by publishing in National and International Journals.
- Encourages the students to enroll into varied research activities.

Assistant Professor
Educational qualification and experience:
- Master Degree in Nursing.
- Total 7 years of experience with minimum of 3 years teaching.
- Registered in State Nursing Council.

Job Summary
Assistant Professor usually works under Professor and HOD of the particular department of specialty depending upon her/his specialization and the requirement of the institution and assists in Administration, Teaching, Guidance, Counseling and Research activities. She/He is also responsible for co curricular, extracurricular and developmental activities of the college. Responsible for the completion of all the prescribed, allotted syllabus for a particular year.

Departmental Administration
Assistant Professor is responsible for:
- Contributes to the development and implementation of the philosophy and policies of the total education program.
- Participates in formation of educational objectives of the program.
- Utilizes opportunities through group action to initiate improvement of the educational program.
- Overall planning, organization and execution of her/his department with the help of lecturers and Public Health Nurses, in consonance with the philosophy and objectives of the University of Health Sciences. She/he is accountable for all the activities of her/his department.
- Plans, organizes and implements class room teaching program at all levels in her/his specialty or in allotted area.
- Makes arrangements for part-time/guest lecturers.
- Plans, organizes and conducts in service education for her/his department faculty.
- Maintains intra and inter departmental harmony for the smooth functioning of educational programs.
- Develops desirable interpersonal relationships with the students, parents and the community at large.
- Finds resources for the development of educational programs in the institution.
- Participates in budget preparation.
- Participates actively in professional organizational activities.
- Attends conferences and educational meetings.
- Keeps the students informed of their progress/time to time.
- Recommends for approval of leave on health grounds.
- Develops desirable functional relationships with the other teaching institutions and clinical/field areas.
- Participates in student welfare programs, Seminars, workshops, CNE programs.

Teaching
- Identify the learning needs and curricular needs of students.
- Prepares master rotation and individual rotation plans.
- Plans, organizes and conducts all class room teaching and clinical teaching in accordance with the learning needs and curricular requirements of students.

- Selects and Organizes the learning experiences for students.
- Measures effectiveness of instruction by use of appropriate devices.
- Analyses and evaluates resources material.
- Uses varied and appropriate teaching methods effectively.
- Equips the department and provides conducive environment for faculty and students.
- Ascertains, selects and organizes facilities equipment and materials necessary for learning.
- Develops evaluation tools both for classroom teaching and clinical teaching in accordance with the objectives of the program.
- Participates in classroom teaching.
- Forward leave applications of students.
- Participates in continuing nursing educational programs of the institution.
- Equips the department with the required items and supplies for teaching learning process and departmental administration.
- Develops audio-visual aids required for the department.

Evaluation
- Performs Evaluation measures.
- Recognize individual differences in appraising the learner's progress.
- Uses appropriate devices for evaluation.
- Measures and describes quality of performance objectively.
- Helps learners for self evaluation.
- Participates in staff evaluation of learner's progress.
- Submits internal assessment of students.
- Preserves all assignments, experience records, test paper etc. till the student gets through the course.

Guidance and Supervision
- Guides and supervises teaching faculty of her/his department both in the classroom and clinical settings.
- Evaluates, guides and supervises students in the classroom as well as in the clinical/field area.
- Counsels students and faculty.
- Advises Principal in relation to student affairs.

Research Activities
- Plans and conducts research for the improvement of student programs and nursing sciences.
- Initiates and participates in studies for the improvement of educational programs.
- Identifies problems in which research is indicated desirable.
- Continues to develop competence in problem solving process.
- Utilizes findings of research.

Records
- Maintains adequate and accurate records.
- The minutes of all departmental meetings.
- Attendance of teaching faculty of her/his department.
- Sub stock registers of the department.
- Students attendance.
- Leave records.
- Cumulative records of the students.
- Final records of her/his assigned class.
- Evaluations records.
- Submits a report of monthly attendance on the last day of every month for facilitating the claim of stipend/scholarships.

Lecturer

Educational qualifications and experiences
Masters Degree in Nursing, Registered in Nursing Council, Should possess 3 years experience.

Job summary

Works under direction of the department head and assists him/her in administration, instruction and guidance activities.

Job Description

Lecturer is assigned to a department depending upon his/her specialization or the institutional requirements. Lecturer is responsible for assisting the Head of the department in all curricular, co-curricular and extracurricular and developmental activities of the department and the institution.

Teaching

- Assist the head of the department in planning, organizing and execution of teaching program in the department.
- Shoulders responsibility for assigned teaching lead.
- Develops lesson plans with suitable audio visual aids and submits to the department after the class.
- Selects and organizes learning experience in accordance with educational objectives.
- Ascertains and selects, organizes facilities, equipment and materials necessary for learning.
- Assists the learners in using problem solving process.
- Utilizes various teaching strategies suitable to the topics under discussion.
- Assists the learners in identifying their needs.
- Develops audio-visual aids for the department.
- Maintain class and clinical attendance (both Nursing and Guest lectures).
- Informs student progress from time to time to the HOD.
- Advises HOD on student affairs.
- Guides and supervises students in the classroom and clinical settings.
- Prepares clinical area suitable for student learning.
- Assists colleagues in completion of work.
- Encourages students to participate in co-curricular and extracurricular activities.
- Helps the students in wholesome development.
- Develops evaluation tools both for classroom teaching and clinical teaching.
- Participates in various institutional and departmental committee meetings.
- Maintains the minutes of assigned institutional and/or departmental committee meetings.
- Evaluates students both in classroom as well as in the clinical/field settings.
- Develops desirable functional intra and inter departmental and inter institutional relationships.
- Develops therapeutic and professional relationships with the community.
- Participates in service and continuing education programs.
- Participates in all developmental activities of the institution.
- Assists in preserving assignments, clinical evaluation, test papers etc. till the student graduates.
- Evaluates and maintains a record of classroom and clinical evaluations of all assigned students.
- Assists in maintaining sub stock registers of the department.
- Participates in professional organizational activities.
- Shares information about learner's needs and achievements with other concerned.
- Measures effectiveness of instruction by use of appropriate devices.

Guidance and counseling

- Counsels students as and when necessary.
- Give guidance with own field of competence.
- Helps the learner to grow in self understanding.

Research

- Plans and conducts research projects either individually or as a group.
- Assists in initiating and participating in studies for the improvement of educational program.
- Identifies problems in which research is indicated or potentially desirable.
- Make data available concerning learners and methods of teaching and evaluation.
- Continues to develop competence in problem solving process.

- Cooperate in initiate group activity in development and evaluation of studies.
- Utilizes findings of research.

Records
- Maintains adequate and accurate records.
- Prepares clear and concise reports.
- Maintains class and clinical attendance.
- Assists the HOD in preparing monthly report of attendance.
- Maintains critical incident records.
- Assists in maintaining cumulative records and final records of students.

Public Health Nurse or Public Health Nursing Instructor
Educational Qualifications: B.Sc. (N) and Registered in Nursing Council

Job description:
- Public health Nurse is assigned to a department and is responsible to the HOD for all the activities.
- Assist the HOD in planning, organizing the teaching program in the department.
- Shoulders responsibility for the assigned teaching load.
- Develops lesson plans and submits to the department after the class.
- Develops/utilizes audio-visual aids for teaching.
- Prepares the clinical/field area suitable for providing learning experience for students.
- Guides and supervises students in both the classroom and in the clinical/field areas day/night.
- Utilizes various teaching strategies appropriate to the topics under discussion.
- Maintains the class and clinical/field attendance of students.
- Maintains the attendance of guest lectures.
- Assists in the preparation of evaluation tools both for classroom teaching and clinical/field teaching.
- Appraises students both in classroom and in the clinical/field areas.
- Counsels students as and when necessary.
- Helps the students in the wholesome development.
- Advises HOD on students affairs.
- Participates in various institutional and departmental committee meetings.
- Develops desirable intra and inter departmental and inter institutional relationships.
- Develops therapeutic and professional relationships with the clients and the community.
- Participates inservice and continuing educational programs.
- Participates in professional meetings.
- Acts as an advisor to student welfare committee such as student welfare body, recreation, N.S.S. etc. and check the accounts, keeps the records up-to-date.
- Encourages students to participate in co-curricular and extracurricular activities.

Records
- Maintains classroom and clinical attendance of students in the department,
- Assists in cumulative records, final records of students, various registers of the department and, assists in classroom and clinical/field evaluations.

Tutor/Clinical instructor
Educational qualification and experience
M.Sc(N) or B.Sc(N) with 1 year experience or Basic B.Sc.(N) with post basic diploma in clinical speciality Registered in Nursing Council.

Job summary
Works under direction of the department head and assists him/her in Teaching, Clinical instruction and guidance activities of students.

Administration

- Assisting in the administration activities of the department under HOD.
- Supervises students' health, welfare and security.
- Supervises the living condition of students in the hostel.
- Assist in teaching of other categories of personnel in the hospital and community.
- Assists in the procurement of college supplies and equipment.
- Assisting in the library work.
- Assisting in maintaining departmental records.

Academic activities

- Responsible for planning and implementation of teaching program.
- Supervises clinical teaching program activities in hospital/community health setting.
- Maintains classroom equipments, supplies and teaching aids.
- Demonstrates the Nursing Procedures in the college laboratory and clinical area and supervises return demonstration of procedures.
- Evaluates student's assignments and performance.
- Preparing teaching materials and implementing it under the guidance of other teachers.
- Helping the students with extracurricular activities.

Guidance and Counselling

- Guides the students in curricular, extracurricular and Co-curricular activities
- Counsel the students and guide them in solving their problems.

Records and Reports

- Maintains and supervises Admission Register, Class attendance, Clinical attendance, Hostel attendance register
- Prepares critical incident reports
- Assists the HOD in maintaining the necessary records and reports of the department.

Job description of Teaching faculty in School of Nursing

Principal

Education and Professional experience:
M.Sc. Nursing with three years of teaching experience or B.Sc. Nursing (Basic)/Post Basic with 5 years of teaching experience. Registered in State Nursing Council

Job summary

In Government settings, Principal is the administrative head of the School of Nursing will be responsible to the Medical Superintendent or District Surgeon of the hospital. Once the financial control of school handed over to the principal, he/she shall be directly responsible to the Directorate of Medical Education and Directorate of Health and Family Welfare services. In private settings Principal will be working under the Management authorities. As the head of the school she/he will be responsible for the implementation of the INC syllabus and school administration. Assists the Board in formulating Educational Policies, Objectives, Plans for implementation of Curricular, Co-curricular and Extracurricular activities. Organizes Workshops, Conferences, Seminars, Faculty Developmental or CNE activities. Assists the Indian Nursing Council, State Nursing Council and Board in maintaining standards in Schools of Nursing.

Duties and responsibilities

Administrative

- Preparing and assisting in revision Educational Policies and Objectives of the Educational Program.
- Preparation of prospectus in consultation with the controlling authority.
- Advertising and calling for the candidates for Diploma in General Nursing and Midwifery training Program.
- Scrutinizing applications, Preparing merit list and calling them for interview.

- Participate in total planning of the school with controlling authority.
- Conducting interview through the committee and selecting candidates and informing them.
- Planning for Orientation program for new students and staff.
- Delegation of work load and departments to each tutor along with teaching materials.
- Communicating with other departments, agencies or individuals in connection with the program.
- Maintaining students records, admission register, results, registers of teachers etc.
- Countersigning records of each department, library and hostel after annual verification by the concerned in charge of the department and the warden in case of the hostel.
- Providing the supply of audio-visual aids, teaching materials as requested by the concerned department in charge.
- Placing indents with the government for stationery, uniform for certain category of class IV employees in Government School's and in Private schools coordinating with Management and Government authorities for coordinating school's activities.
- Purchasing furniture, equipments, books and journals as per requirement of the office, hostel and Nursing department.
- Authorizing repairs of vehicles and purchase of oil, petrol and minor parts of replacement.
- Sending proposals yearly for new items costly equipments etc. to the authorities.
- Maintaining income and expenditure registers.
- Seeing that monthly pay bills are sent in time, so also T A bills or any other type of bills
- Preparing school budget.
- Assisting the auditors to prepare budget and filing taxes.
- Monitoring the office-timings and other rules of service are observed.
- Writing annually the confidential report of staff and teachers.
- Holding meetings with teachers, staff of office, hostel staff, students and their committee.
- Representing the School and the profession on various committees. welfare of staff and students.
- Preparing and furnishing reports as required by the state and Indian Nursing Council and the controlling authority.
- Organize annual functions and other functions of the school.
- Supervising teaching staff and giving them guidance in teaching.

Teaching
- Responsible for the smooth implementation of the prescribed syllabus.
- Arranging for theory and practical work for each group, with the help of tutor/clinical instructors to meet the educational objectives.
- Contacting agencies, institutions, for arranging field visits, clinical experiences etc. such that students will get the best possible or maximum experience within the scheduled time.
- Initiating changes in curriculum keeping within the guidelines of the syllabus.
- Cooperating with the state council/board to conduct examinations by providing all facilities.
- Guiding students in filling examination forms, registration fees and seeing that they are submitted to the council in time.
- Teaching the subjects.
- Guides the faculty in preparation of Master Rotation Plan and Clinical Rotation Plan.
- Preparing and displaying weekly/monthly class, schedule, clinical experience of rotation plan etc. in consultation with tutors.
- Maintaining records of examination results.
- Communicating to the council any relevant information regarding students.
- Encouraging teachers to experiment with newer methods of teaching and to find out newer clinical areas which would provide the best possible exposure of students, to that clinical area.
- Encourage and supporting co curricular and Extracurricular activities.
- Issuing transcripts to students.

Miscellaneous
- Encouraging faculty members to take up further studies, attend Seminars, Workshops and participate in professional activities.
- Participating in activities of the professional organization.
- Encouraging students to actively participate in SNA activities and to join TNAI as a life member.
- Arranging graduation and lamp lighting ceremonies with the assistance of teaching faculty.
- Meeting visitors and discussing issues, pertaining to the school program.
- Meeting parents or guardians of the students as and when necessary.
- Preparing for the cooperation with inspectors from the state level bodies or national council.

Vice principal

Educational Qualifications and Professional Experience:

M.Sc. Nursing or Basic B.Sc. Nursing or Post Basic B.Sc. Nursing with 3 years of teaching experience, Registered in state Nursing council.

Job Summary

Assists the principal in administration, teaching, Curricular, Co-curricular and Extracurricular activities

Administration

Assists the Principal in:
- Developing educational Policies, Objectives of the program.
- Curriculum development, planning, implementation and evaluation.
- Co Curricular and Extracurricular activities.
- Supervises teaching of new entrants into teaching.
- Guides tutors in implementation of curriculum.
- In INC, Board, State Councils inspections.
- Suggests the INC, Board, State Councils related to modifications in educational policies and in academic activities.

Teaching
- Teaches to the students in various subjects.
- Adapts New teaching methods with appropriate Audio-Visual Aids.
- Selects, Plans and organizes learning experiences.
- Implements innovative strategies in evaluation strategies.
- Guidance and Counselling.
  - Counsels the students and teaching faculty to adapt specific problem solving strategies.
  - Guides the faculty to utilize resources in implementing curricular, co curricular extracurricular activities.
- Promotes holistic development of students and teaching faculty.
- Maintains and supervises records and reports adequatly in the organization/school guides the faculty in maintaining Records and Reports of School of Nursing.

Tutors

Educational Experience and Professional qualification

M.Sc. Nursing/Basic B.Sc. Nursing/Diploma in Nursing Education and Administration with 2 years of professional experience

Responsibilities
- Teaches the allotted subjects.
- Prepares time tables under the supervision of Principal and Vice principal.
- Preparation of course outline and lesson plans of subject/subjects assigned.
- Plan clinical rotation and clinical teaching.
- Supervises the students in clinical experiences.
- Assists in Curricular, Co-curricular and Extracurricular activities.

- Plan teaching/demonstration, setting up of laboratory for the assigned subject.
- Plan, construct, administer and evaluate tests/exams.
- Prepare students for Board exams.
- Give and evaluate student assignments.
- Participate in working of various committees.
- Plan and arrange external lecturers, educational visits.
- Plan and organize the community health field for both urban and rural areas.
- Maintain and order supplies.
- Guides the students in Professional activities.
- Counsels the students and suggests problem solving techniques.
- Supervises Mess, Hostel and health activities.
- Maintains records and reports pertaining to students and the school.
- Assists in inspections of institution.

LABORATORY EQUIPMENT

Fundamentals of Nursing – laboratory (Basic Principles and Practice of Nursing)
This lab will have facilities for practice of Fundamentals of Nursing and Advance Nursing Practice

A. Equipments

S.No.	Items	Quantity
1	Patient cots - Adult	6
	- Child	2
	Bed side lockers	8
	Stools/chairs	2
2	Manikins for demonstrating Nursing Procedures	
	Adult male	3
	Adult female	3
	Child	2
	New born	2
	CPR	1
3	i) Trays different sizes	
	- 24" × 16"	6
	- 14" × 10"	6
	- 11" × 9"	6
	- 8" × 5"	6
	ii) Trays with cover – Assorted Sizes	6
4	i) Bowls	
	- 16" diameter	6
	- 10" diameter	6
	- 4" diameter	12
	- 2 -3" diameter	12
	ii) Bowls with cover	
	- 6" diameter	
	- 4" diameter	
5	Enema can	
	- 1 lt. capacity	4
	- ½ lt capacity	4
6	Kidney trays of assorted sizes	15
7	Measuring jugs	
	- 1000 ml	6
	- 500 ml	6
	- 250 ml	6

S.No.	Items	Quantity
8	Basins: Assorted size basins	12
9	Catheter dish with cover	4
10	Knife dish with cover	6
11	Feeding cups	6
12	Douche can	6
13	Sputum mugs	6
14	Bed pans	6
15	Urinals - Male	6
16	Funnel - 4" diameter	6
	- 2" diameter	6
17	Jars with covers	
	- 12" × 8"	2
	- 6" × 4"	2
18	Dressing Drums	
	- 8" × 4"	2
	- 12" × 9"	2
19	Tub for sitz bath	1
20	Sauce pan with lid	
	- 1 lt capacity	2
	- 2 lt capacity	2
21	Kettle	
	- 1 lt capacity	1
	- 2 lt capacity	1
22	Trolleys with upper and lower shelves	1
23	Pint measure	2
24	Galli posts	2
25	Mugs	2
26	Bottle brush	2

B. OT-Instruments

S.No.	Items	Quantity
1	Cheatle forceps	18
2	Sponge holding forceps	8
3	Artery clamps	
	- Straight 6"	6
	- Curved 6"	4
4	Dissecting Forceps	
	- Toothed	6
	- Non toothed	6
5	Mosquito forceps	4
6	Kockers	4
7	Scissors	
	- Surgical 8"	4
	- Bandage	4
	- Mayo's cutting scissors	4
8	Tissue forceps	4
9	Sinus forceps	4
10	Biopsy forceps	4
11	Liver biopsy needle	4
12	Alice forceps	4
13	Probe	4
14	Groove director with probe	4
15	Mouth gag	4
16	Tongue depressor	4
17	Tongue holding forceps	4
18	Nasal speculum	4
19	Aural speculum	4
20	Retractors	
	- Single hook	2
	- Double hook	2

S. No.	Items	Quantity
21	Bladder sound	2
22	Male urethral dilator	One set
23	Packing Forceps	
	- Nasal	2
	- Oral	2
24	Ear irrigation syringe	2
25	Ear speculum	3
26	Shaving set	2
27	Safety razor with blades	2
28	Bard Parker Knife Handle	2
29	Surgical blades different sizes	One set
30	Catheters	4
31	Airway	4
32	Laryngoscope	
	- Small	2
	- Big	2
33	Proctoscope	1
34	Infusion set	6
35	Otoscope	1
36	Ophthalmoscope	1
37	Tracheostomy set with various size of tracheal tubes	One set
38	Head mirror	2
39	Tuning fork	4
40	Infusion set	4
41	Oxygen cylinder with stand	2
42	Oxygen mask	20

C. Glass-ware

S.No.	Items	Quantity
1	Measuring cups	
	- 240 ml	6
	- 120 ml	6
	- 30 ml droppers	6
2	Undine	2
3	Eye bath-cup	2
4	Pippets	2
5	Glass connections	
	- Different types eg: Y.T.L.	6 each
6	Wolfs bottle	2
7	Conical flasks	2
8	i) Ounce glass	6
	ii) Dram glass	6
9	Thermometers	
	- Oral	6
	- Rectal	6
	- Bath	2

S.No.	Items	Quantity
	- Room	2
	- Lotion	2
10	Pulse meter	4
11	Urinometer	6
12	Lactometer	6
13	Haemoglobinometer	6
14	Specimen Glasses	6
15	Test Tubes	2 dozen
16	Glass sides with cover	2 boxes
17	Bottles 500 ml. capacity for lotions and mixtures	10
18	Atomizer	2
19	Manometer	2
20	Glucometer	2
21	Head Mirror	1

D. Syringes and Needles

S.No.	Items	Quantity
1	Syringes - 2 ml - 5 ml - 10 ml - 20 ml	12 12 12 12
2	Tuberculin syringe	6
3	Insulin syringe with needle	6
4	Needles - all sizes	One dozen each
5	Lumbar Puncture Needle	2
6	Trochar Canula for abdominal paracentesis	2
7	I V canulas different types and sizes	12
8	Biopsy Needle - Adult - Children	2 2
9	Sternal Puncture Needle	2

E. Suture Material

S.No.	Items	Quantity
1.	Needle holder - 6" - 7" - 8"	6 each
2	Suture cutting scissors	6
3	Suture needle - straight - curved	6 6
4	Suture thread - silks - cotton	2 packets 2 packets
5	Catgut - silk - cotton	6 tubes 6 tubes
6	Catgut tube Breaker	2
7	Suture Clip	1 packet
8	Suture Clip applier and remover	2

F. Rubber Goods

1	Mackintosh roll	
	- Full bed length	5
	- Draw Mackintosh	5
	- Extra Mackintosh for treatment and dressing	12
2	Hot water bag	5
3	Ice cups	
	- Ice collar	6
	- Corrugated rubber sheet	4
	Gloves different sizes	5
5	Catheters	
	- Urinary catheter	6
	- Folley's catheter	6
	- Nasal catheter	6

S.No.	Items	Quantity
	- Plain catheter - Rectal catheter	6 6
6	Finger stalls different sizes	6 sets each
7	Air Rings	6
8	Mucus Sucker	6
9	Breast Pump	2
10	Nipple Shield	2
11	Gastric lavage tube	2
12	Ryle's tube	6
13	Flatus tube	6
14	Blakemore sange staken tube	6
15	Rubber tubes with different diameter and size	
16	Rectal syringe with nozzle	2
17	Ring pressories(all sizes)	2 each
18	Douch nozzle different sizes	2

G. Miscellaneous Items

S.No.	Items	Quantity
1	Mortar and Pestle	6
2	Nelson's inhaler	6
3	Wooden shock blocks	2 pairs
4	Spirit lamp	6
5	Test tube stand	6
6	Test tube holder	12
7	Sterilizer small	2
8	Portable autoclave	1
9	Torch	2
10	Nail Brush	6
11	1) Adult weighting scale 2) Baby weighing scale	2 2
12	Back Rest	2
13	Splints different sizes	12
14	Bandages different sizes	One dozen each
15	Adhesive tapes	2
16	I V stand	2
17	Tape measure	6
18	Bucket with cover	6
19	Comb	6
20	Microscopes	2
21	Sphygmomanometer A - Regular B- Electronic	 6 2
22	stethoscope	6
23	Soap with soap dish	12
24	Dust bins	6

S.No.	Items	Quantity
25	Over bed table (Heart Table)	2
26	Screens/bed side curtains	2
27	Three way adapter	2

H. Solutions

S.No.	Items	Quantity
28	Dettol Solution	1 bottle
29	Phenyle Solution	1
30	Methylated spirit	1
31	Benedict's solution	1
32	Tr. Iodine/Betadine	1
33	Tr. Benzoin	1
34	Nitric acid	1
35	Acetic acid	1
36	Sulphur powder	Half kg
37	Ammonium sulphate crystals	Half kg
38	Vaseline 1 jar	
39	Glycerine	1 bottle
40	Liquid paraffin	1
41	Potassium permanganate crystals	200gm
42	Boric solutions	1 bottle
43	Hydrogen peroxide	1
44	Sodium bi carbonate powder	200 gm
45	Litmus paper strips red and blue	2

I. Linen

S.No.	Items	Quantity
1	Mattress - Adult - Child	06 02
2	Mattress cover - Adult - Child	 18 12
3	Bed sheets - baby cot sheets	30 12

S.No.	Items	Quantity
4	Draw sheets	12
5	Pillows - large - small	12 6
6	Pillow covers - Large - Small	 24 12
7	Sand bags with covers	6
8	Blankets	12
9	Bed spreads	12
10	Towels - Bath - Hand - Surgical - Packing - Towel clips	12 12 12 2 6
11	Sponge cloth	12 each
12	Hot water bag cover	12
13	Ice cap covers	12
14	Air ring/cushion covers	6
15	Gowns - mask	12 each
16	Patient's clothes - Male - Female - Baby dresses of different sizes - Diapers different sizes	 12 sets 12 sets 6 sets 12
17	Trolley cover	5
18	Dirty linen bag/box	1
19	Leggings	2 pairs
20	Perinneal sheets	5
21	Triangular bandages	12
22	Many tailed bandaged	12
23	Eye shields	5
24	Dusters	24
25	Slings	6
26	'T' Binder	2
27	Screen curtains	2 sets

Equipment in Medical- Surgical Nursing Laboratory

S.No.	ITEM	DESCRIPTION	QUANTITY
	Furniture		
1.	Intensive Care Unit Bed	198 X 90 X 60cms	01
2.	Hospital Semi-Fowler Bed, General,	198x90x60cms	03
3.	Stretcher on Trolley, with 4" wheels	80"x22"x32	03
4.	Instrument Trolley With S.S. Top	24"X18"X32"	01
5.	Curved Instrument Trolley With S.S. Top	44"X14"X33"	01
6.	Dressing Trolley With S.S. Top	30"x20"x32")	01
7.	Cylinder Trolley		01

S.No.	ITEM	DESCRIPTION	QUANTITY
	Manikin		
8.	NASCO nursing skill manikin		01
9.	Patient Care/CPR Manikin		01
	Model		
10.	Eye model		01
11.	Ear model		01
12.	Ostomy model		01
	Charts		
13.	Snellen chart		02
14.	Pain scale assessment		01
	Instruments		
15.	Digital Clinical Thermometers	**Thermometers**	05
16.	Rectal Thermometers	„	10
17.	Forehead Thermometers	„	05
18.	Oval clinical Thermometer	„	05
19.	Hypo allergic paper tap	Medical Disposable	05 Roll
20.	Hypo allergic transparent tap	„	05 Roll
21.	Scalp Vein Set (22 G, 23G, 24G Blister pack)	„	05 Each
22.	Levin Tube (Feeding tube)		04
23.	Infusion Set Regular Molded - Standard		02
24.	Syringes with needles, 2ml,3ml, 5ml, 10ml	Disposable syringes	15 Each
25.	Insulin syringe with needles, 1 ml	29G × O.5"	15
26.	Ryles tube	Ryles tube	
		FG ; 08, and 10 and 12 and 14 and 20 and 22	05 Each
27.	Stomach tube	FG 08&09&10&12& 13&18&20&24	
28.	Rectal tube	Rectal tube FG : 18&20& 22&24&28&30&32	05 Each
29.	I.V cannula with wings with port	14G and 16G, 17G and 18G and 19G and 20G	05 Each
30.	Suction catheter	(FG): 08,10, 12,14,16	05 Each
31.	Gibbsons catheter,	(FG): 10. 12, 14, 16, 18	03 Each
32.	Nasal oxygen catheter	FG 4 and 6, 8 and 10	05 Each
33.	Urethral catheter	FG: 08, 10, 12, 14, 16, 18	03 Each
34.	Nelaton(Urinary) catheter	FG : 08, 10 and 12, 14 and 16, 18, 20	05 Each
35.	Foley balloon catheter	FG: 12 to 22	03 Each
	Diagnostic Equipments		
36.	Aneroid sphygmomanometer		10
37.	Blood Pressure Monitor Aneroid	8" Desk Model	05
38.	Sphygmomanometer Stand Model	95-135 cm	05
39.	Digital B.P. Monitor,		05
40.	Stethoscope		10
41.	Stethoscope	Dual Head	10
42.	Weighing Scale Square	Capacity:130 Kg	03

S.No.	ITEM	DESCRIPTION	QUANTITY
43.	Weighing Scale, Round		03
44.	Height Measuring Stand, with Weighing Scale		02
45.	Hammer, Neurological		02
46.	Hammer, Percussion,	Taylor Model	03
47.	Hammer, Queen Square Pattern		01
48.	Tongue Depressor Wooden		05
49.	E.N.T examination set		02
50.	Tongue depressor		05
51.	Nasal speculum		05
52.	Laryngeal mirror		03
53.	Laryngoscope handle standard (Brass)		02
54.	Laryngoscope handle standard (steel)		02
55.	Macintosh laryngoscope blade (single use)	Plastic 2, 3, 4	03
56.	Resuscitators set (with size # 4 face mask)	Rubber	03
57.	Color Blindness Book		02
	Surgical instruments		
58.	Medicare Blood Lancets	Stainless steel	Small box of 20
59.	Surgical blades		10
60.	Scissors One Pc.	Packing 4" Care Straight/Ang	05
61.	Iris Scissors	4", 4 1/2", Dlx	02 Each
62.	Dressing Scissor Straight/Curved	5", 6" , 7",8",10" Dlx Blunt sharp	05 Each
63.	Mayo Scissor Straight/Curved	5 1/2", 6 1/2", 7 1/2"8 1/2"	02 Each
64.	Metzumbum (Tonsil) Scissor Strait /Curved	6, 7, 8 Dlx	02 Each
65.	Kilner scissor 4 ½" Dlx		02
66.	Suture scissors		02
67.	Bandage scissor	5 ½ ,6 ½ , 7 ½ "Dlx	02 Each
68.	Tailor scissor	stainless steel handles 8" to10"	02 Each
69.	Black braided silk sutures ½ circle rounded body	suture size 1 to 4-0	04 Each
70.	Black braided silk sutures ½ circle taper edge	suture size 2-0	02
71.	Black braided silk sutures 3/8 circle cutting suture	suture size 4-0	02
72.	Black braided silk sutures 3/8 circle reverse cut suture	suture size 3-0 and 4-0	04 Each
73.	Black braided silk sutures 3/8 circle microprint spatula suture	Suture size 8-0	02
74.	Black braided silk sutures precut standard length	Suture size 3-0 and 4-0	04 Each
	Orthopedic instruments		
75.	1.5 mm cortical screw		05
76.	2.0 mm cortical screw		05
77.	Mini Straight Plate For 2.0 mm Screw		05
78.	Mini L - Plate for 2.0 Screws		05
79.	Mini T - Plate for 2.0 Screws		05
80.	Straight Reconstruction Plate for 2.7 mm Screw		05
81.	T Plate for 2.7 mm Screw		05
82.	Kirschner Wire with Trocar Tip	0.8 MM to 3.0 mm diameter	03

S.No.	ITEM	DESCRIPTION	QUANTITY
83.	Stainless Steel Wire	16 SEG to 30 SEG	02
84.	External fixation ring type posts	MALE	01
85.	External fixation ring type posts	FEMALE	01
	Hospital Wear		
86.	Surgical Gloves: Latex	6" to 9"	15 Each
87.	Examination gloves : Latex	6" to 9"	15 Each
88.	Disposable Cap		100 in one box
89.	Non Toxic nuisance dust mask,	Yellow and Green	50 In one box
90.	Mackintosh sheeting	Medium size	05
91.	Disposable drapes		10
92.	Urine pot male light with out cover		03
93.	Urine pot female light with out cover		03
94.	Urine pot large with cover and female attachment economy	2 in 1; 1000 ml	02
95.	Bed Pan Pontoon Type with Handle and cover.	2 in 1	02
96.	Kidney tray	8"/200 mm	10
97.	Kidney tray	10"/200 mm	10
98.	Kidney tray	12"/300 mm	10
99.	Enema can/Douche can with cover transparent type	pp 1000 ml	02
100.	Eye Wash cups with stand	White	05
101	Steam inhaler		10
	Sterilizers		
102.	Instrument sterilizer (Electric)	14"x6"x4"(STD)	03
103.	Instrument sterilizer, Non electric	18"x8"x6"	02
104.	Autoclave, 'P'-Type Lock System	12"X12	01
105.	Suction unit with glass jars	overflow valve system	01
	Rubber Goods		
106.	Hot water bag both sides ridded		05
107.	Ice bags round		05
108.	Ice bags oval		03
109.	Air cushion	30 cm to 45 cm	05 Each
110.	B.P.Armlet Bag cuff (adult size)	27-34 cm or up to 13.38 inches (midpoint)	03 Each
111.	B.P.Armlet Bag, cuff (large adult)	35-44 cm or 13.7 inches to 17.3 inches	05 Each
112.	B.P.Armlet Bag, long short	Green and black	02
113.	B.P Bulb with knob		05
114.	Self Retaining Catheter (Malicot)	FR 12 to 18FR	05 Each
115.	Corrugated Drainage Sheet,	size 30 cm × 15 cm (approx)	05
116.	Douche Tube, Red,	137 cm × 8 mm	02
117.	Eye/ear ulcer syringe	100cc	05
118.	Ryles tube	16 FR to 24 FR	03 Each
119.	Rectal tube		03
120.	Syringe and Needle destroyer		02

Midwifery/Obstetric Nursing Laboratory

S.No.	Item	Quantity
A.	**Models**	
1	Stages of development of embryo	2 sets each
2	Female bony pelvis	4
3	Foetal skull	2
4	Female dummy (Zoe model)/obstetrical training manikin – dummy with doll	1
5	Placenta	2
6	Full size foetus	4
7	New born baby	2
B.	**Charts or Posters**	
1	Breast changes in Pregnancy	1
2	Uterine changes in pregnancy showing height of uterus at different terms of pregnancy	1
3	Stages of labour - First stage - Second stage - Third stage	1 1 1
4	Breech presentation - complete breech - Incomplete breech - foot breech - Shoulder presentation	1 1 1 1
5	Face presentation	1
6	Brow presentation	1
7	Twin pregnancy	1
8	Placenta previa - different stages	1
9	Caput succedaneum, cephalo haematoma	1
10	Congenital malformations of new born - Cleft lip- Cleft Palate - Spina bifida - Hydrocephalus - Anencephaly	1 1 1 1
C.	**Instruments**	
1	Vaginal speculum - Sims - Cusco's	2 different sizes 2 different sizes
2	Cervical dilators all sizes	One set
3	Anterior vaginal wall retractor	2
4	Uterine vulsellum	2
5	Sponge holding forceps	2
6	Ovum forceps	1
7	Uterine flushing curette	1
8	Uterine sound	1
9	Mucus sucker	6
10	Pelvimeter	1
11	Foetoscope	2

S.No.	Item	Quantity
	Midwifery Kit for Home Delivery Total no of kits-4 Each kit will contain following items:	
1	Bowls medium and small	2 each
2	Kidney tray medium, small	2 each
3	Enema can with tubing	1
4	Foetoscope	1
5	Artery forceps	2
6	Thumb forceps Toothed – no toothed	1 each
7	Cord cutting blade/scissors	1
8	Cord ties	1
9	Mucus sucker	1
10	Cotton swabs	
11	Mackintosh	1
12	Glove	2 pairs
13	Mask	1
14	Apron	1
15	Rubber catheters	1
16	Spring balance color coated	1
17	Syringe with needles 2cc – 5cc – 10cc	1 each
18	Shaving set	1
19	Sprit	1
20	Soap with dish	1
21	Hand towels	1
22	Measure tape	1
23	Old news papers	
24	B.P. Apparatus	1
25	Urine testing material–Test Tubes, Test Tube holders, Benedict's solution, 1% acetic acid, Sulphur Powder, 10% & 40% Sodium Hydroxide, Alcohol, Hydrochloride, Barium Chloride, Ammonium Sulphate Crystals, Fouchets reagent (To Test for Sugar, Albumin, Bile Salts and Bile Pigments, if necessary).	6 each and solutions

Paediatric Laboratory Equipment

S.No.	Item	Quantity
1	Paediatric cot with side rails	3
2	Paediatric Models or Mankins Baby dolls Newborn dolls Infant dolls	2 each
3	Incubator Radiant warmer Phototherapy Unit	1 each
4	Aprons	10
5	Masks (Disposable Packs)	2
6	Gowns (Disposable or cloth)	10
7	Latex/Latex-free Gloves	15 pairs

S.No.	Item	Quantity
8	Gauze, Bandage, Binders	Sufficient quantity
9	Linen: Bed Sheets -Top Sheets, Bottom Sheets, Blankets, Draw Sheets, Counter sheets, Pillow Covers, Small Towels and Big towels, Bath blankets, Slit/dressing towel, Dusters,	10 each
	Rubber Goods	
10	Mucous suckers	5
11	Bulb Syringe	5
12	Suction catheter	5
13	Nasopharangeal catheters	5
14	Small mackintosh	15
15	Big mackintosh	15
16	Hot Water Bag	5
17	Ice cap	5
18	Urinary Catheters different sizes	5 each
19	Mouth Gag	5
20	Ambu Bag	2
21	Breast Pump	5
22	Ryles tubes	10
	Enamel Appliances	
23	Trays — Big, Medium, Small	10 each
24	Bowels — Big, Medium, Small	10 each
25	Kidney Trays — Big, Small	20 each
26	Basins — Big, Small	10 each
27	Buckets	10
28	Jugs	10
29	Feeding Cups	10
30	Measuring Cups—10 ml, 1 ounce, 50 ml, 100 ml, 200 ml, 500 ml	3 each
	Steel Appliances	
31	Glasses (Different Sizes)	5each
32	Spoons (Table spoon, Tea Spoon, Fork, Katori spoon)	5 each
33	Droppers	10
34	Formula Feeding Preparation containers	10
35	Feeding Cups, Feeding bottle and teat Belcroy feeder	10 each
36	Trolleys (Dressing, Medicine)	6
37	Surgical Instruments – Scissors, Artery forceps, Dissecting Forceps (Toothed, Non- toothed), Umbilical cord cutter, Cheatle forceps, Surgical blade, Needle (Curved , Straight), Dressing Tray (Small, Big), Sponge holding forceps	10 each
	Diagnostic Appliances	
38	Neonatal laryngoscope	3
39	ET Tube	3
40	Pulse oxymeter	3
41	Spirometer	3
42	Stethoscope	10
43	B.P. Apparatus	10
44	Monitor	1

S.No.	Item	Quantity
45	Thermometer: oral Thermometer: rectal Thermometers digital (not mercury) Thermometers Tympanic	15 5 5 5
46	Knee hammer	5
47	Tunic fork	5
48	Nasal speculum	5
49	Torch light	5
50	Tongue depressor	5
51	Height Measuring Scale Measuring inch tape	1 10
52	Weighing scale (infantometer) Adult weighing scale Electric weighing scale (infantometer)	3 2 1
53	Restraints Mummy restraint Elbow restraint – plaster of paris and gauze Extremity restraint Abdominal restraint Jacket restraint Mit/finger restraint	5 each
54	Mortar and pestle	10
55	Minim glass /funnel Ounce glass	10
56	Plastic measuring cups & soufflé cups Syringes (2ml, 5ml,10ml, 20ml, 50ml)	10each
57	Medicine cards	2 Boxes
58	Butterfly needles	2 Boxes
59	Nebulisers	3
60	Medicine slab and spatula	10
61	Humidifier	3
62	Metered dose inhaler with medication canister airway	3
63	Oxygen mask, Oxyhood, Oxygen tent, Oxygen Cylinder, Suction Apparatus	1 each
64	Baby Bath–Tub, Hydrometer	2
65	Soap dishes with Soaps	10
66	Containers for Baby oil, Powder, Spirit Cotton swabs, Gauge piece, antiseptic solution	Adequate
67	Adhesive plaster	5
68	Collecting device–plastic Disposable urine bag or collector (Hollister, U-bag , double chamber)	1
69	Colostomy irrigation Irrigating can with tubing Clamp Catheter IV stand	3 each
70	Suction Apparatus	1
71	Play Material—age wise toys, Posters–Colors, Shapes, animals, flowers, fruits, vehicles etc.	Adequate
72	Models to show all the procedures Video tapes for medical systems examination Health education materials: chart, flip chart	

Nutrition Laboratory

S.No.	Item	Quantity
1	Gas stoves with cylinders/pipe line tubings	6
2	Gas lighters	6
3	Pressure cookers of different sizes Small size (3 litres) Medium Size (5 Litres) Large cooker	 3 3 3
4	Steel cooking vessels big, medium and small sizes	12
5	Cutlery set	1
6	Ladles (wooden spoons/spatulas)	12
7	Juice squeezer	1
8	Water reservoir	1
9	Sauce pans with handle medium and small size	6
10	Spoons–serving spoons Tea spoons Table spoons Dessert spoons Soup spoons Rice serving spoons	6 24 12 12 12 4
11	Bowls Different sizes	25
12	Soup bowls	36
13	Forks	36
14	Sieve	2
15	Tongs	6
16	Knives	6
17	Peeler	6
18	Vegetable cutters	6
19	Vegetable cutting plate	6
20	Water filter/aqua quard	1
21	Flasks	2
22	Frying pans	6
23	Tava	6
24	Vessel holders (chimta)	6
25	Mixer with accessories	1
26	Glasses for drinking water (steel)	24
27	Glasses for drinking water (glass)	24
28	Kitchen weighing scale	1
29	Chapathi making plate and rolling pin	6
30	Measuring scoops	2 sets
31	Napkins	24
32	Glass bowls	24
33	Tea strainer	6
34	Egg beater	6
35	Toaster	2
36	Microwave with appropriate cooking vessels	1
37	Dinner set (12 persons)	2
38	Tea set (12 persons)	2

Community Health Nursing Laboratory

S.No.	Item	Quantity
1	Eligible couple and Child register	1
2	Diary	2
3	Community bags	12
4	One Table for four students	12
5	Chairs	50
6	Sterilizer	1
7	Infant weighing scale	5
8	Salter scale	1
9	Spring balance	1
10	Weighing machine	2
11	Sphygnomanometers	5
12	Stethoscopes	5
13	Dari/mats for health education purpose	2
14	A V Aids on different topics in the form of posters, Flip charts, Flash cards, Pamphlets and Hand outs	Many sets for varied topics
15	Community bag, should contain following articles: The bag should have separate compartments for clean articles, urine testing kit and hand washing kit Assessment articles: Thermometer, Tape measure, Stethoscope and Foeto scope Hand washing articles: Soap dish with soap, Hand towel, Nail brush	1 each 6

Water proof bag

Urine testing kit:
- Test tubes,
- Test tube holder
- Spirit lamp
- Dropper
- Benedict's solution in a bottle (for testing Sugar)
- Glass syringe
- 1% Acetic Acid in a bottle (for confirming Albumin)
- Sulphur Powder (in a container)
- Hydrochloric Acid, Barium chloride, ammonium sulphate crystals. Fouchets reagent, 10% and 40% Sodium Hydroxide in Bottles (if Necessary to test Bile salts, bile pigments)

Dressing kit:
- Bag of sterilized dressing
- Antiseptic in a bottle
- Artery forceps
- Dissecting forceps non toothed
- Dissecting forceps toothed
- Small bowl
- Small kidney tray
- Suture cutting scissors/dressing scissors

Medicines :
- Labeled medicines for essential treatment for minor ailment

Anatomy and Physiology Laboratory

S.No.	Item	Quantity
A	1 Adult human articulated skeleton with hanging facility in a glass cupboard with locking facility	2
	2 Few sets of disarticulated adult human skeleton	2
B.	**Models**	
	1 Full size human body showing all muscles and arteries	2
2	Human torso: - Male	2
	- Female	2
3	Skin cross section	2
4	Heart and large blood vessels	2
5	Heart with detachable parts on a stand	2
6	Eye with different sections	2
7	Ear with different sections	2
8	Human brain with spinal cord	2
9	Lungs and trachea	2
10	Larynx	2
11	Digestive system: - Stomach - Small intestine - Large intestine	2 2 2

12	Female reproductive system:
	- Uterus on stand
	- Ovaries
	  • Macroscopic structure
	  • Microscopic structure
		2
		
		2
		2

13	Male reproductive system	2
14	Urinary system, Kidney: Macroscopic structure, Microscopic structure	2 2
15	Joints and ligaments Wrist, Ankle Elbow, Knee Shoulder, Hip	2 2 2
16	Teeth	2
C.	**Charts**	
1	Skeleton System	2
2	Muscular system: Showing different muscles of the body	2
3	Joints and ligaments	2
4	Nervous system: - Brain - Spinal cord	2 2
5	Cardiovascular system	2
6	Respiratory system	2
7	Lungs	2
8	Trachea	2
9	Larynx	2
10	Digestive system	2

S.No.	Item	Quantity
11	Oral cavity	2
12	Teeth	2
13	Stomach, pancreas and spleen	2
14	Small intestine	2
15	Large intestine	2
16	Liver and gall bladder	2
17	Kidney macroscopic structure	2
18	Kidney microscopic structure	2
19	Skin	2
20	Eye	2
21	Ear	2
22	Female reproductive system	2
23	Menstrual cycle	2
24	Male reproductive system	2
25	Endocrine glands	2
Charts	**On First aid**	
26	First aid for burns	1
27	Cardiac pulmonary resuscitation: - Adults - Children - Infant	 1 1 1
28	First aid charts for emergencies such as fracture, drowning, wounds, poisoning, bites	1 each
29	Bandaging (Spiral, Finger)	

Computer Laboratory

S.No.	Item	Quantity
1	Computers (PC) with latest configuration and should be on local area network	10
2	Server	1
3	Internet facility	
4	Laser printer	2
5	Softwares: statistical package, MS offices, windows operating system, hospital management system, nursing management information system, online search softwares like CINHAL, MEDLAR.	

Audio-visual Aids

S.No.	Item	Quantity
1	Xerox machine (Photocopy machine)	1
2	Overhead projectors	5 (one in each class room)
3	Flannel boards in each class room+ notice board	4
4	Slide projectors	2
5	White board	For each class room
6	Chalk board	For each class room
7	Tape recorder	2
8	Television	2
9	VCR and CD player	2
10	Wet specimens of all organs	

S.No.	Item	Quantity
11	L C D	1
12	Film projector	1
13	Epidioscopes	3
14	Mobile screen for projectors	2
15	Printer	2

Equipment in Microbiology Laboratory

S.No.	Name of Equipment	Quantity
1	Bright Field Microscopes	10
1a	Simple Microscopes	20
1b	Compound Microscopes	15
1c	Dark Field Microscopes (to test Acid -Fast bacilli)	05
2	Glassware for measuring as well as for pouring of the media; slides etc.	50
3	Weighing Machines	10
4	PH meters	10
5	Stoves	05
6	Autoclave Machine for sterilization	01
7	Incubators and refrigerators for the storage of prepared media	01
8	Freezers	01
9	Water baths	01
10	Containers and buds for specimen collection inoculation loops & straight wires	Adequate
11	Bunsen Burners	05
12	Safetyhoods	01
13	Incubators for inoculated media	01
14	Antibiotic disc to test susceptibility	01
15	Centrifuges	01
16	ELISA machines	01
17	Spectrophotometer	01
18	Hot-air oven	01
19	Soap solutions Disinfectants Hand driers Washing areas Buckets with appropriate colored bags To separate hazardous waste from non-hazardous	Adequate

Classification of equipment: Broadly classified into 3 types:
- Preparation (Pre-diagnostic)
- Cultivation (Diagnostic)
- Disinfection (Post-diagnostic)

All the equipments are to be tested periodically for the assessment of quality and performance.

It is preferable to place the equipment separately according to the classification in different rooms.

Equipments required for preparation—These equipment are mainly required for the preparation of wide range of media that supports the growth of the test organisms.

Equipment required for cultivation—These equipment are required for the cultivation and identification of the organisms.

Equipment required for disinfection—These equipment are required for the disinfection of the used media and specimen disposal, e.g. Soap solutions, Disinfectants, Hand driers, Washing areas, Buckets with appropriate colored bags (To separate hazardous waste from non-hazardous), Hot-air oven, Autoclave machines , Incinerators Outside the lab to disinfect hazardous waste.

Along with the previously motioned equipment, an ideal lab must also have the following:
- A separate counter where the specimen are collected and catalogued based on the type of specimen, patient details, hospital details etc.
- It should also have proper warning at the entrance which displays the level of biological hazard.
- The lab must be air-conditioned and the temperature must be maintained at 25°C.
- First-aid kit (should be available in all laboratories).
- Adequate supply of personal protective equipment such as gloves, masks, hair nets, spare lab-coats, etc.
- A computer with details of the previous and present patient specimen being processed.

COLLEGE COMMITTEES

Each college has to formulate the following Committees and describe their composition and responsibilities. Each committee will have one chair person and 2 to 3 members. Chair person and members will be selected among teaching faculty by the Principal and Vice Principal in faculty meeting based on their interest qualifications, experience.
1. College Council Committee
2. Coordinating Committee
3. Curriculum Committee
4. Research Committee
5. Students welfare Committee
6. Discipline/Anti ragging Committee/Joint Consultative Committee
7. Guidance and Counseling Committee
8. Health Committee
9. Library Committee
10. Hostel Committee
11. Mess Committee
12. Recreation Committee
13. Sports Committee.

Student's Welfare Body
Nomenclature: The general student body of College of Nursing, of a specific City is designated as Student's Welfare Body, College of Nursing, particular City.
Aim: To contribute to the whole some development of students.

Objectives
- Encourage students to participate in extracurricular activities and stimulates to develop physically, intellectually and socially.
- Enhances cooperation and collaboration among students.
- Assists in maintaining discipline among the students.
- Develops desirable amicable relationships with other collegiate welfare bodies and University welfare body.
- Brings out a college magazine periodically.
- Upholds welfare funds.
- Along with alumnae, strives towards continuous overall development of the college.

Activities
- Commemorates National events.
- Celebrates College day, Hostel day, Sports day, Teachers' day etc.
- Organizes fresher's party and farewell parties.
- Celebrates important festivals like Diwali, Ramadan, Christmas.

- Organizes educational and recreational excursions and picnics.
- Arranges guest speeches to enrich students knowledge educationally, culturally and intellectually.
- Participates in cultural activities during college function.
- Exhibits and improves talents and potentialities in socio-cultural activities.
- Conducts debates and competitions periodically.
- Provides recreational and educational facilities for advancement such as magazines, journals, video cassettes etc.
- Participates in intra collegiate, inter university and inter professional events.
- Brings out college magazine regularly.
- Boosting up students welfare funds through patrons, fees, cultural activities etc.

Membership
- Open to all students
- Patronship—open to any interested person
- Hon. Members—Teaching faculty
- Annual subscription to be paid which is liable to change according to University guidelines.

Ex-Office
- President of the student welfare body
- Principal, College of Nursing.

Executive Committee
- Vice President
- General Secretary
- Joint Secretary/Treasurer
- Chair person of Recreation Committee
- Chair person of Hostel Committee.

General Body
Consists of all regular members of Students Welfare Body
Election of the Office Bearers
Executive Committee will decide the date for receiving nominations and elections of office bearers from regular members. General Secretary will give information to the General body regarding the venue and date of election a month ahead. Elections will be conducted in the last week of March
For the post of Vice-President, Chairpersons of Hostel committee and Recreation Committee, Students' Canteen Committee and Health Committee candidate should have been regular member at least for a period of two years. For the post of General Secretary, Joint Secretary/Treasurer candidate should be a regular member for at least one year

Policies relating to nominations for Elections
Only regular members are eligible for nominating and voting for office bearers:
- No member is allowed to nominate more than one candidate for one post.
- No member is allowed to second a candidate after proposing.
- No member is allowed to second more than one candidate for one post.
- Voting will be done on ballet system.
- A committee consisting of Vice-President, General Secretary, faculty advisor for student welfare and one member of the teaching faculty will be responsible for counting the votes and announcing the results within 24 hours after holding elections.

Functions of the Executive Committee
- Plan annual programs for student welfare
- Prepare the budget
- Formulate bye-laws
- Vice-President will put up to the Principal for passing bye-laws

- Responsible for organizing extracurricular activities, National functions and College functions for the student welfare.
- Responsible for holding general body meetings and have power for demanding co-operation from members for any purpose concerned with student welfare.
- Draw attention of the faculty advisors in such matters as effect general interest of the student welfare.
- Disciplinary action against any student who breaks the rules of the institution will be taken by the Principal. on the recommendation of the executive committee. But the final decision will be taken by the Principal.
- Hold monthly executive committee meetings and general body meeting every 3 months.

Meetings

The Executive Committee will meet every month, at least 2/3rd of the executive members should form the quorum for an executive meeting. The General Body of students welfare will meet every 3 months. The date and venue will be fixed by the executive committee. At least 2/3rd of the regular members should forum the quorum for a general body meeting.

Responsibilities of Executive Members
Vice-President
- Functions as Chief Executive Officer of student welfare
- Prepares agenda for the meeting
- Presides over the meeting of the executive committee and general body
- Have peer to call for any emergency meeting of the executive committee and general body meeting at short time notice of 24 hours
- In the event of disorder in the house, have powers to either dissolve the meeting or adjourn the meeting.
- Signs the minutes of the meeting after being passed by the house
- Votes for University election
- Plans and executes all the student welfare activities in consultation with the faculty advisor.

General Secretary
- Arranges for the executive committee meetings once in a month and general body meetings once in 3 months
- Assists President in the preparation of agenda for the meeting
- Writes minutes proceedings for both meetings and maintaining records
- Read minutes of the previous meeting before the commencement of every meeting and present to Chairperson for confirmation after being accepted by the house
- Conducts correspondence connected with student welfare
- Puts up notices for information to the general body for meetings connected with student welfare
- Extends invitations to patrons, Hon. members and of the student welfare as and when deemed necessary
- Prepares and present annual report to the General body
- Votes for University elections.

Joint Secretary/Treasurer
- Collects subscription and maintain a record for plan of budget
- Incur expenditure and maintains accounts
- Submits annual report of income and expenditure
- Acts in the absence of General Secretary
- Plans and participates in income generating activities
- Gets the accounts checked by the faculty advisor and an accountant every 3 months
- Votes for University election.

Chairperson of Hostel Committee
- Attends executive committee meetings
- Prepares and gives a report on hostel committee meetings
- Takes the decision of student welfare regarding hostel and discusses in the hostel committee meetings.
- Supervises and maintains the sanitation in hostel.

Chairperson for Recreational Committee
- Attends executive committee meetings
- Prepares and gives a report of recreation committee meetings
- Arranges magazines, cultural activities etc. according to the student welfare body decision
- Takes main role in organizing sports, games and cultural activities.

Chairperson of student's canteen
- Attends executive committee meetings
- Prepares and presents a report of canteen committee meeting
- Takes main role in the arrangement of refreshments for all activities connected with student welfare.

Chairperson of Health Committee
- Attends executive committee meetings
- Prepares and presents a report of Health Committee meetings.

PROFESSIONAL ORGANIZATIONS

International Council of Nurses (ICN)

The International Council of Nurses (ICN) is a federation of more than 130 national nurses associations (NNAs), representing the more than 13 million nurses worldwide. Founded in 1899, ICN is the world's first and widest reaching international organisation for health professionals. Operated by nurses and leading nurses internationally, ICN works to ensure quality nursing care for all, sound health policies globally, the advancement of nursing knowledge, and the presence of worldwide of a respected nursing profession and a competent and satisfied nursing workforce.

Vision

A vision is a compelling image of the preferred future that sets out a group's or organization's highest aspirations in clear, powerful, confident language. When people really take a vision seriously, it becomes an inspirational 'force' in their lives that pulls the present toward the envisioned future, acting as a self-fulfilling prophecy. A vision's power lies in its ability to motivate and align efforts. When people are committed to a vision, they will stretch themselves and their organisations to make it happen. Visions raise people's personal aspirations and provide a focus for collective activity. They create a 'big picture' of where we are going that makes day-to-day activity more meaningful.

For a vision to truly be a force in people's hearts, it must:
- Be legitimate
- Be shared
- Express people's highest aspirations for what they want to create in the world
- Stretch beyond the limits of current realities
- Conceivably be achievable within a specific time frame. It can be a powerful force for guiding and motivating our efforts if we take it into our hearts, keep it before us, and use it actively in our planning and decision-making.

Goals: To bring nursing together worldwide, to advance nurses and nursing worldwide, to influence health policy.

Core values: Visionary Leadership, Inclusiveness, Flexibility, Partnership and Achievement.

The ICN Code for Nurses is the foundation for ethical nursing practice throughout the world. ICN standards, guidelines and policies for nursing practice, education, management, research and socio-economic welfare are accepted globally as the basis of nursing policy. ICN advances nursing, nurses and health through its policies, partnerships, advocacy, leadership development, networks, congresses, special projects, and by its work in the arenas of professional practice, regulation and socio-economic welfare.

Professional Nursing Practice: International classification for nursing practice (ICNP), Advanced nursing practice, Entrepreneurship, HIV/AIDS, TB and malaria, Women's health, Primary health care, Family health, Safe water

Nursing Regulation: Regulation and Credentialing, Code of ethics, standards and competencies, Continuing education

Socio-economic Welfare for Nurses: Occupational health and safety, Human resources planning and policy, Remuneration, Career development, International trade in professional services. Our partnerships and strategic alliances with governmental and non-governmental agencies, foundations, regional groups, national associations, and individuals, assist ICN in advancing nursing worldwide.

Affiliates: Council of International Neonatal Nurses (CINN), European Federation of Nurses Associations (EFN), International Federation of Nurse Anaesthetists (IFNA), International Federation of Perioperative Nurses (IFPN), International Skin Care Nursing Group (ISNG), International Society of Nurses in Cancer Care (ISNCC), World Federation of Critical Care Nurses (WFCCN).

ICN STRUCTURE

Council of National Representatives (CNR)

1 voting member of each member association

ICN Board of Directors

15 members elected by the CNR

ICN Personnel

Functions of the Board: The Board serves as the agent of the Council of Representatives (CNR) and establishes and carries out policy consistent with the framework established by CNR. Functions include those designated by the constitution and those common to all Boards of Directors and are related to setting and monitoring of policy. The implementation of policy and general management of ICN are the responsibility of the Chief Executive Officer and ICN staff. Members of the ICN Board of Directors are elected to represent nurses and nursing worldwide. They are not the representative of any country or region.

State Nursing Council

Functions

- Regulation of training program of the diploma, Graduate and Post Graduate Courses.
- Supervision of the practice of the profession by its Member.
- Granting recognition to the training institutions and periodical Inspection there on, as the Council is governing authority of physical and clinical facilities in almost all the nursing courses conducted in the institution.
- Proscribing syllabus and curriculum for various nursing courses and conducting qualifying examination there for.
- Registration and granting certificate to qualified persons to practice their profession and to watch and take action against practice of profession by quacks and check mal-practice as well and to take action.

State Nursing Councils in India

- Andhra Pradesh Nurses, Midwives, A.N.M. and Health Visitor Council (Council Act published for general information Gazette dt: 28-1-1965).
- Assam Nurses Midwives and Health Visitor Council
- Bihar Nurses Registration Council.
- Chattisgarh Nursing Council
- Delhi Nursing Council.
- Directorate of Health Services, Meghalaya Nursing Council.
- Gujarat Nursing Council
- Haryana Nurses Registration Council.
- Himachal Pradesh Nurses Registration Council
- Jharkhand Nurses Registration Council.
- Karnataka Nursing Council
- Kerala Nurses and Midwives Council.
- Mahakoshal Nurses Registration Council (MP).
- Maharashtra Nursing Council.
- Mizoram Nursing Council.

- Orissa Nurses and Midwives Council.
- Punjab Nursing Council
- Rajasthan Nursing Council
- State Medical Faculty and Uttaranchal Nurses Midwives Council
- Tamil Nadu Nurses and Midwives Council
- Tripura Nursing Council.
- Uttar Pradesh Nurses and Midwives Council.
- West Bengal Nursing Council.

1. Karnataka State Nursing Council

It was constituted in the year 1971 under the authority of Karnataka Nurses, Midwives and Health Visitors Act of 1961. The First council was nominated by Government with different members representing various constituencies under section 3 of the Act, all together consisting of 22 members. The Council is an Autonomous Statutory Registration body for qualified Nurses, Midwives, ANM's and Health Visitors.

Functions

1. Regulation of training program of the Diploma, Graduate and Post Graduate Courses.
2. Supervision of the practice of the profession by its Member.
3. Granting recognition to the training institutions and periodical Inspection there on, as the Council is governing authority of physical and clinical facilities in almost all the nursing courses conducted in the institution.
4. Prescribing syllabus and curriculum for various nursing courses and conducting qualifying examination there for.
5. Registration and granting certificate to qualified persons to practice their profession and to watch and take action against practice of profession by quacks and check mal-practice as well and to take action.

The Council is as per the Act headed by President and Vice-President of the Council and both are duly elected by the members of the council under section 5 of the Act.

The Council meets under the Chairmanship of and take decision on the matters covered by its statutory functions. The expenditure of the Council will be met with the fees charged for Registration and Renewal.

2. Kerala State Nursing Council—The Nurses and Midwives Act, 1953 - Act X of 1953

It is expedient to provide for the registration and training of 1 (nurses, midwives, health visitors and auxiliary nurse-midwives) in the State of Kerala. Registration of Nurses, Midwifes, ANMs, HV, Dais.

"Institution" means any association which maintains or controls an establishment for training nurses or midwives or both and which is recognized by the Council.

Establishment, incorporation and constitution of the Council – The Government shall, by notification in the Gazette, establish a Council to be called the Kerala Nurses and Midwives Council for the purpose of carrying out the provisions of this Act.

The Council shall consist of the following members, namely:
a. The Director of Health Services, the Professor of Gynecology, Medical College, Trivandrum, the Professor of Gynecology, Medical College, Kozhikode, the Professor of Gynecology, Medical College, Kottayam, the Assistant Director of Health Services (maternity and Child Health), the Superintendent, Women and Children's Hospital, Trivandrum and the Superintendent Women and Children's Hospital, Kozhikode, to be ex-officio members.
b. One member elected by the members of the Medical Council from among themselves.
c. Three registered nurses nominated by the Government, two of whom shall be Superintendents of nursing schools and the third shall be the Matron - Superintendent of a Major Hospital.
d. Six members elected by the registered nurses from among the nurses registered in Part A of the register of nurses, of whom at least one shall be a member of the Trained Nurses Association of India registered in the State of Kerala, one a member, of the Kerala Government Nurses Association and one a nurse working in a private hospital in the State.

e. Three members elected by the registered midwives of whom one shall be from among the midwives registered in Part A of the register of the midwives, and two from among the auxiliary nurse-midwives registered under this Act

f. One member elected by the registered health visitors from among the health visitors registered in the register of health – visitors

    President and Vice-President – (1) The Government shall nominate one of the members of the Council to be its President. (2) The Council shall elect one of its members other than the President to be its Vice – President.

Registrar—The Government shall after consulting the Council appoint a Registrar who shall be the Secretary to the Council. The duty of the Registrar to keep separate registers for nurses, midwives, auxiliary nurse midwives and health visitors. The registers shall be in such form and shall contain particulars as may be prescribed by rules. Each register shall be divided into two parts A and B, Part A containing the names of those [nurses, midwives, auxiliary nurse-midwives or health visitors] who are eligible for registration under clause (i) of sub-section (1) of section 20 and Part B containing the names of those (nurses, midwives, auxiliary nurse midwives or health visitors) who are eligible for registration under clause (i) of sub-section (1) of section 20.

Registration—every person who has undergone specific course of training and passed examination as may be prescribed by rules for the purpose of conferring a right of registration as a (nurse, midwife, auxiliary nurse-midwife or health visitor) under this Act, every person who, within the period of one year or such other longer period as may be fixed by the Government, from the date of commencement of the Nurses and Midwives (Amendment) Act, 1964 proves that he had been in regular practice as a nurse or midwife, for a period of not less than three years preceding the first day of April, 1964, shall be eligible for registration under this Act; renewal has to be made 3 year once.

    Admission to register of persons registered in any State in India – on payment of such fees as may be prescribed by rules, any person who proves to the satisfaction of the Council that he has been registered as nurse, midwife, auxiliary nurse-midwife or health visitor in any other State in India may be registered as a nurse, midwife, auxiliary nurse-midwife or health visitor Refusal of registration and removal and re-entry – (1) Subject to such conditions as may be prescribed by rules, the Council may, after giving an opportunity to the person concerned to appear and to be heard, and after holding an inquiry in the manner prescribed by rules refuse to enter in the register the name of any person or may order the removal of the name of any person from the register. (2) The order passed under sub-section (1) shall be in writing and shall be served on the person concerned in the manner prescribed by rules

Annual list of nurses and midwives—(1) The Registrar shall in every year on or before the date to be fixed by the Council cause to be published in the Gazette a full or supplementary list of names of all (nurses, midwives, auxiliary nurse-midwives, health visitors and dhais) registered under this Act.

    Penalty for dishonest use of certificates—any person who—(a) dishonestly makes use of any certificate of registration issued under this Act to him or to any other person; (b) Procures or attempts to procure registration under this Act by making or producing or causing to be made or produced any false or fraudulent declaration, certificate or representation, whether in writing or otherwise Willfully make or causes to be made any false representation in any matter relating to the register of certificates issued under this Act, shall be punishable with fine which may extend to two hundred and fifty rupees.

    Nurses or midwives not registered under this Act not to practice—(1) No person other than a (nurse, midwife, auxiliary nurse-midwife, health visitor or dhai) registered under this Act shall practice or hold himself out either directly or by implication as a practicing (nurse, midwife, auxiliary nurse-midwife, health visitor or dhai).

    Penalty or unlawful assumption of title of registered (nurse, midwife, auxiliary nurse midwife, health visitor or dhai).

    Penalty for instrumental manipulation by 1(nurse, midwife, auxiliary nurse-midwife, health visitor or dhai).

    Power of Council to make regulations—the conduct of any examinations which may be prescribed by rules as a condition of admission to the register and any matters ancillary to or connected with such examinations including the course of training which the candidates appearing for the examinations shall undergo; the approval of any institution for the purpose of such training and the granting of diplomas to candidates passing the examinations.

3. Tamil Nadu Nursing Council

It is the earliest Nursing Council in South–East Asia. Nursing Training and practice was passed by the legislature on 7th May, 1926. It was known earlier as Madras Nurses and Midwives act, 1926. It was amended as per Nurses and Midwives act VII of 1934, and act XXVI of 1960, till now they are following the same. The Council is an autonomous statutory registration body for registering qualified Nurses, Midwives, ANMs, MPHWs, HV as per the provisions of the act.

Philosophy—Quality Assurance

A well planned and systematic pattern of all actions stipulated in the statues of Tamil Nadu Nurses and Midwives Council.

Purposes

To excelling Nursing education in Tamil Nadu.

To produce adequate competent nurses to practice within the frame work of legal and ethical component.

Implementing the syllabus and regulation framed by Indian Nursing Council, New Delhi, so as to impart the uniform standard of nursing education throughout India.

Recognizing the institution approved by the State Government which are fulfilling the guidelines and norms/minimum requirements of INC.

Registering the qualification of the candidates passed out from institution within the State obtained by the recognized examining bodies. (i.e. University - for Collegiate program, Boards - Diploma program).

Tamil Nadu Nurses and Midwives Council Section 11(2)(c) of Tamilnadu Nurses and Midwives Act III of 1926 a) Recognition rule 36,37,38 b) Registration rule 32.

Registration

Within state, from other states and foreign verification.

Recognition

Regulation of training programs and granting recognition to the nursing institutions in Tamil Nadu, Puducherry and Andaman and Nicobar Islands.

All the candidates who have possessed recognized nursing qualification obtained from the recognized examining bodies, i.e. University/Boards should register their qualification under this Council as per the Act to become a registered Nurse/Midwife/Auxilary Nurse Midwife/Health Visitor. So as to practice their profession legal and safe manner by obtaining Registration Number by this Council.

Revoking

Monitoring the professional ethics.

Regulation and surveillance of professional conduct and take action against practice of their professional by quacks and check malpractice.

Challenges ahead to improve the quality in practice.

Nursing Home Act.

Re-Registration Act.

Banning of unauthorised institutions.

Banning of unauthorised courses.

Current Involvement

Nurses Census

Web site – Profile of Nursing Institutions recognised by INC

To Maintain Uniform Standards in Nursing Education in Tamil Nadu, e.g. Preparing the records.

4. Delhi Nursing Council, New Delhi

The Delhi Nursing Council was established under the Delhi Nursing Council Act, 1997 (Delhi Act No.3 of 1999) received the assent of the President in March 1999. The act was published in Delhi Gazette in March 2001.

Purposes

- Regulation of registration and renewal and training of Nursing Personnel (Nurses, Midwives, auxiliary nurse midwives, female health workers, female health assistants, Supervisors) and matters connected with

Objectives

- To regulate and control registration of Nursing Personnel
- To exercise powers of licensing and supervision
- To give recognition to training institutions
- To grant affiliation and withdraw recognition under the provision of act (Section 24&25)
- To conduct examination (Section 22)
- To look into the grievances of persons on filling of appeals(Section 23)
- To deal with offences and to enforce penalties for dishonest use of certificates (Section 27)
- Provides verification of registration antecedents to nursing personnel registered

5. Maharashtra Nursing Council, Mumbai

The council shall be a body corporate and governed by:

a)	Maharashtra Nurses Act. 1966 (modified upto 30/11/1996)
b)	Maharashtra Nursing Council Rules, 1971 (modified upto 01/06/1993)
c)	Maharashtra Nursing Council By-Laws, 1973 (modified upto 31/05/1993) amended time to time.

Constitution of the Council

Under the Maharashtra Nurse Act 1966 chap. II sect. 3(3), the Council comprises:

	Ex-officio Members
1.	The Director of Health Services
2.	The Director of Medical Education and Research
3.	The Superintendent of Nursing Services, Government of Maharashtra
4.	The Assistant Director of Health Services (Nursing)
5.	The Director of Higher Education or his nominee not below the rank of Deputy Director
6.	The Superintendent of Nursing Services of the Municipal Corporation of greater Bombay.
	Elected Members
1.	Five Registered Nurses from each of five regions.
2.	One head of Private and Municipal affiliated institution.
3.	Five Matrons of affiliated institutions.
4.	Five Sister Tutors and Clinical Instructors of the affiliated institutions, from each of five regions.
5.	One Member, from the Maharashtra Medical Council.
6.	One Member from IMA
7.	One Professor and lecturer of the Recognised Colleges of Nursing.
8.	One head (Principals) or Recognised Colleges of Nursing
9.	One Member from Trained Nurses Association of India (Maharashtra state branch)
	Nominated Members
Four Members, to be nominated by the State Government out of whom one shall be public Health Nurse and three shall be, from amongst the Medical Practitioners or Teachers or in Nursing Colleges.	

Functions

1. To maintain the Registration of nurses and their renewals.
2. To hear and decide appeals from any decision of the Registrar.
3. To prescribe Code of Ethics for regulating the professional conduct of Nurses.
4. To reprimand a registered or an enlisted nurse or to suspend or to remove him/her from the register or the list, as the case may be or to take such other disciplinary action against her/him as may, in the opinion of the council, necessary or expedient.
5. To held examinations and to make all necessary arrangements for conducting such examinations.
6. To prescribe the courses of training leading to the examinations held by the council, and to charge fees for such examinations.
7. To prepare publish and prescribe textbooks and to publish statements of prescribed courses of study.
8. To grant certificates and diplomas and marks of honour.
9. To award stipends, scholarships, medals, prizes and other rewards.
10. To recognise institution for the purpose of training and giving instruction for the courses leading to the examination held by the council or to cancel such recognition.
11. To regulate the conditions under which institutions for the nursing of the sick, maternity or child welfare may be affiliated to the council.
12. To provide for the inspection of recognised and affiliated institutions and to require such institutions to furnish such information as may be necessary.
13. Subject to the approval of the state government, to receive donations and to determine the conditions of acceptance of donations
14. To exercise power and perform other duties and functions as are laid down this Act or as may be prescribed.

Rajasthan Nursing Council, Jaipur

Rajasthan Nursing Council is an autonomous statutory registration body for registering qualified Nurses, Midwives, Auxiliary-Nurse-Midwives/Health workers as per the provisions of the Act.

Functions

1. Recognition of nursing institution as per the Act.
2. Registration of qualified nursing professionals and maintenance of state Registers.
3. Development of inter linkages and reciprocities with corresponding Councils in other States of India.
4. Regulation and surveillance of professional conduct and take action against practice of their professional by quacks and check malpractice.

Trained Nurse's Association of India

The Association had its beginning in the Association of Nursing Superintendents which was founded in 1905, at Lucknow. At the Annual Conference held in Bombay in 1908, a decision was taken to establish Trained Nurse's Association. The Association was inaugurated in 1909. In 1922, the Association of Nursing Superintendents and Trained Nurse's Association were amalgamated and called "The Trained Nurses' Association of India (TNAI)". The Association has established within its jurisdiction the following organizations: Health Visitors' League (1922), Midwives and Auxiliary Nurse-Midwives Association (1925), Student Nurses Association (1929-30). In 1974 the TNAI became a member of the Commonwealth Nurses Federation (CNF). The organization was composed of nine European Nurses holding administrative posts in hospitals. The movement gathered momentum and soon nurses, other than nursing superintendents, were seeking to share in:

- Upholding in every way the dignity and honor of the nursing profession
- Promoting a sense of esprit de corps among all nurses
- Enabling members to take counsel together on matters relating to their profession
- The Association has established within its jurisdiction the following organizations:
  - Health Visitors League (1922)
  - Midwives and Auxiliary Nurse-Midwives Association (1925)
  - Student Nurses Association (1929-30).

In 1912 the TNAI got affiliated with the International Council of Nurses (ICN). The TNAI as a national body can give a broad support to local or state organizations of Nurses.

The Trained Nurses Association of India is the national body of practitioners of Nursing at various levels. The main idea behind the establishment of the Association was to uphold in every way the dignity and honour of the Nursing profession and to promote team spirit, apart from enabling the members to represent their grievances and express their point of view to concerned quarters in events of problematic situations. While the stress is on orientating the members to the real needs of the profession, the regular activities of the Association are organised in such a way that those associated with them have a sense of participation in all the programs of direct professional relevance along with treating the Association as a major source of inspiration and provider of title delights of life occasionally. While members at some of the Branches and Units are more active in their participation in the TNAI activities than those at others, the Association has undoubtedly come to be recognised as a major link between the vast number of Nurses in various parts of the country, and even some abroad.

Rapport with Government of India

1. (i) Government Recognition as Service Association: The Association is considered to be on a par with other service organisations. A copy of the letter from the Ministry of Health, Government of India to all the State Governments communicating recognition of the TNAI as a Service Association on par with other Associations is given.

    (ii) Issue of Railway Concessions: In 1991 Railways granted concession to TNAI members and the Association was authorised to issue certificates to members for getting concession 25 per cent and it is available in second class only. This in a way is serving as a financial relief to many Nurses. Students are given 50 per cent concession for educational trips.

2. Affiliation with Government Committees and Councils:

    The Government of India has all along appreciated the importance of TNAI as the National Association of Nurses and following the formal recognition in 1950, it was involved in all governmental endeavours in the field of Nursing and given the opportunity to put across its point of view on all matters of consequence. This was largely due to the great interest of Rajkumari Amrit Kaur in nursing, the first Minister for Health in independent India.

    The committee and investigative bodies launched by the Central Council of Health to study problems and prospects of the profession consult the Association on various matters and give weightage to its viewpoint. The contribution of TNAI to the findings of Bhore Committee and Mudaliar Committee as well as to other similar bodies has been considerable. Its views have been considered as the most authentic for the nursing profession in processing the findings of such official committees.

    TNAI played an important role in the High Power Committee on Nursing and Nursing Profession (Report: 1987). The Central Council of Health (CCH) has also been drawing on TNAI's experience for its recommendations on various aspects of the profession. It can derive ample satisfaction from its role in setting of norms and professional standards in our field of activity in cooperation with the CCH.

    The Indian Nursing Council (INC) which was actually mooted by the TNAI has been doing work in the field of Nursing Education and establishment of professional norms at different levels. The TNAI is associated in most of its activities and its links with the INC have given rise to a number of endeavors for the promotion of Nursing education and other aspects of the profession.

3. Affiliation with Other Organizations:

    It is an associate member of many other associations and societies doing welfare activities in their own fields. These societies are: Indian Red Cross Society, Indian Public Health Association, Association for Social Health, Indian Hospital Association, Federation of Delhi hospital Welfare Societies, Tuberculosis Association of India, Indian Leprosy Association and National Institute of Public Cooperation and Child Development. These associations and institutions too involve themselves in the activities of TNAI on a reciprocal basis.

    The TNAI takes part in the activities of important social organisations devoted to the welfare of women, especially National Council of Women in India, National Federation of Indian Women and All-India Women's

Conference. The Association is invited to all important deliberations of such bodies and effort is made by the TNAI representatives to keep these organisations informed of the problems of practising nurses.

In 1936 Nurses' Auxiliary of the Christian Medican Association (CMA), from 1954 Christian Nurses' League (CNL) was affiliated to TNAI affiliated to Catholic Nurse's Guild of India.

4. Affiliation with International Council of Nurses (ICN):

A Landmark was TNAI's affiliation with International Council of Nurses (ICN) in 1912. Both ANSI and TNAI united for this purpose. TNAI was among the first eight National Nurses' Associations (NNAs) in 1930. The 'Nursing Abroad' program of ICN assisted Indian Nurses in their work and study abroad. In recent years the ICN sponsored a Socio-Economic Welfare Project (1989-91) through which about 300 Nurses from different parts of the country received Training in Leadership Development and Management Skills.

Around 1974 the TNAI became a member of the Commonwealth Nurses Federation (CNF). The association with CNF has been fruitful in many ways.

Affiliation with Scholarship Funds

One of the ways in which the TNAI carries out its educational objectives and is the Trustee for various scholarships.

Kapadia Memorial Scholarship Fund: This fund was created in 1946 by the School of Nursing Administration

Margaret Jehan Scholarship Fund: To provide a scholarship for nine months every year to enable a nurse, preferably from Hospital for Women and Children in India, to take the Sister Tutor's Course at the Delhi Postgraduate School of Nursing.

Ajmer Minto Sister's Scholarship Fund: Scholarship of Rs. 900 per year is awarded to a candidate for four years for doing B.Sc. (Hons.) Degree Course in Nursing in the College of Nursing, New Delhi. The selection of the candidate is made by the College of Nursing and recommended to TNAI for award of the scholarship.

Lady Linlithgow Scholarship Fund: This scholarship is given for the training of nurses for administrative and teaching posts in hospitals and schools of nursing in India.

Rajkumari Amrit Kaur and Miss Adranvala Scholarship Fund: To establish a scholarship for Public Health Nursing, but now a grant out of the income from interest of this fund is to be awarded to a nurse for research, in any aspect of nursing.

Tata Memorial Scholarship Fund: A scholarship has to be awarded to a nurse for post-basic or postgraduate studies in College of Nursing, New Delhi.

Lady Minto Nursing Scholarship Fund: This fund was created from India's share of the funds of the Lady Minto Nursing Association.

Military Nursing Service Scholarship Fund: For awarding scholarship for higher studies in Nursing to any nurse of the Military Nursing Service.

Florence Nightingale Fund for Research in Nursing: This fund was entrusted some time in 1942-43, to the Trained Nurses Association of India by the Indian Red Cross Society. In the early years the income was utilised for scholarships for study in U.K, but in view of the high costs for the courses to be undertaken in U.K, it was decided to use the income for research in Nursing.

Rules for Scholarship in India

a. Courses of Study: Teaching and Administration, B.Sc. (N) Post-Basic and M.N. degree programs, Public Health Nursing or any other post-certificate course given in an institution recognised by the Indian Nursing Council.

b. General education: The candidate should meet the requirements of the institutional, but ordinarily, it would be 10+2 or an equivalent examination.

c. Professional education: Registration as a General nurse and Midwife. In case of men nurses, evidence of having training in a special subject instead of midwifery.

d. Professional experience: A minimum of two years bedside nursing experience in an institution for Ward Administration course; three years experience for a Tutor's course, and five years for a course in Nursing Administration. In all cases the requirements of the institution should be met.

e. Applications: Applications will be invited through The Nursing Journal of India in December/January every year.

f. Selection: Selection will be made by the Committee appointed for this purpose as per the information obtained from the application form and confidential reports from head of the institution.
g. Scholarship: The student will receive the scholarship through the head of the institution to which she/he is admitted for study.
h. Agreement: An undertaking to continue in service for two years within three months of completion of the course or to refund the amount paid to her/him in case of default will have to be executed by the student on the prescribed form.
i. General: The candidate should be a member of the TNAI for at least three years, preferably a Life-Member. The candidate will have to seek admission directly in the institution she/he proposes to join and a!so make her/his own arrangement for getting leave from the institution in which she/he is employed.

The information of the award will be communicated to the candidate by the Secretary of the Scholarship Committee to whom the Selection Committee will give report. The Secretary of the Scholarship Committee will request the Hony. Treasurer, TNAI, to make payment to the institution after the student has joined it.

The Secretary, Scholarship Committee, will submit an annual statement on whether the Students who had secured the scholarship continue to hold posts in institutions for the period required in the agreement. A report on their work will also be called or from the institution in which they are employed.

Union Activities

To move into the trend of Union activities which seems to be necessary to better conditions for Nurses and at the same time, to maintain the dignity and standard of the Nursing profession it suggests the following policies:
a. TNAI members should approach Union/State Governments and other employing agencies to form Grievances Committees, which should include representatives of various cadres of Nurses and employees in each hospital, block or district. These Committees should solve all local problems, personal or professional, wherever possible.
b. A State level committee, including a TNAI representative, should be formed to act as arbitrator in cases referred to by the local Grievances Committee.
c. TNAI members should encourage and assist the organization and work of State Government Nurses Service Associations which will be recognized as negotiating bodies by the employers. A Nurse must be an active member of both TNAI and State Government Nurses Service Association. As TNAI members, Nurses may obtain information, assistance, advice and moral support from other States and the national TNAI for the Government Nurses Association.
d. This is an essential step to prevent Nurses from joining other unions.
e. Where the State Government Nurses organisations already exist, the TNAI should initiate dialogue with them, assure them of cooperation and assistance whenever their objectives are in line with those of the TNAI and create opportunities for joint activities and action through local and State Executive Committees.
f. Where any organisation is frankly anti-TNAI every effort should be made to clarify the reasons and misunderstandings which exist. If this fails and any TNAI member, who is an officer of the other organization and yet is obviously working against the TNAI, steps should be taken to suspend the member from the TNAI by the State Executive with the approval of the national TNAI Council.
g. The State Government Nurses Association and State Branch, TNAI, should agree that as a last resort where the issue involves the welfare of the members of the profession as a whole or the improvement of Nursing services to the community.

Conditions under which a strike by Nurses may be approved or even carried out by TNAI Branches or local groups:
• Where grievances exist, they should be thoroughly investigated by the Government Nurses Association and reported to the local or State TNAI Executive.
• The State Branch Executive, TNAI, should also know all facts regarding the situation and be satisfied that justice requires some action.
• All possible approaches through legal efforts should be made to the authorities for correction of the situation.

- If no action is taken by the authorities despite all efforts, the situation should be put before the members of the Government Nurses Association for vote regarding strike.
- At least two months warning should be given before the date set for the strike.
- During the two months period the following actions should be carried out:
  a. Efforts to persuade the authorities should continue
  b. The public should be informed through the Press
  c. About the grievances of the Nurses stressing the ultimate effect on the care of patients and the public. The efforts already made, Assuring the public that in the event of the strike arrangement will be made to provide Nursing care for all seriously ill patients and emergency cases, asking for support from the press and public, plans should be made by the Government Nurses Associations and TNAI for the methods to be used in carrying out the strike, informing all members on what their action and behaviour should be as professional people. The plan for providing emergency Nursing care should be carefully made and published.
- It must be clearly understood that the TNAI and its members will not support any strike controlled or voted by any union or organisation which includes employees other than Nurses. It must be planned, voted and carried out with the above stipulations in a dignified manner and with the assurance that the public understands and will support the Nurse's demands and that the Nurses will make every effort to prevent harm to patients.

Revision of TNAI Membership Fee

S. No.	Category	From 1.04.2009 (Rs.)
1.	Trained Nurses	3000
2.	Retired Nurses(Provide Certificate)	1100
3.	Religious Sisters (drawing no salary)	1000
4.	HV/ANM/MPHW	1650
5.	SNA to TNAI (for student)	2000

Annual Membership Fee (with NJI)

1.	Trained Nurses(India)	1100 (Rs.)
2.	Trained Nurses(Foreign)	165 (Rs.)
3.	LHV/ANM/MPHW	50 (Rs.)
4.	Journal for Student Nurses	150 (Rs.)
5.	SNA Unit Subscription per student	100 (Rs.)

Life Membership Fee (Foreign)

1.	Trained Nurses	$275 (USD)
2.	Add Postal Charges(Subject to change)	$50 (USD)
3	[Airmail:1 year; Surface Mail:3 years]	$50 (USD)

NJI for non-members

1.	India (Inclusive of postage)	1100
2.	Foreign (Inclusive of postage)	$165 (USD)

Indian Society Of Psychiatric Nurses (ISPN)

ISPN started in 1991 with a motive of enhancing the advanced knowledge and skills in the field of Mental Health Psychiatric Nursing.

To provide platform for discussion and deliberation on evidence based practice.

To create awareness and to translate the research findings in MH nursing practice.

ISPN was registered under the co-operative society act in 1991 at Bangeluru, Under the guidance of Dr. K. Reddemma. the life membership fee is increased to Rs. 760 and the associated life membership fee for Rs. 510.

Nursing Research Society of India

The Nursing Research Society of India was established in May, 1986 to promote research within and around nursing environment. It is registered under the societies Act XXI of 1960 with Registrar of Societies Delhi. Administration (Certificate No. S/18421 dated 2nd December, 1987).

Aims and Objectives

1. Support the development of Nursing Research activities in the universities and Nursing health care institutions to provide nursing care standards.
2. Provide a platform to Nurse Scientists to exchange views on Nursing Research.
3. Promote and sponsor Scientific meets, Seminars and Conferences to advance Nursing Research.
4. Create Public interest in the contribution of nursing in promotive, preventive and restorative activities, contributing to health and family welfare.
5. Establish a Nursing Research Journal of India and bring out other documents pertaining to innovations in Nursing.

Records and Reports Maintained in Nursing Educational Institutions

Administrative Records

- Administrative Manual specifying Educational Policies, Organizational Policies, Educational Objectives, Job Responsibilities, Vision and mission of organization
- Affiliation record of National council (INC) and State Nursing Council, Government order and proceedings (G.O), Universities or Board
- Personal files/Curriculum Vitae of teaching staff along with Photostat copies of certificates along with registration certificates and Non teaching staff Curriculum Vitae
- In private organizations Trust registration, Governing Council members details
- Admission Register specifying number of admissions
- Blueprint of College building/School, Clinical Areas – Hospital and community, Land document
- Organization, structure (Line of Authority)
- Financial Aid Records (Optional/if any) or Grant in Aid record
- Transportation facilities – Bus/Van registration, Driving License
- Staff attendance and leave register
- Audit Report for 3 years
- Budget – Income and Expenditure of three years, Salary register, Account Register along with cheque book, Petti cash details
- Student welfare record
- Registers related to Staff Developmental activities, Faculty Development Programs
- Records of educational programs organized for teaching faculty and students both in the institution as well as outside
- Staff assessment – Confidential Reports of all the staff
- Clinical areas Particulars – Bed strength, Occupancy (In Patient), OPDs, Department Staff list
- Transcripts
- Stock Registers, Furniture register

Academic Records

- Course syllabus, Course out line, Course content Record
- Time tables, Weekly Schedules, Clinical rotations
- Cumulative record
- Minutes of Committees reports and Faculty Meetings
- Students attendance (Theory and clinical; Hostel)
- Leave register
- Disciplinary proceedings
- Record of affiliation (Clinical - Hospital and Community facilities)

- Record of clinical visits, field experiences, Midwifery Record book
- Student hand book
- Master Rotation plan and Clinical Rotation plan for each year and entire course
- Study Guides for all Departments
- Recreation Reports
- Records of extracurricular activities of students both in the school as well as out side.

Committees Record

- Curriculum committee
- Evaluation and quality improvement
- Simulation and technology
- Student awards and scholarship
- Recognition and events
- Advisory committee
- Research Committee
- Student academic progress
- Ethical committee
- Staff development/Faculty Development committee
- NCC, NSS Committee
- Hostel and Mess Committee
- Health Committee
- Student Welfare Body
- Disciplinary/Anti Ragging Committee
- Library Committee
- Recreation Committee
- CNE cell.

Examination Records

- Marks lists issued by University/Board
- Evaluation forms
- Invigilators and examiners orders from Universities or Board
- Clinical assessment
- Internal Assessment register
- The record for academic performance
- Annual reports (Records of the Achievements of the institution prepared annually)
- Performance Appraisal record.

Extracurricular Tecords

- Athletic Council Records
- Sports and cultural records.

S.N.A

- Meetings Reports
- Program record
- Treasures record
- Presidents record
- Minutes of the S.N.A meeting
- Student Alumni
- Committees record.

Library

- Books and Journals Inventory
- Borrowers record/Issue register

- Purchasing of books
- Stock Register
- Borrowers fine
- Furniture Record.

Laboratory and Audio-visual Aids Registers
- Resources
- Models and specimen
- Records for the individual lab
  - Fundamentals of Nursing, Medical Surgical Nursing, Pediatric Nursing, OBG Laboratory and Nutrition
- Equipment record
- Purchasing record
- Loss and damages
- Audiovisual Aids.

Student health record
- Individual student health record

Hostel Records
- Rules and regulations
- In and Out records
- Visitors record
- Roll call
- Mess record
- Maintenance record/Stock register
- Furniture Record
- Staff Attendance record
- Furniture record
- Mineral Water plant.

LIBRARY FACILITIES IN NURSING EDUCATIONAL INSTITUTIONS

Library has to be located in the centre of the Institution with adequate Library staff

Library Staff
- The Chief Librarian—has to possess Post Graduation in Master of Library and Information Sciences
- One Assistant librarians (The number will be depends upon Strength of the Staff and students)
- Four Library assistants
- Attendants (The number will be depend upon Strength of the Staff and students)

Facilities
- Internet with adequate number of computers accessible for both staff and students
- Adequate seating, Ventilation, Lighting facilities., Conducive environment for reading and gathering the information
- Separate sections like Reading section separate for staff and students, Reference section, Journal section and General section where books will be arranged subject wise, the books in all subjects procured as specified by the university or Board syllabus, and other resource books
- Drinking Water facility (Mineral Water Plant)
- Rest rooms (Bathrooms and Toilets separate for ladies and gents)

Functions of Librarian
Librarians manage information and resources and help people to locate and utilize information. Most librarians work in either user services, technical services or administrative services.

General Duties

Librarians keep current on resources and literature and select publications for the library's collection. They require a knowledgeable command of numerous information sources to select material appropriate to a library's needs. A Librarian categorizes, prepares and catalogues these materials. Librarians also recommend material and help individuals to find the information that individual needs. They analyze and organize collections by subject. They educate individuals on how to use the library systems to find the information they need. Librarians may also provide special programming or classes and also they participate in grant writing and fundraising. Librarians may specialize in:

User Services: Librarians help the individuals to find and use library materials and resources.

Technical Services: Librarians work behind the scenes, obtaining and classifying resources for the library. Some might work with or develop computer information storage and retrieval systems.

Administration Services: Librarians in administrative services oversee the management of the library and the staff.

The chief Librarian will classify the books subject wise, catalogue system will be maintained, which will give authentic information like the searching options like position of books in library, number of available copies/ List has to be made—The number of books along with title and author, books has to be bounded periodically, issue register has to be maintained by the librarian.

Records and Registers maintained in Library

- Stock register, i.e. Accession Register –the available books in the Library and their detailed information will be available
- Books Issue register – when the students and staff taking the books from library they have to enter in Books Issue Register or Borrowers Register
- Journals Register—detailed information of available Journals will be maintained in register
- New Borrowers Membership Register – students who are taking new admission/appointment in the college has to take the library membership and to utilize the library facilities
- Visitors Register – When reader from out side wants to utilize library resource has to enter name and in and out time in the visitors register
- Stock register of furniture's and equipments details – Its gives the details of Library furniture & equipments.
- Staff Attendance and Leave Register
- Personal files (Curriculum vitae along with Photo copies of certificates)
- List of books and journals register
- Journals will be ordered through generally on jrnls@sbc.co.in, kmrajiv@totalit.co.in, rhino1@vsnl.com, santoshmuddi@yahoo.com

Stock verification: Yearly once stock verification has to be done by librarian one Teaching staff will assist the librarian for stock verification., usually it will be carried out in the academic year end.

Principal or the Administrator has to subscribe National and International journals in all related fields, so that the students will have the access to refer and gather the information from books, journals, internet. The different university/board question papers also has to be kept as per subject and year wise from the current to previous.

Library services will be available for at least 12 hours in a day to enable the staff and students utilize the library.

Borrowing Facility: This service is being provided for the benefit of user community. The members of the library can borrow books for a period of 15 days. Two borrower's tickets will be issued to students and can borrow two books at a time. Ten tickets will be issued to the Faculty and Research Scholars to borrow the books from the library and return the same after period of 15 days. The users are requested to return the borrowed books to the library on or before the due date to avoid the penalty of Over Due Charges. Students are requested to obtain the NO DUE CERTIFICATE from the library at the end of the Academic Year. The administrator of college or school will not issue hall ticket before examination unless the student submits no due certificate to the office, in order to maintain the books in library properly and to avoid missing of the books. Journals will not be issued to students, they have to sit and gather the information in sitting referral or reading section.

Reference Service: The Library is extending reference and referral services to the users of the library. Most of the reference oriented Text books and General books have been kept in reference and active stock area for reference only by the users of the library. Users are going to be informed about the availability of their required books in other libraries to the librarian.

Orientation Program: The Librarian has to organize, the Library Orientation Program to create an awareness among the fresh students of the institution about the proper utilization of the library and its resources and services; to give first hand information about the library and to provide them a closer acquaintance and more familiarity about the various aspects of the library system. This program is an educative and informative and also bridges the gap between the library staff and user clients. This Program briefs about the physical arrangement and organization of the collection of the University Library, its functions and services both traditional and Information Technology related services like CD-ROM, Fax, Internet and E-Journals Consortium of UGC Infonet. Briefing will be followed by demonstration of Information Technology related services and Tour of the Library (covering all the sections of the library), Rules and Regulation and Do's and Do not's will be briefed to the students. This program enhances the usage of the library to the optimum level.

Books Display Program: The Library is being practiced a unique system of making arrangements of books display program in the library based on important personalities, events, dates and on other rare occasions. the library books on such aspects will be displayed in the library to create awareness among the users about the availability of the various resources.

Inter-Library Loan: The books of one library will be sent to various other libraries on Inter Library Loan as per the request from other institutions. The library also used to get some books on Inter Library Loan basis from other libraries as requested by the users of the institution.

Text Book Loan Facility: The library has to maintain this section for the benefit of students belongs to SC/ST and Other Economically Weaker sections. Five text books will be issued to each student for a period of one academic year in the cognitive subjects. At the end the students has to return the borrowed books and to obtain NO DUE CERTIFICATE from the Library.

CD-ROM Service: Users of the Library especially the Research Scholars can avail this facility. Research Scholars can browse CDs related to their subjects which gives the bibliographical information along with abstracts of journal articles, seminar papers, conference proceedings, book reviews etc. This facility helps them to collect the entire information about the quantum of literature available related to their topic within short span of time.

OPAC Facility: To provide first hand information about the availability and location of the books, journals and other documents of the library, Online Public Access Catalogue facility is being proposed to extend for the benefit of the user community.

Binding Facility: Most of the important reference oriented books and journals will be bounded suitably to enhance the life span and utility of such documents by the user group.

Bibliographic Services: The Library is providing this facility for the benefit of the users by informing about the availability of abstracting and indexing journals and reference oriented documents.

Photostat Copy Facility: The library members can avail the Xerox facility within the library building. The responsibility of providing Xerox facility has been entrusted to a private agency.

Cubicles for Research Scholars: The library has 24 Cubicles/Study rooms which are meant for the benefit of Research Scholars. The each cubicle will be allotted to one Research Scholar. Research Scholars are requested to submit their application for cubicles directly to the concerned Assistant Librarian through the Head of the Department.

Generator: To provide an un-interrupted power supply to the users the Library has acquired 80Kv Generator set. The power connectivity facility has been provided to all the sections of the library.

Participation in Research activities, Publications, Journals and in News Papers

In Under Graduate Program in Nursing, final year students in their curriculum have Nursing Research and Statistics subject with 45 hours Theory and 45 hours Practicals. The course is designed to enable students to develop an understanding of basic concepts of Research and its process and Statistics. It is further structured to conduct/participate in need based Research studies in various settings and utilize the Research findings to provide quality Nursing care. The hours for practical will be utilized for conducting individual/group Research project. Nurse Educator has to motivate the student to select the Research problem in the area of interest of students., and help him/her by suggesting the resources where and how to do review., teach the student to utilize all the steps in Research process, Statistics knowledge will help the students in Analysis chapter, selection of statistical methods in interpreting the research findings which can be communicated through publishing it either in journals are in news Papers. In Post graduate Nursing students will have Research and Statistics, in First Year in some Universities they have to select the need based research or area of interest in the specialized field and submit the synopsis under guidance of Research Guide, in Second year depth of study will be conducted by utilizing the steps of research and using suitable Statistics both Descriptive and Inferential Statistics to discuss and interpret the findings, after Post Graduation, the educator has to motivate the student to communicate research findings to the professional fraternity by publishing in National and International journals, as per guidelines of Journal editors. Educators can also motivate the students to write articles, do the case studies and publish them, and a weapon to increase the awareness of the Public. Interested general Health topics based on the theme, can be prepared and sent to News Papers, and Radio programs to increase the awareness of Public to utilize by adopting Healthy Practices, thus Nurses are essential moderators in Public Health Programs.

Teacher has to motivate the students to become members in Professional Organizations to avail it's benefits through it's functions and strengthen the associations as life members.

BUDGETING

Definitions

- A course of action based upon an estimate of assumed income and expenses.
- A plan of operation where one reviews their income and expenditures, often in the effort to create a strategy in order to achieve some financial goal or goals within a specific period of time.

Aims

- To create a plan of action and balancing between income and expenditure.
- To make necessary adjustments in order to achieve a financial goal.
- To help organizations to keep track or control of their finances.
- To allocate funds to various areas where they are needed and help to keep spending under control.
- It allows a business or organization to predict the financial outcome for a period of time if they undertake a certain project or plan, which can aid in decision making.
- To gauge their financial performance throughout the year and adjust spending to ensure a certain amount of profit can be maintained.
- Budgets are only useful tools as long as they are followed and used to make necessary adjustments.
- For a budget to be a valuable resource, it must be followed as closely as possible.
- The budget is the most important tool of legislative control in the educational institution.

Principles to be followed in the Process of Budgeting

- Planning—A budget is ultimately the plan for the operations of an organization for a period of time. Many decisions are involved and many questions must be answered. Old plans and processes are questioned as well as new plans and processes. Managers decide the most effective ways to perform each task. They ask whether a particular activity should still be performed and, if so, how? Managers ask what resources are available and what additional resources will be needed to achieve organizational goals?
- Preparation of Budget – Budget plan is prepared under the direction and supervision of the administrator or financial officer or Budgeting Committee in the organization, Budget plans has to be prepared and interpreted consistently throughout the organization in the communication of planning process, Budget necessitates a review of the performance of the previous year and an evaluation of its adequacy both in quality and quantity while developing a budget, the provision should be made for its flexibility.

- Requirement—Budget should have a provision, based on sound financial management by focusing on requirement of the organization and council norms or University requirement.
- Objectives and Policies—Budget has to focus on objectives and policies of the organization. It must flow from objectives and give realistic expression to the way of realizing such objectives.
- Resources—Budget should ensure the most effective use of scarce financial and non financial resources
- Delegation for different courses—Budgetary process requires consistent delegation for which fixed duties and responsibilities are required to be allocated to managers at different level for framing and executing budget.
- Fixed Targets—Setting budget target, requires an adequate checks and balance against the adoption of too high or too low estimate. utmost care is a must for fixing targets.
- Control—Once a budget is finalized, it is the plan for the operations of the organization. Managers/ Supervisors/Administrators have authority to spend within the budget and responsibility to achieve revenues specified within the budget. Budgets and actual revenues and expenditures are monitored constantly for variations and to determine whether the organization is on target. If performance does not meet the budget, action can be taken immediately to adjust activities. Without constant monitoring, an organization does not realize it is not on target until it is too late to make adjustments.
- Interdepartmental Coordination—Budget should include coordinating efforts of various departments establishing a frame of reference for managerial decision and providing a criterion for evaluating managerial performance. Different units in the organization need to coordinate the varied tasks they perform to achieve organizational goals.
- Communication—In the budgeting process, Managers/Supervisors/Administrators in every department justify the resources they need to achieve their goals. They explain to their superiors the scope and volume of their activities as well as how their tasks will be performed. The communication between superiors and subordinates helps to affirm their mutual commitment to company goals. In addition, different departments and units must communicate with each other during the budget process to coordinate their plans and efforts
- Activities—Budget requires that program activities should be planned in an advance.
- Publicity—The main stages of budget process includes executive recommendations, legislative consideration, action and budget execution has to be open.
- Clarity—The budget has to be understandable to all team members (Governing body, administrators and Management (Private Institution) and sanctioning Authorities and to all faculty members
- Comprehensiveness—The budget should contain expenditure and revenues on a gross basis reflecting all activities without exception and should show surplus, available for debt retirement or deficit to be met by revenue legislation and borrowing.
- Budget unit—All receipt should recover into one general fund for financing all expenditure.
- Detailed specification—Receipts and appropriation should be expressed in detailed specification; transfer to items should be permitted only in exceptional cases.
- Prior authorization—Budget execution should stay strictly within the legislative authorization and should be checked by an auditing agency reporting to the legislatures.
- Periodicity— Appropriation should be authorized for a definite period of time. An appropriation not used at end of the period should generally lapse or to be reappropriated with the specific amount and purpose should be detailed.
- Accuracy—Budget estimates should be as accurate as possible and there should be no padding of expenditure estimates or providing for hidden reserves by underestimating revenue, all the receipts has to be saved and maintained.
- Appropriate—Budget period must be appropriate to the nature of organization or activities or service and the type of budget.
- Evaluation—One way to evaluate a manager is to compare the budget with actual performance. Did the manager reach the target revenue within the constraints of the targeted expenditures? Of course, other factors, such as publicity and general economic conditions, affect a manager's performance. Whether a manager achieves targeted goals or not is an important part of managerial responsibility.

Classification of Budget—I

- Manpower budget — e.g. wages and other benefits provided for regular and temporary employees by the managing authorities.
- Capital expenditure budget — e.g. purchases of land, building, major equipments of considerable expense and long life, evaluate investments and assets of an organization.
- Operating budget — reviewed in order to decide how to properly allocate funds and determine, typically within the fiscal year, the total profits, e.g. the cost of supplies, minor equipment, repairs and overhead expenses.
- Cash budgeting—deals with the cash-flow: the money going in and out of the business over a period of time.

Classification of Budget—II

- Incremental budget—is based on estimated changes in present operation, plus a percentage increase for inflation, all of which is added to previous year budget, e.g. Sanctioning of Increments for the employees by the managing authority.
- Open ended budget—is a financial plan in which each operating manager presents a single cost estimate for what is considered optimal activity level for each program in the unit, without indicating how the budget should be scaled down if less funding is available, e.g. Sanctioning of specified amount for each college by the managing authority in the beginning of academic year, without specifying how it has to be scaled down further for which programs has to be used. It is the discretion of administrator how it has to be utilized, but she/he is accountable to present the statement to the authorities.
- Fixed ceiling budget—is a financial plan in which the uppermost spending limit is set by the top executives, before the unit and divisional managers develop budget proposals for their areas of responsibility, e.g. For organizing work shop, the management of Nursing Educational Institution will sanction fixed amount and various committee heads has to give detailed proposal of their respective committee.
- Flexible budget—consists of several financial plans, each for a different level of program activity. it is based on the fact, that operating conditions rarely conform to expectations, e.g. Management will release a specified budget for an academic year's expenses, it is the administrators' discretion on where and how it has to be utilized qualitatively, like in the same educational institution all Diploma, B.Sc and M.Sc. (N) Programs will be organized, Principal can decide based on the felt needs and demanding needs of the respective programs.
- Rollover budget—is one that forecasts program, revenues and expenses for a period greater than a year, to accommodate program that are larger than annual budget cycle, e.g. Sanctioning of sponsoring students for improvement of their professional education and which in turn is helpful for the organization as per their agreement they may work further.
- Performance budget—is based on functions, which allocate functions, not division, e.g. Provision of direct nursing care, in service education, quality improvement, nursing research and Continuing Nursing Educational programs etc.
- Program budget—is one where costs are computed for a total program, i.e. group total costs for each service program, e.g. MCH, FP, UIP etc.
- Zero base budget—requires the nurse manager to examine, justify each cost of every program both old and new, in every annual budget preparation.
- Sunset budget—is designed to self destruct within a prescribed time period to ensure the cessation of spend in by a predetermined date.
- Sales budget—is the starting point in a budgetary program, since sales are basic activities which give shape to all other activities sale budgets are complied in terms of quantity as well as of value.
- Production budget—aims at securing the economical manufacture of products and maximizing the utilization of production facilities, e.g. buying of audiovisual aids.
- Revenue and expense budget—is expressed in financial terms and takes the nature of a Proforma income statement for the future. It may be prepared in a detailed form or in an abstract statement showing the items of profit and loss under classified headings, e.g. Administrator will submit budget plan for present academic year.

- Capital expenditure budget—is prepared for assuring planned timely capital investment in the business or an organization to ensure the availability of capital at the right time over longer period, e.g. Keeping Amount in College account, administrator utilizes as and when necessary.
- Cash budget— is prepared by way of projecting the possible cash receipts and payments over the budget per each academic year, amount will be given to the administrator in advance and uses the amount whenever needed. Principal submits the expenditure detailed report at the end of every month, facilitates further sanctioning of amount like, sanctioning petti cash Rs. 2000/- every month to the administrator to meet the small expenses in the institution.

Features of Budget

- Flexible in nature
- Synthesis of past, present and future
- Product of joint venture + cooperation of executive/department heads at different levels of management eg: In Nursing Educational Institution the Principal/Administrator, University authorities, Government officials like DME in Government set up., in Private settings Management along with Administrator of Institution and financial committee members jointly discusses and releases fund to meet the requirements of the institution.
- Budget has to be in the form of statistical standard laid down in specific numerical terms
- it should have support of top management throughout the period of its planning and supplementation and implementation

COST BENEFIT ANALYSIS (CBA)

Definitions

"Helping to appraise or to assess, the case for a project, program or policy proposal; an approach to making economic decisions of any kind".

"Whether explicitly or implicitly, weighing the total expected costs against the total expected benefits of one or more actions in order to choose the best or most profitable option. The formal process is often referred to as either CBA (Cost-Benefit Analysis) or BCA (Benefit-Cost Analysis)"

"Cost-Benefit Analysis (CBA) estimates and totals up the equivalent money value of the benefits and costs to the community of projects to establish whether they are worthwhile".

"Benefits and costs are often expressed in money terms, and are adjusted for the time and value of money, so that all flows of benefits and flows of project costs over time (which tend to occur at different points in time) are expressed on a common basis in terms of their "present value." Closely related, but slightly different."

"A process by which you weigh expected costs against expected benefits to determine the best (or most profitable) course of action"

"To evaluate the total anticipated cost of a project compared to the total expected benefits in order to determine whether a proposed project is worthwhile for a company or team"

"Cost-Benefit Analysis (CBA) estimates and totals up the equivalent money value of the benefits and costs to the community of projects to establish whether they are worthwhile"

"The analysis of an opportunity to demonstrate the benefits in cost saving in order to receive management commitment and support to implement."

Principles of Cost Benefit Analysis

- A common unit of measurement
- CBA Valuations should represent consumers or producers valuations as revealed by their actual behaviour, The valuation of benefits and costs should reflect preferences revealed by choices which have been made. Eg: Improvements in transportation frequently involve saving time. The question is how to measure the money value of that time saved. The value should not be merely what transportation planners think time should be worth or even what people say their time is worth

- Benefits are usually measured by market choices—Consumers will increase their consumption of any commodity up to the point where the benefit of an additional unit (marginal benefit) is equal to the marginal cost to them of that unit, the market price. Therefore for any consumer buying some of a commodity, the marginal benefit is equal to the market price. The marginal benefit will decline with the amount consumed just as the market price has to decline to get consumers to consume a greater quantity of the commodity. The relationship between the market price and the quantity consumed is called the demand schedule. Thus the demand schedule provides the information about marginal benefit that is needed to place a money value on an increase in consumption
- Gross benefits—The increase in benefits resulting from an increase in consumption is the sum of the marginal benefit times each incremental increase in consumption. As the incremental increases considered are taken as smaller and smaller the sum goes to the area under the marginal benefit curve. Some measurements of benefits require the valuation of human life .People voluntarily accept increased risks in return for higher pay. These choices can be used to estimate the personal cost people place on increased risk and thus the value to them of reduced risk
- The analysis of a project should involve a with versus without comparison—The impact of a project is the difference between what the situation in the study area would be with and without the project.When a project is being evaluated the analysis must estimate not only what the situation would be with the project but also what it would be without the project
- Cost Benefit Analysis involves a particular study area—The impacts of a project are defined for a particular study area, be it a city, region, state, nation or the world.The nature of the study area is usually specified by the organization sponsoring the analysis. The specification of the study area may be arbitrary but it may significantly affect the conclusions of the analysis
- Double counting of benefits or costs must be avoided—Sometimes an impact of a project can be measured in two or more ways eg: when an improved highway reduces travel time and the risk of injury the value of property in areas served by the highway will be enhanced. The increase in property values due to the project is a very good way, at least in principle, to measure the benefits of a project. The property value went up because of the benefits of the time saving and the reduced risks. To include both the increase in property values and the time saving and risk reduction would involve double counting
- Decision Criteria for Projects—If the discounted present value of the benefits exceeds the discounted present value of the costs then the project is worthwhile. This is equivalent to the condition that the net benefit must be positive. Another equivalent condition is that the ratio of the present value of the benefits to the present value of the costs must be greater than one. From the set of mutually exclusive projects the one that should be selected is the one with the highest net present value. If the funds required to carry out all of the projects with positive net present value are less than the funds available this means the discount rate used in computing the present values is too low and does not reflect the true cost of capital. The present values must be recomputed using a higher discount rate. The magnitude of the ratio of benefits to costs is to a degree arbitrary because some costs such as operating costs may be deducted from benefits and thus not be included in the cost figure. This is called netting out of operating costs

Cost-Benefit Analysis in Health Care

"The analysis of health care resource expenditures relative to possible medical benefit."

This analysis may be helpful and necessary in setting priorities when choices must be made in the face of limited resources. This analysis is used in determining the degree of access to or benefits of health care to be provided.

Clarity of the medical decision - making process demands that cost - benefit analysis has to be separated and differentiated from risk - benefit analysis as well as from determinations of efficient and cost - effective medical care during medical decision-making.

'Risk-Benefit Analysis' weighs the potential for undesirable outcomes and side effects against the potential for positive outcomes of a treatment and is an integral part of the process of determining medical necessity in the delivery of quality medical care.

'Efficient Medical Care' is correlated to the timeliness of delivered medically necessary services and supplies that are delivered at the least cost and are consistent with the applicable standard of care.

'Cost-Effective Medical Care' is a method for comparing several intervention strategies using common units of cost and benefit.

Techniques of Cost-Benefit Analysis

Cost-effectiveness analysis—Examination of the cost and the outcomes of the alternative means of accomplishing an objective, in order to select the one with the highest effectiveness relative to its cost.

Economic impact analysis (EIA)—analyzes the effect of a policy, program, project, activity or event on the economy of a given area. The impact area can be a neighborhood, community, region or nation.

Fiscal impact analysis—A projection of the direct, current, public costs and revenues associated with residential or nonresidential growth to the local jurisdiction(s) in which this growth is taking place

Social Return on Investment (SROI) analysis—A principles based method for measuring extra-financial value (i.e., environmental and social value not currently reflected in conventional financial accounts) relative to resources invested. It can be used by any entity to evaluate the impact on stakeholders, identify ways to improve performance and enhance the performance of investments.

Benefits of CBA

- A cost benefit analysis finds, quantifies, and adds all the positive factors
- Improves organizational policies
- It identifies, quantifies, and subtracts all the negatives, the costs. The difference between the two indicates whether the planned action is advisable
- Increases staff morale, due to using these modern tools to support the organization
- Adding staff
- Introducing technologies and facilities
- Upgrading existing system, modifying work flow, implementing new procedures.

Demerits of Cost Benefit Analysis

Potential Inaccuracies in Identifying and Quantifying Costs and Benefits—Human error often results in common cost benefit analysis errors such as accidentally omitting certain costs and benefits due to the inability to forecast indirect causal relationships.

Increased Subjectivity for Intangible Costs and Benefits—The amount of subjectivity involved when identifying, quantifying and estimating different costs and benefits. Since some costs and benefits are non-monetary in nature, such as increases in customer and employee satisfaction.

Inaccurate Calculations of Present Value Resulting in Misleading Analyses—Evaluation method estimates the costs and benefits for a project over a period of time, it is necessary to calculate the present value. This equalizes all present and future costs and benefits by evaluating all items in terms of present-day values, which eliminates the need to account for inflation or speculative financial gains

A Cost Benefit Analysis Might Turn in to a Project Budget—Misappropriating costs and setting unrealistic goals when approving and implementing a project budget. This can put a project manager in an unfavorable situation when he or she attempts to control costs in order to maintain the expected profit margin.

CAREER OPPORTUNITIES IN NURSING

The term "nurse" is a generic label usually applied to all nurses working within the health care industry; however, there are different groups of nurses, each of which has its own level of education, clinical experience and respective title. The specific career opportunities in nursing available to each group can vary greatly and the choices often depend upon the type of education like certificate programs like MPHA, MPHS, LHV followed by Diploma Holders, Graduates, Post Graduates, Doctorate Program etc. which the nurse has earned.

Doctorate in Nursing

Nurses who earn a PhD in nursing have obtained the highest level of education in their field. PhD nursing programs will prepare nurse researchers and nurse scientists to better address the health care needs of individuals and their families, as well as the communities in which they live. These individuals are often more focused on academic and research activities rather than direct patient care and they are usually affiliated with teaching hospitals, research facilities and universities. These nurses are certified by the national organizations as Higher Education in Nursing with additional qualifications.

Nurses who are interested in Education and Research also can do PhD program in other related disciplines like Women Studies, Child Development, Adult Education, Behavioural Sciences etc.

M. Phil in Nursing

Nurses who are interested in Research and obtain higher degree can do M. Phil in Nursing or M.Phil in related disciplines.

Advanced Practice Nurse(Postgraduate In Nursing)

An advanced practice nurse (APN) is a Graduate in Nursing who chooses to further their education and obtain a master's degree by specializing in Clinical Nursing Specialities. Advanced practice nurses are considered as expert clinicians eg: Nurse Anesthetists, Nurse Practitioners, Nurse Midwives and Clinical nurse specialists are all APNs. These nurses are certified by the national organizations as Higher Education in Nursing with additional qualifications. MSc(N) has specialities like, Community Health Nursing, Pediatric Nursing, Obstetric Nursing, Medical-Surgical Nursing speciality with subspeciality like Cardiothoracic Nursing, Neuro Nursing Psychiatry etc.

Registered Nurse(Graduate Nurses Or Diploma Holders)

Graduates in Nursing or Diploma Holders are registered nurses who enjoys the most flexibility within the health care industry and bed side Nursing. Although RNs typically specialize in patient care according to the department for which they work, such as pediatrics, they can also sub-specialize. For example: A nurse trained in Pediatrics might further specialize in the field of pediatric oncology. Registered nurses generally continue their education and broaden their experience through further studying higher courses by inservice education or using their personal time and resources for further improvement in their Professional education. Aside from hospital jobs, registered nurse can find work in private settings and clinics, schools, Community settings as Public Health Nurses (Graduate Nurses) to provide Homecare services.

Multi Purpose Health Assistants(MPHA), Multi Purpose Health Supervisors (MPHS), Health Visitors (HV)

MPHA, MPHS, HVs will be providing health care services within the Community.

CAREER LADDER

Definitions

- The term "career ladder" is a metaphor or buzzword used to denote vertical job promotion
- "Structured sequence of job positions through which a person progresses in an organization"
- "A sequence of jobs within an organisation or department, starting with the most junior and ending with most senior, through which an employee can advance in the course of their working life"

In Human Resources Management, the ladder typically describes the progression from entry level positions to higher levels of pay, skill, responsibility or authority. frequently used to denote upward mobility within a stratified promotion model. Because the ladder does not provide for lateral movement, it is assumed to be a singular track with the greatest benefits at the top.

Nurses work hand in hand with doctors so they can help to treat a patient. Medicine has evolved into different fields, it has created so many nursing career opportunities. For example: Oncology is a field of Medicine that deals with patients who are suffering from cancer. Nurses who decide to specialize here may administer chemotherapy, counsel patients and work with doctors to create the right treatment plan depending on what stage of development is the cancer. Nurses who are interested in perioperative nursing otherwise known as OR nurses assist the surgeons both directly and indirectly during an operation. They help prepare the patient before and after the operation as well check on the equipment to be used by making sure they are sterile. Given that there are different types of surgeries done on patients, nurses have to specialize again to be part of the working team. Sickness is not the only reason that a patient may end up in the hospital as accidents take place in the work area or on the road. If the person has a neck or a head injury, it is up to the otorhinolaryngology nurses to help the patient. To get this job you must have a resident nurse with a diploma or have a degree either in AD or BSN. These individuals may find work also in hospices, clinics and home care agencies.

Kids get sick and it is up to the paediatric nurse to help them get better. But paediatrics also has other specializations such as oncology and hematology if ever the child is either suffering from cancer or a blood disorder. Anaesthesia is given to a patient prior to surgery. For that, you will a nurse that specializes in perianaesthesia to help the patient go to sleep and slowly bring them back after the operation. The difference between an anaesthesiologist is that he or she will be the one to administer the anaesthesia. The nurse simply helps the patient to make sure they are comfortable.

Soon to be mothers need the help of prenatal nurses in preparation for motherhood. This is done by telling them what to anticipate especially if this is their first child and giving them general health advice for them and the baby. Cancer prevention is important so this can be detected and removed during its early stages. For that, individual to undergo a few tests and the ones work these machines are called radiology nurses. They are the ones who operate the X-rays, sonograms, mammograms, ultrasound and a bunch of other machines. There are

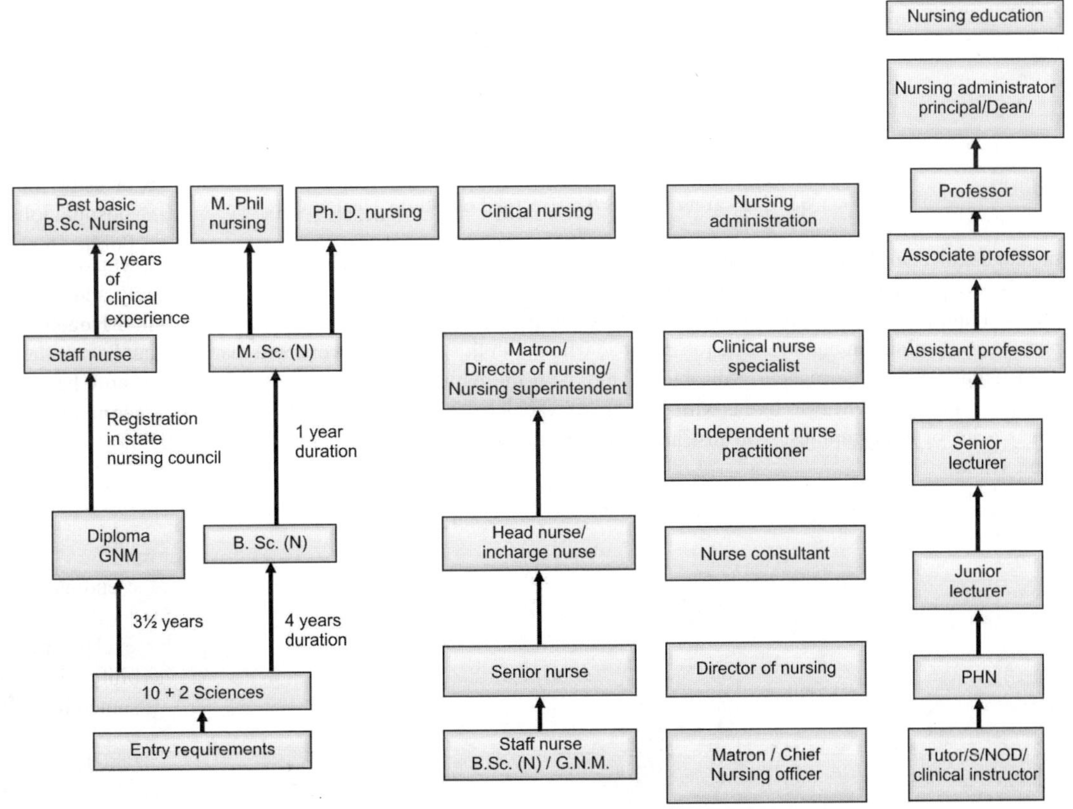

Model of Career Ladder

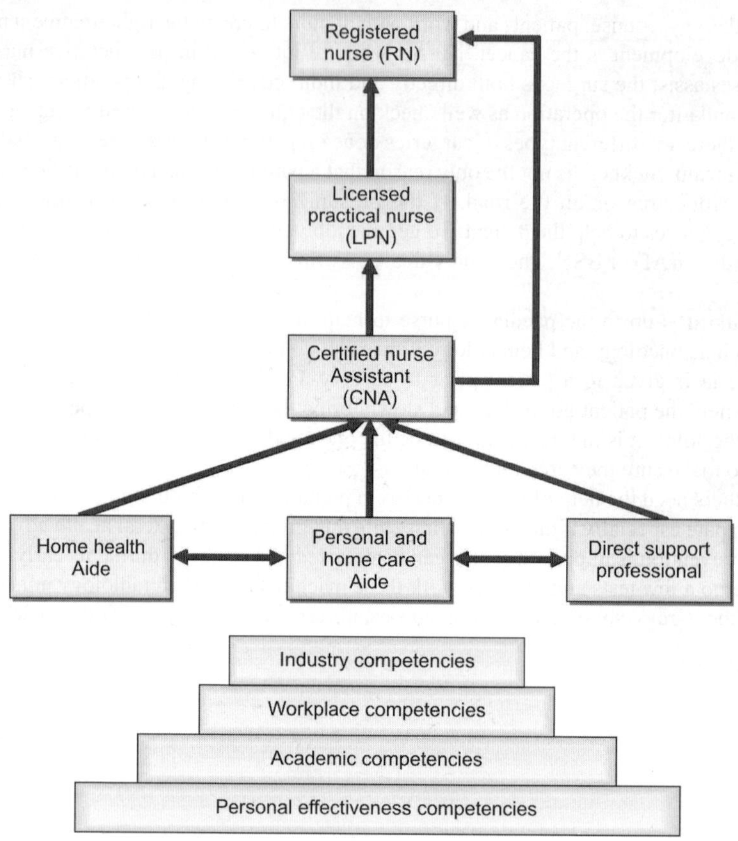

Sample career Ladder/Lattice for Long-term Health Care

mental health disorders and problems that patients face. Aside from the psychiatrist who will help you out, you can also see psychiatric nurses. These individuals are trained to handle patients suffering from anxiety, addiction, physical and sexual abuse, personality disorders and depression. Close to cardiac and otorhinolaryngology nurses is rehabilitation nursing. The job of those who are in this field is to work with patients that have either been temporarily or permanently disabled. They help the patient deal with the fact that they now have a handicap and the only way to live is with the help of wheelchairs, crutches and prosthetics. A career in nursing opens a lot of opportunities. You just have to specialize in something in order to make the most of your profession.

QUESTIONS

- Accreditation (5M, NIMS, May 2010; 5M, NTRUHS, Nov, 2010)
- Anecdotal Record (5M, MGU, Nov, 2009)
- Career Ladder (5M, NTRUHS, June, 2010)
- Career Opportunities (5M, NIMS, May 2010)
- Cumulative Record (5M, MGRUHS, Aug, 2008)
- Describe the principles and types of Budgeting. Explain Cost Benefit Analysis (10+5M=15M, NTRUHS, May, 2010)
- a) Enumerate purposes of budget, b) Explain features of a good budget (15M, RGUHS, 2006)
- Evaluation of Nursing Education in Programs (7.5M, RGUHS, Oct, 2009)
- Explain the accreditation process of the educational institutions in India (5M, RGUHS, Oct, 2008 and 7.5M RGUHS, Oct, 2009)
- Explain the administrative aspects required to run School of Nursing (10M, NIMS, Sep, 2010)
- INC (5M, NIMS, Sept, 2010)
- List out the records maintained in Institution (8M, NIMS, Oct, 2010)
- Nurse as educator- 4M, Line of Authority- 4M, Records & Reports - 4M (NTRUHS, July, 2008)
- Nurse Participation as a committee (5M, NTRUHS, July, 2008)
- Opportunities in Nursing (5M, NTRUHS, June, 2010)
- Professional Organization (5M, NTRUHS, Dec, 2007)
- Records in school of nursing(5M, RGUHS, Aug, 2010)
- Records maintained in a School Of Nursing (5 M, MGRUHS, Aug, 2006 & Feb, 2009)
- Registration, Licensing & Certificate (5M, NTRUHS, July, 2008)
- Role of a Departmental Head (5M, NTRUHS, June, 2010)
- Role of a Nursing Teacher(5M, NTRUHS, June, 2009)
- The Need For Curriculum Change (15M, NIMS, Oct, 2008)
- What are the steps taken by INC to maintain uniform standards for B.Sc(N) course in India (15M, NIMS, Oct, 2006)
- What is Budgeting (3M, NIMS, Sept, 2010, 5M, NIMS, May, 2008)
- What is Job Description (2M, NIMS, Sept, 2010)
- Why norms and guidelines are necessary for management of Nursing educational institutions (2M, NIMS, May, 2010)

Curriculum

INTRODUCTION

Curriculum is a Latin word, 'currere' means 'the race, the path, lap or course or runway' which one takes steps to reach a goal applied to a course of study. If the teacher is the guide, the curriculum is the path. Curriculum is the total structure of ideas and activities. The curriculum in a literal sense, "A pathway towards a goal". Curriculum is the crux of the whole educational process. Without curriculum, we cannot conceive any educational endeavor (Figs 3.1 and 3.14).

Education finds its effect and results through implementation of its curriculum by the school. Curriculum is actually what happens during a course i.e. ,lecture, demonstrations, field visits, the work with the clients and so on.

Pedagogically curriculum means the course of the studies to be pursued by the students or the written description of course content to be imparted through organisation of its entire work. The course of study means the specific content of education, the details of the study (Method of Teaching, Lesson Plans, Assignments & Evaluation strategies), which the students has to study to obtain different certificates or degrees from the educational institutions.

Definitions

- "A systematic and planned series of intended learning conceived to be imparted through selected, planned, organized and sequential learning experiences for a defined group of learners to attain the stated aims of a specific educational program"
- "A tool in the hands of the artist (teachers) to mould his material (the pupil) in accordance with his ideals (Thoughts/Knowledge) in his studio (school)"—*Cunningham.*
- "All the experiences of pupil which has undertaken in the guidance of the school"—*Blond's encyclopedia, 1969*
- "A curriculum is an attempt to communicate the essential principles and features of an educational proposal in such a form that is open to critical scrutiny and capable of effective translation into practice"—*Stenhouse, 1975*
- "All the learning activities which are planned and guided by the school, whether they are carried out in groups or individually, inside and outside the school"—*Kerr, 1968*
- "The curriculum is the manifestation of many composite parts and factors which together enable the achievement of nursing educational goals that have been fully identified, selected and articulated"— *Bevis, 1982*
- "A systematic arrangement of the sum total of selected experiences planned by a school or a defined group of students to attain the aims of a particular educational program"—*Florence Nightingale, International foundation*
- "A composite of the entire range of experiences the learner undergoes under the guidance of the school"—*Lambertson and Eleanor*
- "A series of sets of intended learning learnt by group of learners as a consequence of education"
- "It is a complex of more or less planned and controlled conditions under which students learn to behave in various ways. In it, new behavior may be acquired, present behavior may be modified, maintained or eliminated and desirable behavior may become both persistent and viable"—*Kearney and Cook*

- "A curriculum is the offering of socially and scientifically valued knowledge, skills and attitudes made available to students through a variety of arrangements during the time they are at school, college or university"— *Bell, 1973*
- The curriculum is primarily "an aid in the process of adjusting the child to the environment in which he function from day-to-day and in the environment in which he will organise his activities later"—*KG Sayyidain*
- "All the planned learning experiences of the school is by its very nature a cooperative problem, best solved by the teachers and the students working together".

Concept and Meaning

- It includes all the learning experiences, which a learner has, regardless of when or how they take place under the guidance of the school
- The systematic arrangement of courses designed with specific objectives for the students
- The courses offered within the school, e.g. GNM program; Basic B.Sc. (N); Post Basic B .Sc. (N) and M.Sc. (N) program
- The courses studied by an individual learner
- Total educational programe of the school i.e., learning activities and learning experiences occur within or outside the classroom
- The traditional concept of curriculum is, the teacher will focus his/her efforts and attention in making students to learn the subject content and course of study according to the prescribed syllabi, in a rigid, set pattern, to enable them to pass a set of examinations. The learners were given specific knowledge and skills which would fit them to become a mature and successful adult. Learner was prepared to live in the future as foreseen by the teacher and the parents
- New concept of curriculum, through education the learner lives in the present world and to adapt himself/herself to it. The teachers will prepare the learner to adapt for future world also, in which he and his contemporaries will live
- Textbooks and subject matter are not fixed rigidly. The student learns much more, the environment also provides learning experiences for him. The school provides materials to suit felt needs of students, for the development of the learner's intellect, personality, social life and cultural enrichment
- According to the best modern educational thought, curriculum does not mean only the academic subjects traditionally taught in schools, but includes the sum total of experiences that a learner receives through the manifold activities that exists in the schools, classroom, library, laboratory, workshop, play grounds and in the numerous informal contacts between teachers and learners which helps balanced personality of the students – Kothari commission
- Curriculum refers to "the totality of activity and experiences planned by the school with a view to achieve the objectives of education. Thus a curriculum is the instructional and educative program, through which the learners will achieve their goals, ideals and aspirations of life"
- Curriculum directs the teaching, learning experiences of nursing educational program
- Curriculum is the sum total of the school's efforts to influence learning and behavior of the child whether in the classroom, school, library, laboratory, workshop in the play ground or out of the school. In fact, the curriculum has been described as 'the environment in motion'
- It provides formal and informal contacts between teachers and learners in educational institutions, the curriculum touch the whole life of students at all points and helps in development of balanced personality and intellectual development of the learner
- Curriculum is the blueprint or plan of the school that includes the experiences for the learners to have
- It reflects the pattern of life – A careful selected pattern, covers the entire range of activities and experiences
- It is a tool in the hands of the teachers to give training to children in the art of living
- It helps to inculcate the standards of moral action, which are essential for successful living in society, for getting true satisfaction out of life
- Three facets of curriculum are: Goals/purposes of education, Process of Curriculum and Evaluation of products

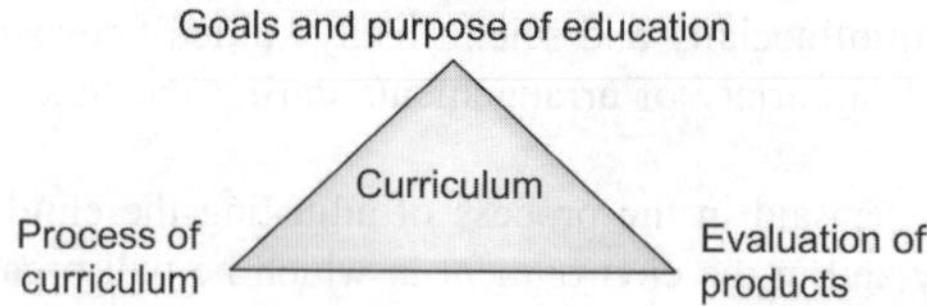

- Curriculum includes course of studies, curricular activities, methods of teaching. In-addition to the regular programs, extracurricular activities are direct products of the situations which arise out of the teachers'deliberate planning

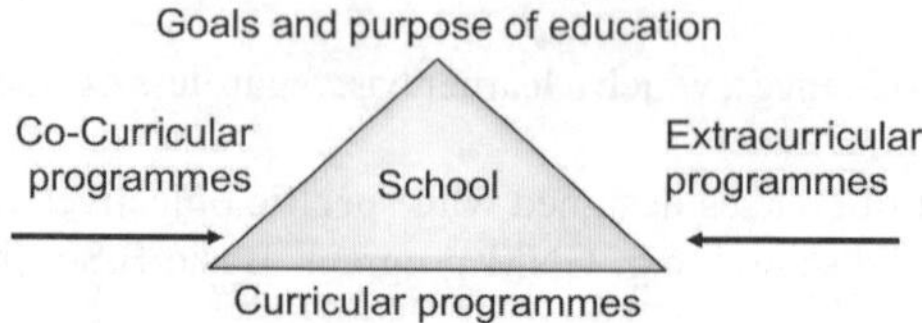

- Intellectual development of the learner is conceived as a mastery of subject matter achieved primarily through teachers' exposition, drills, tests, problemsolving, creative thinking etc. The primary purpose is to build a store house of information, skills and values which may be useful to the individual in his future life, e.g. subjectmatter curriculum, formal lecture classes
- Growth of the learner is interrelated viz., emotional health, personal and social adjustment, skill in group interaction, physical health, etc. all contribute and are essential to intellectual effectiveness. Therefore, the curriculum must give consideration to curricular, cocurricular and extracurricular activities, e.g. emphasis on the inclusion of subject matter and directed learning experiences with establishment of effective communication skills, interpersonal relationship skills and use of group techniques
- Development for effective functioning in all areas of living is important. Therefore, the school has a responsibility to provide learning experiences for the student's development to function effectively by fulfilling citizen role in the nation, etc.
- The essential purpose of a school of nursing is to prepare a practitioner of nursing. Therefore primary emphasis in the curriculum will be on nursing and related fields, development of a nurse who will be interested in the health and related aspects of the community. The school must provide the opportunities for the development of knowledge, skills and attitudes which make this possible
- In nursing education today, we have a convergence of all of these approaches in curriculum development.

The Curriculum of Nursing Includes
- Learning opportunities
- Subjectmatter
- Knowledge
- Skills
- Values
- Attitudes
- Learning activities that the faculty plans and implements in all settings: classroom teaching and clinical experiences includes laboratory, hospital, public health for a particular group of students at a specified time period
- Curriculum is a plan of logical sequence of correlated and integrated subjects which students may pursue in the attainment of a given goal
- In reality two curricula in each instance:
  - Planned by the faculty
  - Experienced by each student
- If the curriculum provided is broad, varied and flexible in learning opportunities, the curriculum selected and experienced can be highly appropriate for each individual learner.

The Four Cs of Curriculum Planning.

Cooperative: A program prepared jointly by a group of faculty will be less liable to error than one prepared by a single faculty, e.g. in universities, Board of Studies (academic), a group of senior faculty will meet and formulate the guidelines of different Nursing Program.

Continuous: The preparation of a program is not a one shot operation, provision should be made for its continuous revision to meet the felt needs of present era.

Comprehensive: In an approach which accepts the interaction of all the program components must be defined with the requisite precision cover all areas.

Concrete: General and abstract considerations are not a sufficient basis for drawing up a program. Concrete professional tasks must constitute the essential structure of a relevant program.

Nature of Curriculum

- Curriculum is the outward expression of the ideas and aspirations of a specific training programe
- It is ongoing and continuous
- It is flexible to meet the changing demands of society and health scenario of a country, advancement and trends in health fields in terms of scientific and technological pattern
- It is oriented towards societal aspects, life situations and health
- It meets the needs of group of learners
- It deals ideal and realistic approach
- It is dependent on the philosophy and objectives of the respective educational program
- Geared to shift its emphasis in terms of the national health policy, goals and consequent demands in nursing
- It is dualistic in nature, e.g. involves both the minds of the learners and the course content, two theories i.e. theory of values and theory of knowledge, stated in two ways in terms of subjectmatter and children's activities, intimately connected with the achievements and aspirations of the people
- It is prepared by the traditional authority like INC, Board of members in University
- It is based on the interests, abilities, aptitudes and needs of learners
- Curriculum is influenced by political, economic, philosophic and scientific factors
- A flexible curriculum where planning is done in terms of developing needs and the abilities of learners against the background of the needs of the society, usefulness of various knowledge and skills, the logical and psychological nature of learning
- The school should take responsibility of developing its' own Curriculum
- The complete curriculum includes objectives, materials, methodology and organization.

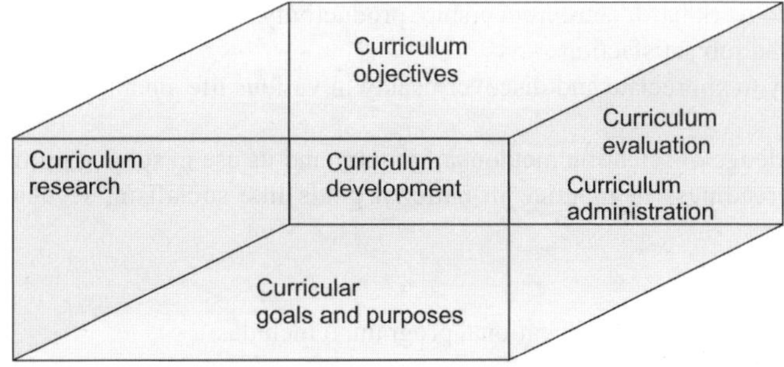

Fig. 3.1: The cubical form of curriculum process

Aims/Objectives/Purposes

1. To equip the learners by bringing the desirable behavioural changes within them.
2. To cope with and handle life situations realistically, rationally without sacrificing the humane principles.
3. Helps in
   - Development of health personnel at all levels

- Preparation of respective health team members specifically for the tasks they will be required to perform in their respective job positions
- Student's participation in curriculum development
- Achieves in educational objectives.

4. Curriculum is intended
   - To draw, cultivate, excite and inspire the holistic development of each student
   - To create an atmosphere in which students will learn to think; where faculty and students will be critical enough to be objective, constructive, truthful to solve the problems, reason out and develop the power of thought
   - To establish values through intimate acquaintance with the Humanities, Arts, Natural Sciences, Social Sciences and Theology
   - To shape the character of students i.e., integrity, honesty, judgment, cooperation, friendliness and goodwill
   - To create a community of scholars where research, curiosity, free enquiry and advancement of knowledge takes place
   - To prepare the pupil for citizenship in a democratic society where liberty, freedom, law, justice and responsibility will observed
   - To meet the needs of students with a wide range of ability, aptitudes and interests
   - To discover the landmarks of human achievement
   - It makes good decision and judgments in a socially desirable direction.

Need and Significance of the Curriculum

"The child of today is the builder of tomorrow". A well-designed curriculum, if it is effectively implemented, the learner will be equipped with inner potentialities and become instrumental to build up Nation. Curriculum is basic for the holistic development and increases the abilities of the learner in total, e.g. esthetic, emotional, ethical, intellectual, physical, social, material, spiritual, language abilities, communication skills and vocational skills, etc.

Functions of the Curriculum

- Relates various learning experiences in curriculum to produce the maximum cumulative effect among learners to attain the objectives of educational program
- Gains mastery over the subjectmatter, develop concepts, inculcate skills, attitudes, values and habits conducive for the all round personality development which are needed for social living and further learning
- It makes the man socially effective and happy in various social settings by meeting varied social needs, e.g. friendliness, co-operativeness, compassion, self-discipline, constructive criticism, self-control, humor, courage, love for social justice, honesty, truthfulness, independence, courtesy, fearlessness, vocational skills, willingness to work hard, entrepreneurship, productivity, cultural heritage, cultural diversity, social systems of living and job satisfaction
- Increases the ability to appreciate and discover beauty in various life situations and integrate it into one's own personality
- Promotes the knowledge of scientific methods of inquiry and its use in solving problems
- Appreciation and readiness to practice in national goals like socialism, secularism, democracy and non-violence.

Components of Curriculum

Curriculum is planned for a particular educational program. It includes:
- Philosophy
- Objectives
- Duration of learning experiences
  - Theoretical
  - Practical
  - Clinical components (supervised Clinical Nursing practice, i.e. lab, clinical)
- Courses of study, placement, sequences and learning situations (includes task analysis, selection, planning and organization of learning experiences)

- Instructional methods
- Program of evaluation
  - Evaluation methods
  - Plan and schedule of evaluation
  - Results of evaluation.

Areas of study from where the components of nursing curriculum will be drawn:
The Nursing education program offered by the school, keeps pace with scientific and technological advancement in the field of health and related areas, for such preparation, the Nursing curriculum requires to draw its components from:
- The Natural sciences/fundamental sciences like Biology, Microbiology, Bio-Physics, Chemistry, Pharmacology, etc. gives the information like facts and principles
- The Humanities, Behavioral Sciences like Psychology, Sociology, Fine arts, etc. provide the insight and background for the development of the art of nursing
- National Health Policy goals, country's health scenarios, job responsibilities and resources, man power requirements and availability demographic trends, epidemiological trends, socioeconomic factors, sociocultural trends on issues, lifestyle issues and standards of living
- Professional Nursing areas where by the student nurse will learn the subjects like Fundamentals of Nursing, Community Health Nursing, Pediatric Nursing and Midwifery and Practice Nursing skills
- The organized instruction constitution includes:
  Teaching-learning Activities
  - Classroom instruction – Follows curricular outline and course content (Varied subjects).
  - Planned instruction and demonstration – Procedures, simulation techniques in labs.
  Supervised Clinical Nursing Practice
  - The Planned Clinical instruction – Clinical Areas – Hospital (General and Specialities) and Community oriented nursing practice (Rural & Urban).
  - Community and task analysis to assess the needs of community, nursing components of the National health policy goals and planning tasks to meet their needs.
  - Provision for correlation and verification of theory and clinical practice.
  - The recommendations made by the relevant health related committees report.

According to KA Feithwood (1981) Curriculum Encompasses
- Educational philosophy
- Values and objectives
- Organizational structure
- Materials
- Teaching strategies
- Student experiences
- Learning outcomes.

Main components:
- Program of studies – Languages, Behavioral sciences – Theory
- Program of activities – Learning experiences in clinical areas
- Program of guidance – To solve their educational, personal, professional and vocational problems.

According to Agnes S. Robinson (1971), the components of curriculum are:
  - Philosophy
  - Goals and objectives (Behavioural and programe)
  - Content
  - Processes
  - Resources, course statement
  - Conceptual framework
  - Planning, organization, implementation and evaluation of learning experiences in classroom, lab, in the hospital and in community; extracurricular activities and co-curricular activities, and sports and games, NCC, NSS, cultural activities.

Levels of Curriculum Planning

Goodland describes curriculum in 3 levels:

a. Societal curriculum:

The curriculum which is planned for a large group of students in a specific program, e.g. B.Sc (N).

It is planned by Councils outside the University, e.g. Indian Nursing Council, National League for Nursing.

They determine criteria which shall be used in the accreditation of schools, general curriculum content—It's sequence and the pattern of implementation, which are likely to prepare the type of nurse practitioner needed to meet society's needs. There is a significant relationship between curriculum and the nature of the society which supports it and to the relative stability or fluidity of the culture. In the periods of social change, many issues and problems arise, then according to the need, the curricula undergo change. The Government should provide financial resources for training projects and for research. It aids for enhancing of curriculum.

Curriculum planning at the societal level can be helpful to schools as they are contributing for societal' welfare, through stimulating, initiating and supporting curriculum studies. Guides, which have been developed by outside groups and experts, can be planned so that they are sufficiently flexible to apply to different situations. The base of organization curriculum planning and implementation in each situation still has to be determined by the faculty of each school.

b. The Institutional curriculum:

It is planned by faculty for a clearly identified group of students who will spend a specified time period in a particular institution. It is one speaks of a curriculum in a particular school. Cooperative planning through curriculum committee within the school is obvious of one looks at the broad base of facts, principles, understandings, skills, habits, attitudes and appreciations that are required to prepare the student to function as a modern professional nurse in a democratic society. More active participation of individuals in group affairs generally brings about change and improvement, but also because the teacher has a right to participate and the desire to find opportunity for the growth of students and their capacities through contributive and constructive sharing of social progress. Voluntary and intelligent co-operation of all concerned is needed. It requires a high degree of self-discipline, integrity of personal character and an ability to co-operate with others.

c. The Instructional curriculum:

It consists of the content (subject matter and learning activities) planned day by day and week by week by a particular teacher for a specific group of students. The curriculum is made in the classroom, for it is the teacher who largely determines the educational fate of their students by what and how they teaches. It may serve as a valuable guide to the teacher and the student in the development of a course. The way in which the curriculum is interpreted in the particular situation will influence the importance and the amount of individual teacher planning. The curriculum is conceived to include all the planned learning experiences of the student, it includes:

- Essential facts, information, concepts, meanings, principles
- Activities that is necessary for the development of skills, habits, attitudes, ideals and appreciations
- Methods that is useful in teaching, supervising, guiding and evaluating results
- All the content planned by the teacher, experienced by the students to achieve the desired behavioural changes implicit in the educational objectives
- Nursing curriculum comprises not only subjectmatter, but also activities, methods, school and classroom, organization, clinical nursing experience, measurement and even the teacher herself/himself
- The curriculum consists of the tools, which the teacher may use to effect behavior changes in the life of the student
- The teacher must select from the abundance of available situations those that are appropriate to the needs of the student
- The teacher is part of the curriculum since she/he is involved in the situations that are responsible for the development of students
- Teacher selects the objectives, the learning activities and the aspects of physical and social environment that serves in the development of the student's personality

- Nurse educators are concerned with providing the specific type of learning environment which will enable the student to learn the needed skills of nursing and provide complete and continuous nursing care to the patient
- Educational objectives must be prepared to meet immediate social needs
- Cooperative planning is essential in the development of the curriculum.

Factors Influencing Curriculum Planning

- University Council (INC i.e., National councils and State council), Government Requirements and approval to organize curricular activities related to current Nursing Program
- Principal's/Administrator of Nursing Educational Institution and their Professional background
- Recent Findings of Nursing Research
- Interdepartmental decisions
- Circulars/Government Orders/Felt needs of society/University orders
- Governing body rules
- Programed instructions
- Management instructions (applicable for Private Institutions)
- Study projects
- Committees Recommendations
- Learners' requirements
  - Health
  - Family
  - Vocation
- Religion and culture
- Employment opportunity
- Social, civil and economic aspects
- Psychological aspects
- Teachers availability and their professional background, their commitment towards professional welfare and subjects to be studied
- Environment within which education takes place
- Availability of Resources
- The world of knowledge
- The learner and nature of their growth and development
- A clear conception of what makes a good life
- Curriculum planning must take into account the characteristics of past, contemporary and future society
- Needs and interests of both individual and society
- It has to recognize and encourage diversity among the learners
- Curriculum planning makes provision for all aspects of teaching-learning situations like suggested activities, content, resources, measuring devices and characteristics of the learners for whom it is intended
- Curriculum planning should also make use of approaches other than subject area approach
- It must provide flexibility to allow teacher – learner planning
- Curriculum planning reflects a balance among cognitive, conative and affective domains of the learners
- It should include provision for reflective thinking, values, enhancement of self-concept and self esteem
- Cooperative planning and development are most effective in cooperative settings
- Teacher held responsibility in curriculum planning and implementation
- Needed integrated set of experiences
- It must provide opportunity for concurrent and terminal evaluation of aspects of curriculum
- Adequate preparation of teachers to meet the changed requirements of the curriculum
- Sufficient supply of teaching aids and equipment is needed for the implementation of the programe
- Receptivity of the community for new curriculum
- Adequate preparedness of the students to accept the new curriculum with its additional requirements of energy, money and time

- Adequate availability and interested teachers for teaching, clinical supervision and guidance, adequate clinical facilities availability and permission from clinical authorities for effective implementation of the curriculum.

Factors Influencing Curriculum Development in Nursing Education

Nurse educator needs to understand the fundamental principles and practices involved in curriculum development. It will enable the teacher to understand the importance of preparing themselves to function efficiently in curriculum development (Fig. 3.2).

a. Philosophy of Nursing education:

Education is, "the deliberate and systematic influence exerted by the mature person (Teacher) upon the immature (Learner) through instruction, discipline and the harmonious development of all powers of the human being— Physical, social, intellectual, esthetic and spiritual according to their essential hierarchy, by and for their individual and social efforts and directed toward the union of the educator and with his creator as the final end".

Philosophy of education may be defined as "the application of the fundamental principles of a philosophy of life to the work of education". It offers a definite set of principles and establishes a definite set of aims, objectives and background for the selection of subject content. It offers criteria for intelligent interpretation of educational ends and means. Main purpose of education is to bring about changes in the behavior of the student, to determine what changes are desired, involves value judgments and is influenced by the underlying philosophy of the curriculum.

Instruction and development of powers are the means, to prepare the student so that he/she can attain the end for which he/she was created.

b. Natural bonds:

There is a natural association between the spiritual life and education as well as between the ideals and the cultural standards of the adult generation.

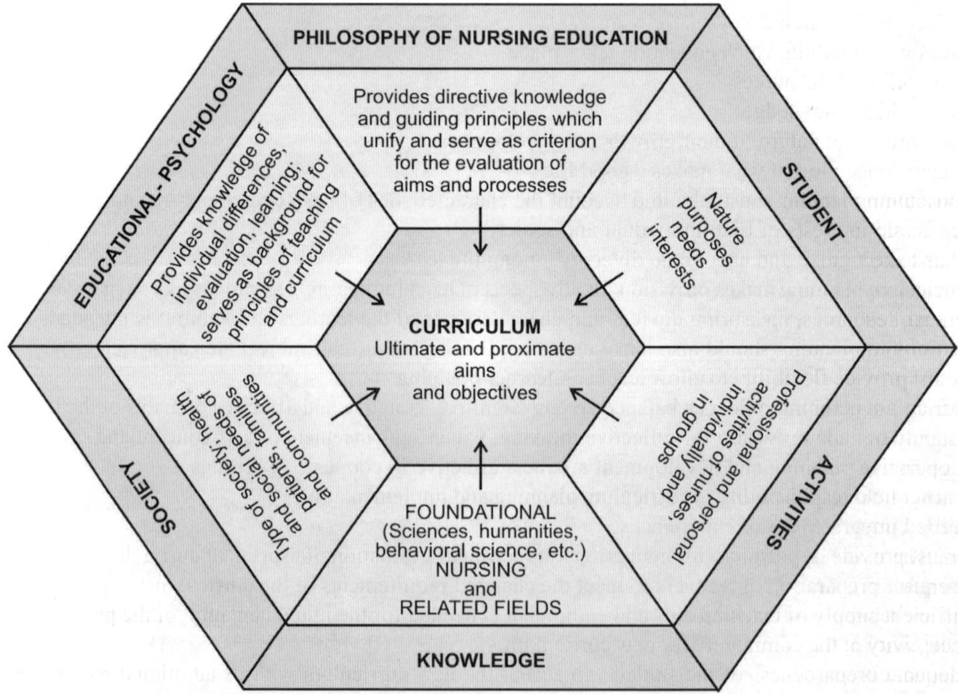

Fig. 3.2: Major factors of the development of a curriculum

c. Logical bonds:

Ideals are determined through the philosophy. Once ideals have been established, it may be said to follow logically that a system of education must be set up in order to perpetuate them. The core or heart of any given system of education is found in the ideals it sets out to attain.

d. Social bonds:

Education aims at perpetuation of social institutions which are based on philosophy of life and the progress of society. History is the authentic method of recording, in the interest of man's activities and the progress of human society.

e. Cultural bonds:

Culture includes the sum total of people's accomplishments but the ideals and the virtues after which they strive. The very essence of culture is to be found in the ideals towards which it aspires. Philosophy determines ideals and culture in all its phases, including philosophy is transmitted through the institution of education.

f. Human bonds:

Psychology is the basis for education, it will help in development of the personality of the learner . Knowing the individual student and the ideal that will best serve as a model for his education. The teacher must give herself/himself totally to the work of education. Students' mind and heart must be in it. Teacher's wisdom and knowledge should manifest in her/his deeds.

g. Religious bonds:

Education realizes its finest expression in religion. Religion has an extraordinary penetrative influence, as the omnipresence of God is a strong deterrent from evil.

The interdependence of a philosophy of life and the theory of education, which every teacher must recognize clearly and understand if she/he fulfill her/his obligation properly, takes on a real meaning.

h. Educational psychology:

It provides us with data on problems of learning through experimentation, it provides us with data from which the principles of learning are developed; thereby it forms the basis for development of principles and methods of teaching. Educational objectives are the educational ends—the results will be achieved through learning. The information obtained through educational psychology applied to nursing education, through research and experience, provides information and principles which serve to help in the selection, organization and the evaluation of learning experiences in the curriculum.

i. Society

To educate nursing students who ought to possess sound judgment are intellectually and morally enlightened and professionally equipped so that they are capable of caring for the sick and functioning efficiently in health programs and thereby contributing to the health and the welfare of society .Therefore a study of the nature of the society of which she/he is a part and of the health needs of society serve as an important guide in the selection of educational objectives and the development of a curriculum in nursing. Nursing is one of the social institutions concerned with health, a fundamental need of all people and consequently cannot be conceived of today apart from the society in which it functions.

Man is a social being, society is natural to man, he should not forget that he has an individual personality and dignity of his own. Society exists for man, man does not exist for society. Man's personality is developed through social means and his destiny achieved by living in the midst of society. Individual needs others, to help him to develop his personality completely. This social need is first met by family (primary group) and secondary groups, it lays the foundation for social solidarity. The social attitudes developed throughout the nation. The nation is bound together by ties with common ideals. As the instrument of education for society, the curriculum will necessarily reflect the ideals, the knowledge and the skills that are believed to be significant or that are related to the common activities of the members of society. Therefore the curriculum is interwoven with the whole social fabric that sustains it. The democratic way of life has to be protected, preserved and developed, continued emphasis toward shaping the human personality is essential. According to the changing needs of society the curriculum also has to be modified.

j. Health needs:

The nurse educator needs to know society's health needs and resources, the changing social pattern of family life. A study of the social changes and their influence on the family provides data, which are essential to the development of a curriculum. The expansion of public health facilities, enlargement and extension of hospital services, prepayment plans for hospital and medical care and other similar extensions of health services have created the need for an enormous increase in the supply of nursing care required to meet these demands. Nursing is inextricably tied up with the social culture in which it is carried on, nursing is affected by the society in which it flourishes and the School of Nursing must prepare the number and the kind of nurses essential to fulfill the nursing needs of society.

k. The student:

Meeting the student needs requires the inclusion of certain activities in the curriculum. If the student nurse is young and inexperienced in living away from home and unprepared to meet the environmental challenges of his/her new life, he/she may develop emotional tensions and anxieties that will disturb his/her scholastic achievements and his relationship with others. Guidance programes in School of Nursing will assist the student to help them to overcome their difficulties and in adjusting with scholastic environment e.g. Organizing orientation programs to each new learning situation. The student is considered as a whole individual whose ability is to learn and to adjust is conditioned not only by his/her intellectual capacity, but also by their emotional make-up, attitudes, social relationships, physical and psychological conditions.

l. Life activities:

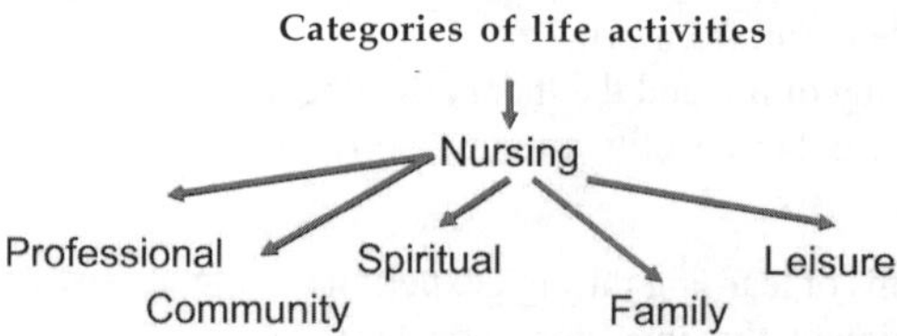

Activities: The Nursing Professionals will engage in both Professional and Personal activities.

Effective Preparation for Life Activities
- The growth of the student in individual capacities and in social participation.
- The nursing curriculum should provide opportunities for the total development of the learner
- Factors affecting life activities
  - Changes in the health of the nation
  - Changes in nursing functions
  - Changes in nursing program requirements
  - Changes in socio-economic factors
  - Political forces
  - Technologic resources.
- The primary purpose of the curriculum in nursing
  - The preparation of the student to function as a nurse
  - Increase preparation of the student for family functioning
  - To become fully prepared to participate in the life activities, to become a better person and a better citizen as well as a good nurse for having studied in the Nursing Educational Institutions
  - The preparation of a nurse to carry out activities necessary to fulfill his function as a professional nurse in a democratic society.

A curriculum in nursing education strives to develop student's understanding and responsibility in dealing with all the spheres of life.

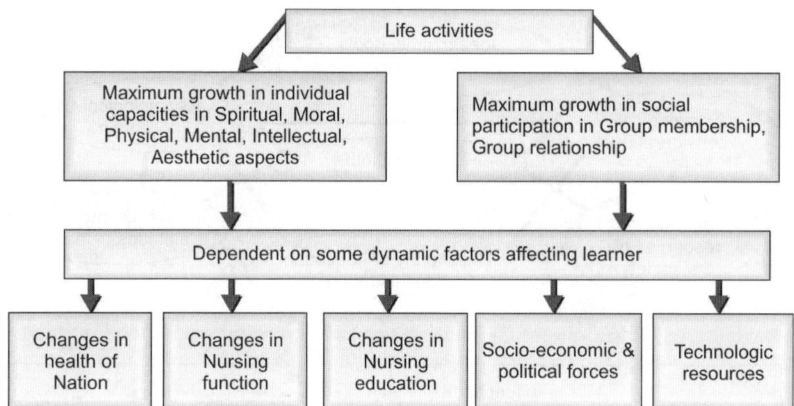

Fig. 3.3: Factors and life activities

m. Knowledge:

It is substantive dimension of the educative process. Knowledge is the stock in trade of all schools curricula which consist of:

- Subject matter courses in which mastery of content is not pursued as the end, but is used as a resource
- Change in every phase of life is probably the greatest challenge to education today.

Nature of Knowledge

- Descriptive knowledge: Statements about things that can be perceived directly or in principles. It includes— Facts, Laws, Rules and Theories. It describes about the facets of life.
- Normative knowledge: Knowledge is organized into specific branches or fields generally referred to as 'disciplines', e.g. Rules, Norms, Standards, Moral or Esthetic choices.

"A discipline is a collection of parts of systematized knowledge arbitrarily selected and bound together in a manner suitable for learning, mental training and research". Knowledge is organized around basic concept, which form the structure of discipline. The discipline is the way of learning.

Phases in Curriculum Development

Phase	Steps
Development phase	Planning and developing
Implement phase	Management and implementation
Evaluate phase	Assessment of teaching and learning process

Connecting links between these fields and humanities are:

    Art and literature

    History

    The natural sciences and mathematics.

Main modes of intellectual activity:

- The logical, e.g. reasoning activities
- The empirical, e.g. facts of experiences
- The moral, e.g. ethical issues, Values, Judgments
- The esthetic, e.g. statements of preferences, Evaluation strategies.

Social sciences

Philosophy

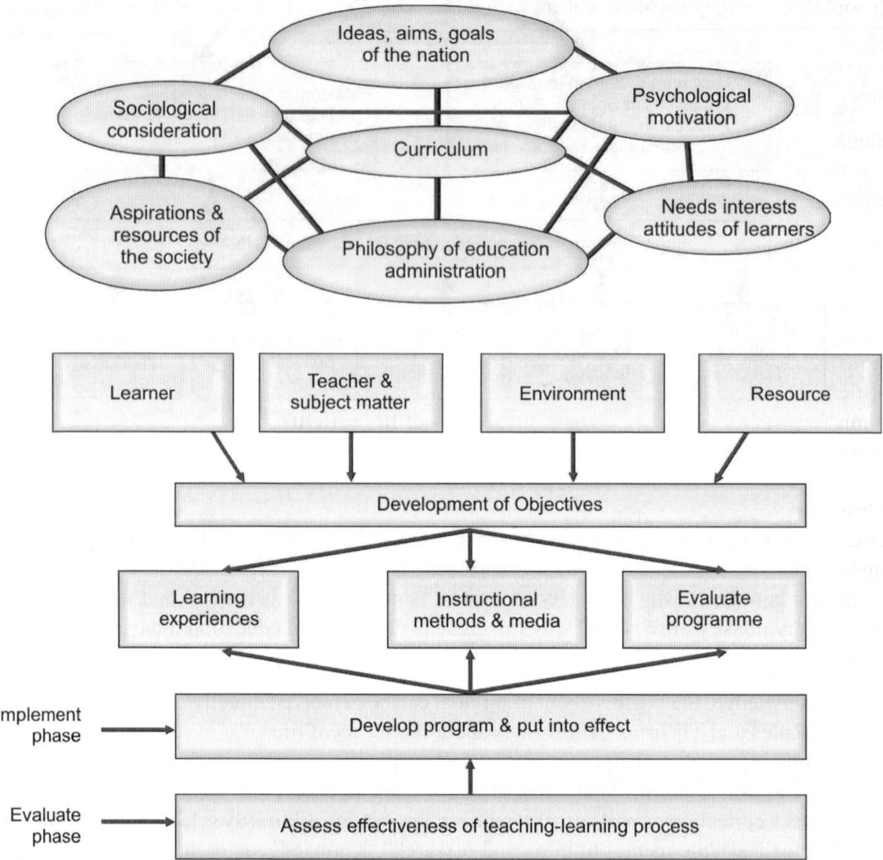

Fig. 3.4: Flow chart showing relationship of factors and phases of curriculum

Determinants and Foundations of Curriculum

The development of curriculum depends largely on three fields:

- Philosophy
- Sociology
- Psychology.

The knowledge of three fields will help them to satisfy their lives within the context of the society. Curriculum is organised in terms of stages and it's sequence—Instruction, Motivation and Learning.

a. Philosophical determinants

Philosophy is a powerful determinant factor of aims (why) of education, but is also equally a strong deciding factor of contents and methods (what and how) of education

- It aims at the all-round personality development of an individual
- It is based on the philosophy of the nation
- It reflects the ideals and aspirations of the people
- It inculcates the desired ideals of life in the youngsters
- It helps in the development of proper philosophy of life
- It is in accordance with the aspiration level of the individual learner
- It enables the learners to learn the desirable cultural values, intellectual virtues, social norms, moral doctrine and Worthwhileness
- It helps in the development of personal and national character
- It frames the structure of knowledge.

The philosophical foundations of education includes:
- Child centeredness (Naturalistic philosophy)
- Need centeredness (Pragmatic philosophy)
- Activity centeredness (project and basic curriculum).

b. Sociological determinants

Schools are the social institutions specially set up for the preservation and transmission of culture and knowledge by society. Schools seek to discharge this function through the curriculum.

Sociological considerations that guide the curriculum development are:
- National ideology and it's change
- Educational philosophy
- National goals and aspirations
- Religious doctrine
- Scientific and technological advancement
- Economic planning and its' efficiency
  - Need for modernization
  - Social change
  - Culture and it's change
- Core values and needs of Society in any Nation
- Demands of modernization
- Family life and ways of living
- Democracy
- Faiths, beliefs and attitudes of the people
- Cooperation
- Media exposition
- Population explosion
- Regional and national imbalances
- Education for fellowship and leadership
- Creative and purposeful activities
- Cultural and political factors
- Knowledge.

The characteristics of the curriculum, i.e. determined by sociological foundations of education are:
- To realise the social aims of education
- Makes education as an effective media of social control
- Keeps in mind the social changes and meets the social needs of the community
- Dynamic, flexible and progressive
- Transmits the ideals and values that the society upholds and considers to be inherited by the new generation
- Related to social interests and problems of the society
- Enables the youngsters to participate efficiently in social life
- Inculcates in learners respect for different vocations and professions and creates dignity of labour
- Develops desirable social attitudes
- Aids them in promoting the social progress
- To develop each individual to the optimum possible level
- Aims at educating for the vacation and vocation
- It is functional and socially utilitarian

Principles
- Integratedness: Knowledge is unitary. Logical integration of different activities and subjects to become a meaningful whole, is felt as a dire educational need
- Life centeredness
- Social-utilitarianism.

c. Psychological determinants
- Knowledge of
  - The nature of the learner
  - Learning process
  - Conditions facilitating optimum learning
  - Needed personality development of learner
- Intelligence, development capacities
  - Curriculum has to be child centered, learning experiences should be provided in accordance with the psychological development of the learner i.e., ability to grasp
  - Interests of the learner.

Curriculum committee
- Policy Makers and Developers
- Administrators/Program Coordinators
- Principals
- Advisory commitee
  - Board of Nursing in Educational Boards and in Universities
- Educational Researchers
- Teacher/educators
- State departments of education
- Parents
- Students
- Project directors
- Authors
- Testers/Evaluators
- Accreditation authority, e.g. Councils
- Lobbyists
- Philanthropists.

Purposes
- Review the data regarding curriculum needs
- Investigating specific curriculum problems
- Developing plans for specific curriculum implementation
- Steering faculty planning and coordination
- Articulating instructional programs between teams, grades (academic year), subjects and schools
- Planning and organizing staff development activities relating to curriculum needs, Conducting curriculum research and experimentation
- Developing innovative proposals
- Working on problems submitted through the communication channels of the council
- Preparing curriculum plans in new areas or courses evaluating existing programs
- Searching literature, practice and research for information relative to any aspect of curriculum and instruction
- To secure feedback regarding established or proposed curriculum practices
- To ensure representation of the central administration, community, parents and students served
- Acts as a liaison between the school's curriculum council and the community and students' advisory councils
- The quality of arrangements made to relieve problems and proposals from the constituent units and the opportunity given to these units to review recommendations made to them
- Creation of alternative schools for particular purposes
- Identification of problems for research
- Review of feedback from various sources on the curriculum and instructional program
- Helpful in curriculum planning—Selecting General and Specific objectives for each academic year, subject, section, school, subdivisions or other basis of organization

- Designing appropriate learning opportunities to achieve goals
- Assigning of responsibility for particular programs and students
- Procuring needed materials
- Scheduling instructional groups and facilities
- Defining student evaluation procedures
- Planning for and conducting evaluation of particular instructional programs and indeed, the entire curriculum plan for which the team is responsible
- Interdisciplinary, intra-disciplinary or simply a planning group for grade or departmentalized teaching, the decision will be taken in particular curriculum domain
- Curriculum implementation will be decided, e.g. what instructional models has to be used (when and how), individualized self-teaching, guided independent study and method of teaching.

Weaknesses of Structured Committee Approach

- Participation of each committee member may not take place, had not been accompanied by a clarity of their roles each member has to play, 'between decisions that involve general wisdom and those that require expertise'
- The curriculum development becomes a piecemeal operation
- It may arise a faculty division of labor
- Failure to articulate programs between grade levels or different levels of schooling
- Securing appropriate representation in curriculum committee is often a problem
- Individuals selected are neither interested in curriculum development, nor trained in the requisite skills. Sometimes they are not even representative of their group
- Over simplification of the task
- The time required to develop, try out and implement a plan may be under-estimated
- Too often there is no plan and thus no resources set aside for implementation.

Curriculum Construction

Nursing curriculum planners always consult with:
- National health policy goals, recommendations of health related committee reports, e.g. High power committee, Kartar Singh committee, Bhore committee, INC, etc.
- Obtain a feedback from different categories like Clientele, Peers and Colleagues, Non-nurse members of health team, Controlling officers, Supervisors and Superiors, Opinion leaders of community etc.

The success of a curriculum depends on certain principles:
- The purpose and educational objectives of the program—The objective should be stated in clear, unambiguous, behavioral, observable, measurable, feasible and achievable terms.

    To enhance the capacity building of learner to perform the appropriate and relevant demanded to fulfil professional responsibilities.
- The students and teachers should have a clear perception of the expected results.
- Learning experiences should be related to the theoretical, practical and clinical components (Hospital and Community field) and Teaching-learning content should be selected accordingly.

Grading of content can be done
> E – Essential or must learn
> D – Desirable or useful to learn
> S – Supportive or nice to learn

Teachers have to decide in planning the theoretical courses, clinical experience and community based clinical experiences for their students and also when they are evaluating their progress.

Principles

- Conservation: 'Nations live in the present, on the past and for the future'. Hence the past, present and future needs of the community should be taken into consideration.

- **Selectivity:** The selection of the curriculum content is based on Societal and National needs at present and requirement of specific course or program.
- Forward Looking: Today's children are future citizens of tomorrow. Their education should enable them to be progressive minded persons. Education should give them a foundation of knowledge, feeling, which will enable them to change the environment where change is needed.
- Creativity: The curriculum should exercise creative and constructive power. The education should discover and develop special interests, tastes and aptitudes among learners. It should meet the needs of today and of the future.
- The Activity and Experience: The curriculum should be taught in terms of activity and experience, rather than of knowledge to be acquired and facts to be stored. Growth and learning takes place only where there is activity. Experience along with instruction is required to meet the needs of the various stages in Professional growth. Curriculum should provide varied experiences/activities by keeping in mind with learners' progress and interests.

  Class rooms, workrooms and laboratories not only direct the natural active tendencies of youth, but also involve course, communication and cooperation.

  The learner needs experience rather than instruction, he must play, explore and physically active, if he has to derive a daily satisfaction out of his attendance at school. The curriculum must ensure the activity of body and mind. The methods of teaching are based on specific principles, e.g. Kindergarten, Montessori, Project method are based on the principle of activity.

- **Preparation of Life:** Education must equip the individual for life, hence curriculum must include the activity which enable the child to take his part effectively and amiably in the activities of the community when student becomes an adult, teacher has to prepare the child that he is capable of facing the various challenges of the complex problems of the future.
- **Linking with Life:** The community needs and characteristics should be kept in view while framing the curriculum.
- **Child Centredness:** Teacher can help the learner to live carefully and richly, his life at that stage at which he is. The child automatically prepares himself for the next stage by living well and truly life at one stage, by living fully in the environment.
- **Maturity:** Curriculum should be adapted to the grade of the learners and to their stage of physical and mental development.
  - In the early childhood, 'wonder' predominate, so these elements should be included in the subjects
  - At a later stage, the child is interested in practical things, so the curriculum should orient the practical problems
  - At the senior stage, students are interested in generalisations, accordingly curriculum should provide such activities. The experience should be provided within the comprehension level of the students
- **Individual Differences:** Individuals differ in qualities like taste, temperament, skill, experience, aptitude and innate ability. Therefore it should be adapted to individual differences. Curriculum should be flexible, not to be rigid.
- **Vertical and Horizontal Articulation:** Each year's course should be built on what has been done in previous years and at the same time should serve as basis for subsequent work. Entire curriculum should be coordinated, e.g. First Year B.Sc.(N) the child will learn Fundamental Sciences like Psychology, Sociology, Anatomy, Physiology, Biochemistry etc. which forms as basis for professional growth of child, where the normal physiological functioning will be studied, later in Second and third year B.Sc.(N) Medical- Surgical Nursing, Pediatric Nursing where the disease aspects will be studied.
- **Comprehensiveness and Balance:** Every aspect of life, e.g. Socio-Economic relationships—Social activities, Occupation etc. is given due emphasis.
- **Loyalty:** Curriculum should teach a true sense of loyalty to the family, the school, community, country and the world at large. It should enable the child to understand that there is unity in diversity.
- **Flexibility and need basedness:** Curriculum should meet the special needs and circumstances of the learner
- **Core or Common Subjects:** Broad areas of knowledge, skill and appreciation with which all the learners must

be made conversant and these find place in the curriculum. Core subjects, e.g. Mathematics, Science, Crafts, Language, Basic subjects have to be included.
- Leisure: The curriculum should prepare the child for the use of leisure time. Literature, art, music, sports, NCC, NSS, etc. as per learners' interest, encourage them to occupy the leisure part of education. The capacity to enjoy leisure greatly determines a man's capacity to work.
- Sensitivity: Curriculum should be sensitive to the feeling of the students' community and nation.

Stages of Curriculum
Torres and Stanton described the four stages in curriculum process:

1. The Directive stage
It lays foundations for all other stages by
- Identifying the beliefs, knowledge and concepts which forms the basis of the curriculum
- Formulation of theoretical framework in the selection and sequencing of content, done by
    - Systematic gathering of information from the literature
    - Exploration of common beliefs about the nature of nursing
    - Formulation of philosophy of the curriculum

2. Formative stage
- Overall design of the curriculum will takes place based on philosophy of educational institution, Program and the nature of nursing
- Objectives (general and specific) will be formulated
- Content mapping.

3. Functional stage/Implementation stage
- The curriculum assumes more practical form, i.e. implementation
- Teaching methods and learning experiences will be planned and executed (theory and practical/lab and clinical).

4. Evaluative stage
- Input evaluation—How much the students gain the knowledge in the course, e.g. problem-solving abilities, Strengths achieved during programe
- Evaluation for continued learning. It provides feedback for students which areas he is good or the areas which he need improvement in learning
- Concurrent and Terminal evaluation—Internal Assessments (Tests, Assignments,Study Guides), Final (Theory and Practical, Viva) examinations
- Output evaluation—Achievement of the characteristics identified in the directive stage
- Evaluation for curriculum revision—It involves assessment of the total curriculum package and present needs of community in Nation and in Globe.

Curriculum Planning and Development
- A process in which participants at many levels make decisions about the purposes of learning, teaching-learning situation
- It is the process of gathering, reviewing and analyzing, sorting, selecting, balancing and synthesizing relevant information from many sources in order to design those experiences that will assist learners in attaining the goals of curriculum
- It is the orderly study and improvement of schooling in light of stated objectives.

Characteristics
- It is a continuous process
- It takes place at many levels
- It involves many groups, decisions about a variety of planning and issues
- It is ultimately concerned with the experiences of the learners.

Steps in Curriculum Construction

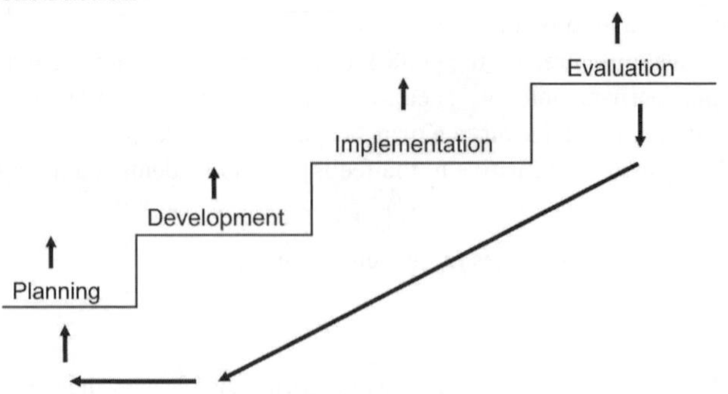

Fig. 3.5: Steps in curriculum construction

- The subjects and activities in the curriculum should be towards capacity building of students in the areas of creation, construction, observation, investigation and problem - solving
- Periodically the teacher has to evaluate the curriculum to meet the up-to-date with the modern trend and changes in the health field
- Curriculum should be prepared from social point of view, society is not static and so curriculum development is an ongoing activity
- Development of nursing curriculum is educational Institutions' responsibility. It will be based on philosophy, resources, need and other conditions
- The core content will be common to all the curriculums in the state or country prescribed by a statutory body, e.g. Indian Nursing Council, Universities, Boards
- The subject matter and experiences in a particular school for their students and is developed by its own curriculum committee (Principal, Administrator, Senior teaching Faculty).

Fig. 3.6: Interrelationship between phases and steps

1. Planning

- Determine the needs and purposes, identification and analysis of existing situation
- Formulate the philosophy of nursing educational program
- Formulate Objectives based on community needs, resources availability, nursing roles, demands placed on nursing profession, philosophy and purposes of the educational program
- Involve the influential personalities in preparing curriculum construction e.g. Nurse educators, Nurse administrators, Nurse leaders and Nurse practitioners
- Constitute a committee for curriculum preparation
- Decide the philosophy and policy of the organization, e.g. student recruitment, type of educational programe, method of teaching, group involved, duration of the period, staffing requirement e.g. Teaching, Supervised clinical practice, Teaching-learning activities, Selection of learning experience – theory and practice, instructional time, e.g. supervised clinical and community nursing practice, self-activity, self-study, co-curricular and extra-curricular activities, learning methods and materials etc.

2. Development phase

Preparation, Organization and sequencing of:

- Theoretical Instruction Hours
- Practicals/clinical Hours
- Supervised clinical practice

- Master Rotation plan, Clinical Rotation plan for total batch, specific group of students and Individual student rotation plan
- Preparation of teaching-learning materials, AV aids
- Curriculum committee reviews the progress, identifies constraints, assess needs for modification and formation of other standing committees for management of the curriculum.

3. Implementation phase

- Actual conduction of teaching-learning activities (learner centred, socialized methods)
- Conducting practical sessions in laboratory - institutional settings and in Clinical Fields (Hospital and Community)
- Refinement of teaching-learning methods
- Assessment of student performance
- Student guidance and counselling services
- Health services
- Curriculum committee meeting
- Necessary action need to be carried out.

4. Evaluation phase

- Assess
  - The level of students' learning which is manifested through knowledge, skills, attitudes eg: Concurrent and terminal evaluation, Practical examination and Viva
  - Teaching-learning process
  - Effective use of AV aids
  - Students activities undertaken in the community and institution settings
  - Effectiveness of educational experiences.

Curriculum Organization

a. Articulation

Poses three problems in its nature

- Interdisciplinary problem.
- Correlation of Theory with Laboratory and Clinicals (Hospital and Community)
- Nature of the relationship between the school and the current life outside the school.

Team teaching is effective to overcome the problems. There are many opportunities to talk and plan their teaching around common areas and themes and cooperate in an interdisciplinary approach.

b. Continuity

The conditions whereby the learner will move smoothly from stage to stage and from class to class in an educational system. School will plan the activities whereby the learner will meet the needs e.g. to adjust to the transition of the student from home environment to school environment and fully engaged with curricular, co curricular and extracurricular activities, whereby the learner will have the continuity in the educational practice.

c. Balance

A balance has to be sought in the curriculum provided by the school subjects to be offered, required and programs of studies to be recommended, time allotments for various subjects and activities like theory classes, demonstrations, clinical, Leisure time activities(Extracurricular), Co-curricular, the use of books and other educational media, etc. More significant dimension of balance is that curriculum actually selected by and/or experienced by each learner. If the curriculum provided is restricted and inflexible, there is little opportunity for the selection of learning experiences and individuals suffer from a poor and ill balanced curriculum. In the ideal situation balance is achieved in the individuals' own curriculum as he or she becomes competent in each of the areas for which provision is made in the curriculum.

Patterns of Curriculum Organization

1. Student centred curriculum

Programe has the students' view. Education is life and since life is ever changing, there could be flexible curriculum.

In this, the student need something, perceive something, do something and get satisfaction from the resulting experience. The whole learning process would become vivid and hence more valuable. It is related to learners' interest, hence learners have to be active; activity is built around psychological problems. The program is flexible, democratic and community related. The student centred plan is in accordance with interests and problems of the learners, without any regard to the boundaries of subject matter so that correlation is really possible. It lacks balance, as it leans away from content and the central core of educational materials and the learner is interested in play and not enough in study. Too many transitory interests and topics included and the principle of continuity in the curriculum is violated.

Characteristics
- The interests of the learner will facilitate his learning, hence the program is more life related.
- Cooperation, common interests, working together are unifying elements brings about growth in life-related skills.
- Learners are active partners in the curriculum, individual needs are essential ingredients of the curriculum.
- Flexibility in nature – content, areas of learning, use of instructional materials.
- Suitable resources has to be organized e.g. reference books, news papers, journals, excursions, libraries, films, audio tapes and TV etc.

2. Correlated curriculum

Two or more subjects often exist in a school, side by side with no apparent connection. In some cases, these points are 'natural', e.g. mathematical formulae needed for solving problems in physics or chemistry, Basic Principles and Practices of Nursing or in Nursing Foundations – Calculation of Drugs and Solutions.

Correlation necessitates cooperative planning, mutual help and understanding among the various teachers before any cooperative project can be undertaken.

While teaching Nursing subjects, Theory has to correlate with Practical demonstration and Clinical posting of the students in specific wards.

Limitations
- It is very difficult to break through the logical arrangement of the various aspects of the subject arrangement of human experience
- Correlation of subjects will be only casual and teaching cannot be sufficient to integrate human experience
- There is a likelihood of the attempts at correlation being largely forced with little reference to real sequence in human experience
- Attempts at correlation usually come from the teachers
- There is a limit, beyond which it is not possible to provide all experiences

3. Integrated or fused curriculum

It means 'blended together. A pouring together of subjects and students might provide a stronger base for learning, e.g. postbasic B .Sc. (N) program, all the subjects which basic students learned in four years, will be studied within two years as they had preliminary training in diploma course.

4. Core curriculum

It is a concept
1. According to John Dewey's "Philosophy of experimentalism" gave concepts of core curriculum.
   - Focus of learning upon fundamental human activities
   - Learning viewed of continuous reconstruction of experience
   - Problem-solving.
2. Basic democratic values and the dynamic changes in political and social ideas, cultural factors.
3. Acceptance of cognitive theories of learning. It is a dynamic, organic process.
4. Elements

- General education aspect of all teaching, regardless of social status or vocational choice of the student
- All students can benefit by it
- Problem-centred
- The process of learning is important, e.g. in preparation for living in a democratic society, the learner should get first hand experience in the fundamental processes of democratic living
- Cooperative pre-planning by teachers. Teachers pool their ideas to develop resource units
- Teacher- pupil planning daily in the class-room
- The emphasis in core is on total growth of the pupil (socially, intellectually, physically, emotionally and spiritually)
- The core pattern is flexible
- The utilization of learners' ideas, allows for adjustments within the broad framework of the unit under consideration
- As special need arises, the program can be adjusted, e.g. the teacher can give a short break at anytime, when she feels that the pupils need it, instead of waiting for a bell
- A long block of time at a stretch is desirable
- The core pattern is oriented towards guidance and counselling.

5. Basic education curriculum

It is a vital, dynamic, meaningful curriculum related to the life with experiences of the learner.

Mahatma Gandhi's Views

- Education for life through living. Productive, socially useful and creative work in it, in which the students participate regardless of caste, creed or social status. Learners will live and work in the educational environment which prepares them to maintain social order
- Basic crafts, e.g. spinning, weaving, agriculture, dairy farming and cottage industries
- The principle of correlation with the craft and knowledge
- An activity curriculum for productive learning is based on 'learning by doing' principle
- Self-sufficiency, Education is free and compulsory for all
- Mother tongue as the medium of instruction
- Parents and the community are a means of establishing a close relationship between education within the school and outside. They will be involved in school activities as much as possible, so that the school is an expression of the aspirations of the community.

6. Subject centered curriculum—The traditional concept of curriculum

Type of curriculum content is organized in terms of subjects. It includes different branches of knowledge according to the level of understanding at various stages.

- The school has a major role in transmitting cultural heritage from one generation to another through the medium of various subjects
- The learner's cognitive functioning pattern follows the adult's functioning
- Various disciplines or subjects would allow for the accommodation of the expansion of knowledge
- It has an integral order and it can be presented in a sequence
- Subjects can be presented in suitable units or branches
- The teacher has focused his effort and attention on making students learn the items in the subjects and courses of study according to fixed syllabi in a rigid set pattern to enable them to pass a set of examinations
- The learner was given knowledge and skills which would fit him to become a mature and successful adult
- He was prepared to live in the future.

Limitations
- It is bookish
- It is narrowly conceived
- It stresses knowledge aspect
- It does not adequately reflect life activities.

Subject-centered curriculum	Student-centered curriculum
1. It is structured around subject	1. It is centered around learners
2. It aims at increasing the knowledge of subjects	2. It aims at promotion of knowledge of the learners
3. Subject matter is selected and organized before the actual teaching-learning situations	3. Subject matter is selected and organized according to teaching-learning situations
4. The teacher is the controller and director of curriculum structure	4. Curriculum is initiated and organized by the learners
5. Emphasis is on teaching facts and presenting information for the sake of possible future use	5. Emphasis is on matters, which are useful for the present and future also
6. Stress is on the teaching of specific habits and skills as separate aspects of learning	6. Stress is on integrated learning of habits and skills
7. There is uniformity with respect to learning situations	7. Variability of exposure is advocated
8. Education is viewed as schooling and stress is laid on the teaching of the subject	8. Education is viewed as an allround growth and development of the learner
9. The subject matter is organized before it is presented in the class	9. Subject matter is planned with the cooperation of the learner
10. Instruction is imparted for the sake of knowledge	10. Instruction is imparted for the sake of improving the life of the learner
11. Facts are considered more important	11. More importance is given to the process of acquiring facts
12. Memorization of facts is given prominence	12. Stress is laid on building skills
13. Subject-based curriculum regards education as schooling	13. Education is regarded as a process of learning for progress
14. Education is confined to a general pattern of instruction.	14. Education is regarded as a means to prepare the learner to be a socially efficient individual.

Subject curriculum	Experience curriculum
It is in terms of subjects, centered around subject	It is in terms of experience
The subject-matter is selected and organized before the teaching situations	All learners during learning-teaching situation select and organize cooperatively the subject-matter
It stresses the teaching of facts, imparting information for its own sake or for the possible future	It stresses the practical aspects of life
It is isolated from life	Emphasis is on correlation with life
There is no correlation of subjects	It stresses correlated knowledge
It is rigid and uniform.	It is flexible, it caters to individual needs.

EDUCATIONAL OBJECTIVES/LEARNING OBJECTIVES

Introduction

'If you are not certain of where you are going, you may very well end up somewhere else (and not even know it)'.

Education is a process, the chief goal of which is to bring change in human behavior. Every individual should have access to a type of education that permits maximum development of his potential and strengthen his abilities/capacities.

In planning effective curriculum, the objectives of the different courses of study has to be clearly defined and laid down, so that the courses are well guided. Any work or simple activity or assignments etc. everything in the curriculum has to be done with a purpose or goal oriented; one should have in mind, what he has to achieve and what efforts are required to achieve the goal or objective. The fulfillment of the task becomes easy, when he know the purpose or goal. For any educational program has to be effective the purposes and objectives are to be clearly stated so that it is easy to select the right subject matter, the clinical experiences and the right methods to evaluate the students' achievements and the teaching-learning process. Direct relationship between the clarity of purposes of the school, objectives and the effectiveness of the program. Before formulating the objectives of nursing educational program, the needs of learners, need of organization, society, community at large, nation to be considered. The learners have to be trained specifically for the tasks they have to perform, taking into account the circumstances under which they will work. So it is essential to prepare the objectives before planning of the curriculum, if it is modifying automatically the objectives of the program also has to be modified accordingly.

It is imperative for the planners to have a clear understanding about the behavioral outcomes expected in the students for whom the curriculum is being developed. Thus the objectives are desirable outcomes of intended actions through the mode of education. The active participation of teacher and learner in the teaching-learning situation is maximally needed.

Definitions

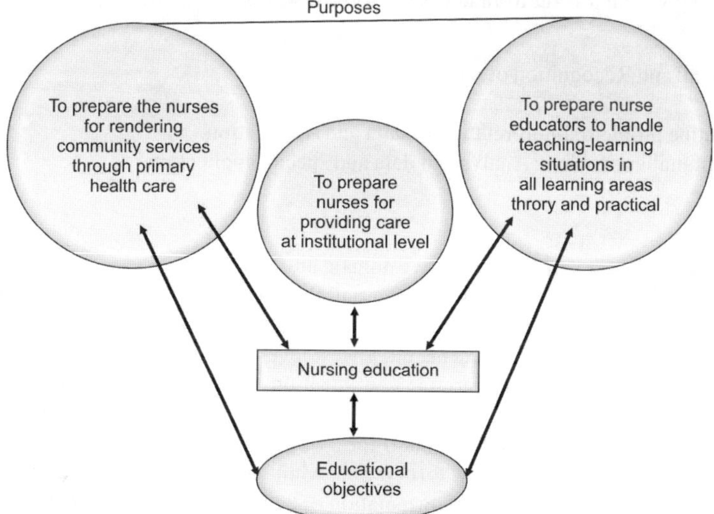

Fig. 3.7: Purposes of educational objectives

'The result sought by the learner at the end of the educational program, i.e. what the students should be able to do at the end of a learning period, that they could not do before hand' – JJ Guilbert.
'Desired end results or goals are expected or anticipated end results'.
'Objectives are the behaviors to be displayed by a learner', aims are for the teacher and the objectives are for the learners—It is 'learner centered or behavior centered and subject centered' which will be achieved through the support and guidance of the teacher.
'The statements of those changes in behavior which are desired as a result of specific learner and teacher activity which is a two-way process'.

Importance and Meaning

The words, 'aims'/'goals'/'objectives'/'targets' are often interchangeably used in relation to the educational purposes of a school programe (Fig. 3.7). The educational objectives are expressions of what a teacher has the hope with their teaching, their students will be accomplishing his goals. In education process, the learners should be able to demonstrate the possession of a large quality of facts, concepts, greater ability to manipulate in more complex ways and greater ability to do things based upon complex manipulative abilities. Educational objectives are policy statements of direction and provides foundation of the entire educative structure. These are statements, which express specifically and in measurable terms, an attitude that will be developed cognitive or psychomotor skills that the students would be able to do as a result of a prescribed treatment method or mode of instruction. Educational objectives are broader and they are related to current educational system, schools' philosophy and relevance to health needs of society is the essential quality of educational objectives.

Taxonomy of Educational Objectives

A systematic organization of objectives into three domains to help the teachers in precise formulation and evaluates the results of a system of education (for both terminal and concurrent evaluation), it helps the students to prepare for examinations to obtain the desired end results.

1. Categories in the Cognitive Domain (Intellectual Skills and Knowledge)

McGuire (1963) described the levels in cognitive domain.

    a. Recall of facts: Remembering the facts, principles, processes, patterns and methods necessary for efficient performance of a professional task.

    b. Interpretation of data: The process of application or use of ideas, principles, methods to deal with a new phenomenon or situation.

    c. Problem solving: Relating to diagnosis, treatment, organization, etc. Problem solving includes finding solutions for a problem arising from new situations. It serves as a guide.

Levels

1. Knowledge, Recall and Recognition of meaning.
2. Generalization.
3. Solving of a routine problem, Interpretation of data and Application.
4. Solving of an unfamiliar problem: Analysis of data and special application.
5. Synthesis.
6. Evaluation.

Bloom (1956) described the categories in cognitive domain are:

Knowledge: Remembering of previously learned material. It represents the lowest level of learning outcome.

Comprehension: The ability to grasp the meaning of material. The learning outcome goes one step beyond the simple understanding of material and represents the lowest level of understanding.

Application: The ability to use learned material in new situation, it requires a higher level of understanding.

Analysis: The ability to breakdown material into its component parts. A higher intellectual level as it requires an understanding of both the content and the structural form of the material.

Synthesis: It is the ability to put together to form a new whole learning outcomes in the area and stress to creates behavior, with major emphasis on the formulation of new patterns or structures.

Evaluation: The ability to judge the value of material for a given purpose. The judgments are to be based on definite criteria.

Taxonomy of educational objectives (Bloom's taxonomy)

Objectives	Mental process or abilities
Knowledge	Recall Recognize
Comprehension	See relationship Cite example Discriminate Classify Interest Verify Generalize
Application	Reason Formulate Establish Infer
Analysis	Predict Analyze
Synthesis	Synthesize
Evaluate	Evaluate

Cognitive objectives and associated words

Objective	Associated action verbs
Knowledge	Define, State, List, Name, Write, Recall, Recognize, Label, Underline, select, Reproduce, Measure
Comprehension	Identify, Justify, Select, Indicate, Illustrate, Represent, Name, Formulate, Explain, Judge, Contrast, Classify
Application	Predict, Select, Assess, Explain, Choose, Find, Show, Demonstrate, Construct, Compute, Use, Perform
Analysis	Analyze, Identify, Conclude, Differentiate, Select, Separate, Compare, Contrast, Justify, Resolve, Breakdown, Criticize
Synthesis	Combine, Restate, Summarize, Precise, Argue, Discuss, Organize, Derive, Select, Relate, Generalize, Conclude
Evaluation	Judge, Evaluate, Determine, Recognize, Support, Defend, Attack, Criticize, Identify, Avoid, Select, Choose

2. Conative or Psychomotor Skills or Domain of Practical Skill

It deals with the routine actions carried out by the student. The student is able to perform a practical act automatically and with a high degree of precision and efficiency, having effective control over the practical skill (Table 3.8).

Three levels are described:

a. **Immitation:** The student, exposed to an observable action makes an attempt to copy it step by step, guided by an impulse to imitate, he needs a model.

b. **Control:** The student is able to demonstrate a skill according to instructions and not merely on the basis of observation. He also begins to differentiate between one set of skills and another and be able to choose the one required, he starts to adapt at handling instruments.

c. **Automatism:** A high degree of proficiency is attained in using the skill, which now requires only a minimum of energy.

3. Domain of Attitudes or Affective Domain (Communication skill)

Behavior representative of feeling or conviction. An objective dealing with emotions or feelings indicated by words, e.g. interest, appreciation, enthusiasm, motivation and attitudes. These are reflective of the values.

A persistent disposition to act either positively or negatively towards a person, group, object, value or situation. It refers to interpersonal relations. Three levels are identified:

a. **Receptivity or attention:** Sensitivity to the existence of a certain phenomenon; willingness to receive.

b. **Response:** Sufficient interest in the phenomenon noticed to do something about it.

c. **Internalization:** Perception of a phenomenon affecting values. This enables you to adapt your attitude to the other person as if you were experiencing the same phenomenon yourself , e.g. On the death of a child, Nurses' attitude to members of their family will show them that you care about their grief and are ready to help them to get over from the situation.

Components of a Complete Statement of Objectives (Fig. 3.9)

1. **Condition:** Behavior can be displayed under certain condition. The condition will favor the learner to display the desired behaviour. It relates to the aspects of

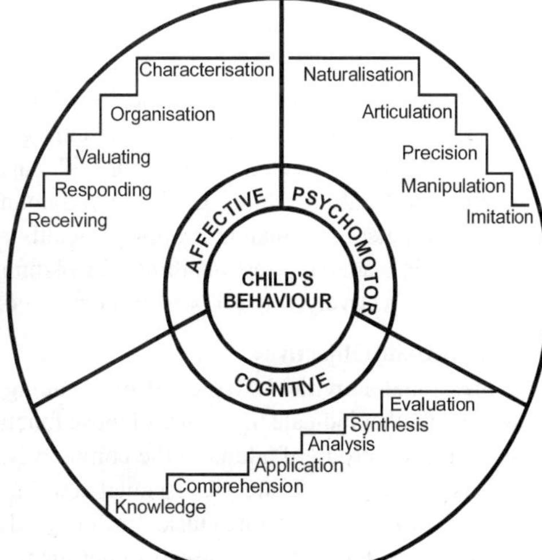

Fig. 3.8: Objectives of cognitive, affective and psychomotor domain

circumstance, e.g. a learner will be attending a workshop, then only he will be able to explain the concept of title of workshop.

2. **Behavior:** Manifested in action, what the student must perform. An objective in behavioural terms indicates what behavior, a learner should display after going through the unit eg: After studying Psychology (I year) and Psychiatry (III year) classes, the learner will be able to distinguish normal and abnormal behavior.

3. **Standard/Criterion/level:** Acceptable level of performance expected from the student. It relates to the aspects denoting the extent to which learning has taken place. While stating objectives,

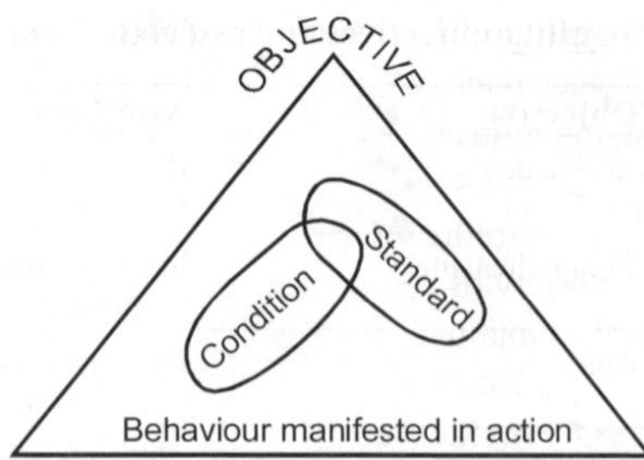

Fig. 3.9: Components of stated objective

teacher has to set some 'norms' for the behavior to be displayed. The learner must know, to what level they should be able to perform (time, accuracy, minimum number of correct, responses etc.). The standard of objectives also depends on the level of the learners, You are writing for and also what we want them to achieve, e.g. a standard set for 1st year student for a procedure is not the same as we expect from a final year student of the same program.

Data Necessary for Formulation of Educational Objectives

Health needs, demands and resources of society, Services to the patient (list of tasks), Services to the community (list of tasks), The profession itself, The students, Progress in sciences, Scientific methods, Statement of the school's philosophy, Level of professional competence to be attained, The students' background, level of education, Statutory minimum requirements, Teaching, physical and clinical resources available, Future demands on nursing in terms of advanced technology and increased use of them in therapeutic services, Expected responsibilities for different nursing positions and relevance to the professional tasks of the personnel to be trained.

Types of Educational Objectives

1. **General objectives or Professional functions:** Correspond to the functioning of the types of health personnel trained in an establishment. The course objectives must be in harmony with the general curriculum objectives of the programe of the school. For example:

   a. Providing preventive and curative care to the individual and the community in health and sickness.

   b. Health education of the public will depend on the population's general level of education.

   c. The graduates of the new baccalaureate nursing programe will be prepared to function as a generalist with beginning competencies in a specialized area of nursing.

   The graduate will be prepared to function in a variety of settings and be able to:

   - Obtain health histories and make general health assessments
   - Provide safe and competent care in emergency situations and acute illnesses
   - Provide supportive care to persons with chronic or terminal health problems
   - Provide health teaching, guidance and counseling
   - Assist persons to maintain optimal health status
   - Provide leadership responsibility for planning and evaluating nursing care
   - Work effectively with all persons concerned with health care problems.

2. **Intermediate Objectives**

   a. Professional activities: Arrived at by breaking down professional functions into components (activities) which together indicate the nature of those functions. For example, planning and carrying out blood sampling session for a group of adults in the community.

   These components are professional activities which in turn can be broken down into more specific acts that are called, "professional tasks" as long as they can be measured against given criteria. Sometimes, there can be several intermediate levels rather than a single one. Intermediate objectives reflect the health needs of a population living in a given context. It acts only a means or working instrument and not an end in itself. It was drawn up as a basis for choosing instruments of evaluation for measuring the skills of students.

b. Institutional objectives: The graduate of the new baccalaureate nursing program will be prepared to function as a generalist with beginning competencies in a specialized area of nursing. For example: The graduate will be prepared to function in a variety of settings and be able to:
  - Obtain health histories and make health assessments
  - Provide safe and competent care in emergency situations and acute illnesses.

c. Specific or Instructional Objectives/Professional tasks.

Instructional objectives are descriptions of performance the instruction is expected to produce:
  - Defining objectives help to identify the terminal outcomes of instruction in terms of observable performance of learners, these outcomes are to be presented in behavioral terms.

I. Professional tasks and specific (instructional) educational objectives (Fig. 4.10):

Corresponding to (or derived from) precise professional tasks whose results are observable and measurable against given criteria.

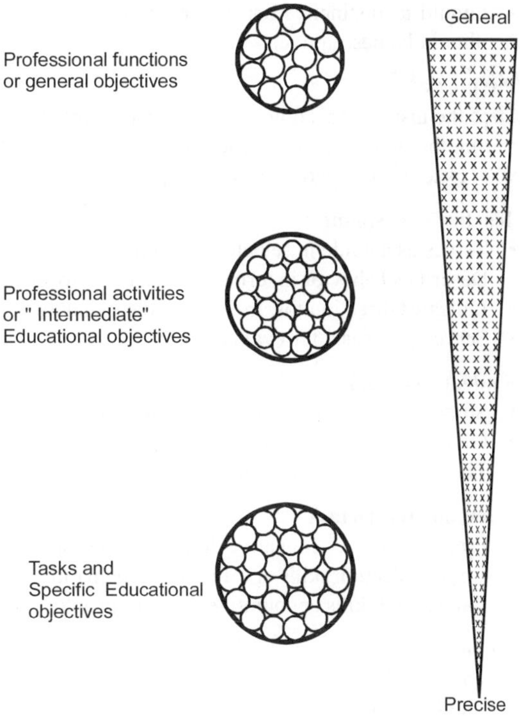

Qualities—Logical (The objective must be internally consistent) , Feasible (It must be ensured that what the student is required to do can actually be done, within the time allowed and with the facilities to handle), Observable (Unless there is some means of observing progress towards an objective, it will be impossible to tell whether the objective has been achieved), Measurable (The objective must include an indication of acceptable level of performance on the part of the student. The existence of a criterion for measurement will make it easier to choose or to construct a valid evaluation mechanism), Relevant free of any superfluous material but cover every point relating to the aim in view, Unequivocal: "Loaded words" (words open to a wide range of interpretations) should not be used, to avoid any possibility of misunderstandings.

General

Professional functions or general objectives

Professional activities or " Intermediate" Educational objectives

Tasks and Specific Educational objectives

Precise

Fig. 3.10: Relationship between professional acts in the health field and educational objectives

For example:

Many Interpretations	Fewer Interpretations
To know	To write
To discuss	To identify
To understand	To differentiate
To really understand	To solve
To appreciate	To list
To believe	To compare
To have faith in	To contrast

Characteristics
- Should be written in behavioral terms (what the students must do)
- Should reflect the condition (under what circumstances)
- Should reflect the standard (with what degree of skill)
- Should be reasonable in number of behavioral changes expected out of the teaching unit should not be too many or too less usually 4 to 5 behavioral objectives are stated for a unit
- Should be consistent with unit theme and related to each other and to the unit
- Should be approximately of some level of generality or specificity

- Should be distinctive but not completely independent
- Should be descriptive.

Purposes

State the instructional objectives in clear, simple language has advantages for both teacher and students. After stating the objective the teacher will be clear about the purpose of the lesson/unit and the student will know what exactly are expected to achieve/perform (Fig. 3.11).

Teacher's viewpoint

- Serves as a guide in selection of important/vital content and desirable subject matter
- Describes behavior in terms of student performance
- Indicates direction towards which the behavior is to be geared
- Serves as a basis for evaluation.

Student's viewpoint

- Students know the worthiness of the program in terms of cost (time, energy and money)
- Give direction to the students towards in-depth study
- The expected achievement at the end of the course.

Components of a task

- Practical skills or cognative domain (initiation)
- Communication skills or effective domain (attitudes) feelings (conviction)
- Intellectual skills or cognitive domain (problem-solving)

Elements

- To act/task
- The content
- The condition
- Criteria.

II. The objectives are classified into:

Teacher centred objectives: e.g. to develop teaching skills, to use Audio-Visual aids effectively in teaching situation. Student centred objectives: e.g. to understand the subject in-depth.

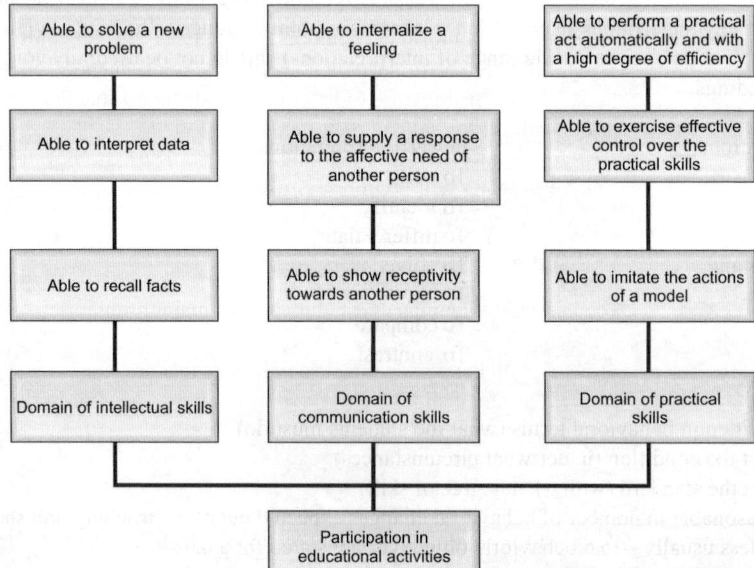

Fig. 3.11: Schematic representation of purposes of educational objective

Abbreviate, Accent, Act, Add, Administer, Aid, Alphabetic, Allow for, Alter, Analyze, Answer, Apply, Appraise, Arrange, Articulate, Assist, Ask, Assemble, Attempt, Attend, Audit, Avoid, Begin, Bend, Bisect, Blow, Bring, Build, Calculate, Calibrate, Care for, Categorize, Change, Capitalise, Chart, Check, Choose, Circle, Cite, Clarify, Classify, Clear, Clean, Close, Collaborate, Color, Collect, Combine, Communicate, Compare, Compile, Complete, Compliment, Compute, Conclude, Conduct, Connect, Construct, Contrast, Contribute, Control, Convert, Cooperate, Correct, Create, Criticize, Decide, Decrease, Deduce, Defend, Define, Delimit, Demonstrate, Derive, Describe, Design, Designate, Detect, Determine, Develop, Diagram, Differentiate, Direct, Discover, Discriminate, Display, Dissect, Distinguish, Divide, Do, Draw, Edit, Effect, Encourage, Enumerate, Enunciate, Establish, Evaluate, Examine, Exchange, Execute, Explain, Extract, Extrapolate, Facilitate, Fill, Find, Follow, Formulate, Furnish, Generalize, Generate, Get, Give, Guide, Hold, Identify, Illustrate, Implant, Implement, Increase, Indicate, Induce, Infer, Inform, Insert, Integrate, Isolate, Justify, Label, Lead, List, Locate, Maintain, Make, Manipulate, Map, Match, Measure, Meet, Mobilize, Modify, Move, Name, Note, Narrate, Obtain, Omit, Operate, Oppose, Order, Organize, Outline, Paraphrase, Participate, Perform, Pick, Place, Plan, Point, Position, Practise, Predict, Prepare, Present, Prevent, Prognose, Protect, Provide, Persue, Put, Raise, Read, Recite, Reassure, Rearrange, Record, Reconstruct, Recount, Reduce, Regroup, Relate, Remove, Reorder, Reorganize, Rephrase, Replace, Request, Reset, Resolve, Respond, Restate, Safeguard, Select, Send, Separate, Serve, Set, Share, Simplify, Solve, Sort, Speak, Specify, Start, State, Store, Structure, Suggest, Supply, Support, Synthesis, Tabulate, Take responsibility for, Teach, Tie, Time, Trace, Translate, Treat, Use, Utilize, Verify, Wash, Weigh, Work and Write.

LEARNING EXPERIENCES

Introduction

Learning is a multifarious job, which the child starts soon after the birth and continue throughout the life till the death. The child learns first at home and in the safe environment. The individual will face learning situations in their life. Some of the activities, the child will learn by observation during his childhood. Mother is a first teacher for the child. Parents and family members has to teach the child, how to handle the situations. As the child grows he will be going to the school. In school, the teacher has to select suitable content, activities, methods and devices of teaching in order to make best learning. Keeping in view the aims of teaching on one hand and the children, their varied needs, capacities and interest on the other hand, Teacher has to create learning situations in which the various powers of the learner are exercised leading to the balanced development of his personality in a integrated and harmonious manner (the 3 domains like cognitive, conative and affective domain).

In nursing education, optimum learning situations have to be provided. Inquiry and discovery are needed. The learning situation should develop potentials in a student nurse and enable the student to achieve the goals and influence their behavior in positive directions. The elements of identification and levels are important in order to create teacher-learner relationship. The various learning experiences during the course of study within the program and over the time period will help him to perform tasks satisfactorily.

Definitions

Learning is, 'any relatively permanent change or modification of behavior that results as a result of practice or experience'—*Murthy and others*.

'Every modification in behaviour to meet the environmental requirements'.

'It is the process by which behaviour is originated or changes practice or training'.

'It is an episode in which a motivated individual attempts to adopt his behaviour so as to succeed in a situation which he perceives as requiring action to attain a goal '– *Pressy*.

Experience

It is the lesson one learns as a result of or from his/her interaction with people in various and varied situations and/or with the environment. The word, 'experience' comes from 'experiri' meaning 'to try out' it means anything lived or undergone.

Learning Experience

Deliberately planned experiences in selected situations where students actively interact and participate, which result in desirable change of behavior in the students. All the learning experiences planned and guided by the faculty to achieve their stated objectives, the learning experiences must be selected in relation to the desired objectives. The learning experience is a mental or physical reaction for seeing, hearing or doing the things to be learnt and gains meaning and understanding useful in solving new problems. Learning experiences are reaction of the learner where he will learn in effective manner. The learner has to be active in order to learn. Teachers should provide some activity in which the learner can react in a desirable manner. Learning experience must be carefully planned to bring specific change in learner's behavior.

For example: Applying nursing process principles in rendering qualitative care.

Teachers have to create formal or informal learning situations, which increases the learner's ability. The teaching methods employed by the teacher directly influence the effectiveness of the student.

Teaching-learning Unit

Unified learning experience involving comprehensive problems or projects which are important to the students in nursing, thus permitting inclusion of knowledge component in a course selected, structured and unified in comprehensive problems or projects by focusing on objectives.

Objectives of Learning Experiences

- The sources which influence the selection of learning experiences and the experiences selected in and of themselves determine in some degree the way in which the curriculum will be arranged or organized.
- In educational program, the teacher should make an effort to provide appropriate experiences both in hospital and in community health field, to the learner so that the changes in the behavior of the learners take place in the right direction as outlined in the objectives of the program.

1. Imparting the knowledge

Knowledge, which has imparted in a way so as to facilitate effective learning on the part of the learners. Educational pedagogists have attempted to formulate some general procedure for the conduct of the course.

a. *Preparation:* A learner has to be prepared to receive new knowledge.

b. *Presentation:* The teacher has to select the subject matter according to the needs, abilities and mental level of the learners has to be arranged in a logical sequence. Teacher has to introduce the lesson and announces the aim clearly, proceeds to present the new knowledge marks the actual commencement of the lesson.

c. *Comparison of association:* The facts or ideas presented should be compared or associated with one another. It enhances the process of assimilation and sharpens the mental faculties of children and involves high mental process than mere memorizing and recollecting.

d. *Generalization:* When mind has comprehended a new place of knowledge and compared it with the old, arrive at a general idea underlying various ideas and formulating some laws or principles especially in an inductive lesson. It develops the independent thinking of the pupils.

e. *Application:* When a rule, formula or principle has been evolved, it should be tested and verified by applying it to new situation. The ability to apply the knowledge in the form of generalizations to new problem situations explicitly as well as implicitly. The individual can identify and explain the relevant principles.

2. The acquisition of skills

Skill includes a wide range of activities like capabilities, cultivation of habits, etc. For example Carrying out Nursing Procedures like conduction of labor, bed making.

Steps in skills

- Preparation
- Presentation
- Statement and formulation of rules
- Practice—Demonstration and return demonstration
- Correction and application.

3. Development of esthetic sense or taste (Appreciation):

It aims at aesthetic development in the learners, provide them with emotional experience and stability in them. The teacher provides conducive environment for the success of an appreciation.

4. Motivation:

Motivation is the vital aspect to gain mastery over the knowledge for the students as well as for the teachers and administrators so that the teaching will be effective and results in effective learning.

Criteria for Selection of Learning Experiences

- To bring desirable behavioral changes in the learner
- To achieve the desired objectives
- Learning experience selected should be consistent with the educational philosophy of the school and lead to the fulfillment of proximate aims or objectives or goals
- Learning experience has to be varied and flexible enough, keeping in mind the learners' ability and background to undergo the desired change of behavior and not going beyond their particular stages of development, e.g. a first year student, who has no knowledge of growth and development of the child, should not be posted in pediatric ward or well baby clinic to monitor growth and development, this will be beyond his stage of development in learning
- Provide sufficient opportunity to practice or self-activity, the kind of behavior implied in the objective so that the transfer of knowledge remembered, skill acquired and desirable attitudes become habitual, e.g. students have to apply the skills in application of nursing process, in caring of clients, students have to be encouraged the principles and steps of nursing process for every client in all settings which will develop the skill, knowledge and right attitudes towards 'Nursing process'
- Learning experience should provide opportunity for the development of independent thinking and study, decision-making, good judgment, intellectual resourcefulness, selfdiscipline and sound integrity of purpose as well as the mastery of many different kinds of knowledge and skill. For example when nursing a client with unconscious, the student is allowed to take decision (under guidance) how and when to maintain Glasgow Coma Scale
- Learning experience should be adapted to the needs and concern of the student so that the learner will obtain satisfaction from behaving in the manner implied to the objective
- Learning experiences are arranged in a manner that provides continuity, sequential developmental, logical, correlation and integration of theory and practice which will facilitate effective learning, e.g. maintenance of body temperature, to meet this goal, the student has to learn the physiological process of temperature, practice the procedure in the laboratory, in clinical field student has to get an opportunity to meausre and record temperature applying cold applications (if need arises) and meeting the needs of the client this will provide for continuity, completion and integration of theory and practice
- Learning experiences are selected and arranged to give the appropriate emphasis and weightage according to the relative importance of the various learning experiences and contents, e.g. if the teacher post the first year student in OPD, he will learn what are the types of data to be collected, in 2nd year he/she will try to observe and identify the diagnosis with appropriate data and guides the client to solve his problems
- Learning experience is consistent with the aims of democratic society
- Learning experiences are structured so that, the central and the contributory objectives of the unit and the course will be attained
- Encourage and promote motivation at appropriate times and in a manner that will stimulate the curiosity of the students and challenge them to continue expenditure of effort
- Planned with full awareness of proceeding and forthcoming learning for the particular group of the students
- Provide variety of learning experiences with selected content
- Learning experience has to involve all the senses in the learning process to achieve maximum learning
- By learning experience maximize the responsibilities of the learner
- Utilize the resources and media in organizing learning experience
- Improvise the suitable materials when situation arises to meet the needs of the client
- Create interest and desire for more learning
- Learning experience should be planned ahead of time so that the learner will be prepared to meet his need, reinforce those experiences, which are provided in the coming week

- Provide learning experience, which will provide deeper and broader understanding and increased skill for the students.
- Learning experience in one area of instruction is related to (interdependent) other areas of learning, e.g. knowledge of Anatomy and Physiology, Basic Sciences, Behavioral Sciences in 1st year will help the students to understand 2nd and 3rd years subjects like Medical-Surgical nursing, Pediatric nursing and Psychiatry Nursing
- Provide learning experience in chronological order, place the events in terms of time in which they occur, e.g. place the student in advanced clinical areas in 3rd or final year; 1st year student can be placed in Medical, Surgical wards to practice basic nursing principles
- Use maxims of teaching in planning learning experience e.g. simple to complex, concrete to abstract etc.
- Learning experiences are planned and evaluated cooperatively by the teacher and the student so that the varied experiences, which are provided, will be effective, interesting and useful
- Provide the students with the opportunity to practice the behaviors sought.

Components of Learning Experience (fig. 3.12)
1. Learning situation
2. Learning activity
3. Learning experience–Theoretical and clinical/practical
   It is concerned with the decision about the content of subject matter and clinical practice

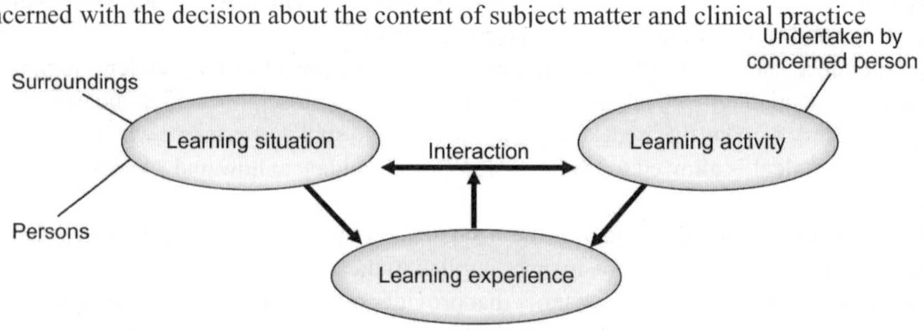

Fig. 3.12: Components of Learning Experience

Principles to be Followed in Selecting Learning Experiences
To decide the learning situation and activities, the teacher has to keep certain principles in mind are:
- Purposes and objectives in view
- Learning activities related to life situations where the students are expected to practice after being qualified
- Integration of learning experience between theory and practice
- Identified tasks and their expected jobs
- Focus of selecting learning activities should be:
  - Needs and demands of learners, community, national and the world population
  - Community oriented and hospital oriented
  - Levels of prevention
  - Nursing care practices at all three levels of health care
  - Values in nursing
- Development of student's logical and analytical thinking.

Maxims has to be Followed While Providing Learning Experiences for Group of Learners
- Easy to difficult
- Simple to complex
- Concrete to abstract
- Particular to general
- Analysis to synthesis
- Whole to parts
- Empirical to rationale

- Psychological to logical
- Actual to the representative.

Principles Used in Implementing Teaching Activities

Principle of aim: It serves the goal for the teacher. It makes teaching and learning, interesting and effective, e.g. providing pediatric experience for the learner. In this example is to develop the skills in rendering care to the children of different ages.

Learning by doing: The learner is active by nature; he has certain urges which impel him to action. For example: all the Nursing procedures will be learnt and practiced by student is by following the principle of " learning by doing" "learning by repetition" "learning through positive reinforcement".

Principle of linking: With actual life and other subjects; theory and practicals should be integrated and linked with each other.

Principle of planning: Teaching is always has to be well-planned. Planning involves selection, division and revision.

Principle of interest or motivation: Interest is like a "petrol" that drives the "mental engine".

Principle of sympathy and kind atmosphere: The teachers' kindness and sympathy is a stimulating dose for the slow learners. Teachers should avoid scolding, nagging and rebuking. In this way the teaching becomes a mother of pleasure for the teacher as well as for the student.

Principle of flexibility and cooperation: The plan should have scope to make necessary changes. Teaching should be flexible to meet the unexpected situations of any, in providing learning experience.

Principle of diagnostic and remedial teaching: Teaching should be diagnostic and remedial, once the learners' difficulties has to be identified and guide or suggest the students, how to overcome it, by clarifying their doubts with constructive criticisms, encourage them to implement steps to resolve the problem, they should not be left as they are, the teacher has to be a moderator and do follow-up to assess the outcome of her/his suggestions. Learning difficulties should be discovered early, to avoid them taking root into the learning habits of the pupils.

Principle of looking ahead: Open-mind teacher is always forward looking. She/he is ever prepared to discover new possibilities for widening learner's knowledge and range of experience. Good teaching is over looking forward to their improvement in the light of new experiments in the field of pedagogy.

Principle of creativity: The ideal teacher will make the creative learner by introducing new materials. Good teaching open up the fields of investigations and enables the learners to make original contribution to the existing store of knowledge.

Systematic Exposition

curriculum and subjects must be systematically presented in the form of 'Course plans', 'Unit Plans' and 'Lesson Plans'.

Clear Understanding

Mechanically the teachers should not teach lessons. She/he has to make clear the content of the lesson taught to be clear to the students. After completion of each sub-heading, pose questions to the learners, care to be taken all corners of classroom has to be covered when asking responses from the group, to enhance alertness and to promote interest among learners. Important points has to be reinforced by repeating the content, She/he should proceed to the next part, only if the previous parts are clearly understood by them.

Provision of Correlation and Integration of Learning Experience

The teacher has to teach the lesson as a whole and not in isolated parts. Definite link must be maintained between the various parts of theory with the practicals. So whenever new topic starts, teacher has to review the previous class by questioning and get the feed back, to assess the level of understanding and to reinforce on points where they are weak, correlates the content in a meaningful manner, promotes long lasting memory for students in their mind. Teacher always acts as a 'mentor' and inspires for the all round personality development of learners and felt glad whenever their children/learners achieved higher goals and appreciates the child by showing their concern.

Principle of Revision and Fixation

The careful teacher shall always serve the course or lesson/units in hand before proceeding to the next unit, "Law of Revision and Law of Reinforcement" has to be followed in their teaching. Teachers should assure themselves that the learners have grasped and fixed in their mind. Curriculum characteristics has to be kept in mind while selecting and organizing learning experiences:

- Primary focus (General and Specific Objectives of Lesson Plan has to be kept in mind)
- Target population/Specific group of learners whom at that moment they are teaching or being served
- Primary settings for learning (Classrooms and Clinical Areas (Community, Hospital and Educational Institutions)
- Role of Nurse and their concern (Nursing practice)
- Problem solving process
- Objectives of Nursing Practice – Prevention, promotion, treatment and rehabilitation
- Health care delivery system
- Evaluation of nursing practice.

Areas to be Selected for Learning Experiences

To fulfill the educational objectives, learning experiences in terms of theory and practice has to be selected. The selection of these areas is dependent on statutory norms, type of programe, educational objectives, the health profile and health needs of the country.

Relevant Areas from Which the Topics have to be Selected

As per the Curricular guide lines (Statutory Bodies/Professional Bodies), University/Board requirements and the objectives of Course, Unit and lesson plan, Learners' background and Schools' Philosophy, The Nursing College/School Administrator/Principal has to organize faculty meeting and allot the subjects based on educational background to the faculty. Periodical meetings will be conducted to assess the teaching activities, to identify the problems encountered by teachers with specific programs.

Variables in the Learning Process

1. The learner student
   - He/she is the centre of teaching-learning process.
   - The conditions affecting learning are: Physical factors—Age, maturation, sex, and fatigue

   Psychological factors: Mental set, motivation, readiness of the individual to learn, self effort, attitude towards learning, cooperative mindedness.
2. The learning material (content)

   The teaching technique should be according to the mental level of the trainees. Teacher presents teaching content in a language that could be understood by the learners. The preparation and presentation of learning materials, e.g. Lesson plan with appropriate Audio Visual Aids is of great importance in teaching and learning process, both the instructor and the trainee has to understand the content of the lesson.
3. The learning methods

   Comprehensive learning (whole learning) is better than part learning. Modes of learning—Self-evaluation, Periodical revision, Repetition, Trial and error, Energy spending towards learning, Using successful methods in learning based on maturity and age.
4. The methods of instruction
   - It affects the learning process
   - Includes instructional objectives, lesson plan, trainee and trainer activities, active participation of learner (accelerates the absorption of learning) AV aids (for faster learning and help to retain what has been learnt)
   - Remedial instruction helps backward trainees
   - For intelligent, gifted learners will have intellectual and difficult skills should be provided to exploit their abilities to enhance their learning, which benefits both individual and society
   - Results of performance of trainees has to be communicated as early as possible
   - To help them to improve in case of deficiencies
   - To develop interest for success and better results.

5. Environment:
   - Provision of conducive environment for learning is essential i.e., in school, campus, outside and hostel
   - Facilities have to be provided to learn and to practice
   - Develop and create a healthy congenial environment which can bring about good qualities and character in the trainees and this helps them later in their life to become good craftsman and better citizens.
6. Psychological factors:
   In teaching-learning process both the teacher and the trainee should have cordial relationship which provides security and comfort to the learner and aids in increase the attention. It helps for improving self-expression, self-assertion and satisfaction. The better learning conditions like discipline, positive attitude of instructors, ability of the administrators involvement of all these connected are equally important.
7. Instructional media for learning:
   It helps in choosing appropriate methods, strategies and media for making instruction a congenial process. It makes the learner for easy learning, remembers for longer. All these leads to planned systematic use of learning media for learning. Thus the teaching-learning model and media gets the top priority in the instructional process.

   The media which provide a variety of learning experiences are: Textbooks, Supplementary and reference books, Journals, magazines, Newspapers, documents, clippings, Programed materials, Motion picture films, TV programs, Radio programs, Recordings (tape and disc), Audio-Visual aids and Multimedia kits.

Levels of Learning Experience

1. Direct experience: Immediate sensory contact with the actual object. It is useful educative experience where the learner will have the opportunity to see, handle, taste, touch, felt, smelled. It gives first hand information, e.g. Lab practice and demonstration, Clinical Practice in the clinical area
2. Vicarious experience: Create the actual situation through rearrangement of the reality. We can bring the world to the classroom, e.g. Model, specimen, film, television, radio, pictures, records and photographs.
3. Symbolic experience: These are offered through verbal symbols (oral or written). These experiences occur at the conceptual level. In teaching-learning process, the content and objectives of education are symbolized by circles and the activities of instructors and learners by rectangular. In each relationship, between the instructor and the trainee and between the trainee and the content, different kinds of learning may take place at the same time.

Experiences Leading to Learning Experience

Learning experience should be planned thoughtfully, leads to desired learning. Curtaining learning experience can be planned for instructional planning, so that it increases the curiosity and interest in learning among the learner, mechanical or routine way of learning will be avoided.

For example:

Thinking	Speaking	Editing	Displaying
Discussing	Reporting	Scripting	Charting
Conferring	Reading	Interviewing	Creating
Constructing	Painting	Writing	Outlining
Lettering	Exhibiting	Mapping	Drawing
Taking notes	Graphing	Showing	Demonstrating
Photographing	Collecting	Dancing	Researching
Travelling	Singing	Working	Audio-recording
Experimenting	Judging	Evaluating	Observing
Organizing	Observing	Organizing	Programming
Summarizing	Watching	Experimenting	Problem-solving
Video-recording	Imagining	Visualizing	

Role of Instructor in Selection of Classroom Teaching Activity for a learner in Nursing Educational Programe

- Nurse Educator will allot the topic to teach student-teacher well in advance and give sufficient time for the student to prepare content for lesson plan and appropriate Audio-Visual aids
- The student-teacher has to prepare the outline for the topic and get approval from the concerned teacher/supervisor along with instructional objectives (general and specific) for the lesson plan
- Maxims of teaching and Principles of learning has to be kept in mind while planning learning experience
- Student-teacher ought to do broad review/search and organize the content related to topic by using varied resources (like Library—Text Books and Journals: National and International), Web search and discussions with experts, peer group and personal experiences to quote suitable examples in appropriate time
- Arrange content in accordance with the planning by fulfilling Instructional Objectives
- List teaching activities to enrich students' abilities, decide teaching method
- Analyze and organize the elements of topic and related skills into effective learning experience
- Choose and prepare learning aids based on the specific objectives
- References have to be given at the end of the lesson plan as a bibliography or list of references
- Teacher/Supervisor has to provide guidance to student – teacher from the time of allotment of the topic to the presentation of the topic to the group of learners in a classroom
- Provide learning experience, evaluate, verify the achievements of the objectives
- After the teaching session, the supervisor will have reflective session by asking the student teacher to narrate the experience about her/his preparation and the difficulties faced, problems notified and the methods adopted to overcome the barriers
- The teaching session will be evaluated by supervisor based on certain standardized criteria viz., student - teacher voice and content presented, communication and interaction skills, Audio-Visual aids and it's presentation, Group participation, Questioning pattern, time maintenance to cover the topic and feedback from the selected audience etc.

Organization of Learning Experiences

Once learning experiences are selected, teacher has to organize the experiences. Organizing involves identification and grouping of activities to be performed along with establishment of authority, responsibility and relationships.

In organizing learning experience two aspects are necessary:

1. Grouping learning experience under subject headings: Select the learning experience according to criteria, organize the learning experience, so that the student will receive maximum benefit. The individual school of nursing can make their own choice based on their philosophy and objectives of the organization. The practice of grouping them under subject methods is a method of organization, e.g. Basic Sciences applied to Nursing, Anatomy, Physiology, Microbiology, Physics, Chemistry and Behavioral Sciences applied to Nursing: Psychology, Sociology, Community Health Nursing, Nutrition, Personal and Environmental hygiene, Health Education and Communication skills.

Nursing specialities: Nursing Foundations, Medical-Surgical Nursing, Pediatrics Nursing, Maternal and Child Health Nursing, Psychiatric Nursing and Obstetric and Gynecologic Nursing.

2. Placement of the selected learning experience covering sequencing and integration: Placement of learning experience in the total curriculum is 2nd step in organization of learning experience. All the elements of the curriculum should be related to one another. The learning experience should be so organized that they continuously reinforce each other and broader and deepen the understanding and skills of the learners. Vertical organization of learning experience refers to the relationship existing between different levels of the same subjects and skills. Criteria which can serve as guide for effective organization of the subject matter and the learning experience in the curriculum. Sequence in the placement of learning experience content for gradual progress from simple to complex, concrete to abstract, normal to abnormal, e.g. in 1st year, the student learns about nutrition, this knowledge will help the student in 2nd year, to understand dietary modifications, planning of therapeutic diets according to disease conditions and meet the nutritional needs of different clients.

- The development of the ability to shoulder accountability. It will start early with the student's accountability for looking after his own health by following sound health habits and hygiene and maintaining a personal record
- Thereafter being accountable for health maintenance and providing basic nursing care to two-third patients during 1st year program
- Being accountable to render comprehensive nursing care for several patients in subsequent years of his educational program
- In the final year of the program learner is made accountable for the management of an entire nursing unit
- Integration—A state of wholeness, harmony and relatedness. To blend things into a harmonious whole. The integration process takes place only in the student. Hence, teacher has to provide the opportunity to learner to integrate his various learning experience with new ones. Learner has to analyze nursing care situations and problems, apply the principles learned to provide qualitative nursing care. Integration of theory into practice is essential, e.g. Learning about Microbiology in 1st year will make the learner for better understanding of communicable diseases in further years. They have to integrate earlier learning to the later learning
- Learning about 'blood chemistry' in Bio Chemistry and involves integrated learning of functions of blood and CVS and Pathology in Health Deviation/Diseases
- Relatedness—Theory has to be related to practical. The student whatever he/she learnt in classroom has to correlate the knowledge into clinical practice, then only learning will be comprehensive, e.g. Learning Body Mechanics in First Year and applying the principles of Body Mechanics in carrying out Nursing Procedures will further help the learners while rendering nursing care to meet the felt needs of the client and their families.

General Plan for Curriculum

Teachers has to prepare general plan of the whole curriculum, where the placement of subject matter along with clinical experience will be included (Master Rotation Plan). This will give a clear picture as to how, in which year and in what stage are the subject matter going to be taught and the relevant clinical experience to be offered. The nursing programes in India must follow the statutory requirements laid down by the INC. the clinical experiences can be arranged in an educationally sound, sequence and the subject matter in connection with the related clinical experience can be charted with each experience. The general plan covers the number of hours in theory and practice, co-curricular activities, tasks, examination and vacation.

The general plan includes:
- Total duration of the program i.e., Total hours of instruction—Theory, Clinical practice, laboratory work, evaluation, co-curricular activities (Core content), Defining different courses of study—Theory and Practicals
- Course outlines of individual theoretical course of study denoting total units, titles, contents, allotted hours, objectives for each unit (unit plan)
- Guidelines for practicals in general and clinical nursing specialties (Clinical Rotation Plan)
- Communication skills
- Teaching—Practice teaching, Clinical teaching—Ward teaching, Demonstrations, Health teaching, Case studies, clinical Presentations, Ward management, Internship etc.
- Rotation plan—Master rotation plan, Individual course and unit plan, Guidelines for co-curricular activities.
- Instructional methods and media for theory, practical and laboratory work
- Scheme of evaluation includes Concurrent, Terminal and Evaluation tools
- For each of the practice based courses of study a minimum one third of the total hours has to be devoted to practical work in each subject particularly because nursing education should have heavy component of clinical experiences both in Hospital and Community set up.

Correlation Chart

Indian Nursing Council has prescribed guidelines and syllabi for the different courses of studies in a specific nursing program must be followed as minimum requirement to fulfill.

A correlation committee (consists of the teachers incharge of each class) to look into the total correlation of the student program and plans regularly as well as to see to the organization of classes, etc. in accordance with the objectives. This committee also looks after the preparation of timetable, planning clinical rotation plans, obtaining permission from the authorities for clinical experience and organizing both clinical and teaching block etc.

The preparation of the correlation chart gives a portrayal of the extent of correlation achieved in the total curriculum in relation to the different courses of study and the various subjects and clinical experience offered in the program. Teachers can attempt to achieve the maximum possible while planning, the chart shows what subjects will be taught each week (or month) and each year. The concerned subject teacher has to prepare outlines for teaching each subject.

Teaching System

Common methods which will be used in nursing practice are: The teaching block system, The partial block system, study day system and daily classes.

Teaching Block (study block or clinical block)

The teaching and clinical experiences in curriculum are organized in blocks i.e., the entire programe is divided into specific blocks according to the speciality. Before posting the students in the clinical area the related theory can be taught in a study block.

Advantages

- Students can concentrate on the learning of the subject matter, as they are withdrawn from the clinical postings.
- All the students in the whole class have to attend so necessity of repeat classes is thereby eliminated.
- Planning of curriculum becomes easy and correlation is made easier.
- When teachers are posting all the students in clinical area after study blocks, clinical administration becomes easy, the students are not withdrawn from the ward or clinical work for a stipulated specific some part of the day, the experience not being interrupted. The quality of student's practice can be ensured enriching their experience at the same time.
- When the students are posted in the clinical area, give assignments like ward teaching, group discussions, case study, health talks, etc. arrange bed side clinic/ward clinic, clinical conferences, case presentations, etc. all these will help in learning, efficiency in teaching, review and evaluation.

Partial block system: The postings of the students in the clinical area either morning or afternoon or evening based on availability of clinical instructors and requirement of the course or philosophy of the organization. Students may have theoretical classes either in the morning or afternoon depending upon availability of faculty, time and objectives. Daily theoretical instructions are required to spread over a greater length of period to cover the courses of study.

Study day system: One day in a week can be completely planned for theoretical instructions/classes for all the batches. Other days, half a day in clinical area another half day in classes or weekly two days totally they will be taken for the classes. The students are free from clinical responsibilities for a total day. Teaching can be organized more easily in a correlated manner. The student will enjoy the student status and their withdrawal does not hamper the smooth running of ward. The qualified Registered Nurse will takes the responsibility of rendering client care services.

Daily classes: The classes will be arranged regularly each day. Students will attend clinicals mornings or afternoons then theory classes will be taken accordingly.

Team nursing or clinical blocks: Total students of the college will be posted for clinical duty; completely looks after ward's work. Depending upon students' number, the number of wards will be taken under control of college and will held responsibility for total clients care. Final year student will act as team leader under him/her III, II and I year students will work. They will be called as one team, under each team few clients will be allotted. The clinical supervisor will be supervising the teamwork. Each shift will be handing over and other shift will take over the charges. During handing over time, teaching faculty will be monitoring the reporting, Thus 24 hours care will be taken completely by the students only.

Curriculum Plans

The general curriculum plan shows the subject to be taught (Theoretical Instruction hours and respective hours of clinical experiences) throughout the entire program, Vacation, Examinations briefly drawn in graphical representation.

Master Rotation Plan

'Overall plan of rotation of all students in a particular educational programe, showing the placement of the students belonging to total program (4 years in B.Sc. (N) and 3 and half years in GNM courses) includes both theory and practice denoting the study block, clinical blocks, team nursing, examinations, vacation, co-curricular activities etc.

It is prepared well in advance for the whole year so that it gives a complete and clear picture about students placement either in theory or clinical field during an academic session. For each year, it can be prepared separately and for total program one can be prepared so that every faculty will be aware of students' postings. Teachers should follow the respective University or Board syllabus as a guideline for preparing either master rotation plan or clinical rotation plan.

Purposes

- Availability of an advance plan before implementation of curricular activities during an academic year for the entire program
- All concerned are aware of the placement of students in clinical fields
- Coordination becomes more effective when theory, practice correlates and integrity exists
- Helps the students and teachers to prepare themselves for working in the areas
- Any modifications are required based on situations concerned, collaboration between the faculty and service staff can be made for smooth running of organizational activities and meeting the objectives of educational programe
- Assessment of curricular program is more effective
- The faculty members and nursing service staff are in a position to make tentative advance plans for their leave or vacation without jeopardizing the teaching-learning activities.

Principles to be Followed While Preparing Master Rotation Plan

- Plan in accordance with the concerned curriculum plan/syllabus for the entire course/program
- Plan in advance for all students in all years of program.
- Plan the activities by following maxims of teaching
- Post the students based on university syllabus and availability of concerned required specialities
- Select areas that can provide expected learning experience
- Plan to build on previous experiences
- Acquaint the clinical staff/clinical supervisor with clinical objectives and rotation plan
- Provide each clinical experience of same duration to all the students
- Rotate each student through each learning experience or block
- Plan for all students to enter and leave at the same time schedule.

Staff Involvement in Curriculum Planning

Curriculum committee consisting of members who actively participate in the development or construction of a curriculum for their school. The members may be drawn from various disciplines i.e., Teaching Faculty in Nursing Educational Institution. Curriculum committee main responsibility is to organize all learning experiences planned by individual tutors into an integrated whole. A learning experience is something in which the student actively participates and brings change in his/her behavior. The individual teachers analyze their own subjects in order to help and contribute to the correlation of teaching with other subjects. The school administrator has to explain/orient all the staff about the philosophy, objectives of the organization; responsibilities of each staff. When there is an appreciation and common understanding among the staff members of the school, there is bound to be a greater appreciation by their service, staff has to plan scheduling of classes and field work clinical experience of the students. Teachers will maintain harmonious curriculum in order to meet the national health.

The school should keep a close connection with the clinical fields (hospital and community) wherever possible continuity of service should be maintained by the school in these fields, which will bring in cooperation, understanding and a sense of appreciation of the program offered. A better organization and planning of learning experience will be the resultant effect.

Faculties are accountable for implementing the program that enables the students to learn. Its goal is always concerned with fostering of ability of their students in carrying out of the necessary service to the society in the future.

The important aspects of curriculum planning are: the selection and organization of learning experience for the students who are undergoing a program. The careful selection of the experiences and their organization is built on the student's past knowledge and previous experience and according to the levels of the students. Progress in complexity to higher levels of learning and comprehension in the practice of nursing, is the aim. It should exhibit an inner relatedness among the various subjects and also their relationship to the clinical instruction and practice of nursing.

PLANNING AND ORGANIZATION OF CLINICAL EXPERIENCE

Introduction

Planning of clinical experience is a component of learning experience at basic level. The syllabi formulated by University/Board will acts as a guideline for fulfilling the minimum requirements.

To bring change in human behavior, the learning experience must be organized as to have cumulative effect. Clinical experience is an integral part of learning where the student will be actively participate to obtain skills in clinical practice by applying the principle of 'learning by doing'. The time, the student spends and learns in the clinical fields is an important and integral part of the total school program. The teacher's responsibility is to provide conducive environment for the expected desired behavior.

The faculty has to plan the clinical experience, keeping the objectives in view so that it will provide the needed learning at a particular stage in the course so that the student will be posted in right clinical area at the right time. The teacher has to orient the students why they are posted in the particular clinical area; so the teacher has to complete the theoretical component early, before posting the students in the clinical area. Teacher has to inform to the students about the postings early, what are the requirements they have to fulfill in postings, what type of desired learned behavior they have to develop, everything she/he has to explain judicious decision making and greater efforts are need to plan the clinical experience as well as plan for supervision and better learning. The clinical experience and rotation plan should be well-organized and interrelated to achieve the effectiveness in the overall objectives of nursing program. One of the objectives of school of nursing is, 'understanding of the psychosomatic and social factors that affect the client and ability and inclination to aid the patient in adjustment to and possibly in improvement of the health status'.

Factors to be considered while providing Clinical Facilities

- Philosophy and objectives of an organization (School Philosophy) and an educational program
- Health care delivery system
- Nursing Philosophy—Nursing Theories and Models—Clinical Nurse practitioner—Functions of the nurse
- Levels of prevention, Health promotion, curative and Rehabilitation activities
- Methods of delivering Nursing care
- Legislation establishing independent nursing regimens and independent practice
- Standards for practice—structural process outcome and evaluation tools
- Availability of infrastructure i.e., community—sub centers, primary health centers, CHC, hospitals with speciality facilities/institutions–general hospitals, specialties, number of patients in a clinical setting and student strength
- Health agencies like Rehabilitation centers, Hospitals, Nursing homes, Clinics, subcenter and primary health center
- Equipments and supplies
- Clinical Instructors availability
- Budget
- Field visits.

Principles in selection of learning experiences in Clinical area
- Learning experience should provide an opportunity for students to practice the type of behavior implied in the objective
- Students must have time and opportunity to analyse the problems of specific patients, recognizing the emotional and social problems, which affect the physical status and interrelationships of various aspects of health
- Provide learning situations to assist in making and carrying out plans for the present and continued regimen of care
- The activities sought must be within the range of possibility for the students concerned
- Students should acquire mastery of essential information and basic concepts for effective health teaching.

Organization of Clinical Learning Experiences
Objectives can be attained only by learning experience through reinforcement and repetition. An effectively organized educational program provides opportunity for fulfillment of 4 important criteria.
1. Continuity: The relationship existing between the different levels of the same subject and skills required. It refers to the vertical relation of major curriculum events.
2. Sequence: It emphasizes the importance of having each successive experience build upon the preceding one, but go more broadly and deeply into the matters involved.
3. Integration: The horizontal relationship of curriculum experience.
4. Correlation: The theory has to be correlated to practice, e.g. to develop skill in mechanical ventilation, the students need to have knowledge of physiology of respiration, anatomy of the respiratory tract and in practical experience, the learner should have the opportunity to operate a ventilator, observation of a client who is on ventilator, documentation and reporting of the progress, etc. For example: A student is taught Basic nursing/Nursing Foundation in the first year, but the same subject is continued in the 2nd and 3rd years in greater depth like Medical-Surgical Nursing and other specialities sequence is the placement of the content in a gradual progress from simple to complex and comprehensive. Sequence goes beyond continuity.

Teacher has to provide the opportunity for the students to teach the clients in each successive clinical experience, student has to assume an increasingly broader responsibility for recognizing the local health problem and making contacts with other individuals or agencies for putting efforts in the solution of the problem.

Some questions has to be answered before planning clinical experiences of educational value:
- What is the background of the student, when he comes to the professional education?
- What experiences he should receive to meet the objectives?
- How long students can be posted (duration of clinical experience as per norms—INC and University or Board?
- What experience does the ward can offer to the student?
- What is the student expected to gain from clinical experience?

Learning experience should be consistent with the philosophy of the school and lead to the achievement of terminal goal of the program. The teacher should clearly understand the philosophy of institution, program and concerned hospitals where students will be posted. The teachers has to state behavioral objectives to get desirable knowledge, skills and attitude and select those experiences, which are appropriate in achieving the stated objectives. Learning experience should provide opportunity for the development of independent thinking, good judgment, self-discipline and integrity of purpose.

Planning Clinical Assignments
The students' future competence as a Nurse Practitioner depends to a large extent upon the quality of instruction provided during clinical practice periods. Responsibility for planning the clinical assignments rests squarely with the clinical supervisors, e.g. assigning clinical responsibility, planning for ward-teaching, health-talk, case presentation, bedside clinic/ward clinic, ward conferences, etc. recognize what else must be dealt within the situation, besides the particular experience being planned.

Orientation of Students to the Clinical Area

The clinical supervisor has to orient the students to the clinical area, staff and objectives, expectations from the student, assignments to be completed, duration of posting, activities to be performed and adhering to the clinical rotation plan etc.

Matching the Right Student with the Right Client

The teacher has to identify the ability of students when planning their clinical assignments. The less able student should be helped to move toward the level of performance expected of all students in the group i.e., posting the students in clinical area based upon their clinical requirement, e.g. Posting III year B.Sc. (N) student in ENT ward to render nursing care for the clients with ENT disorders.

Planning for Continuity of Care

The first day of learning experience, the student has to assess the client, observe the client clinical findings and collect the history, document the history, reviews the chart of the client, formulate/identify the Nursing diagnosis and plan the care by utilizing the principles and steps of Nursing Process. On the second day, he can provide complete care and meet holistic needs. By the 3rd day, he may help the client and his relatives to gain knowledge about client's condition and needed assistance by family (the activities,which family has to carry out in rendering care to the client to attain optimum health), which includes implementation of Nursing care activities as per long-term goals, short-term goals.

Providing adequate Clinical Supervision

The teacher has to supervise the student's tasks in the clinical area as Nursing is practice discipline , strict clinical supervisory practice is essential, while posting the students in clinical areas, INC norms related to teacher student ratio has to be followed strictly to teach effectively.

Coordinating Classroom Teaching and Clinical learning

It is facilitated by formulating units of study, which are sufficiently broad reasonably they can find suitable clients for students' assignments.

Recording Results to Help with the Planning of Future Clinical Assignments

The teacher should maintain the records and document students' performance in clinical area. Cumulative records has to be maintained, which has to be submitted at the time of pre finals and final examinations, The documentation should meet the purposes of the course and reflect the strengths and weaknesses of each student.

Clinical Rotation Plan

In nursing education-rotation refers to "regular, successive and recurrent posting of various groups of nursing students belonging to different classes in specific nursing fields i.e., OPDs, speciality wards, OT, delivery room, clinics, community health fields – clinics, out reach centers, subcenters, health centers, schools etc."

The school should select the clinical fields for the purpose of providing clinical practice at the outset of the program. The learning situations are where the students are practicing nursing procedures, carry on care related activities.

Factors to be Considered in Planning Clinical Rotations

- The objectives of the course have to be clearly stated
- Number of students in each class
- Number and size of departments, agencies, areas, teaching units or wards where students should be given opportunity for practicing clinical skills/clinical experience
- Presence of students of other programes in the same ward/field
- The agency, concerned authority
- The duration of clinical experience in each area as per INC and University /Board norms

- The number of teaching faculty available for clinical supervision. This is particularly important because the students need supervision and guided experience to enable them to learn the right way of performing a nursing procedure or make the appropriate nursing interventions for the clients assigned to their care
- Indian Nursing Council and University/Board requirements or norms
  Although the individual schools have the freedom to organize the clinical experience the way they choose, but all must meet the minimum prescribed by the council
- Number of staff nurses employed to provide nursing services in the hospital/field
- Sectors that are solely dependent on student services during day and night (try to give students, student status), sequence of experience required, select wards depending on learning experiences to be provided
- Adhere to rotation plan.

Basic Principles in Planning Clinical Rotation

- The clinical rotation plan must be in accordance with the total curriculum plan
- It has to be prepared in advance
- Theoretical instructions should precede as closely as possible with clinical experience, simultaneously the ward teachings, case presentations, bedside clinics etc., can be conducted and supervised
- The teacher and student ratio will be 1:4 or as prescribed by INC or according to the types of patients nursed eg: in critical care unit 1:1
- Select the type of learning experience from simple to complex
- Clinical supervisors must be familiar with the rotation plan; a copy of rotation plan should be available in each area
- The students should be posted where they will get maximum supervision from clinical supervisors and qualified nursing staff
- Each student should get all the experience on rotation wise
- Over crowding in clinical area should be avoided
- Avoid overlapping of work
- All students should enter and leave the particular clinical area at the same time and they should complete the assignments in time
- Continuity in clinical care is needed.

Individual Rotation Plan

To make sure that each student in a particular block posting undergoes experience in each area. The objectives of the experience are discussed with the students so that they can gain maximum, during the time of their clinical placement. The student has to maintain a log book or a cumulative record book of daily experience in the area of posting. The individual rotation plan is prepared by the subject teacher in consultation with principal and faculty. The clinical supervisors has to rotate each student into the assigned area related to the specific course of study, e.g. Third-year B.Sc. (N) students will be posted for Psychiatry, Pediatrics, Obstetric and Gynec experience.

Needs of the Students in the Clinical Area

- The students need to identify the objectives for their respective clinical placement. Orientation of objectives, assignments, work allotment, clinical area, staff has to be clearly explained by the teachers, before placing them into the clinical area
- Facilities made available to each student for the practice of good nursing, where he can correlates theory with practice
- Guidance and supervision should be provided to each student
- Assignments should be given based on level of learning acquired by each student
- Make the student to perform the activities independently or practicing alone. The teacher has to protect, guide the student until they can obtain proficiency in acting independently and appropriate decision making
- Students must have the opportunity to work in a team
- Teacher has to observe the performance discuss and evaluate the activities

- Provide accessibility of library or to the reference materials which are meaningful to the clinical areas of their placement
- All the staff has to recognize the student participation and purpose of posting, they have to give cooperation with the students for their effective learning
- Students should have an opportunity to practice high standards and qualitative nursing care. Appropriate prioritization of values is required.

Responsibilities of the Nursing Staff in Clinical Area

The success of the clinical experience will depend to a great extent on the standard of patient care being practiced in the clinical area. No amount of teaching in the classroom can equal the benefit the students derive from observing the consistent practice of good nursing.

- The standards of nursing care services they render
- Role models they present have a paramount place in shaping the students, for their future professional roles and in giving them the right direction in nursing. Cooperative planning, collaboration of experiences between hospital staff and school staff, they must share the responsibility and accountability of preparing the student nurses, so that they become good professional nurses and great advantage for the students placed in their units
- To demonstrate a high standard of patient care
- To create an atmosphere which encourages learning
- To assist the nursing faculty in preparation of the clinical rotation plan
- To ensure that the student receives maximum learning experiences
- To have well-organised and accurate nursing record system
- To participate in orientation programe of students
- To make evaluation reports in connection with students' clinical experience
- To guide, supervise and evaluate the students' performance wherever feasible
- To participate and cooperate in clinical teaching programes through daily report, nursing rounds, daily conference, and ward clinic
- To hold periodic joint conference with nursing faculty concerned with students clinical experience
- To cooperate in maintaining record of practical experience.

Faculty Role in Clinical Postings

- The teacher has to prepare objectives for clinical experience
- Based on objectives, clinical experience has to be planned in advance to provide specific planned learning experience
- The teachers have to see as far as possible the students will have adequate theoretical background to benefit from the experience making it meaningful
- If necessary for some of the topics provide spot clinical teaching and such teaching has to be repeated to each group of students as they rotate, e.g. conduction of delivery
- Plan the course outline and so that theory can be correlated to practice
- Get permission from clinical authorities; place the necessary material required for client care, plan the assignments, evaluation tools
- Ensure that each student is aware of the objectives and assignments and criteria for evaluation
- Place and guide the students to get required clinical experience
- Orient the student to the clinical area, ward staff, policies, philosophy of the organization where they were posted
- Participate in teaching, supervision and evaluation of students in the wards
- Arrange ward-teachings, ward-discussions, and case presentations
- Criticize constructively the students' activities, which improves their performance
- Help the students for effective charting of records and reports
- Depend upon nature of posting evaluation methods, tools will be offered. For example performance evaluation, audit etc.

Implementation of the Curriculum

Planning is essential for good teaching, but planning itself does not effect mastery of teaching, is dependent on many factors. The teacher by virtue of her/his maturity, knowledge, understanding and experience is accepted as authority in the area being studied. A good teaching plan is a creation of mind that has sound ideas and understanding. The teacher understands the philosophy, objectives, curriculum pattern in that school, based on these factors the teacher will plan the learning activities for the students. The responsibility of the teacher to implement the courses whereby she/he can achieve the course objectives, whenever feasible the students should be involved in planning, implementing as well as evaluating their learning experience. The total curriculum (Fig. 3.13) (theory and practical) is divided into various courses of study.

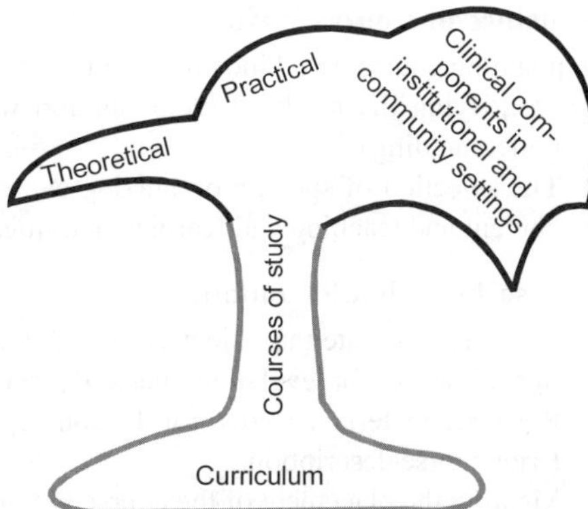

Fig. 3.13: The curriculum tree

COURSE PLANNING

Introduction

The key to successful teaching is course planning. It serves as a guideline for the teacher as well as for the students in creating the conducive atmosphere for worthwhile learning and purposeful activities. Good teacher install in her/his students urge to learn and the sincerity of purpose in all activities.

Levels of Course Plan

1. Pertains to organizing both content and learning experience within a unit or a subject i.e., at the level of a course of study, at the level of unit.
2. Deals with designing the pattern for the entire program at the programe level.

Principles

- State the objectives in behavioral terms, which has to be achieved
- Establish sequence in order of succession, the content materials has to be organized, e.g. In teaching bed making, plan teaching of simple open bed first, admission bed next followed by postoperative bed, fracture beds, renal beds etc.
- The teacher should keep in mind
  - What should the students learn from the course?
  - What should be the sequence of topics/units?
  - How much time has to be allotted?
- Ensure logical and psychological continuity to organize continuity into fewer units, easy understanding and repetition. Organize the course focusing around the students, it should be adopted to the level of the students, individual differences has to be allowed, should encourage logical memory and problem solving; combining logical and psychological requirements
- Provide cumulative learning by reinforcement
- Plan for integration (plan related courses horizontally)
- Unity curriculum:
  - To reduce unmanageable the bulk of specialized subjects and bring some unity into atomized specialization. Focusing centre determines the ideas that will stand out of the ideas put together. It also reduces the unit to manageable size and serves as a centre of organization
- Select an approach that is acceptable to all teachers
- Provide variety in modes of learning, e.g. group discussions, independent study modules, problem solving approaches that facilitate better learning, thought provoking assignments should be given.

Structure of Course Plan

In planning course, two kinds of planning are involved:

1. Identifying the kinds of elements and which specific learning has to be organized (knowledge and understanding).
2. The selection of specific organizing centers on which learner's entire development be focused (specific content and teaching and learning activities to be involved in the learner's inquiry).

Course Plan should contain

- Objectives—State the objectives or outcomes to be achieved through the given course
- Specifications for level of learner and placement within the curriculum
- Resource materials needed for the course
- Brief course description
- Mention the placement of the course within the curriculum
- Organize the organization, content topic wise, unit wise or lesson plan wise
- Describe the resource materials and methods of teaching
- Prepare the plan of learning activities for students, (e.g. assignments)
- Mention place, length of experience, experience record/Cumulative record, observations, procedures, plan for rotation with field experiences, supervised and guided practice
- Evaluation measures—Describe the procedures for ongoing concurrent and terminal evaluation
- Bibliography.

Process of Organizing Learning Experiences

- The concerned faculty for teaching the course and administrator of the program will discuss and agree on the general scheme of organization of the course and its smooth implementation
- Agreement should be made regarding the general principles of organization i.e., continuity, sequence and integration
- The basic units should be include
- Flexible plans should be developed which can be handled by each teacher
- The plan should be used for particular activities in a particular course.

Teacher's Role in Course Planning

- The extent, to which a teacher will plan courses individually, will vary from institution to institution and teachers' abilities and background, teaching skill
- The general objectives, general areas of subject matter, evaluation measures for each course will be determined at the institutional or faculty or instructional level has to ensure continuity and progression in learning, to avoid gaps and nonproductive repetition in subject matter context and to provide the reinforcement of previous learning. It depends on:
  - Teacher's own self-appraisal
  - Attitude towards their students teaching and learning
  - Knowledge and skills related to the area of teaching
  - Composition of learner's group
  - Teacher's insight and skill sound ideas and understanding and known conditions.

At the Instructional Level, Teachers Plan:

- Basis for planning
- Units of work
- Select materials and learning activities
- Set up working groups
- Arrange the teaching-learning environment

Planning is essential to good teaching, but itself does not affect mastery of teaching; "teachers make plans; plans do not make teachers". The teacher's efforts are foccussed on achievement of goals and to uplift the learner's development.

Teacher-student Planning

The learner is the center of the whole educative process; he/she is the life of the teacher's efforts. The student's internal mental activities are the primary causes of learning, the teacher is only the secondary proximate cause. Hence, education in the school must be a cooperative act—a joint enterprise between the student and the teacher to achieve the desired goals.

Planning for effective teaching and learning is based on sound educational psychological principles i.e., the objective worth and subjective worth of the material to each student.

Appropriate student involvement in planning will help students to learn more, to acquire not only deeper understandings, but also to plan worthwhile experiences, to take wise decisions by themselves and to learn many other important processes. It will affect the attitudinal set of the learner.

Cooperative planning for learning is a significant motivating factor because the student is immersed existentially in the purpose and the implementation of the learning situation.

To the degree to which learners are involved in the planning and the evaluation of their activities will assume responsibility for their own activities. As practitioners, nurses are expected to be able to plan effectively and to act in nursing as well as in other realms of life. If we wish to develop nurses who can plan and act, then we must educate our students for activity by making them active in the total process, include planning. The teacher's concept of learning and of the function of teaching will be important factors in their decision.

The teacher, by virtue of her/his maturity, knowledge and experience, is a recognized authority in the area being studied. As a member of the faculty she/he has an overview of the objectives, the content and the learning activities of each course, as well as the method of their organization in the particular curriculum pattern in that school. Therefore, she/he has a responsibility to plan and to implement courses in such a way that not only will the objectives of the courses that she/he teaches has to be achieved, but also they will contribute to the attainment of the general objectives of the curriculum.

The factors which will influence student involvement in planning, executing, evaluating for learning experiences includes:

- The nature of the course
- The teaching-learning situation (hospital or community)
- Maturity
- Experience level of the learners in her/his class.

UNIT PLANNING

Introduction

The teacher has to recognize the content of the textbook on the subject into suitable units. 'Unit' is developed psychologically in the student as a means of integration; unitary teaching necessitates the interlocking of ideas in order to achieve full understanding.

Definitions

"A large sub-division of the subject matter, wherein a principle of a topic or a property is central to the well-organized matter, planning the unit is known as 'unit planning'.

A unit consists of " A comprehensive series of related and meaningful activities to achieve the educational objectives by providing significant educational experience that would result in appropriate behavioral changes among the learners".

Characteristics

1. Unit planning recognizes that learning takes place most effectively in terms of whole rather than of fractions. The concept of wholeness, must be interpreted in terms of:
   - The maturity of the learner
   - The possibilities of the proposed learning situation
   - Activities for making significant changes in the behavior of the learner
   - Total situation
   - Recognized objectives of the group
   - Relationships of the proposed activities to the present level of the student.

2. Learning is developmental therefore it provides for vertical and horizontal organization of learning experiences All learning experiences are continually related to the over all aims of the course and the curriculum, e.g. In Nursing courses, the knowledge component of the course may be acquired in the classroom and from clinical settings. At the same time that the student is gaining knowledge and understanding, she/he will be developing the intellectual skills in implementation of steps in Nursing Process - Assessment, Nursing diagnosis, identification of principles, selection of treatments relevant to the nursing functions, implementation of nursing activities and evaluating or estimating expected outcomes.

3. Unit planning recognizes that learning takes place most effectively when there is an understanding and acceptance of goals to be achieved and when there is full and active participation in planning for the attachment of these goals, e.g. Many of the decisions which the teacher ordinarily makes by herself/himself might be shared on a group learning basis.

4. Unit planning recognizes the necessity for providing for individual differences in the rates of learning and interests. Therefore, a variety of assignments, e.g. projects, field trips, conferences and other similar activities are planned by and for individual and groups.

5. Unit planning recognizes that true learning renders the learner increasingly skilled in self-direction, therefore opportunities are provided for the student steadily and gradually to assume more responsibility for the selection, organization and evaluation of many of her/his own learning experiences. In nursing education, especially in the clinical situation, the student faces real nursing problems which she has to solve. She/he can be helped to organize and apply as his/her knowledge and her clinical learning experience in the solution of the problems at hand.

6. Unit planning provides a sound basis for evaluation: Setting up of goals in terms of change of behavior, e.g. attitudes, understandings, abilities and skills, etc. provide a basis for evaluation of learning outcomes.

Criteria of a good Unit

- The needs, capabilities and interests of the students should be kept in view
- A variety of experience should be planned for better learning, e.g. field trips, experiments, demonstrations, projects etc.
- The previous experience and background of the students should be taken into account
- The length of the unit should be based on interests of the students
- Provide an opportunity for new experiences
- Familiar and related topics should be included in the unit
- It should be related to social and physical environment of the students; help, anticipate and satisfy some of the future needs of the students
- Unit should be a part of sequence that permits growth of learner from year to year
- Unit planning should be the result of cooperative planning of teachers and students
- Signifies the unity or wholeness of learning activities related to some problem or project
- Psychological principle, 'learning by whole' is followed
- Importance has to be given to integrate learning outcomes
- Represents both subject matter and learning experience as well
- Organizes the subject matter into units of experience
- Organizes similar type of subject matter
- It achieves a set of specifications and objectives
- Teacher should have mastery over the subject content, so that she/he can identify the difficult units
- The time availability for completing all units has to be considered.

Activities Involved While Planning and Developing Teaching-Learning Units

1. Selection and statements of objectives: To bring desirable change in behaviour which are manifested result of specific teaching-learning activities.
2. Selection of content—Facts, concepts, principles, which are required to objectives of the unit Information, generalizations, subject matter are organized into knowledge.
   - Sources for its knowledge component – textbooks, references, periodicals, journals
   - Audio-visual aids

- Educational resource–study of a client at home, hospital or clinic or any situation
- The content and learning experience for a unit vary according to the type of unit, objectives and the field of study
- Primary emphasis in nursing course is placing scientific principles along with the development of clinical skills
- Pretest has to be administered to test the knowledge, understanding and skills in the area
- Study guide has to be prepared by the teacher in advance and give to the students to workout earlier as it orients, reviews the topics related to unit and familiarizing the student for the topic.

3. Distribution of time and the allotment of time.
4. Organization of content of the unit to meet the desired objectives keeping in mind the curriculum, policies, administrative pattern. Subject matter or learning experiences has to be organized for student development to:
   - Produce a cumulative effect, i.e. accumulation of results of experience in a desirable manner
   - Reinforce the subject content
   - To create a broader and deeper understanding of knowledge base
   - To develop, refine and strengthen the skills already acquired.
5. Selection of teaching and learning activities
   - Tracing out and utilization of available education resources and flexibility according to the needs, providing opportunities for students to practice the behaviours they are expected to develop as a result of participation in these activities.
6. Teacher's expertise: Teacher's expertise plays a pivotal role in shaping the students in the desired manner and moulding them with positive attitudes.

   The teacher should have the knowledge:
   - Of the subject that she/he is teaching
   - Teaching-learning process
   - Learners for whom she/he is planning the course and the unit
   - Her/his positive attitude towards teaching and her/his students together with her/his experience in teaching.
7. Selection of methods of evaluation: To find out how effective the teaching learning activities have been.
8. To ascertain the extent of student learning ongoing and terminal plans are necessary.
9. Selection of reference material: Reading of relevant books, articles, journals is necessary. The school should have a good library equipped with books, journals, periodicals, reference materials which will aid in the teaching-learning process. Teacher should give the list of references to the students for their self-study according to their needs and levels.
   To update the knowledge regularly the teacher also should make use of library.

Types of Unit Planning

1. Caswell and Campbell classified the types of units into 2 main groups:
   a. Subject-matter units
      - Topical unit
      - The generalization unit
      - The unit based on significant aspect of environment or culture.
   b. Experience units and process units
      - Units based on center of interest
      - Units based on student purpose
      - Units based on student need.
   c. Resource unit
2. According to Smith
   a. Adaptation units
   b. Survey units.

- Subject-matter Units—"An arrangement of the materials and the conditions of learning planned and developed to result in the desired products of learning".
  "A body of subject matter, together with a group of implementing activities, every item of which is focused on a central cluster of ideas".
- Adaptation Units— "A comprehensive and significant aspect of the environment, of an organized science, of an art, or of conduct which being learned results in adaptation in personality".
  Adjustment may be to an aspect of the environment, of an organized science, of an art (expression) or of conduct (behaviour).
- Survey Unit and Generalization Unit—"A certain subject matter content is used to develop a general comprehension of that particular phase of the culture covered by the unit."
  In generalization unit–materials of instruction, subject matter, learning activities are centered on understanding of the principle and the law or the generalization.
- Experience Units (Center - of - interest Unit)— "It is the basis for the activity programs emphasized in elementary grades".
- Student-purpose Unit—It is based on a series of activities which the learner carried out in order to achieve a given end objective. Culmination occurs when the learner achieves the purpose setup. It must be planned continuously as it develops, e.g. Nursing care plan.
- Student Needs Unit—It is based on needs which the student recognizes as essential activities and subject matter are selected in relation to student needs. The unifying force is the student's requirements.
- Process Unit - Units are planned on the basis of thought processes, e.g. problem-solving.
- Unit of Discovery and Verification - used in clinical situation. It essentially involves-
  - A problem, which the student faces.
  - Suggested ideas by the student for the solution of the problem.
  - Testing out of ideas, by the student to see which if any will solve the problem.
- Normative Units—It studies the problems, which are concerned with situations in which action is impeded by a difference of social views, interests and values.
- Unit of Criticism—More rigorous examination of hypothesis, principles, policies and programes of action.
- Resource Units—"A compendium of suggested activities and materials, accompanied by statements of significance, scope, objectives, educational resource materials and suggestions for everything used by teachers in their preparation for teacher-student unit planning". Resource units are constructed by faculty groups.

Characteristics

- Offers innumerable suggestions, but do not restrict; they provide plenty of margin for teacher ingenuity
- Indicates the scope of a particular area of knowledge, thereby helping the teacher to view it as a whole
- Contains behaviorally defined objectives useful for teacher in goal setting and evaluating
- Take into account the principle of individual differences by suggesting a wide variety of activities geared to different levels of learning.

Purposes

- Used as a basis for developing a teaching unit
- Provide improvise education for the teacher that construct and implement them
- Lay a ground work for good teaching through the extensive preplanning which they entail
- Stimulate teacher activity by offering a variety of suggestions and materials
- They can be substituted for textbooks
- Excellent source of information for beginning teachers
- Help the teacher to assist students in setting definite attainable goals
- They emphasize evaluation and offer various approaches.

Factors to be Considered While Planning a Unit

- Objectives with specifications
- Learning activities
- Content analysis
- Testing procedures.

Steps in Unit Planning

1. Content analysis by means of terms, concepts, facts, principles, laws, situations, processes, generalizations, relationships and conclusions etc.
   - It helps the teacher to have a thorough knowledge about the subject matter
   - It gives self-confidence since she has mastery over the subject matter
   - Missing points will be avoided.
2. Objectives with specifications can be realized through the content analysis
3. Learning activities: Individual differences and psychology of the pupil will be considered in choosing learning activities
4. Testing procedures: Types of evaluation tools and techniques are mentioned through which the teacher would get evidence of the achievements of objectives on the part of pupil.

LESSON PLANNING /DAILY PLANNING

Introduction

Planning is essential not only in teaching, but in all spheres of human activities. To have effective performance every intelligent individual plans out his work. A teacher has to create learning situations and it demands a thorough planning of the teaching program. Therefore planning must be done in advance. Daily lesson plan directs the daily work towards the overall goals of the course. It is pre-teaching or anticipatory teaching. Daily lesson plan is to guide the teacher in her/his teaching activities/work. It should be adopted to her/his needs at all times. Teacher must be aware of the specialized and personal, professional growth. For this, planning with foresight is very essential. To teach, the teacher must use experience already gained as starting point of work.

Lesson planning is an important part of planning of daily teaching. It describes the brief outlines of the main point of the lesson. A teacher has to prepare a more detailed, written plan. Even an experienced teacher must make mental note of what he is going to teach in the class and how he is proceeds with the lesson. The teacher's mental visualization of classroom experiences and activities put down in black and white.

A good lesson plan indicates clearly what has already been done in what direction, what the teacher intends to do in the form of stating general and specific objectives, group of learners, Audio-visual aids, Total time allotted for the session, place where the session will be conducted, content-selecting and arranging the subject matter and techniques to be employed by the teacher, Teaching-Learning activities, i.e. what the learners has to do, how the learner is engaged in various activities, what activities are to be pursued, the immediate work which the students has to be taken up, kinds of evaluative devices followed by list of References/Bibliography.

Definitions

"A statement of the aims to be realized in clear and specific means or methods which they are to be attained during the period, the class spends with a teacher".

" It is a plan of action of a teacher, which includes the working philosophy of the teacher, her/his knowledge, information about and understanding of learners, her/his comprehension of the objectives of education, knowledge of the material to be taught and her/his ability to utilize effective methods".

"It is the core and heart of effective teaching, where the teacher's mental and emotional visualization of the classroom experience as she/he plans it to occur".

"A plan prepared by a teacher to teach a lesson in an organised manner".

"A plan of action and calls for an understanding on the teacher's part about the students' knowledge and expertise about the topic being taught and his/her ability to use effective methods".

"Lesson plan is the title given to a statement of the achievements to be realized and the specific meaning by which these are to be attained as a result of the activities engaged during the period".

A Lesson plan is a Plan of Action, it Includes:

- Working philosophy of the teacher
- Information and understanding of learners
- Comprehension of the objectives of education
- Knowledge of the material to be taught
- Ability to use effective methods of education.

Purposes

- It ensures a definite objective for the day's work and a clear visualization of that objective
- It forces consideration of goals/objectives, the selection of subject matter, procedures, planning of the activities and the preparation of tests of progress
- It keeps the teacher on the track to ensure steady progress and a definite outcome of teaching and learning procedures
- Ensures selection, presentation of subject matter and interpretation
- Enables to chose and adopt effective method of teaching
- Enables to evaluate the teaching sessions
- Helps to review the subject and gives up to date knowledge
- It helps to clarify the ideas
- It helps the teacher to delimit the teaching field, keeps boundaries within which the teacher has to work, and thereby saves the time and labour
- It bids the teacher to be systematic and orderly encourages good organization of subject matter and activities by preventing haphazard in teaching
- It makes the teacher to look ahead and plan a series of activities for modifying the learners' attitudes, habits and abilities in desirable direction
- It encourages proper consideration of learning process and learning procedures.
- When it is well-planned, interest of the students can be maintained
- It is a best technique to judge the outcome of instruction
- Serves as a check on unplanned curriculum
- Provides a sensible framework to help the work, directing along the lines of syllabus at a suitable rate
- Continuity is assured in educative process, needless repetition is avoided
- Gives the teacher greater confidence, self-reliance, assurance, ease and freedom in teaching, she will not forget any point that should be explained to students, prevents him deviating from the topic
- With lesson plan, the teacher can enter the classroom without anxiety as she understand and prepares to carry it in the classroom
- Helps the teacher to select and organize the material, which he wants to present in the class
- Ensures definite association and link between various lessons and units or past and future lessons
- Helps the teacher to devise the desirable teaching to judge whether the desired objectives are being achieved.
- It stimulates the teacher to think of related material, illustrations and audio-visual aids to make more relevant, lively, meaningful, effective and inspirational.
- Provides guidelines for the teacher in teaching-learning process.
- Provides awareness of structure, content with which the teacher is involved in the direction to achieve the objectives.
- Relates the learning structures with teaching activities.
- Enables the teacher to organize classroom teaching activities by considering the individual differences of students.
- Develops the reasoning, imagination and decision-making ability of the teacher.
- Facilitates microteaching.

Teacher Competence

- To use:
  - A wider variety of teaching materials and learning activities in the classroom through a wider acquaintance with resources.
  - Courses of study more effectively as resource materials.
- Ability to construct better lesson plans with the greatest economy of time.
- Ability to make constructive preparation for cooperative planning of activities with learners.

Components

- Preparation of a subject matter
- Effective presentation
- Efforts of the participants.

Steps

1. Preparation or introduction: Exploration of the student's knowledge which helps to lead them onto the lesson. The teacher needs to prepare the students to receive new knowledge. She/he can introduce the lesson by testing previous knowledge of the students by questioning. It arouses interest and curiosity to learn new matter. Introduction should be brief and to the point.
2. Presentation: Aim of the lesson should be clearly stated before the presentation of the subject matter, which helps both the teacher and the students to have a common pursuit. In the teaching-learning process, both learner and the teacher should be actively participate. The teacher has to present the topic in enthusiastic manner so that the learner will be motivated and get interest to learn.
3. Comparison or association: Quote examples, associate facts with example, so that learners can understand very easily and arrive at generalizations on their own.
4. Generalizations: It involves reflective thinking. The knowledge, which will be presented by the teachers, should be thought provoking, innovating and stimulating to assist the students to generalize the situation.
5. Application: The students make use of the knowledge acquired in and at the same time tests the validity of the generalizations arrived at the students, whatever they have learnt in the theory has to apply in clinical field to make learning more permanent and worthwhile.
6. Recapitulation: Teacher has to ask suitable, stimulating and pivotal questions to the students on the topic. The answers will give feedback to the teacher regarding the efficacy of the methods of teaching clarification, etc. are needed or not.

Prerequisites for Making Good Lesson Plan

Teacher must possess:
- Good knowledge about the students' interests, traits and abilities
- Mastery over the subject matter
- Principles of teaching and learning
- Awareness of individual differences among students
- The knowledge of the students about the topic what they already possesses
- Adequate training in the topic
- Organization of material in a psychological and logical fashion
- Fully conversant with new methods and techniques of teaching the subject
- Ensures active pupil participation.

Essentials of a Lesson Plan

Successful teaching depends upon
- It should be written and should have clear aims
- A flexible plan should be clear and specific
- A teacher, who is free to change it as the lesson develops based on the needs of the children is required.
- Should cover the exact scope
- Should follow maxims of teaching
- The new ideas must be related to those held by learners
- It should clearly show the relationship between what has been taught before and what has to follow.
- It should contain the suitable subject matter
- Enables the teacher to know the most desirable types of teaching method
- Provides continuity in the teaching process
- Illustrative aids have to be prepared
- Learners must be given enough scope to be active
- The plan should meet the needs of students of varied capacities

- It includes summary and assignments
- Provide list of reference books
- Prepare tests for judging the outcome of teaching.

Elements

The teacher should adapt the daily plan to her/his own needs, she/he should use a guide in forming the plan.

a. Objectives:
1. The plan should state clearly the outcomes to be achieved, including both the central and the contributory objectives.

    The contributory objectives should be stated in terms of the understandings and the abilities that are necessary for the attainment of the central objective for each class session and for the unit. Central objectives focusses on general purpose of the lesson, what the teacher intended to teach, the central aim of the specific session of lesson.
2. Student-teacher centred objectives
    a. Student-centered objectives
    b. Teacher-centred objectives
        - General
        - Specific
    Related to previous work.
3. The plan should relate each class session to the previous work of the course. The desired objective in all learning is unity and understanding.
4. A well-organized course requires each day's work to fulfill some specific function in the realization of the course. Therefore, each class session should bear a definite relation to the previous one, e.g. by summary or review of past work, by well-chosen and directed questions and by student reports.

Selection and Organization of Subject Matter
The plan should provide for the selection and the organization of subject matter or the knowledge component and other such materials.
1. Learning activities:
    - The teacher chooses learning activities. It should be varied sufficiently to allow for individual differences in the group
    - Teacher should make her choice in view of the maturity of the group and the character of the subject matter, e.g. laboratory problems/exercises, nursing care plans.
    - In setting up the learning situation, the teacher starts the activities into motion to stimulate activity by questions, recollection of experiences, performance of experiments, solution of problems.
2. Teaching activities: The teaching techniques which will most directly help the teacher to obtain the objectives should be used.
3. Types of illustrative materials—Audio-visual aids and instruction media.
4. Assignments—The plan should use assignments to project the immediate work into the next situation Unity and continuity can be maintained only by directing the student's attention to the next step.
5. References: The teacher will have ready references to be used in directing the student's assignment and resource material for the study.
6. Evaluation: Some type of evaluation should be planned for each lesson; teacher supervisor will write comments after observing and practice teaching lesson by student teacher.
7. Format of lesson plan:
    Title of the course
    Unit
    Topic
    Name of the student-teacher
    Duration
    Date and time
    Place

Group of Students
Method of teaching
Audio-visual aids
Previous background of trainees
Student-teacher objectives
    General
    Specific.

Development of the Daily Class Plan

- Lesson plan should act as a guide; it creates a sense of assurance for the teacher. Since self-confidence allows greater freedom, the teacher is better able to direct student-learning activities. Teacher surely facilitates teaching of the student first and teaching of the subject matter second
- The teacher must be master of the daily plan
- Plan should be used as a basis for continuous growth and development
- The teacher should change her/his lesson plan according to the learning situation
- The teacher should adapt the daily plan related to the student needs and abilities
- Special work—Daily plan should provide for students who require special work
- Daily class plans—The new teacher should use more detailed daily plans. Later, as she/he gains experience, self-confidence and briefer forms may be used.
- Enthusiasm—If the teacher has an air of confidence, approaches the class positively, speaks in a natural, conversational tone, asks questions in an easy manner, creates immediate interest by means of an introduction, stands in a central position and fulfills fundamental requirements, for making a satisfactory presentation, the teacher should use good motivational techniques.

FORMAT OF LESSON PLAN

Time	Specific objectives	Content	Teaching-Learning activity	Evaluation

Common Problems in Daily Class Planning

1. Providing for emotionalized controls: Reemphasize the favorable attitudes in the form of appreciations grow out of satisfying experiences.

   An individual may gain knowledge and acquire abilities, but it is what the individual values that determines the direction of her/his actions. 'Values' of some kind are bound to grow out of the student's experiences with both the teacher and other students, hence, teacher should be interested in choosing activities from which students likely to develop positive aspects related to values of life.

   Attitudes, appreciations, interests are concomitant outcomes of teaching-learning activities. They are an outgrowth of activities in which students are concerned with getting understandings and abilities.

2. Providing for individual differences in abilities and interests: There will be individual differences in intelligence, abilities, previous experience and ideals among nursing students is common.

   The teacher's problem is to select those learning experiences, which will meet the student's needs. different procedures may be used in meeting the individual needs of students, e.g. individual projects, group projects, directed study, laboratory work, differentiated assignments, programed materials.

3. Providing integration of learning experiences: Provide the right kind of learning opportunities at the right time, which will help to facilitate the integration of student's learning experiences in a logical, sequential manner. Integration refer to the organization of content and activities so as to facilitate comprehension in the learner. Assignment motivates each student to self-initiated and self-directed study and asking question at the right moment, stimulates the student to creative thinking.

4. Providing for the evaluation of outcomes

   Purposes
   - To discover what learning products have been attained
   - To determine what progress has been made toward the attainment of other learning products

- To discover what skill has been gained in the use of learning products
- To reveal what difficulties the learner is encountering in her/his learning.

5. Helping students towards independent study:

"Study is an act or process of acquiring by one's own effort knowledge of some subject".

"Planned effort on the part of the learners in solving a problem, in getting knowledge or understanding or in acquiring certain abilities".

"Directing study means providing opportunities for students in class and outside of class to develop increasingly the attitudes and to acquire the skills which will enable them to engage in independent or self-directed study".

Aids to Effective Study

1. Ability to read with comprehension, speed and to outline, organize and summarize what has been read.
2. Ability to take lecture notes—Brief, intelligible, comprehensive, well-organized heading, sub-headings and its content, lists for easier reading.

   Notes: listen, select, evaluate and then summarize in her/his own words. Notes taking stimulates concentration and attention.
3. Ability to concentrate and discipline oneself to study,
4. Ability to determine the relative importance of memorizing, analyzing and reviewing.
5. Ability to plan and organize study time.
6. Certain environmental conditions to be met.

   If a point has been missed, the student should not stop taking notes to check it, instead, he/she should leave a blank space after the lecture has been finished and refer it and then correction can be made.

   Notes should be directly written in permanent form, so as to eliminate copying. mere re-copying of notes is a waste of time. Frequent review of notes facilitates unity and continuity by relating each lecture to the previous one and to the total unit.
7. Concentration—It consists of many specific habits and develops and associated with specific material. It is the result of control and direction of attention. The mind is constantly attending to something. Direction of the mind's activities results in concentration.

Aids to Concentration

- The student should have a definite purpose or goal and should set up objectives
- She/he should develop regular habits, work at certain times and in certain places
- Habits of positive attack on studies also should be developed. If effort is put forth, interest will follow
- Student will work under pressure:
  - Time should be set for the accomplishment of a certain paper, chapter or assignment
  - Intensive effort to work rapidly
  - Persistent well-directed work, results in maximum efficiency.
- The student should achieve an alert questioning attitude, criticize what is read and look for new meanings and new relationships
- The more information a student has about a subject, the more likely she/he is to be interested, the more interest he/she has, the easier is to attend
- Concentration can be aided by observing the proper length and distribution of study periods
- The student should compete with herself/himself to improve quality and rate of achievement
- She/he should train herself/himself to ignore distractions and to persist with studying inspite of them
- A familiar place of study is immediately suggestive of work and stimulates the proper reaction through conditioned response.

TYPES OF LESSON PLAN

A. Knowledge Lesson

To impart knowledge in a systematic manner, a set procedure has to be followed.

1. Preparation: "It ensures revision"—bringing back to consciousness of old knowledge with which the new is to be related. The assimilation and identification of a new idea by the mass of ideas already in the mind. It directs our attention to-mature the learner's mind and the mode of its approach to new ideas.

Preparation helps the teacher to ascertain what ideas on a particular topic his learners' possess and what further knowledge they require to satisfy their purpose, before he/she decides the next step in the teaching process.

2. Presentation: The teacher has to teach new facts, Illustrates the new procedure
   - Liberty should be given for the learner to suggest solution for the problem
   - For clear exposition, various devices can be used, e.g. questions, illustrations, explanations, exposition, Audio-visual aids, demonstration, etc. new knowledge may be explained, revealed or suggested.
3. Association or comparison: The teacher helps the class to analyze the new knowledge or experience and to compare and contrast it with the old and build up old one into a new and complete unity (association).
4. Generalization: The whole lesson is drawn together—A summary is made, a general rule formulated. Integration and arranging in pattern is essential. The goal of generalization is systematization, orderliness and unification and the means hitherto for comparison and abstraction. Generalization completes the process of inquiry by providing the answer to the problem with which it began.
5. Application: The teacher should seek an application both in the setting of problems and in the acquisition of further knowledge. Induction process should be followed deduction process.
6. Systematization or recapitulation: A revision or repetition of the knowledge learnt in the lesson. It helps the learners to come to some conclusion with reference to the wider significance of the proble Ways of Recapitulation—Sectional revision at convenient sections of the lesson for revising the main facts taught therein. Revision at the final stage of the lesson (feedback).

B. The Skill Lesson

To learn various skills is a human need. The use of the muscles is not only good for the body, it is also good for the mind. 'No impression without expression' clearly speaks the value of skill.

Methods of Teaching Skill
1. Demonstration—Thorough and neat in execution to express.
2. Verbal instruction—If the teacher has the clear mental imagery to describe the movements in details and the learner has sufficient experience to grasp them

Steps for Teaching Skill
- The teacher has to create interest among learners—By showing good specimens of articles, encourage the learners to observe or participate in visiting museums, exhibitions and workshops
  - Giving assignments for the learners to do the projects, i.e. execution of plan, preparation of Audio Visual aids different varieties, encourage the learner to formulate clear aim /objectives for every lesson plan is essential
- Presentation
  - Motivate the learner to demonstrate the process, while carrying out the procedure, she/he may verbally explain the process with the help of diagrams and blackboard sketches.
- Practice—Repetition of the activity that the teacher has demonstrated
- Proficiency in the skills depends on the success of individual practice. The learner will certainly need much guidance
- Practice makes men perfect when the proper movements and the correct usages are repeated. Hence the importance of proper supervision during practice is essential
- Statement of rules—Rules restricts activity and endangers freedom and spontaneity.

Types of Skills
1. Mechanical skill —For example utilizing body mechanics while practicing fundamentals of nursing preocedures to prevent strain over the muscles.
2. Manipulation skill—For example surgical manipulation for simulator-based surgical skill.

C. The Appreciation Lesson

It aims at developing the aesthetic sense of the learners, enable the pupils to appreciate beauty expressed in color, form, sound or other excellence especially art, science, literature.

To develop the emotions as against the acquisition of skill or knowledge.

Steps in Carrying out Appreciation Lesson

1. Preparation: The teacher's first task is to provide and repeat experiences from which the learners derive emotional pleasure. Teacher has to motivate the learners for enjoyment, provide suitable environmental conditions and suitable material available. There should not be any distraction. Difficulties of students must be appreciated by teacher and then treated in a preceding lesson.
2. Presentation: Teacher should make use of every device, which will assist the vividness of appeal and enable the learner to enjoy the lesson to the maximum extent. Appreciation cannot be forced, the learners can be helped to appreciate through various techniques: proper atmosphere, good presentation, good expression and his own interest.
3. Contemplation: Critical appreciation or intellectual discussion is concerned that should only be attempted at higher levels. It should be dealt from whole to parts.
4. Application: Appreciation should seek an immediate application in the stimulus, it may provide for creative exercises.

Essentials of a Well-delivered Lesson

- Plan should be well-designed, well-prepared, well-written in terms of good confidence
- Clear about the objectives of lesson plan
- Have complete mastery of the subject matter
- Use audiovisual aids systematically, effectively and productively
- See that the learners are well-seated, good ventilation, clean blackboard properly placed
- Introduction should be interesting; time is 5 to 7 minutes for introduction for the whole class 30 to 45 minutes
- Adopt right methods of teaching and involve active participation of learners, be clear about the thoughts and expressions. Give challenging situations to them
- Use blackboard systematically and timely; writing on blackboard should be legible, clear and bold. Prepare a neat blackboard summary with the help of the learners
- Ask questions to the group, should be definite, clear, stimulating, thought provoking
- Learning activities should inspire self-learning among the students, they should give them sufficient time to think, to reason, to analyze, to synthesize and to deduce
- Periodically check whether the pupils are coming along, give time to the pupils to clarify their doubts and mistakes should be corrected
- Lesson should be related to the actual life. You should have the appreciation of the functional correlation between subject-matter and the problems of life (needs of life)
- Budget the time according to the steps of the lesson
- Pay individual attention to the pupils where needed, careful about back-benchers
- Be natural do not put your hands in the pocket or lean on the chair or table. Avoid playing with the chalk, have neat and tidy work habits
- Attend to pupils work habits also, pay attention to defective reading, writing and standing postures
- Have adequate command over spoken language for effective smooth and flawless expression. Be clear, concise in the use of language. Avoid verbatim; be economical in the use of language
- Recapitulation and application to new situations
- Maintain the discipline of the class. Competition and cooperation in a rational way is needed
- Teacher has to provide intellectual, moral, emotional integrity, a model of creative and responsible leadership to direct the learners' activities
- Do not be too rigid and mechanical.

Critical Observation of Lessons

1. Teacher's personal appearances and movements:
   - Command of language
   - Voice (rhythm, speed, volume, pitch should be taken into consideration)
   - Interest in the subject and pupils
   - Alertness.

2. Mastery over subject-matter:
   - Preparation
   - Selection
   - Suitability
   - Division of sections and their arrangement.
3. Method:
   - Type adopted
   - Presentation
   - Learner's involvement in the lesson
   - Range of activities provided and their productivity
   - Amount of originality shown in the presentation of lesson
   - The extent to which interest is created
   - Skill in questioning and dealing with answers
   - Clarity of thought and expression, use of audio-visual aids
   - Blackboard work
   - Correlation of lesson to actual life
   - Class-management
   - Neat and tidy work habit
   - Sectional revision.
4. Miscellaneous:
   - Lesson notes
   - Proportioning time to different steps
   - Application and practical work
   - Student's written work
   - Learner's reaction to the lesson.

Approaches of curriculum

a. Knowledge approach: (Subject-area approach) Subjects are selected to transmit the desirable knowledge to the younger generation. Certain disciplines are brought together to form broad-field curriculum or integrated curriculum. Based on need individual subjects are selected as the subjects of study. Teacher centered approach will be used. For example conducting theory classes.
b. Activity approach: Activities are selected to form curriculum. The students engage themselves in different activities and acquire knowledge of different subjects incidentally as by products of their activities. The teacher assumes the role of consultants or directors of activities. Students assume active role. Education becomes learner-centred, e.g. clinical activities.
c. Living approach: Life-centred education. Living is learning. Students learn as they live their learning experiences. Accept the degree of learning will be in proportion to the degree of their active association, acceptance and retention. For example growth and development.
d. Broad fields approach: Organizing the curriculum by combining two or more subject areas into a broader field, e.g. behavioural sciences.
e. Social problem approach: It consists of organizing curriculum around major problems in society, e.g. social pathology
f. Emerging needs approach: It focuses on the personal and social needs that are emerging in the lives of the learners at the present time, e.g. Environmental Hygiene.

CURRICULUM EVALUATION

Definition

Evaluation is "The systematic process for determining the degree to which changes in behavior (of students) are actually taking place"– *Tyler.*

Concept and Meaning

It is a process of assessment, it will serve as the basis for making an assessment about the individual program or the institution. It is a continuous process (Fig. 3.4), helps in making decisions about students, teaching-learning techniques, facilities, objectives to be realized. Evaluation includes measurement but goes beyond in having qualitative considerations and suggesting modifications for deficient areas. Whereas measurement includes a variety of testing procedures that describe output in quantitative terms. It refers to observations and judgments made about what actually happens in the school, what the students have achieved and what else may be included. It determines the value of curriculum, whether it is fulfilling its purposes for which it was formulated.

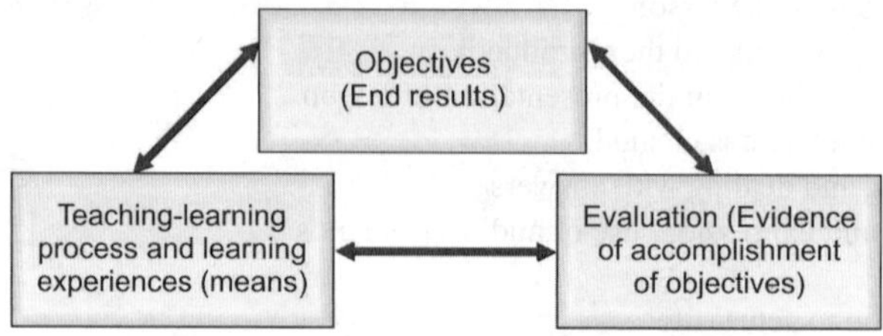

Fig. 3.14: Cycle of process of curriculum

Need

- To measure the extent of achievement of objectives and to clarify objectives
- To assess effectiveness of curriculum implementation
- To identify the cause for defective curriculum
- It leads to whether modification is required for improving instruction and the teaching-learning process
- Determines the students' level of knowledge, skills and attitudes at intervals
- To assess students' performance levels.
- Motivates the students to implement specific efforts for their improvement in performance levels
- To Diagnose difficulties in implementation of curriculum process i.e., with the individual students or group in certain achievement areas or with performance of teachers or in teaching - learning activities
- To identify the remedial measures to promote the situation and to solve the problems
- Helps in gathering information for administrative purposes
- It provides quality control in education
- To provide effective, meaningful, need-based and rational curricular material. As good materials and resourceful information contribute for bringing desirable changes among learners.
- Evaluation helps in modifying the curriculum to meet the growing challenges.

Methods and Techniques adopted—Opinion survey, questionnaire, Schedules, Interview—Individual and Group, Discussions, Observation, Experiments, Practical performance and Anecdotal records.

Levels of Curriculum Evaluation

1. Formative evaluation:

The curriculum developer, himself/herself carries out the task of material evaluation. It is used to improve the materials while they are prepared and developed. Ongoing evaluation to measure the progress made by the students from the moment she/he begins the programming until the time he/she completes it. It gives feedback at intervals in accordance with the progress made or lack of it. Inventories, questionnaires, observational and reporting techniques are used.

- The teacher should not use formative evaluation for certification.
- As the course proceeds, an ongoing evaluation is carried out to establish:
    - How far the learning prescribed has been mastered?
    - What are the attitudes of teachers and their pupils towards the course?

2. Summative Evaluation:

- Persons other than writer or the developer of the curriculum material will do it. For example external examiner from other university
- It takes place after the implementation of the curriculum material

- Is used after a specified period of instruction for certification
- Describe the extent to which the program has attained the objectives
- Provides guidelines for decisions about curriculum revision or modification or shift of emphasis
- Is designed to protect the society by preventing incompetent personnel from practicing
- It assesses overall attitudes of teachers and pupils to the course.

Curriculum Evaluation Plan

1. The rationale of evaluation: It denotes the need for evaluation; the approach and the benefits obtained by an evaluation.
2. Objectives of the evaluation study: Concerned with the specifications of the standards that the curriculum should meet.
3. Curriculum description: Description of curriculum objectives, Philosophy, Content, Procedures and minimum requirement of the learners to entry into the program.
4. Evaluation design: Constraints under which evaluation is developed, evaluation model used, appropriateness of evaluation design, assessment of extent of achievement of objectives, sources of information, methods of collecting information, implementation of curriculum planning, data analysis techniques and budget
5. Evaluation report: The findings of the evaluation program, the extent to which the objectives of curriculum have been achieved and suggestions for further study.

Factors influencing the change in curriculum

1. Societal changes: Population explosion, Population pattern, Urbanization and Consumption of natural resources, health status, health problems (incidence & prevalence).
2. Changes in health care delivery pattern.
3. Maintenance of standards and equality throughout the globe in implementation of educational programs.

Need for curriculum revision

- To restructure the curriculum according to the needs of learners and societal needs
- To achieve maximum extent of achievement of objectives
- To modify the content based on findings of curriculum evaluation
- To introduce latest and update methods in teaching and content, new knowledge and practices
- To meet the standards of statutory body and global requirements.

Management of Curriculum

In the management of curriculum different educational authorities play different roles:

1. Role of faculties and Board of study members in universities/Boards: Helps to propagate the concepts and principles of curriculum development and its implementation and prepares examiners list by considering faculty list submitted by the respective professional colleges evaluation and research on curriculum.
2. Role of Indian Nursing Council: It formulates philosophy, objectives, syllabi, frame-work of all the courses. It will give permission to start, to continue the course and to increase student strength or it can stop the program, if it feels school/college is not having enough facilities.
3. Role of state government: It has an advisory role. Advisory bodies helps in providing necessary guide lines in curriculum construction, preparation of and evaluation materials, examiner lists, techniques of evaluation, research and reconstruction through their education departments. It permits the schools/colleges to start and continue the course. Having responsibility to produce an publish textbooks, teachers' handbooks and other instruction materials to be used in the classroom instruction. It is responsible for the proper curriculum development and implementation in the schools on the basis of leadership provided by the national bodies.

Role of Nursing Education Department

a. Directorate level—Director of Nursing
   - To ensure the educational policies and goals are properly reflected by the curriculum
   - Responsible for the realization of the curriculum goals through its effective implementation
   - Try out is made properly and necessary modifications are carried out
   - Priorities were established to different programs at different levels.

b. Role of educational supervisor
   - Active participants in curriculum development
   - Prepare Guides for curriculum implementation
   - Evaluation of curriculum
   - Curriculum reformers.
c. Role of school organizers/Administrators
   - Curriculum implementers
   - Curriculum evaluators.
d. Role of subject specialists
   - Determiners of the curriculum
   - Framers of the syllabi
   - Writers of textbooks, handbooks.
e. Role of methodology experts
   - Curriculum planners
   - Syllabi makers
   - Textbooks and handbooks writers
   - Curriculum evaluators
   - Curriculum reviewers.
f. Role of Teachers
   The teacher is the heart of the curriculum and he/she determines in a large measure the actual learning experiences that go in the classrooms. The teacher must be acknowledged in curriculum planning he/she should be allowed freedom in planning educational experience for learners.
   Teachers should be given adequate opportunities to carry instructional experimentation in the classroom setting so that they can be active in the selection of learning materials.
g. Role of educational organizations
   Educational organizations play active role in planning, developing, implementing, evaluating, producing instructional materials and evaluation materials, textbooks, supplementary reading materials and reconstructucting curriculum as and when necessary arises.
h. Role of parents
   Parents will be influenced by the curriculum developed. Parents, if they are qualified, involve them in syllabi modification and evaluation.
i. Students' Role
   Students are the clienteles for whom the curriculum is developed. They are the most affected persons by the curriculum. Hence there is dire need to actively involve them in the development and implementation as well.

CURRICULUM ADMINISTRATION

Three phases involved in curriculum administration (Fig. 3.15).

- Curriculum Planning
  It is a dynamic nature of human life and essential feature of administrative programs of instruction and its concomitant effect on the educational scene.
- Curriculum Organisation
  It is a prerequisite of any kind of instructional program. In each course of study, subjectwise, classwise curriculum organization takes place. The detailed syllabi are prepared, as these serve as the bases for writing the textbook.

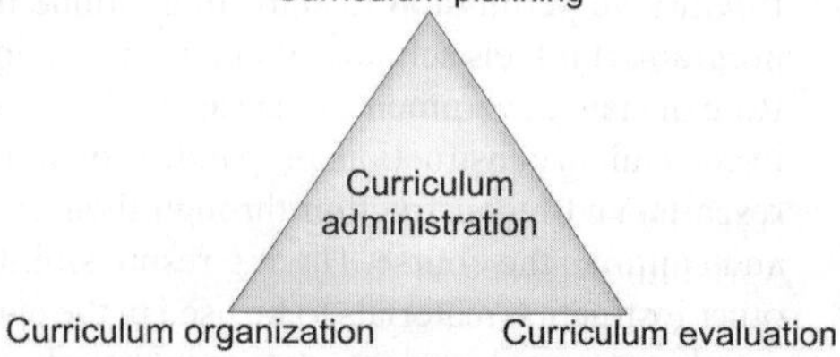

Fig. 3.15: Phases of curriculum administration

Highly centralized and decentralized system of curriculum construction, reconstruction and administration are functional aspects to be satisfied for the effective implementation of curricular program.

Educational machinery of state government has to take chief responsibility of curriculum organization as it develops educational policy and its effective implementation for financing adequately the organization of educational programs in schools and colleges.

Freedom has to be given to implement curriculum at the school.

The effectiveness of curriculum organization depends on—Quality of syllabuses prescribed, Type of handbooks and textbooks prepared, Adequacy of guidance provided to teachers and Institutional aids supplied.

- Curriculum Evaluation

  Educational administration has to take up the responsibility of curriculum evaluation. It provides needed feedback for further revising and reforming the curriculum implementation from time to time.

  Curriculum evaluation is carried out by Supervisory program of classroom instruction, Guidance and direction based on educational supervision, Planning of methods and means for the improvement of effective implementation of the evaluated program.

MINI COURSES

To meet the educational needs and demands of population, innumerable number of educational institutions has grown up but there is no guarantee of employment, even after the completion of long-term courses. The more number of people, the institution numbers are less, it is not coinciding or not fulfilling the felt needs of population. Due to industrialization and privatization, there is an increased demand for skilled workers. Realizing the importance of skilled training, less duration courses in the form of certificate courses or short-term, job oriented courses were started. The government (state and central) is encouraging to introduce mini courses in the universities, e.g. IGNOU, Open Universities, Distance Education training program; even private organizations like: Apollo Hospitals, NIMS, Speciality Hospitals, etc. are encouraged to start mini courses, e.g. certificate course in Neuro-Nursing, Pediatric Nursing.

Objectives

- To provide practical experiences
- To Provide specific skill training
- To develop professional skills
- To become suitable for certain jobs and to fit for promotions
- To widen the knowledge and to provide varied experience
- Useful to the persons who are not afford to take up long-term professional courses
- To acquire educational achievements
- Provides opportunity and easy accessibility to acquire higher qualifications
- Acquaints the learner to enter into various courses based on their interests and aptitudes.

These mini courses are of short duration like 4 to 6 weeks; 6 to 12 months, etc. viz.
- Diploma /certificate course in critical care management, Oncology.
- Apprenticeship courses.
- Computer education courses .
- Type writing and shorthand courses.
- Book binding course.
- Machine repair and maintenance course.
- TV and radio repair course.
- Sericulture course.
- Agriculture training course.
- Land survey course.
- Inservice training programs.
- Extension service programs.

QUESTIONS

- Bloom's Educational Objectives (5 M, NTRUHS, June 2009 & RGUHS, 2009).
- Characteristics and types of attention, explain span of attention & distraction (10M, NTRUHS, Dec, 2007).
- Clinical Rotation in III year B.Sc Nursing (10 M, RGUHS, April 2007).
- Clinical rotation in III year B.Sc Nursing (10M, RGUHS, Oct, 2006).
- Clinical Rotation Plan (5M, MGU, Nov, 2009)
- Clinical Rotation plan for Second year B.Sc. (N) students as per INC syllabus (15M, NIMS, Oct, 2008).
- Co-Curricular activities and their importance in Nursing Educational Institution (15M, NIMS, Oct, 2009).
- Cognitive Objectives (5M, MGRUHS, Nov, 2010).
- Components of Lesson Plan (5M, MGRUHS, Feb, 2009).
- Course planning (10 M, RGUHS, April 2009, M.Sc., & 5M, NTRUHS, Nov 2009, 5M, MGU, Oct, 2007).
- Criteria of a good objective (5M, RGUHS, Aug, 2010).
- Curriculum Committee (10M, RGUHS, April, 2008 and 5M, RGHUS, Aug, 2010).
- Define Curriculum and Write the steps and Levels of Curriculum (5M, NTRUHS, June 2009).
- (a)Define Course Plan (b) Describe the elements of a unit plan (c) Prepare a lesson plan for "Administration of Intramuscular Injection" for first year GNM students (2+5+8 =15M, MGU, Nov, 2009).
- (a)Define curriculum (b) Explain steps in curriculum development (c) Describe organization of learning experience for II year GNM students (2+8+5 M, MGU, Oct, 2007).
- (a)Define Curriculum (b) Explain steps in Curriculum development (c) Discuss the importance of Curriculum evaluation (15M, NIMS, Sept, 2010).
- (a)Define educational objectives (b) Explain educational objectives (c) Describe criteria for the selection and statement of objectives (2+8+5 M, MGU, Dec, 2006).
- Define Curriculum and explain any one step in the development of Curriculum (2+10M, NTRUHS, June, 2010 & 3+7M NTRUHS, July, 2008).
- Define Curriculum, Explain the factors influencing in Nursing Curriculum Development, Discuss in detail about Steps in Curriculum Development (7 + 8M, MGRUHS, Feb, 2009 & Nov 2010) .
- Define Curriculum-, Explain the selection a organization of Learning Experiences (3M + 8M, NTRUHS, June 2009).
- Define curriculum. Explain curriculum planning in nursing educational institution (15M, NTRUHS, Nov, 2010).
- Define Curriculum? Write about the determinants and steps in developing Nursing Curriculum? (15M, NIMS, Oct, 2009 &15M, NIMS, May, 2007).
- Define educational objective, Explain the elements of educational objective, Describe Bloom's taxonomy of educational objective (2+5+8 = 15 M, MGU, Nov, 2009,).
- Define Learning Experience (2M, MGRUHS, Feb, 2010).
- Define Lesson plan (2M, MGRUHS, Feb, 2010 & 5M, Rajasthan UHS, March, 2010) Write a lesson plan for any one Nursing Procedure (15M, NTRUHS, June, 2009).
- Define Objectives and classify the Educational Objectives according to Bloom (5M, NTRUHS, Dec, 2007).
- Describe "Bloom's" taxonomy of educational objectives. How are they useful to a nurse educator? (10M, RGUHS, Oct, 2008).
- Describe the Characteristics of a Good Lesson Plan (5M, MGRUHS, Feb, 2010).
- Describe the steps in curriculum development, Enumerate the principles of curriculum organization (15M, RGUHS, Oct, 2009).
- Develop a lesson plan on Communication for 1st B.Sc. (N) students (10M, RGUHS, May, 2010).
- Differentiate between aims and objectives (2M, RGUHS, Aug, 2010).
- Differentiate between Institutional curriculum - Societal curriculum (5M, MGU, Dec, 2008).
- Discuss the determinants of Attention (10M, NTRUHS, Dec, 2007).
- Discuss the importance of clinical rotation plan in nursing education. What are the factors to be considered while planning a clinical rotation plan? (10M, RGUHS, Aug, 2010).
- Discuss the importance of Unit planning and explain the differences between Unit Planning and Lesson Planning (15M, NIMS, Oct, 2009).

- Explain any one Step in Curriculum Development, Factors affecting Curriculum Development (5+6M, MGRUHS, Nov, 2010).
- Explain any one Type of Curriculum (5M, MGRUHS, Aug, 2007).
- Explain Steps in Curriculum Development, Describe the various Levels of Curriculum with examples (10 M, RGUHS, April 2009).
- Explain steps in curriculum development? describe the various levels of curriculum with examples (5+7M, RGUHS, 2009).
- Explain the advantages of Clinical rotation plan (6M, NTRUHS, Dec, 2007).
- Explain the Curriculum Change, Discuss the selection and organization of Learning Experiences (15M, RGUHS, May, 2010).
- Explain the factors to be considered when selecting and organizing learning experiences for Nursing students (10M, RGUHS, April, 2008).
- Explain the Factors to be considered when Selecting and Organizing Learning Experiences Students. (15 M, RGUHS, April, 2008).
- Explain the factors to be considered when Selecting and Organizing Learning Experiences for students (15M, RGUHS, April, 2008).
- Factors influencing Curriculum (4M, NIMS, May, 2007).
- Factors influencing Curriculum Development (5 M, MGRUHS, Aug, 2006).
- Formulation of Objectives (5M, NTRUHS, July, 2008).
- Lesson Plan (4M, Rajasthan UHS, Feb, 2008).
- Lesson Plan (5M) Discuss the role of Teacher in Nursing Education (6M), Prepare lesson plan to demonstrate administration of 40 units of Plain Insulin to a patient (7M, MGRUHS, Aug, 2006 & Feb 2010).
- Lesson Plan (5M, NTRUHS, July, 2008 &June, 2010; 7.5M, Baba Farid UHS, 2010; 4M, NIMS, May, 2007).
- Master Rotation Plan (5M, MGU, Dec, 2008; 5M, MGRUHS, Nov, 2010; 5M, MGU, Nov, 2009).
- Master rotation plan and its importance in basic B.Sc. Nursing programme (10M, RGUHS, Oct, 2009).
- Master Rotation Plan and its importance in Basic B.Sc. Nursing programme (10 M, RGUHS, Oct, 2008).
- Maxims of Teaching (5M, NTRUHS, June, 2009 &5M, 8M, Baba Farid UHS, 2009 & 2010, 5 M, MGRUHS, Aug, 2007 & Feb, 2010, 5M, MGU, Nov, 2009; 5M, NIMS, Dec, 2009).
- Name the Taxonomy of Educational Objectives (10 M, MGRUHS, Aug, 2008 & 5M, RGUHS, 2009).
- Objective structure (5M, NTRUHS, June, 2009).
- Organization of learning experience (5M, MGU, Dec, 2006).
- Prepare a Lesson Plan for first B.Sc. Nursing students on Urinary Catheterization (8M, MGRUHS, Feb, 2010).
- Prepare lesson plan to educate a group of mothers on prevention of diarrhoea. (5M, RGUHS, Feb, 2010).
- Prepare lesson plan to educate a group of mothers on prevention of diarrhoea (8M, RGUHS, Feb, 2010).
- Principles of curriculum development (5M, MGU, Dec, 2008).
- Principles of curriculum development (5M, MGU, Dec, 2008).
- Principles of Curriculum Development (7M, MGRUHS, Nov, 2010).
- Programmed Instruction, Taxonomy of educational Objectives (4+4M NTRUHS, Dec, 2007).
- Rotation Plan (5 M, MGRUHS, Aug, 2006).
- Selection of Learning Experiences and Learning Outcomes (10 M, RGUHS, Oct, 2008).
- Selection of learning experiences and learning outcomes (10M, RGUHS, Oct, 2008).
- State the Characteristics of Unit Plan (2M, MGRUHS, Feb, 2010).
- Three elements of good Lesson Plan (3M, MGU, Dec, 2008).
- Three elements of Unit plan (3M, MGU, Dec, 2006).
- Types of Educational Objectives (5M, MGRUHS, Feb, 2009 & Nov, 2010).
- Unit Planning (5 M, NTRUHS, June 2009).
- Unit Planning (4M, NTRUHS, June 2009; 5M, RGUHS, Aug, 2010; 5M, MGU, Dec, 2008).
- What are learning experiences, Explain the learning experiences will you select for teaching Fundamentals of Nursing (6+6=12M, NTRUHS, June 2009).
- What are the factors to be considered for developing Curriculum, critically evaluate the B.Sc. Nursing curriculum prescribed by INC (15M, NIMS, Oct, 2009).

- What are the Subjective Determinants of Attention (7.5M, NTRUHS, July, 2008).
- What is a lesson plan? Why should you plan a lesson? Evaluate critically lesson plan format which you are practicing during your course of study (10M, RGUHS, Oct, 2008).
- What is a Lesson Plan? Why should you plan a Lesson? Evaluate critically Lesson Plan format which you are practicing during your course of study? (15 M, RGUHS, Oct, 2008).
- What is curriculum planning? What aspects would you consider in planning the clinical rotation for the B.Sc. nursing four year programme? What criteria would you follow in selecting the clinical facilities for your students? (10M, RGUHS, Oct, 2009).
- What is Learning Experience? How will you select and organize the Learning Experiences for B.Sc. (N) Programme (15M, NIMS, Oct, 2009).
- What principles will you keep in mind while making a Master Rotation Plan (6M, NTRUHS, Dec, 2007).
- Write a Lesson Plan for any Basic Nursing Procedure (11M, NTRUHS, June 2009).
- Write the purposes of Lesson Planning? (5M, NTRUHS, Dec, 2007).

Teaching and Learning Process

CONCEPT OF TEACHING

Interactions between teacher and student is the teacher's responsibility to bring expected behavioral changes within the student's behavior, 'Teaching' is a distinctively 'human activity, imparting knowledge' and the 'learning process' means by which 'the student assimilates the information and share the content'.

Definitions

"Teaching is stimulating and challenging the student to learn, of enhancing has realization of the values of a subject, helping her/him to bring to bear her/his own resources in formulating and pursuing a method of attack on learning the subject (including the relevant skills and attitudes) and guiding her/him in the process".

"Teaching is immediate mastery of particular knowledge or skill".

"It is concerned with growth and development of whole personality of the student–her/his mind, spirit, character and effective behavior".

"Teaching is an intimate contact between a more mature personality and a less mature one which is designed to further the education of the latter"—*HC Morrison*

"Teaching is an arrangement and manipulation of a situation in which there are gaps and obstructions, which an individual will seek to overcome and which he learn in the course of doing so"—*J Brubacher*.

"An interactive process, primarily involving classroom talk, which takes place between teacher and the student and occurs during certain definable activities"—*Edmund Amidon*.

"Teaching is a task of the teacher, which is performed for the development of the child"—*TF Greens*.

"Teaching is a combination of an Art and Science viz.

Teaching is an Art:
- It is an activity, which is practiced with skill.
- It cannot be reduced to any exact sequential series of actions; it involves two dynamic factors:
  - The mind's natural activity of the learner
  - The intellectual guidance on the part of the teacher, with the principal dynamic factor or the propelling force being the internal vital principle in the learner and the teacher being secondary, eventhough a genuinely effective dynamic factor and ministerial agent".

Teaching is a science, as it is based on a body of systematically derived knowledge, converted to principles which guide to its practices".

Principles to be followed in planning learning and educational activities

- The learner's own intellectual progress, the activity whereby his/her mind (assisted by the teacher through instruction and by observation and interaction with others) trace out the connection between facts and principles of knowledge and the particular conclusions in a given field.
- Teacher's knowledge, her/his convictions become an instructive and effective part of the act of teaching; she/he communicates through her/his voice, tone, manner and attitude as well as through her/his words.
- Teaching will be based on the previous experience of the learner.
- It includes teaching to base itself on facts and experiences to realize itself in rational knowledge grounded in principles i.e., to grasp reality in terms of how and why.

Purposes of Teaching

- Immediate mastery over the subject with its related skills is important, but advancement toward growth in all spheres of the human personality is considered
- Development of wholesome personality (changing habits, attitudes, reconstituting ideals and changing interests) of the learner.
- To help students to:
  - Acquire, retain and be able to use the knowledge in relevant fields.
  - Understand, analyze, synthesize and evaluate the knowledge.
  - Achieve skills.
  - Establish habits.
  - Develop attitudes, Abilities/Strengths.
- Focus and implements the steps to solve the problems.

Qualities of a Good Teacher

1. Respect for the student's maturity and sense of responsibility.
   a. Allow the students to select their own topic of interest to be pursued as a term paper.
   b. Avoiding useless repetition and irrelevant material during lectures.
   c. Being so thoroughly prepared for each class period as to make it obvious that she/he was an adult speaking to adults.
2. Stimulating
   a. Ideas presented were have meaning.
   b. Strong, modulus, clear voice.
   c. No embarrassing stuttering or stammering for the proper or correct word, term or phrase.
   d. Pauses were inserted deliberately and yet non-dramatically to allow for some "digestion of complex thoughts" were followed by a few concrete examples or analogies.
3. Assignments: clear and concise
   a. Oral
   b. Written
4. Subject matter content
   a. Lectures with student discussion, e.g. ask questions at the 10 minute break between hours and during last 5 minutes and starting of session.
   b. Organization of subject matter in class or clinical experiences, e.g. before class began, the necessary diagrams, charts or relationships were drawn on the chalkboard or kept ready in workable condition.
   c. Time should not be wasted by teacher in trying to clarify her/his own ideas.
   d. She/he must know:
      - What she/he wanted to say?
      - When she/he wanted to say?
      - How she/he wanted to say?

Factors Intrinsic to the Teacher (Personal Attributes)

1. Mastery over the subject
2. Psychological security and maturity
3. Excellent speech and delivery (good voice quality)
   Voice — Clear
   Distinct
   Pleasant
   Well-modulated
   Lucid.
4. Neatness and poise
   Good esthetic sense
   Correct posture

5. Sense of humor
   No need to resort.
6. Broad interests and wider exposure
   Familiarity in all related fields
   Extra curricular activities.
7. Well-balanced personality
   She/he should know when to smile, laugh or be serious to make the teaching meaningful.
8. Professionally well groomed
   Poised
   Self-confident
   Neat, clean, attractive in her /his personal appearance.
9. Tolerant and fair
   No partiality
   Caters time to listen to student's problems.
10. Kind and patient
    Sincere person
    Intense love for Nursing and for young people
    Gives few words of encouragement
    Empathetic in nature.
11. Teaching qualities — Knowledge of subject matter
    She/he should present her/his lecture with background material by which a student could understand more fully the particular topic being taught.
    She/he displayed evidence that she/he too was a constant learner by her/his frequent presentation of up-to-date nursing topics and trends.
12. Preparation of classes
    She/he should present outlines of the class or present session to the student in advance.
    - Purpose
    - Objectives
    - Content in brief
    - Student should aware of the meaning of the class and the course
    - Understand group's limitations.
13. Clear exposition of subject matter
    - The students should understand the subject being taught
    - She/he brought up a reference that was assigned to read
    - Discussion was encouraged
    - Effective utilization of resources
    - Employs varied teaching approaches
      - Talk to students
      - Talk with students
      - Have them talk together
      - Show students how and why of a procedure (Rational, it will be long lasting in the minds of learners)
      - Supervise them
      - Provide opportunities for practice.
14. Leadership ability as well as a deeper knowledge
    - Teachers should be represented to the students that a professional person to be
    - Her/his personality coupled with his/her deep interest in each individual student was a great source of stimulation and motivation to achieve and become a well-rounded professional being.
15. Exhibits Interest and appreciation in nursing and in Learners
16. Friendly in nature
17. Responsible, systematic, stimulating force, imaginative and creative teacher
18. Ever-loving nature

19. Exemplar, role model
21. Inspirative, encouraging in nature
22. Good motivator
23. Ever change her/his interests, purposes, attitudes, habits, abilities and skills
24. Positive philosopher (optimistic in nature)
25. Good guide and counselor
26. Effective organizer
27. Good administrator
28. Keen observer, supporter and listener.
29. Idealistic in nature
30. Reassurance in nature
31. Maintaining good human relations
32. Good communicator
33. Diplomatic in nature
34. Researcher
35. Dignified in nature
36. Evaluation
    - Evaluation of student for entire course was on:
        - Reference readings
        - Class discussions
        - Speeches
        - Mid-term and final exams
        - Performance in both class and clinical settings.

Role/Functions of the Teacher

Instructional role

1. Planning and organizing courses
    - Selecting objectives
    - Substantiate content and teaching, learning activities, correlating them with other courses in the curriculum
2. Creating and maintaining a desirable group climate which will encourage and enhance learning and will lead to the development of learner self-discipline
3. Adapting teaching and preparing and instructional materials to the varying interests, needs and abilities of the students
4. Motivating and challenging students to pursue and to sustain learning activities which will lead them towards acceptance of responsibility for their own learning
5. Teaching involves many activities
   For Example:
    - Supplying information needed or telling the source of information
    - Explaining, clarifying and interpreting
    - Demonstrating or explaining a procedure, a process or exhibiting materials
    - Serving as a resource person for group activities or group projects or to the individual students
    - Supervising student's performance in classroom, lab setting and other learning experiences
    - Evaluating all the planned learning and teaching activities and student's outcome.

Faculty role

In the case of college or university, the term 'faculty' is used to refer to 'the teaching staff'.

The role Tof the faculty will vary according to the philosophy, objectives and setting of educational institution.

1. Chairwoman, secretary or member of one or more committees
2. Counselor of students in matters (academic and non-academic)
3. Researchers
4. Resource persons to groups outside the institution, other schools, health agencies
5. A representative to professional nursing organizations and other agencies for her faculty or for the institution
6. A public relations agent, she/he interprets the objectives and the policies of institution and helps in recruitment

Individual Role

As an individual he/she plays personal role:

- As a member of a family, a church, a community and a citizen
- Dignified, distinct personality
- Friend and Philosopher.

The Psychology of being a Teacher

'A teacher one never truly teach unless he/she is still learning himself/herself, a lamp can never light another lamp unless it continues to burn its own flame'.

'Teaching is a unique process of socio-psycho-emotional behavior. Environmental factors, such as administrative policy, curriculum objectives, materials and class size, have a unique effect upon each teacher's physical and mental health. However, the factors, which may have the greatest effect on mental health in teaching, are the competencies acquired during the period of preparation in teaching. These competencies affect one's purpose, attitude, efficiency, interest and self-appraisal. These learning factors determine the quality of mental health experienced in teaching. Natural personality and academic professional competencies are dispensable in developing and in maintaining good mental health in the art and science of teaching. The following list is offered as a suggested selection of goals which the conscientious teacher may properly strive to realize all of these aims but the ideals should be kept in mind'.

Competencies contributing to maintain good mental health in teacher

1. Each teacher should acquire and maintain certain qualities which are characteristics of mature personality
   - Good physical health and appropriate health habits
   - Social tact and confidence
   - Ability to work cooperative with other persons.
2. Each teacher should develop a positive philosophy of life and education
   - A code of moral values for directing and appraising personal and social behavior
   - An appreciation of the values and principles inherent in democracy
   - An understanding of the goals, principles and practices involved in democratic education
   - An awareness of the relationship between teaching and learning.
3. Each teacher should possess knowledge of the nature of human growth and development
   - An understanding of the nature and uniqueness of human behavior
   - Recognition of the nature and the function of individual differences
   - An understanding of the personal and social problems and tensions experienced by learners and youth in finding adequacy in living and working with peer associates and adults
   - Recognition that mental health is a learned way of personal interaction with other persons.
4. Each teacher should possess an appreciation and understanding of the meaning and practice of democracy in the classroom
   - Readiness to discover and to respect the worth of each individual
   - Provide leadership and opportunity for cooperative planning, executing and evaluating of curriculum activities
   - Encourage members of the classroom society to formulate desirable citizenship objectives and duties
   - Assist learners in learning, responsibility through participation in socially useful work
   - Provide leadership and practice in individual and group decision making.
5. Each teacher should have an understanding of the objectives and function of each social institutions such as the family, the religious institutions, Government agencies and the school
   - Recognition of the cultural background and the evolutionary process
   - An appreciation of the affect of the institutions on the personal development and social living of young people
   - Recognition that the value of these institutions is based on their contribution to the improvement of the general welfare of people.

6. Each teacher should have knowledge of the ideas, leader and events that produced the heritage of the nation.
   - An appreciation of the ideals and ideas that motivated historic actions
   - An understanding of the leaders who gave direction to the human experiment in social, political, economical and educational democracy
   - Respect and support for freedom of worship, speech, assembly, franchise and education.
7. Each teacher should have acquired academic competency in identifying and understanding the significant issues and trends in contemporary national society.
   - Recognition of the economic, political and sociological issues and trends
   - Understanding of the historical foundations of social issues and trends
   - Recognition of the impact of industrial change on personnel and social living
   - An understanding of the educational requirements for dealing intelligently with such contemporary issues as housing, management labour, local autonomy and federal authority in Government.
8. Each teacher should have knowledge about the life, culture and Government of people in various countries.
   - Understanding of the geographical features of their impact on personal and industrial life
   - Recognition of the similarities in the basic human needs of the people of the world
   - An awareness of the educational impact of the education. Customs, religion, economics and politics in different countries
   - Understanding of the 'conditions, issues and trends' in the neighbour countries
   - An appreciation of the effect of racial and ethnic factors on the personal and social development of young people and on their mental hygiene.
9. Each teacher should have possessed an understanding of the increasing independence among the nations of the world.
   - Recognition of the events, inventions and needs, which accelerated interdependence among nations
   - Awareness of the contribution that education can make to improve world understanding.
10. Each teacher should have understanding and appreciation in the humanities.
    - Appreciation of music and its contribution to creative living and mental health
    - Appreciation of literature and its values in personal and community living
    - Appreciation of literature and its value in personal behavior and in mental hygiene.
11. Each teacher should have an understanding of the moral values and ethics of the teaching profession.
    - Understanding of the history and progress of the profession
    - Acceptance of a code of professional ethics in all relationships with teachers, administrators and layman
    - Understanding of the objectives and services of the local, state and national education organizations
    - Readiness to participate as a contributing member in educational organizations
    - Acceptance of responsibility to share in maintaining and in improving standards of teachers' certification and of teacher employment
    - Acceptance of responsibility to work for improvement in conditions affecting the mental health of all school personnel.
12. Each teacher should possess abilities in effective use of expressive and receptive communication
    - Recognition of the contribution of critical reading to mental health
    - Understanding of the psychological-emotional-social nature and consequences of expressive communication
    - Recognition of the difference between language as a system of symbol and as a way of thought and notion
    - Readiness to listen to one's own language to comprehend its probable interpretation by and effect on other persons.

Principles of Teaching

Successful teaching is based on following principles:

1. The principle of aim—Definite aim should be there for every lesson. It serves as the goal for the teacher. It will make teaching and learning interesting and effective, e.g. at the end of the class, the learners will be able to understand clearly about the topic.

2. The principle of activity or learning by doing—Child learns through self-activity. Learning by doing removes the dullness of the lessons and the students will not get bored, it puts them into life situations. For example: Working out through the projects and demonstrations related to Nursing Procedures

3. The principle of linking with actual life and other subjects, e.g. the students will learn Theory in the classroom, Practice in the lab and in real situations in clinical area, In first year, the students will learn the normative subjects i.e., Anatomy and Physiology that forms a basis to understanding Medical-Surgical Nursing in second year.

4. The principle of planning—Teaching is always well planned. It involves
   a. Selection: is made on the basis of
      • Teacher's aim
      • Teacher's ability to impart the knowledge
      • The child's capacity to receive.
   b. Division: means breaking the topic into convenient units in order to make it more intelligible.
   c. Revision: is essential for assimilation
      • Knowledge is to be fixed in the minds of the learners
      • Revision should take place at each stage and section, better known as sectional revision.

5. The principle of interest or motivation—Learners are naturally interested in those things which are connected with their natural urges or activity. Motivation can secure the desired results. It prepares the mind (mind set) and once it is done, the learners are ready to conduct anything. Motivation sets the mind for assimilation and calls for full attention in the lesson. For example: The teacher has to create interest among the learners while teaching the subject.

6. The principle of sympathy and kind atmosphere—The teacher's kindness and sympathy proves a stimulating dose and easy to approach both for the slow-learners, works miracle for the brilliant student. Teaching should become a matter of pleasure for both i.e., the teacher and to the students.

7. Principle of flexibility and cooperation—The plan of a lesson must provide scope to make necessary changes. Teaching must be flexible to meet the unexpected situations if any, in the classroom and the cooperation of students is required.

8. The principle of diagnostic and remedial teaching—The teacher should suggest remedies for problems and do follow-up to assess the outcomes of his/her suggestions. Learning difficulties should be discovered earlier to avoid their taking root into the learning habits of learners.

9. The principle of looking ahead—An open-minded teacher is always looking forward. He is ever prepared to discover new possibilities for widening learner's knowledge and range of experience.

10. The principle of creativity—The ideal or a good teacher has to make the learners as creative learners. By introducing new materials, good teaching opens up fields of investigation and enables the learners to make original contribution to the existing store of knowledge.

Maxims of Methodological Teaching

1. Proceed from the known to unknown: The new knowledge has to be imparted should be linked with the life and experience already gained by the learners. This forms a link, e.g. The work at school must grow out of the life and experience of the child. A teacher must arrange his/her subject matter and lesson in such a way that each part is properly connected with what has done before. So, for effective teaching, what the learner already knows should be linked up with what he/she is going to know, e.g. the students will learn basic subjects like Anatomy, Physiology in first year, so in second year when teacher teaches Medical-Surgical Nursing, first he/she review Anatomy & Physiology of the affected organ, then only they will discuss about abnormal changes in a specific disease, the concept of Known to Unknown is very helpful for the learner to comprehend subject and easy to remember the changes.

2. Proceed from easy to difficult: Teachers has to take into consideration, the psychological make-up of the learner. Teacher should go from easy to difficult.

3. Proceed from simple to complex: Based on psychological development of the students, the teacher has to proceed from simple to complex, so that the learner can understand the subject very easily.

4. **Proceed from concrete to abstract:** The students learn better from things which they can handle and see. The child picks up concrete knowledge more easily. He understands the abstract through the concrete, e.g. in teaching Anatomy and Physiology, for clear understanding of the subject teacher uses Audio-visual aids like Models, Specimens which enhances effective learning and long lasting memory.
5. **Proceed from the particular to general:** The specific fact must be presented to the children before giving them general rules. Particular is more definite than the general which is indefinite. The study of particular facts should lead the learners themselves to frame general rules.
6. **Proceed from analysis to synthesis:** The teacher should start with analysis so that the complex whole becomes clear. This will help the learner to understand every part and also the relationship among various parts is not sufficient. This should be put in a systematic and elegant form. This is the work of synthesis. Analysis makes the things comprehensible and synthesis later on makes them definite. Synthesis must come at the end. Otherwise analysis will be of no use.
7. **Proceed from whole to parts:** It is based on the result of psychology of learning. Persons always perceive the whole thing first and then pay attention to its parts, e.g. while teaching a poem, the learner should first be given an idea of the whole poem. After this he/she should be made to understand its metre, rhythm, language, etc.
8. **Proceed from empirical to rational:** Empirical knowledge is that which is based on observation and first hand experience about which we cannot give any reasoning at all.
   Rational knowledge is that where facts form part of general system of truth and explained most scientifically. It is always good to begin what we see, feel and experience than with what we reason about, generalize and explain.
9. **Proceed from psychological to logical:** A teacher has two important duties to perform:
   a. The suitable selection and arrangement of subject matter
   b. The study of the learner's nature:
      • Teaching should be done in accordance with the interests, needs and capacities of the learner
      • Teacher has to use psychological approach in teaching
      • Teacher must select the material wisely for presentation, keeping in view the learners
      • The logical approach implies the systematic explanation and arrangement of the matter presented, this will ensure the continuity of the subject matter and help in understanding the same.
10. **Proceed from the actual to the representative:** Real, actual and natural objects appeal to learners more than the improvised or representative objects. Actual things have greater appeal than their representative forms, e.g. If objects like Clinical apparatus shown and it's use if teacher demonstrates, the learner will never forgets in life, enhances long lasting memory.

THE EDUCATIONAL PROCESS

Education is a complex process. Various views about education are Philosophical View: Looks at the purpose and the essential nature of education.

Psychologist's view: At the individual learner, the teaching and learning process.

Sociologist's view: Consider at the social system and at the interaction of learners in groups.

Scholar's view: Clear Vision at the substantive content of learning and respective discipline.

The educational spiral
• The "behavior" will be defined explicitly in the form of "Educational objectives derived from professional tasks"
• An evaluation system will be planned so that better educational decisions will be taken
• A programme will be prepared and implemented to facilitate attainment of educational objectives by the students
• The evaluation process will be used:
  – To measure the extent to which the objectives have been achieved
  – To measure the student's final abilities
  – To assess the effectiveness of programme and teaching.

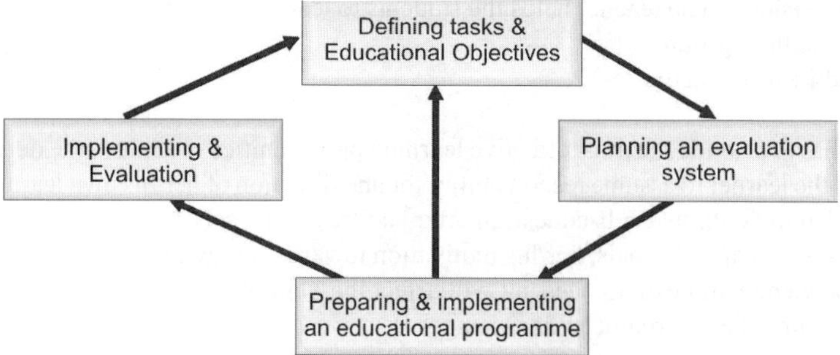

Fig. 4.1: The educational spiral

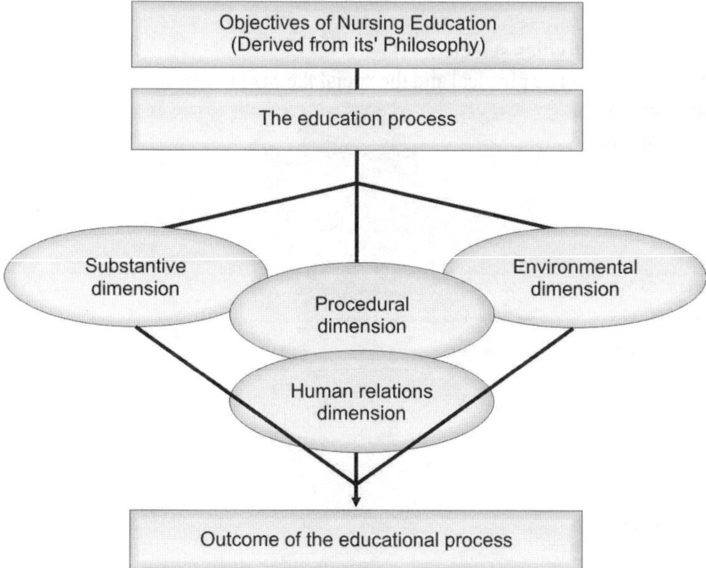

Fig. 4.2: Schematic diagram of components in education process

The members of the health team must be trained specifically for the tasks they have to perform (taking into account the circumstances under which they will work). These tasks only be defined in accordance with a plan in which the nature of the services to be provided is specified, priorities are allotted, the staff needed to provide these services determined etc. Professional training programmes must then be tailored to meet these needs. Defining the professional tasks of health personnel is the basis of educational objectives of training centers is of crucial importance. Thus an educational programme, must be shaped in terms of the goal to be achieved, to meet the population's health needs. Evaluation provides a sound basis for programme planning, therefore an evaluation mechanism must be set up before proceeding to any reform of the programme. This makes it possible to measure the level at the outset (prerequisite level) and the level at the finish and thus to determine whether the change has been positive or not. This process can be represented by "educational spiral" (Fig. 4.1).

Components of Educational Process (Fig. 4.2)

1. **Substantive dimension (the curriculum)**—The curriculum includes all the content (knowledge, values, skills) and the learning activities are planned and directed by a faculty for a specific group of students, with a specific purpose. The nursing curriculum is concerned with providing opportunities for acquiring the essential knowledge, skills and attitudes that will prepare the student to assume the role/responsibilities and functions in nursing at the level for which she/he is being prepared.

2. **Procedural dimension**—The teacher helps the students to learn, it includes:
   - The learner and their group
   - Teaching and Learning activities
   - Teacher.

   The teacher has to provide the most effective learning opportunities to achieve the desired goals and will most likely lead the learner to assume responsibility for and direction of her/his own learning, not only while in school, but also in continued self-education after she leaves the school.

   Many factors, e.g. learner's goals, her/his motivation towards achieving these goals, her/his ability, her/his previous knowledge and experiences, all will affect the kind of learning activities which will be most effective in providing the desired behavior changes.
   - The teacher's personality
   - The teacher's concept in teaching and learning
   - Mastery of the subject she teaches
   - Teaching skills
   - Teaching and learning activities selected.

3. **Environmental dimension**—The physical and the social factors in the teaching - learning situations constitute the environmental dimension.

   The Physical Environment:
   - Classroom
   - Lab settings
   - Hospital
   - Community
   - Health agency
   - Home
   - Lighting and ventilation
   - Equipment
   - Group climate
   - Organizational pattern
   - Administrative policies
   - Leadership
   - The school environment
   - Nursing service status.

   Environmental dimension brings a definite personality pattern, a set of aims, values, social habits, self-image, concept of each one's sense of identity, where she/he belongs? what she/he can do? what are her/his assets and liabilities and needs for self-growth and development? each of which operates in producing the particular psychosocial climate in each teaching-learning situations.

4. **The human relation dimension**
   - The learner
   - The teacher
   - The administrator
   - The group of learners
   - The patient
   - Nursing service personnel
   - Allied health personnel and their interactions.

   The interaction of human relations of these individuals both in the school and in the educational settings, outside the school exerts an important influence on the effectiveness of the educative process.

LEARNING

Definitions

"The relatively permanent change in an individual's behavior or behavior potential (or capability) as a result of experience or practice (i.e. an internal change inferred from overt behavior)."

'Modification due to energies of organism and environment impinging on the organism itself'—*Daniel Bell*

'Learning is modification of behavior through experience'—*Gates*

'Learning involves the acquisition of habits, knowledge and attitude'—*Crow-Crow*

'Learning is a process, which brings about changes in the individual way of responding as a result of contact with aspects of environment.'—*Ruch*

'Learning as acquisition and retention.'—*BF Skinner*

'Learning refers to growth of interest, knowledge and skills and to transfer these to new situation.' —*Encyclopedia of Education Research*

Characteristics of the Learning Process

- Purposeful process: Most people have definite ideas about what they want to achieve. They have goals or clear objectives. Effective instructors seek ways to create new learning situations to meet the trainee's goals. Motivation, the force that impels a person toward a goal, is the instructor's most effective tool to encourage learning. This can be either weak or strong motivation depending on the situation .

- Internal Experience: The instructor cannot learn for the trainee, nor can he or she pour predigested learning into the trainee's head. The trainee can learn only from his or her own experiences. A person's knowledge is a result of their experiences and manner of perceiving them and reacting to them. No two people have exactly the same experiences. All learning stems from experience e.g. by repeated drill, a trainee can learn to repeat a list of words or to recite the principles of leadership. However, trainees can make the list an actual part of their lives only if they understand them well enough to apply the ideas that they represent correctly in real situations.

- Active process: Since learning comes only through experience, the trainee must be actively involved in the experience. This activity can take many forms. Learning is more than simply exposing a trainee to an idea or a skill. Likewise, one cannot safely assume that trainees can apply what they know just because they correctly quote a paragraph from a textbook. The trainee must become actively involved in the learning situation, but just any kind of involving activity will not suffice. The trainee must engage in the appropriate activity. Obviously, learning a physical skill requires experience in performing that skill. The instructor should understand, however, that mental habits are always learned through practice. Even attitudes are developed or modified as an individual reacts emotionally to a stimulus.

- Multidimensional: Learning is multidimensional. It develops new concept. In other words, it is possible to learn other things while concentrating on or practicing the main subject. While practicing drill, the trainees learn teamwork and cooperation.

- Individual process: All trainees do not learn at the same rate. New instructors are likely to be discouraged when they discover that a well-planned lesson does not enable them to teach all the trainees with equal effectiveness. They soon recognize this as a natural and predictable problem because trainees seldom learn at the same rate. Differences in rates of learning are based on differences in intelligence, background, experience, interests, desire to learn and countless other psychological, emotional and physical factors. Instructors must recognize these differences in determining the amount of subject matter to teach, the rate of which they will cover the material and the appropriate time to teach it. Once the slower trainees are identified, it is upto the instructor to bring them up to the level of the rest of the flight. Teacher must identify their weak areas, bring the areas to their attention and show them how to correct them. Teacher may be fortunate and have some trainees who excel. These trainees may be used to help others during their practice. This serves a twofold purpose. The fast learning trainees are relieved from boredom and the slow learning trainees receive the benefit of the peer's expertise.

Characteristics of Learning

1. Learning is Unitary: The learner responds as a total person in a unified way to the 'whole' situation or total pattern. Learner responds intellectually, emotionally, physically and spiritually. She reacts to the whole learning situation rather than to any single stimuli—is coordinated and integrated manner.

Teaching- Learning situation is approached differently by each learner with different goals with the result that each learner responds differently. Learning is individual, though responses are diverse and are made simultaneously to more than one factor in the learning situation. Learning is complex which includes cognitive, conative, affective domains, appreciations and habits. An individual response to the total situation.

2. Learning is individual and social: Learning takes place in response to the environment which includes physical, Social and emotional environment. Each learner is a unique person, they have individualized characteristics in the patterns of living viz. slow learners and fast learners. Learning is influenced by heredity, environment and self determination like learner's intellectual abilities, purposes, aptitudes, abilities etc. everything plays vital role. Teacher must understand individual variations and provide needed assistance based on their needs and abilities.

3. Learning is self active: An individual can learn only through her/his reactions to situations by his own efforts. It is the process of self activity, self direction and self realization. Self development is by self discipline. Teachers through their teaching motivates the learners to study and understand the subject content, teachers act as role models, the students will follow the teacher in many ways in their lives.

4. Learning is Purposive and active: Learning is active in a specific direction, goal oriented, goals are determined directly by motives and indirectly by incentives. Motives are the forces that directs the behavior of an individual. Learning experiences are meaningful when they are related to the individual's interests, intelligent adjustments. Learning is influenced by the intention or will to learn. Man has a will and he can choose the action he wishes to take.

5. Learning includes a progressive organizing and reorganizing of educative experiences: Learning is goal directed, but the activity in the attachment of the goal is also directed.

6. Learning is gradual and developmental process: The organization and the reorganization of experience and behavior are accomplished through the processes of differentiation, integration and precision.

7. Learning is more than a process of differentiation and precision, it is also a process of integration.

8. Learning is Creative and selective: Human be creates the unique things in the world, He/She has own potentialities, abilities, strengths and actualities. With expertized knowledge and skills, he will be able to create purposively whatever he/she intends.

9. Learning is a process of personal choice making, it is the activity in which the learner through his/her own experience, he/she learns only that which he/she chooses to learn. Learner responds to her/his environment

10. Learning is transferable: The teacher will transmit the knowledge, learning also affects the conduct of the individual. True learning takes place only when the learner will acquire the type of knowledge or a skill or change in attitude will takes place.

Characteristics of Informal Learning

- Desire to set own learning pace—Self pace
- Desire to use own style of learning—Personalized
- Learner can keep the learning strategy flexible and easy to change—Tactical
- Learner can fulfil desire to put own structure on the learning project—Empowerment
- Learner didn't know of any class that taught what he/she wanted to know—Complex
- Student wanted to learn right away and couldn't wait until a class might start—Right attitude
- Just in - time
- Lack of time to engage in a group learning program—Flexibility
- Learner don't like a formal classroom situation with a teacher—Casual
- Learner don't have enough money for a course or class—Free
- Transportation to a class is too hard or expensive—Free Transportation to educational centres

Constructivist Learning Environment

Honebein (1996) describes seven goals for the design of constructivist learning environment

- Provide experience with the knowledge of construction process
- Provide experience in and appreciation for multiple perspectives
- Embed learning in realistic and relevant contexts

- Encourage ownership and voice in the learning process
- Embed learning in social experience
- Encourage the use of multiple modes of representation
- Encourage self-awareness in the knowledge construction process.

According to *Vygotsky* (1978), student's **problem solving skills** fall into three categories
- Skills which the student cannot perform
- Skills which the student may be able to perform
- Skills that the student can perform with help.

Scaffolding allows students to perform tasks that would normally be slightly beyond their ability without that assistance and guidance from the teacher. Appropriate teacher support can allow students to function at the cutting edge of their individual development. Scaffolding is therefore an important characteristic of constructivist learning and teaching.

Characteristics of Constructivist Learning and Teaching

Jonassen (1991) noted that many educators and cognitive psychologists have applied constructivism to the development of learning environments.
- Create real-world environments that employ the context in which learning is relevant
- Focus on realistic approaches to solve real-world problems
- The instructor is a coach and analyzer of the strategies used to solve these problems
- Stress conceptual interrelatedness, providing multiple representations or perspectives on the content
- Instructional goals and objectives should be negotiated and not imposed
- Evaluation should serve as a self-analysis tool
- Provide tools and environments that help learners interpret the multiple perspectives of the world
- Learning should be internally controlled and mediated by the learner

Jonassen (1994) summarizes "the implications of constructivism for instructional design". The following principles illustrate how knowledge construction can be facilitated:
- Provide multiple representations of reality
- Represent the natural complexity of the real world
- Focus on knowledge construction, not reproduction
- Present authentic tasks (contextualizing rather than abstracting instruction)
- Provide real-world, case-based learning environments, rather than pre-determined instructional sequences
- Foster reflective practice
- Enable context and content dependent knowledge construction
- Support collaborative construction of knowledge through social negotiation.

Wilson and Cole (1991) provide a description of cognitive teaching models which "embody" constructivist concepts, embed learning in a rich authentic problem-solving environment
- Provide for authentic versus academic contexts for learning.
- Provide for learner control.
- Use errors as a mechanism to provide feedback on learner's understanding. *Ernest* (1995) in his description of the many schools of thought of constructivism suggests the following implications of constructivism, sensitivity toward and attentiveness to the learner's previous constructions.
- Diagnostic teaching attempting to remedy learner errors and misconceptions.
- Attention to metacognition and strategic self-regulation by learners, e.g. Metacognition is knowing about and directing one's own thinking and learning process. The concept was introduced into cognitive psychology in the 1970s (Flavell, 1976) and emphasizes self-regulatory tactics used to ensure success in the learning endeavour (Brown, 1982). The three Metacognition strategies in skills are Planning, Monitoring, and Adjusting. Planning strategies include eliciting purpose from self and the situation, organizing and identifying the steps essential to the learning process.
- Metamotivation is an awareness and control over factors that energize and direct one's learning. The three Metamotivation strategies in skills are Attention, Reward/Enjoyment and Confidence.

- The use of multiple representations of mathematical concepts.
- Awareness of the importance of goals for the learner and the dichotomy between learner and teacher goals.
- Awareness of the importance of social contexts, such as the difference between folk or street mathematics and school mathematics (and an attempt to exploit the former for the latter).
- Emphasis on conceptual interrelatedness and interdisciplinary learning.
- Collaborative and cooperative learning are favoured in order to expose the learner to alternative viewpoints.
- Scaffolding is facilitated to help students perform just beyond the limits of their ability.
- Assessment is authentic and interwoven with teaching.
- Multiple perspectives and representations of concepts and content are presented and encouraged.
- Goals and objectives are derived by the student or in negotiation with the teacher or system.
- Teachers serve in the role of guides, monitors, coaches, tutors and facilitators.
- Activities, opportunities, tools and environments are provided to encourage metacognition, self-analysis and self-regulation-reflection and awareness.
- The student plays a central role in mediating and controlling learning.
- Learning situations, environments, skills, content and tasks are relevant, realistic, authentic and represent the natural complexities of the 'real-world'.
- Primary sources of data are used in order to ensure authenticity and real world complexity.
- Knowledge construction and not reproduction is emphasized. This construction takes place in individual contexts and through social negotiation, collaboration and experience.
- The learner's previous knowledge constructions, beliefs and attitudes are considered in the knowledge construction process.
- Problem-solving, higher-order thinking skills and deep understanding are emphasized.
- Errors provide the opportunity for insight into student's previous knowledge constructions.
- Exploration is a favoured approach in order to encourage students to seek knowledge independently and to manage the pursuit of their goals.
- Learners are provided with the opportunity for apprenticeship learning in which there is an increasing complexity of tasks, skills and knowledge acquisition.
- Knowledge complexity is reflected in an emphasis on conceptual interrelatedness and interdisciplinary learning.
- Collaborative and cooperative learning are favoured in order to expose the learner to alternative viewpoints.
- Scaffolding is facilitated to help students to perform just beyond the limits of their ability.
- Assessment is authentic and interwoven with teaching.

Nature of Learning

Learning means change, it implies a different internal state that may result in new behaviors and actions or new understanding and knowledge. Learning can be undertaken within a formal setting or be spontaneous or incremental.

Learning can change lives—Teacher can gain access to the minds, passions and souls of people. In making such connections, guided by the light of *ethics and morality*, teacher can change lives, lift people and impact organizations. Teaching is a *sacred calling* with *serious responsibilities* and *wonderful opportunities* for those who become able teachers. By incorporating these laws into teacher's leadership, *teach* people through change rather than simply motivating, persuading or pushing-to a more engaged and lasting success.

Learning is both an emotional and intellectual experience—Emotional connection to the teacher or topic opens a door to the mind. Failure to open the emotional door means that information, *no matter how well crafted*, bounces off the door with little impact.

Learning was conceptualized as—(a) increasing in one's knowledge (b) memorizing and reproducing (c) applying (d) understanding (e) seeing something in a different way (f) changing as a person. The first three categories describe learning as a reproduction of information whereas the last three depict learning as knowledge transforming.

Learning as

- An externally determined event/process
- A developmental process
- Student activity/any one in life can learn, learning is never ending process
- Strategies/styles/approaches
- Information processing
- An interactive process
- A creative process
- Is necessary for man's survival and for human progress. It includes acquisition of knowledge, skills, formation of habits, development of perception
- Depends upon intelligence, motivation and needs
- It is a continuous process, both conscious and unconscious

Learning is the key in developing person's potential, 'to learn' is the effective key , it enables the individuals to meet the demands of change. The capacity to learn is an asset for an individual.

Society survives and thrives through learning. It contributes for cohesive society. Collective learning reinforces the informed, conscious and discriminating choices, It helps to enhance the capacity of individuals to create a more fulfilled society.

Types of Learning

1. Ideational Learning/Cognitive Learning—The learner acquires Knowledge, Perceiving, Remembering, Discriminating, Integrating, Abstracting, Generalizing, Evaluating, Imagining, Problem solving and creating etc.
2. Skill/ Conative Learning / Psychomotor Learning—A skill is a refined pattern of movement or performance based upon and integrated with the perceived demands of the situation. Skill is the ability to perform an act. Skill discriminates the situation, it is a process of gradual refinement. It includes content and a sequence of actions.

   The factors contributing to one or more skilled performance are: strength, reaction, time, speed, precision, consideration and flexibility. Skill consists of 2 aspects: form and execution. 1. Form in a skill, refers to the manner in which the movements are carried out. It can be learned best by explanation, description of steps, demonstration, students will learn by imitation and inquisitiveness, purposive learning, activity, i.e. Learning by doing. Attention is required to develop a skill. 2. Execution of skill–The actual performance of a skill, timing, force and coordination are required to execute a skill. A correct theoretical knowledge of execution of skill is required. Accuracy and Speed are required to develop and execute the skill. Practice is an absolute necessity in the development of a skill. Practice, attitude of the learner, interest, theoretical knowledge are required for execution of skill.
3. Emotional learning/Affective Learning—The end products of Affective Learning–attitudes, values and ideals determine the character and conduct of individuals motive power. Thinking, doing, Learning are influenced to some extent by affective state. Control of emotions by will is self control. The teacher has to teach the students how to control the will and maintain self control and how to develop positive attitude, promote the desired responses in relation to the ideals, traits and habits, motivation arises out of appreciation, these are acquired as a result of emotional experiences.

Organisational Behavior

Learning is a part of human condition. Organisations need to carefully manage knowledge and learning. There is mutual benefit gained from the development of the skills which fulfil the goals of organisation as well as meeting the individual's aspirations. Psychological well-being can be enhanced by new experiences or by supporting and developing others. Encouraging creativity is of growing interest in the fulfilment of individual and organisational goals. It is a challenge to find new ways of studying invisible processes and of accurately measuring changes in behavior.

Learning provides powerful processes which can lead to positive outcomes, e.g. Increased competence, understanding, self esteem and morale. Individuals who enjoy learning are more likely to be flexible in times of constant change and therefore more adaptable to organisational turbulence. Learning culture affects organisational effectiveness. Learning is the most powerful, engaging, rewarding and enjoyable aspect of personal and collective experience.

Learning increases everyone's capacity to contribute to the success of organisations. Learning enables the organisation to be more effective in meeting it's goals. It emancipates the organisation through clarification of purpose, vision, values and behavior. Learning produces a wide range of solutions to organisational issues. It helps to achieve a better balance between long term organisational effectiveness and short term organisational efficiency.

Laws of Learning:

Edward L. Thorndike in the early 1900's postulated several "Laws of Learning," that seemed generally applicable to the learning process.

- **Law of Exercise**–The law of exercise stresses the idea that repetition is basic to the development of adequate responses; things most often repeated are easiest remembered. The mind can rarely recall new concepts or practices after a single exposure, but every time it is practiced, learning continues and is enforced. The instructor must provide opportunities for trainees to practice or repeat the task. Repetition consists of many types of activities, including recall, review, restatement, manual drill and physical application. Remember that practice makes permanent, not perfect unless the task is taught correctly. The performer must practice the task regularly in favourable conditions, e.g. gaining clinical skills.

- **Law of Effect**–This law involves the emotional reaction of the learner. Learning will always be much more effective when a feeling of satisfaction, pleasantness or reward accompanies or is a result of the learning process. Learning is strengthened when it is accompanied by a pleasant or satisfying feeling and that it is weakened when it is associated with an unpleasant experience. An experience that produces feelings of defeat, frustration, anger or confusion in a trainee is unpleasant. Instructors should be cautious about using negative motivation. Usually it is better to show trainees that a problem is not impossible, but is within their capability to understand and solve Performer is more likely to repeat the task if their behavior is followed by experiences of satisfaction, e.g. Positive reinforcement.

- **Law of Readiness**–The Law of Readiness means a person can learn when physically and mentally adjusted (ready) to receive stimuli. Individuals learn best when they are ready to learn and they will not learn much if they see no reason for learning. If trainees have a strong purpose, a clear objective and a sound reason for learning, they usually make more progress than trainees who lack motivation. When trainees are ready to learn, they are more willing to participate in the learning process and this simplifies the instructor's job. If outside responsibilities or worries weigh heavily on trainee's minds or if their personal problems seem unsolvable, they may have little interest in learning. Performer is physically and mentally able to complete the task, e.g. appropriate Motivation.

- **Law of Primacy**–This law states that the state of being first, often creates a strong, almost unshakeable impression. For the instructor, this means that what they teach the first time must be correct. If a subject is incorrectly taught, it must be corrected. It is more difficult to un - teach a subject than to teach it correctly the first time. For the trainees' first learning experience should be positive and functionally related to training.

- **Law of Intensity**–The principle of intensity states that if the stimulus (experience) is real, the more likely there is to be a change in behavior (learning). A vivid, dramatic or exciting learning experience teaches more than a routine or boring experience. A trainee will learn more from the real thing than from a substitute. Demonstrations, skits, and models do much to intensify the learning experiences of trainees.

- **Law of Recency**–Things most recently learned are best remembered, while the things learned some time before are remembered with more difficulty. It is sometimes easy for example, to recall a telephone number dialed a few minutes ago is easy, but it is usually impossible to recall a telephone number dialed a week ago. Review, warm-ups and similar activities are all based on the principle that the more recent the exercise, the more effective the performance. Practicing a skill or new concept just before using it will ensure a more effective performance. Instructors recognize the law of recency when they plan a lesson summary or a conclusion of the lecture. Repeat, restate or reemphasize important matters at the end of a lesson to make sure that trainees remember them instead of inconsequential details.

- **The Law of Doing/Experience:** The connection between actually doing something and our brain is a strong one, e.g. clinical Experiences.
- **The Law of Motivation:** When something is worth learning, it is worth learning well, learn how it affects our life, motivate to pick up a skill, e.g. Teacher will motivate the child to do a task, after completion of task immediately she/he will appreciate the learner for accomplishing task.
- **The Law of Repetition:** By repeating the information and principles, we retain the subject matter more strongly and are more easily able to recall the subject, e.g. Learning by immitation.
- **The Law of Association:** Mind works by associating similar classifications of things and applying them to the new field of study, e.g. Application of relevant knowledge whenever problem arises, appropriate steps will be implemented.
- **The Law of Relevancy:** If a subject is not relevant to us in our life, we will unconsciously refuse to learn it. We must know what is relevant and cut out all of the rest that will be of no use to you, e.g. avoid unnecessary steps in carrying out the procedure. Only suitable or appropriate tasks has to be implemented.

Theories of Learning

- Drive Reduction Theory: Hull suggested learning will occur due to the performer's desire to complete the task and only by achieving their drive they will be satisfied. Motivation of the performer is always maintained, this will involve the teacher to formulate the challenging goals allowing continued development to occur.
- Conditioning Theory/Connectionist/Associationist Theories
  It involves the performer developing specific link to a certain cue, known as 'Stimulus-Response Bond (S-R Bond)"
- Learning by Trial and Error
  Slow, laborious and primitive type, e.g. Child will learn by imitation and trial and error method
- Learning by Observation and imitation
  Observation promotes attention, discrimination and recognition. We will learn the skills by observation method only. Learners will follow their role models (e.g. Teachers) in formulating habits.
- Learning by Doing: coordination of muscular responses with sensory impulses, e.g. Nursing Procedures
- Learning by remembering–Memorizing the events, dates etc.
- Learning by insight, e.g. Problem Solving
- Learning is measured by performance of activities, e.g. Teacher observes students' performance in theory and in clinicals
- Operant Conditioning—Developed by *B.F.Skinner*, the S-R bond will be either strengthened or weakened depending what happens after the action has taken place. Often the learner will experience trial and error and through a gradual process of elimination will develop the appropriate response with the correct use of positive reinforcement.
- Theory of Reinforcement—It may take two forms
  Positive Reinforcement: The stimulus will be used to create feelings of satisfaction to encourage the repetition of action, e.g. Appreciation from the teacher, when the learner performs desired task, personal satisfaction from the completion of movement; reward, Praise
  Negative reinforcement: Involves the withdrawal of an unpleasant stimulus when the desired response occurs, e.g. Punishment: May also be used effectively to reduce the likelihood of the actions being repeated, e.g. dropped from the team, however the continual use of punishment may cause some resentment and have an adverse effect so punishment should be used carefully. Disadvantage - may be lack of understanding as to why the skill is being executed in a particular fashion.

Factors Affecting Learning

1. Internal factors/subjective factors

- *Age:*
  Age can influence upon the capability of learning. A child can learn faster and an aged person will have difficulty to learn modern ways of knowledge.

- *Intelligence:*

  Learning depends upon mental faculty of an individual. Intelligence effects a lot on learning, if individual has maximum level of intelligence, she/ he can learn more and easily at maximum level.

- *Attention:*

  If a person does not pay attention towards how to learn a specific knowledge, *skill* or experience, he/she cannot learn easily but, if the individual pays attention the results are vise versa. Attention plays an important role in the education and training process. Without attention, one cannot observe or perceive. Attention was associated earlier with will, judgement, reasoning, etc. But attention is a selective activity of individuals consciousness. Attention is not a power of the mind. It is not static. It fluctuates from one object to another, quickly. It is very difficult to prevent such fluctuations. Only one thing will remain in the conscious mind and all other inattentive activities in the subconscious mind. Unconscious activities cannot be recalled at will. Inattention by trainees is a problem for instructors. Trainees are distracted from instructional activities because of (a) ill health (b) external disturbances (c) bad instruction (d) lack of motivation (e) monotony of activity (f) unhygenic conditions (g) improper seating conditions (h) disinterest etc. Distraction causes a general increase in muscular tension, utilisation of increased energy in work, nervous restlessness and of adopting defence movements.

  Conditions for attention are classified as:

  a. Subjective conditions, e.g. interest, dispositions, moods, urges, needs, habits, emotional state etc.

  b. Objective conditions, e.g. method of presentation, nature of stimulus and its intensity, size, novelty, movement, repetition, contrast etc.

- *Interest:*

  Interest is an inner disposition or tendency of readiness to perceive. Interest therefore elicits attention active attention is conducive for better learning. Closely related to interest is concentration and success in learning is closely related to degree of concentration. Effective learning requires assimilation and interest. Creating interest in learning is a principal function of the instructor as interest forms the prime basis of learning. You do not learn a thing if you have not developed the interest to learn. Therefore in the lesson plans, there is special provision for motivating and creating interest in the trainee. Interest is dependent largely on the need. Interest also leads to better attention and hence to better observation and perception. When interest is keen, one can learn under most difficult situations also.

  Interest should be aroused before learning begins and for satisfactory results it should be maintained throughout the learning period. The instructor by creating proper interest can capitalise the same to procure other values needed for all round development. He should not distract the trainees from their basic interest. Interest should be aroused before learning begins and for satisfactory results it should be maintained throughout the learning period. The instructor by creating proper interest can capitalise the same to procure other values needed for all round development. He should not distract the trainees from their basic interest.

- *Holistic health:*

  Physical (No diseases), Mental Health (Lack of frustration and conflicts, sound mental health) promotes effective learning. If an individual does not have sound mental health or physical health, the individual cannot fulfill the demands of the process of learning due to his weak mental and physical capabilities.

- *Maturation:*

  Learning depends on mental age. Maturation means mental ability or maturity, social maturity and psychological readiness i.e., development of physical factors like sensory and reacting mechanisms. Before learning takes place the sensory, motor and nervous structure should reach a certain level of maturity. Maturation of both muscles and brain are necessary in any skill learning situation. Deterioration of muscular coordination and cerebral cortex tissues in old age brings deterioration in skill learning abilities. Maturation is a natural development of the nervous system and other structures which makes one ready and able to engage in a particular activity, whereas 'learning involves the modification of existing patterns of response. Normal development prepares one, for the neuromuscular systems, for making certain responses.

- *Observation and learning:*

  The ability for observation is a prerequisite for good perception and consequently for learning. Item and conscious observation paves the way for better perception, which in turn results in quicker acquisition of responses to be learnt. Learning process is affected by observation. An individual observes process, behavior and phenomena and later copy them in his/her own way. Thus skill and knowledge are developed by conscious and sometimes unconscious observation. Children learn and acquire habits by observation. Keen observation leads to better comprehension and understanding. Consequently this enables better formulation and visualisation of goals and better visualisation leads to development of insight, which is directed towards achievement of required skills and knowledge.

At the very early childhood, an infant learns through observation, by observing objects and events through vision, hearing and other senses. Experiences gained through the different senses are correlated and the learning through perception occurs. Perception tends inevitably to lead to the formation of concepts. But our perceptual capacity is limited. We do not become aware of everything within the range of our senses, but only of those things or a part of those things, to which our attention is directed.

- *Fatigue:*
Every physical activity involves consumption of energy. Output is proportional to input i.e., achievement is proportional to energy spent as input. Human efficiency is the ratio between achievement and energy spent. Cause of fatigue are loss of energy, loss of oxygen, limited storage of energy, loss of interest, development of dislike etc. Symptoms of fatigue are reduction of efficiency, distraction, jerky movements, cardio-muscular movements, unwillingness to work etc. Physiological fatigue relates to fatigue of muscles due to exertion. This may be due to loss of energy. Thus physical fatigue and loss of energy are directly related. Mental fatigue is caused by loss of interest and monotonous nature of work. When an individual is tired, he/she cannot pay total attention or concentration towards learn something.

- *Insight:*
Insight also plays an important part in learning. Insight is defined as, "a sudden flash of thought or solution in mind that helps one to face a problem solving situation". It involves Gestalten conception of perception. That is, discovering and making use of means and relationships in reorganising the psychological field of observation. Problems that are not within the reach of physical or normal mental tackling are solved by insight. 'Gestalt' is a German word meaning 'Whole'. The basic principle of Gestalt learning is to study everything as a whole and observe meaningful connections between different parts and the whole, when insight into the learning situation is facilitated. Insight is not always available to many and so cannot be depended on. Foresight is a prominent factor for goal seeking behavior. Without clear foresight it is not possible to develop behavior towards the goal. Insight learning is based on the ability of synthesizing the perceived facts and factors. It involves creative and imaginative thinking.

2. **External factors:**
- *Knowledge:*
If knowledge is interesting in nature, any individual can learn it more efficiently.
 Recitation: Recitation is more effective tool of learning, if an individual recite something louder he/she can learn more effectively.
- *Meaningfulness:*
If the material of knowledge is meaningful, the individual will learn it more effectively and easily, meaningless material neither can be learnt easily nor kept in memory on long term basis.
- *Exercise and repetition:*
Single act is learnt in single trial but complex acts require repeated trails. If a material is difficult to learn it can be learnt through exercises or repeated trials.
- *By parts learning:*
If the material is so long it can be divided into small parts, so individual can learn specific knowledge, skill etc. more effectively.
- *Teaching and learning environment:*
Each individual has different environment .The individual internal environment is created by past experience, self attitude, self concept and involves acquired knowledge, attitudes and skills. The influences from the learner's external environment include the learners peer group, family membership, socio-economic status, community and school as well as work situations.

- **Learning Situation**

  Learner should have conducive environmental facilities to learn which will progress learning process e.g. Resources like Textbooks, Lesson Plans, Library resources, good seating arrangements, adequate ventilation, lighting, no sound, etc.

  In nursing education, an effective environment should be created in which the learner knows that people are more highly valued that procedure. Any practice that contributes to the erosion of the self image or self esteem must be open to question. This includes thoughtless remarks by teachers or students about patient and other learners. The student who has a positive self image will react differently to the same environment than student whose self image is negative. The teacher should anticipate situation of this type. The teaching learning environment should be structured to provide opportunities to cope with student individual difference. The physical learning environment may be improved by bulletin boards showing materials such as a copy of the patient's bill of rights, displays that carry different relevant message, pictures of learners teaching patient and other motivating themes, etc.

- **Motivation and Learning**

  Classroom learning is directly proportional to motivation. Motivation leads to attain objectives and goals. Mental and bodily physical activities are dominated by interests. It has been found that our feelings in the form of attitudes, interests and aspirations have a vital relationship to learning. Timely and methodological motivation affect improvement in achievement as it increases the ability of trainees. We learn more effectively when we have the gratification provided by knowledge of reasonable success in our efforts. Positive incentives help in the furtherance of learning while negative incentives has a retarding effect. Favourable learning conditions are created by means of rewards praising, patting, appreciating, awards, scholarship and stipends. The powerful motives are Positive reinforcement e.g. recognition, etc. will motivate the learner to learn effectively, Punishments like fine, marking absent for late coming, making trainees stand in classrooms, scolding, corporal punishment, etc. lead to diminishing 'learning process. The presence or absence of reward can affect learning, generally, reward is more effective in promoting learning than is punishment, the latter does have some effects on learning, it tends to repress a desired response then to extinguish it. Thus instructors should motivate learners so that they should feel that what they learn are going to be useful in their life and they will be benefitted by it by way of higher ability, higher emoluments etc.

- **Clarity**

  "The ability of the learner to clearly see, hear, and understand what is being said." Threats to clarity include small fonts, jargon, slurred speech, obstructions to sight, and ambiguous language. Clarity was found to be the number one factor in improving learning.

- **Task Orientation**

  People tend to learn better when they are engaged in a task. If they spend time with introductions, attendance or other "housekeeping" chores, they have less time to spend on task. Teachers and presenters who keep guiding their students and audience back to the topic have a better chance of achieving their objectives.

- **Student Opportunity**

  Students and audience members should be given the opportunity to engage the material. This could mean that the speaker is quiet at times to allow the listener to digest what they've heard, or maybe there is an activity where the listener writes something or discusses an issue with the person next to them. If a hands-on activity is indicated, be sure to budget adequate time, space and materials for all participants to adequately engage the material.

- **Variety**

  Some people learn better by listening, some by seeing and some by doing. Regardless of their best mode of learning, it would help everybody in audience if you covered the material in a variety of ways e.g. if you are teaching persons how to properly install a protective hearing device, you might wish to show a short video, use a large illustration of an ear, hand out a brochure with text and graphics and have everybody practice. (This might seem time consuming, but each could probably be done in a minute or less). The variety of approaches has a better chance of changing behavior than if the teacher had used a single approach.

- **Teacher Enthusiasm**
  The enthusiasm of a teacher or presenter is contagious. If the teacher show interest in a topic the audience/ learners are more likely to be interested. If teacher apologize for how boring a topic is, do not expect learners to stay awake or listen to you any more.

TEACHING LEARNING PROCESS

Teaching and Learning Process is the heart of education. It depends on fulfillment of educational objectives or goals. It is the most powerful instrument of education to bring about desired changes in the students. The teacher, the learner, curriculum and other variables are organised in a systematic way to attain some predetermined goals.

Teaching is a complex and abstract concept, it is a system of directed and deliberate actions that are intended to induce learning through a series of directed activities designed to induce learning. Teaching is an art and science in which the content is structured and processes used that will enable student learning.

Teaching-learning process is a planned interaction that promotes behavioral change that is not a result of maturation or coincidence. A dynamic process or transaction, which is a complex, cooperative and personal relationship between faculty and student, when viewed from the perspective of the learning paradigm rather than the instructional paradigm, the teaching learning process is a personal interactive relationship that extends beyond the subject matter. Within the interactive relationship faculty relate students with dignity and respect, with the expectation that students will be supported and stimulated to develop intellectual integrity and independent judgment (Hyman 1974). The teacher performs varied roles such as facilitator, learner, guide, coach and mentor acting in partnership with students. The student roles become those of learner inquirer and seeker of knowledge within an active participative student faculty relationship.

In humanistic model the faculty, as senior learner and a student as a junior learner are engaged in the teaching-learning process. According to Diekelmann (1989), both teacher and learner engage in a transformed relationship as a result of meaningful dialogue with one another. The roles associated with these purposes include raising question; nurturing creative drive, caring, assertiveness and ethics, designing ways to engage mental processes; and interacting with students as persons of worth, dignity, intelligence and high scholarly standards.

Teaching is an active process in which one person shares information with others to provide them with the information to make behavioral changes.

Learning is the process of assimilating information with a resultant change in behavior.

Learning is considered as a change in a person that has caused by experience. Learning is a process of understanding, clarifying and applying the meanings of the knowledge acquired. Furthermore, learning is the exploration, discovery, refinement and extension of the learner's meaning of the knowledge–Heidgerken, 1953

Essential aspects of Teaching-Learning Process

Discussion between teacher and student
Interaction between the learner and some aspect of the world defined by the teacher
Adaptation of the world by the teacher and action by the learner
Reflection on the learner's performance by both teacher and the learner.

The process is circular with each step interacting with the preceding and subsequent step.

1. Assessment—Assess the needs of learners and curricular requirements
2. Planning—Establishing objectives, Choose content, select strategies, Prioritize, Order learning experiences
3. Implementation—Teaching environment and teaching guidelines
4. Evaluation of teaching and learning process
5. Documentation.

Assessment—It has three major components; the curricular attributes, the faculty attributes and the student attributes. The program and course objectives, critical learning experience and learning outcomes must be thoughtfully examined. These curricular components provide the foundation for identifying and preparing the appropriate content that is to be taught.

Faculty also need to appraise their own attributes, including their level of content knowledge, their philosophy and attitudes about teaching and the instructional skills they already possess and those want to develop. Faculty should be well informed about various theories of learning and other theories relevant for teaching and learning. Appropriate theories relevant to learning are used as a framework to design the teaching learning process.

Student's personal attributes that are particularly relevant are those associated with successful learning. Student's attributes having significant bearing on the decisions made for the entire teaching learning process include the student's entry knowledge and skills, cognitive abilities, learning styles, motivation to achieve, study habits, readiness to learn the content and preference for instructional methods.

Data about student's personal attributes can be obtained from various sources. Student's entry knowledge and skills can be obtained from a brief review of the course materials and texts used for prerequisite courses; this helps in establishing reasonable expectations of the student. Informal discussion with faculty and students are another excellent source of entry level of information.

Steps
1. Specific learning needs of learners are determined by:
- Asking the learner to identify his/her perceived learning needs
- Consulting with key faculty personnel, e.g. Subject teachers
- Mandatory training requirements
- Assessment of learners includes current knowledge levels, previous exposures or experiences related to the topic, learning styles, readiness to learn, level of education and reading, and comprehending capacities/abilities.

2. Understanding Learning Styles:
Learning style is personal, biological and developmental characteristics that makes identical instruction effective for some students and ineffective for others.

A person's individual learning style explains how he/she processes new information:
- Learns it
- Concentrates on it
- Understands it
- Retains it

To be effective in the classroom, educators must understand learning style differences among the learners. Learning styles involve perceptual strengths and processing styles.

3. Perceptual Strengths:
The four major perceptual strengths are:
- Visual people learn by seeing (30 to 40% of learners)
- Auditory people learn by hearing (20 to 30% of learners)
- Actual people learn by touch (20 to 25% of learners)
- Kinesthetic people learn by doing whole-body or real-life experiences (20 to 25% of learners).

4. Selected Teaching Strategies:
- Visual learners prefer seeing new information (overhead transparencies, charts, diagrams, pictures, videos) and study best with visual aids (flash cards, diagrams, posters)
- Auditory learners prefer hearing new information (lecture, videos) and study best with auditory aids (tape recordings of lectures, audio resources, reciting concepts out loud.)
- Tactual learners prefer hands - on experience and learn best with manipulatives, simulation, demonstration/return demonstration. In addition, tactual learners learn by writing important concepts down several times

Kinesthetic learners prefer learning by doing and learn best by role play activities, Puppet shows, skits and activities involving movement using giant wall charts and flip charts.

5. Processing Styles:

Most people use one of two processing styles to learn:
- Global learner (55% of learners)
- Analytical learner (28% of learners)

The remaining 17% of learners process information either way and show no preference to style.

6. Learners prefer:
- Knowing what they need to know and why they need to know it? then they will concentrate on details
- Introductions to training session that capture their attention such as a funny story, a short story, a quote or an illustration
- Explain while working and soft lights
- Informal seating such as sofas or chairs
- Working on several tasks at one time with breaks in-between
- Snacking while working on tasks
- Following standard directions Assignments that use graphs and illustrations to map out new information.

Analytical learners prefer:
- Having information introduced to them step by step, fact by fact and will listen to facts as long as they are goal directed
- Quiet while working and use bright lights
- Formal seating such as hard chairs and desks
- Working on a single task at one time, completing it and then beginning a new one
- Snacking after completing the task
- Working with peers
- Immediate feedback
- Having copies of assignments, directions, test dates, and objectives written down on paper and passed out to each student.

Planning

Assessment data are used as a foundation for instructional planning. Instructional plans are essential for good teaching; plan to help faculty for better prepare to meet their teaching responsibilities. Instructional plans can be thought of as sketches developed at the course, unit and lesson level.

Instructional planning includes selecting and organizing the appropriate and essential content in a logical to the meaningful sequence, with attention given to the appropriate delineation of the important relationships between facts, concepts and principles. Planning also includes selecting the instructional strategies and designing all of the learning activities. Developing a blue print of all lesson plans before the course begins is beneficial because it ensures that the content will be adequately addressed and allows faculty to examine the variety of instructional strategies and learning activities to be used throughout the course.

1. Establishing Priorities

Determining teaching priorities allows the educator to organize and rank order his/her responsibilities.

Teaching priorities are derived from the previous assessment and are based on both facility needs and staff needs.

Other individuals, such as administrators or regulatory representatives may influence teaching priorities.

Once the educator determines the top teaching need and establishes the broad idea or topic, he/she can then continue with the planning phase of the teaching-learning process.

2. Establishing Learning Objectives
- Learning objectives (behavioral objectives) state what the learner is expected to "know," "do," or "feel" at the end of the educational session
- Learning objectives that state what the learner is expected to "know" fall within the "cognitive domain of learning"

- Learning objectives that state what the learner is expected to "do" fall within the "psychomotor domain of learning"
- Learning objectives that state how the learner is expected to "feel" fall within the "affective domain of learning"

Behavioral objectives or learning objectives describe observable behaviors or performance that a student must demonstrate or perform for the teacher to conclude that learning took place.

3. Choosing Content

The content is the material that the educator will teach and is determined by learning objectives. Sources for content include in-house data, in-house policy/procedure manuals, resources from regulatory agencies, textbooks, handbooks, nursing journals, periodicals, the Internet and suggestions from experts in the field.

Content should be accurate, current and adjusted for characteristics of the learner (age, educational level, employment background, culture and reading level). Time constraints and availability of resources should also be considered when selecting content.

4. Selecting Teaching Strategies

During planning, the educator selects appropriate teaching methods to deliver content to the learners.

A teaching strategy is the way that a teacher delivers information and is based on the learning needs of the people receiving the information.

Teaching strategies are selected based on the particular domain(s) of learning that will be taught.

- Lecture—a strategy that involves active participation by the teacher and allows him/her to convey a large body of information to a group of learners. Lecture is best used with periodic group discussions, visual aides and question/answer sessions. A successful lecturer moves in the room, reflects excitement and is well prepared. Group discussion—a strategy that allows the learners to gain insight from each other and offers a forum for opposing viewpoints in a safe environment.
- Simulation—an approach that mimics a condition a person may have to face and requires the learner to handle the situation as if he/she was actually experiencing the situation.

Understanding the Three Areas of Learning

1. Cognitive Area

   The cognitive area includes intellectual skill, cognitive learning arranged from simple to complex.

   The level of learning required determines teaching strategies and method of evaluation.

   Teaching strategies include lecture, discussion, examples, outlines, question/answer sessions and acronyms. Examples of verbs used for learning objectives include compares, defines, describes, explains, identifies, lists, selects, states and summarizes.

   Knowledge—remembers previously learned material (e.g. a health care provider learns the stages of pressure ulcer development).

   Comprehension—understands the meaning of learned material. (e.g. a health care provider learns how the different stages of pressure ulcer development can be recognized and what to do at each stage).

   - Application—applies newly learned material in new concrete situations. (e.g. a health care provider learns to minimize pressure at certain areas of a resident/patient's body to decrease the later development of pressure ulcers)
   - Analysis—breaks down learned material into components parts and separates important from unimportant. (e.g. a health care provider recognizes which skin conditions are abnormal and reports them to their supervisor)
   - Synthesis—takes parts of learned material and puts them together to form new material. (e.g. a health care provider learns steps to prevent the development of pressure ulcers)
   - Evaluation—judges the value of the learned material (e.g. a health care provider can describe how the knowledge of pressure ulcer development can prevent skin breakdown among residents/patients)

2. Affective Area

   The affective area deals with the expression of feelings/emotions and involves the acceptance of attitudes, opinions or values.

Teaching strategies include case studies, simulation, role-play and discussion.

Examples of verbs used for learning objectives include chooses, initiates, justifies, shares, uses, participates, and follows.

For example: a health care provider realizes the worth and value of pacing and patience while caring for residents/ patients.

3. Psychomotor Area

The psychomotor area involves acquiring skills that require the integration of mental and muscular activity. The psychomotor includes motor skills development. The psychomotor area includes learning arranged from simple to complex.

Teaching strategies include sequencing of sub-skills, demonstration, lab practice and clinical practice.

Examples of verbs used for learning objectives include arranges, assembles, calculates, creates, demonstrates, measures and organizes.

Method of Writing Behavioral Objectives—A behavioral objective is the central point of a lesson plan. It is a description of an intended learning outcome and is the basis for the rest of the lesson.

It provides criteria for evaluation of the learning of content.

A well constructed behavioral objective describes an intended learning outcome and contains three parts.

1. Condition—A statement that describes the conditions under which the behavior is to be performed.
2. Behavioral verb—An action word that infers an observable student behavior.
3. Criteria—A statement that specifies how well the student must perform the behavior.

To write behavioral objectives, the teacher should begin with an understanding of the particular content to which the objectives will relate.

Step 1. Determine the Conditions

The teacher first specifies the conditions or circumstances, commands, materials, directions, etc. that the student is given, to initiate the behavior.

The "conditions" part of an objective usually begins with a simple declarative statement such as the following:

- Upon request the student will . . . (this means the student is given an oral or written request to do something).
- Given (some physical object) the student will . . . (this means the student is actually given something, such as a role play activity, a set of bed linen, that relates to performing the intended behavior).

Step 2. Choose the Appropriate Verb

The verb in a behavioral objective is an action word that implies an observable behavior and the domain of learning that is expected.

Verbs such as "identify," "name," and "describe" are behavioral because you can observe the act or product of identifying, naming or describing.

Verb examples representing each cognitive level of Bloom's Taxonomy are listed below. Bloom's Taxonomy is a method to categorize behavioral verbs based on level of difficulty.

Knowledge: identify, define, label, list, locate, match, select, recall and state.

Comprehension: classify, describe, estimate, discuss, explain, express, measure, summarize and recognize.

Application: apply, arrange, calculate, construct, demonstrate, operate, schedule, sketch and solve.

Analysis: analyze, debate, determine, compare, categorize, contrast, criticize, interpret and differentiate.

Synthesis: arrange, assemble, collect, compose, construct, create, design, develop, formulate, manage, organize, plan, prepare and propose.

Evaluation: appraise, argue, assess, attach, defend and judge.

Verb examples representing affective learning include: accepts, attempts, challenges, defends, disputes, joins, judges, praises, questions, shares, supports and volunteers.

Verb examples representing psychomotor learning include: administers, operates and demonstrates.

Step 3. The Criteria

The criteria are a set of descriptions that describe how well the behavior must be performed to satisfy the intent of the behavioral verb. Usually, criteria are expressed in some minimum number or as what must be, as a minimum.

Putting it all together che condition	The behavioral verb	The criteria
Upon completion of the instructional session, the learner will	Describe	Three signs of normal wound healing.
Upon request, the learner will	Compare	Two non-therapeutic communication techniques.

Implementation

To enhance student achievement, faculty should be flexible when adapting and modifying preselected instructional strategies and or when implementing the predesigned lesson plan. Student's verbal and non verbal responses during the lesson usually provide cues that indicate a need for some further explanation, clarification or additional practice in applying the content. The lesson is planned to give, the lesson you gave and the lesson you wished, you had given provides some insight into the need for flexibility and an awareness of recognizing that the practice of teaching is an ever evolving process.

Environment—An optimal learning environment includes the following: adequate space to accommodate the number of learners present, comfortable chairs and a table or tables (so the learners can take notes), adequate lighting, free from glare or bright sunshine, comfortable temperature, pleasant smell and functioning audio-visual equipment.

Characteristics of an Effective Teacher:
- Is interesting and holds the learner's interest
- Is optimistic, positive and non-threatening
- Presents content that is accurate and current
- Provides positive reinforcement
- Uses a variety of teaching strategies to accommodate a variety of learning styles
- Uses the learning objectives to guide his/her teaching efforts
- Uses time and resources wisely.

Evaluation

Evaluation is the final step of an interactive teaching learning model. Formative and summative evaluations are two common forms of evaluation used during instruction. Formative evaluation is used to determine student progress throughout the course and is often used during a class session. Informal strategies such as questioning, discussion and feedback about student participation and success in attaining the objectives of the learning activities provide faculty with valuable information about student comprehensive and achievement during the lesson.

Summative evaluation is conducted at the end of course and is used to determine the extent to which students have achieved the desired learning outcomes. Strategies used for summative evaluation include Objective type and subjective type of questions like multiple choice, essay and short answer examination; simulation, case studies and formal paper presentation. Faculty may choose to use the results of a combination of formative and summative evaluation data as the basis for assigning student grades.

Teaching:

It is important to have the learner to evaluate all aspects of the teaching - learning process. Evaluation should include consideration of the following–timing, teaching strategies, amount of information, environment and whether the objectives were met. It is also a good time to determine perceived learning needs of the learners. This information will serve as valuable input for future teaching activities. The teacher should use feedback from learner evaluations to modify the present teaching activity and consider the feedback when developing future teaching activities.

Learning:
Learning is measured against the learning objectives selected during the planning phase of teaching-learning process. The best method for evaluating whether cognitive learning occurred is by direct observation of behavior, written tests, oral questioning and self-reporting. The best method for evaluating psychomotor skills acquisition is direct observation of performance. The best method for evaluating whether affective learning occurred is by direct observation of behavior, oral questioning and self-reporting.

Documentation

Records should be kept based on the type and amount of information that may be requested at a later date. Record keeping should mirror requirements by regulatory agencies and follow protocols established by the facility's administrative body.

Often regulatory agencies require documentation of:
- Mandatory education
- Competence and continued competence of skill performance
- Facility-based problems and how they have been resolved through education. At a minimum, the following information should be kept for each education session:
  - Participant information (e.g. name, age, sex, group, etc.)
  - Attendance records
  - Contact hours of instruction
  - A syllabus or course outline (includes objectives)
  - Method of evaluation–Educational records are requested by regulatory agencies, have been used to defend employees or teaching faculty to protect them for legal purposes in case of malpractices.

Teacher- Student Relationship

Teacher will communicate with the student based on the learning situation and environment exhibits themselves as Authoritarian/Democratic/Laisseze-faire leader. Majority of the times, teacher will act as a democratic leader, when the situations are going out of control either Laisseze-faire qualities autocratic leader qualities teacher will exhibit to reach the set goals and set right the problems. Teacher will maintain conducive environment for learning, which is productive, benefit for both, especially to the learner. Teacher will maintain good IPR through effective communication skills. Teacher acts as a Philosopher, Guide, Friend, Role model, Exemplary, Counselor and Manager based on the learning situations of the learner. Teacher has to possess positive attitude towards learner, should have interest in the growth and development of the learners. Learner should have confidence on teacher and develop mutual trust, respect with the teacher. Teacher has to identify strengths/capabilities/abilities and weaknesses of the learner always encourage the student and motivate the child to improve his/her abilities and the inner strengths which will mould his/her personality. Teacher has to assist the learner's growth and ability to meet all his/her felt needs by creating self awareness, self concept and to reach highest need fulfillment of the learner i.e., self esteem and self actualization. Teacher will act as a counselor and helps the learner to meet his/her personal and professional needs. Certain qualities like establishing, maintaining and terminating the either personal or professional relationships when the need completes, ability to share the knowledge and power, having competitive spirits, self control capacity, keeping themselves always busy, away from negative thoughts and attitudes, ability to develop self concept and professional self i.e., ability to derive self satisfaction, implementation of planned actions into practice, appreciation of shared power and willingness to develop and possess positive change, taking steps to improve personal and professional self, willingness to take steps in changing behavior which promotes personal and professional growth, developing willingness to take risks to achieve the set goals, mutual trust, respect, cooperation and developing self confidence, assuming and sharing the responsibilities for achieving group goals. Thus teacher is helding responsible for providing suitable environment and strives hard for molding personality of the learners.

Management of Teaching-Learning Process

For effective Teaching, teacher has to carry out specific activity like Organizing and utilizing the in depth of resources.

Functions/Responsibilities of the Teacher
1. Planning of the Teaching and Learning activities
- Formulation of General and Specific learning objectives
- Observe the curriculum, identify and organize the headings of content and Audio-visual Aids in a logical and sequential way
- Uses the library resources, internet facilities to gather and frame the subject content, prepare the Teaching aids based on experience and critical judgement skills in advance and pre test the aids for the utility. Gets the peer group opinion if feels necessary
- Teacher uses his/her own imagination and creativity in planning the material for the lesson plan
- Identify suitable teaching–learning activities to keep and maintain effectiveness and activeness and live experience for the group of students in teaching and learning situation.

2. Organizing learning activities
- Teacher will organize the content in a sequential and logical manner, teacher always thinks and selects the methods which will keep the learners engaged in a active manner
- Teaching–Learning activities are focused on accomplishing the objectives of the lesson plan
- Teacher will explain the content effectively with the help of audio-visual aids to make teaching and learning activity in a meaningful manner
- At the end of the class and beginning of the next session teacher will review and get the feed back of audience or group of learners whether they understood the topic, if they require still explanation based on the quantity she/he may arrange one on one explanation and clarifying the subject or repeat the class based on the response of group of learners.

3. Leading the group
- The teacher utilizes appropriate techniques in leading the group like motivating, inspiring the group, asking questions, using simple and clear terms while explaining, monitors student responses while teaching, make the group of learners in an active manner. Make the teaching–learning session in an effective, productive, qualitative manner where both the teacher and the learner will be benefitted in a useful manner, based on the situation the teacher will exhibit varied styles of leader
- If the student exhibits positive manner and performs in a better way, even small accomplishment of the activities by the learner also will be appreciated and if possible she/he discusses with the authority to give certain rewards or prizes etc. positive reinforcements for the learner, thus motivates the learner to be rich in knowledge and experiences
- Manipulates the learning material if the need arises, based on the understanding level and need of the students, teacher will organize the material
- Guides, motivates, inspires the students to learn effectively and increase or maximum efficiency in gaining the learning outcomes.

4. Controlling the group activities
- Teacher will apply specific theories and the models based on the subject content and objectives and expected outcomes of the curriculum
- Teacher will be more conscious about their responsibilities and implement the measures for achieving self satisfaction and to achieve learning outcomes
- Monitors the learning system and implement necessary steps to make the learners as a profitable experiences.
- Teaching system has to best utilize the student needs, abilities, attitudes and interests
- Assess the teaching-learning process, get the feedback, based on the need and requirement of the student and course objectives plan the activities accordingly like organizing and modifying the teaching-learning activities, teacher will not leave the students until goal reached. She/he motivates the students to work hard and to reach targets set by the teacher
- Certain times teacher has to use autocratic and Laisseze-faire leadership to achieve the learning objectives, teachers' goal is make the student to achieve their target and fulfill course requirement. All the time democratic leadership may not work out to control total group of learners' their achivements.

ADULT LEARNING

Andragogy

"Art and Science of helping adults to learn"
"An intentional and professionally guided activity that aims at change in adult person"

Elements that influence Adult Learning

- Preparing the learners
- Climate setting
- Mutual Planning
- Identification of Learning Needs
- Formulation of Learning Objectives
- Learning plan design
- Learning plan execution
- Evaluation

Principles of Adult Learning

Assumption or Principle	Andragogical approach to adult learning
Concept of the learner, Level of self directedness	Increasingly self Directed
Readiness to learn	Develops from life tasks and problems
Experience	A rich source for learning by self and others
Orientation	Task or Problem centered
Motivation	Internal incentives and curiosity
Need to know	Learner's perception of what and why of learning important to overall learning experience

Process Design / Elements of Adult Learning

Process Design Element	Andragogical approach to adult learning
Preparing the learner	Supply information, prepare students for participation, Develop Realistic expectations, Begin thinking with content
Climate	Relaxed, Trusting, Mutually respectful, Informal, Collaborative and Supportive
Planning	Mutually by learners and facilitator
Diagnosis of Needs	By Mutual assessment
Setting of Objectives	By Mutual Negotiation
Designing Learning Plans	Learning contracts, Learning Projects, Sequenced by Readiness
Learning activities	Inquiry Projects, Independent study, Experimental Techniques
Evaluation	By Learner collected evidence validated by peers, facilitator, experts, and criterion referenced

Principles of Adult Learning

- Learning is a normal adult activity:
  Human beings will learn continuously throughout their lives. Without teacher the adult will learn by observation, insight. Adults learn at their own pace, reduce threat in the learning environment, without any obligations the individual adult will try to learn.
- Adults with a positive self concept and high self esteem are more responsive to learning:
  The adult want to live qualitative life and productive in varied roles which he has to perform. Adults see them as achievers and therefore wanted to be treated with self respect. They avoid situations which they can not control, they do not want to be told, what they can or can not do, be talked down to or judged. Adults learn best in environment that does not threaten their self-respect, self- concept and self-esteem. For adults learning will take place in a non–threatening environment . Adult learners has to learn in a simulated environment where mistakes can be corrected during practice and self respect will be maintained.

- Adults learn best when they value the role of adult learner and possess skills for managing their own learning.
- Adult learning is dynamic/active and self directed process, after being reoriented to learning, adults can take responsibility for their own learning as they have done with other facets of their lives.
  The adult learner is held responsible for sharing in planning implementing and evaluating his/her learning. This collaborative approach adult learner can become interdependent learners.
- Immediate, descriptive feedback is essential if adult learners has to modify their behavior:
  An adult learner practice new skills, they need feedback about how they are progressing towards objectives. The timing of feed back is important, immediate feedback affects learning the most. The longer the interval between feed back and performance, the less likely is that feed back will have a positive effect on learning. Immediate feedback after performance of skill will facilitate active learning, Adult learning is facilitated by when the learner has clear idea of the behavior to be learned. Objectives that describe the skill and how it has to be demonstrated is important feedback and has to be in terms of stated objectives and be descriptive rather than judgmental.
- Success reinforces changes already made and provides a motive for further learning:
  For the adult learner, meeting established objectives reinforces the newly acquired skill and motivates more learning. The earlier satisfaction and success come in the learning program, the more likely is that further learning will take place. Opportunities have to be created that has built in success factor. Learning activities should be sequenced so that the learner will experience success on the first few skills taught.
- Adult tend to begin learning programs from some anxiety and further stress can interfere with learning Excessive anxiety will interfere with adult learning. Adults do not like to be seen by others that they are upset, so they use most of their energy to mask their emotions. so energy will not be there further to learn for adults. So the educator has to avoid the threatening environments, initial activities has to be planned which will reduce anxiety, create supportive, acceptance environment, provide time for learning new behaviors and achieve desired skills.

The Andragogical Practices Inventory

- Through review of other instruments from past Research
- Development of a Survey item pool based on specific Andragogical Principles and design elements
- Development of a draft Andragogical Practices Inventory (API)
- Panel of expert's review of the API for purposes of establishing content validity
- Revision of survey based on results of the panel review
- Finalization of survey instrument
- Use of instrument in data collection
- Statistical Analysis.

QUESTIONS

- Characteristics of learning (5M, NTRUHS, June, 2010 and 5M,NIMS, May, 2010).
- Define Attitude and explain the factors involved in attitudinal change (15M, NTRUHS, Dec, 2007)
- Define Attitudes and delineate factors in their formation, Change and Measurement (15M, NTRUHS, July, 2008)
- Define Attention (2M, MGRUHS, May, 2010).
- Define Intelligence (2M, NTRUHS, June, 2009 & 2M, MGRUHS, May, 2010).
- Define Learning and discuss its nature (5M, NTRUHS, Dec,2007).
- Define learning Briefly describe the basics of classical conditioning (10M, MGRUHS, May, 2010).
- Difference between learning - Teaching (5M, MGU, Oct, 2007).
- Differentiate between Cognitive domain - Affective domain (5M, MGU, Dec, 2008).
- Differentiate between Teaching – Learning (5M, NIMS, May,2010).
- Discuss the principles of learning. (10M, RGUHS, Feb, 2010).
- Domains of learning (5M, RGUHS, Aug, 2010).
- Elaborate the process of social learning through immitation (10M, RGUHS, May, 2010).
- Explain the methods of Learning (10M, NTRUHS, Dec,2007).
- Explain the role of a Nurse teacher in Nursing Education (10M, NTRUHS, June, 2010).
- Explain the teaching and learning process, Identify the role and functions of a teacher (10M, NTRUHS, July, 2008).
- Factors influencing Learning (5M, NTRUHS, June, 2009).
- Learning Process (5M, MGRUHS, Feb, 2009).
- List four Qualities of an Effective Teacher (4 M, MGRUHS, Aug, 2008).
- List the qualities of a good teacher (10M, NIMS, May, 2007) (b) Explain briefly the principles of teaching (c) Enumerate the teaching methods used in Nursing (5+7+8M, MGU, Nov,2009).
- Methods of Class Room Teaching (5 M, MGRUHS, Aug, 2008).
- Principles adult learning (2M, RGUHS, Aug, 2010).
- Principles of Learning (5M, MGRUHS , Feb, 2009 & Nov, 2010).
- Principles of Teaching (5 M, MGRUHS, Aug, 2006; 5M, NTRUHS, Dec, 2007; 2M, RGUHS, Aug, 2010; 4M,NIMS, May, 2007).
- State Principles of Teaching, Describe Teaching Learning Process (6M + 10M, Rajasthan UHS, Feb,2010)
- Teaching Learning Process (5M, Rajasthan UHS, March, 2010).
- Teaching Module (5M, MGU, Oct, 2007).
- Theories of learning (5M, MGU, Oct, 2007).
- Three principle of learning (3M, MGU, Oct, 2007 & Dec, 2008).
- Types of learning (5 M, NTRUHS, June 2009 and June, 2010).
- What are two main Types of Reading (2 M, MGRUHS, Feb, 2009).
- What is attention? Explain the determinants of attention, What is span of attention? Explain the factors determine span of attention? (15M, NTRUHS, June, 2009).
- With reference to attention, explain the following – fluctuation of attention, span of attention, Division of attention (5M+5M+5M, NTRUHS, July, 2008).
- Write a note on reinforcement on learning (6M, MGRUHS, May, 2010).

CHAPTER

5

Teaching Methods

INTRODUCTION

Teaching Method includes the principles and methods of instruction. All instruction material will be carefully selected and arranged in a orderly fashion. The teaching methods appeal through sensory perception to enhance the understanding of the learner. Progressive methods of teaching provide suitable opportunities for 'learning by doing', 'experimentation' and 'cooperation'. Every teacher must devise their own method of teaching by following broader principles, e.g. Orderly arrangement of subject matter which will save time and energy. A method must link up the teacher and learners in an association/relationship with constant mutual interaction.

DEFINITIONS

'An orderly systematic, organized well planned procedure where skillful teacher broadly review the teaching material, scrutinize and analyze the specific content, arranges the topic in a systematic, logical, sequential way which directs and guides the teacher in their classroom instruction and enhances effective teaching by achieving the specific instructional objectives where by learning output will be maximized'.

'A device implies the external mode or form in which teaching may take from time to time'.

'Teaching method is the stimulation, guidance, direction and encouragement for learning'.

— Burton

MEANING

The procedural dimension in the educative process refers to the methods and techniques, which will be used by both the teacher and the learner to achieve the desired educational objectives. The dimensions like substantive, environmental, human relations and procedural dimensions are interrelated. Knowledge, environment and human relations all affect the procedural aspect of education. Teaching in Nursing encompasses both cognitive and artistic aspects. Teaching skill and technical competency in teaching have effect on student's learning. Art in teaching is necessary which has to be developed. Systematic attention to methods and materials of teaching and learning as well as mastery of the subject matter are essential for the development of artistic teaching.

OBJECTIVES

- Inculcates the desire to do work with the maximum efficiency which one is capable of, 'Work is Worship'
- Develops the capacity for clear thinking
- Provide adequate opportunities for participation and activities in which cooperation and discipline are constantly interlinked
- Expands students' interest
- Provide opportunities to learners to apply practically the knowledge and skill acquired by them
- Teaching method should adapt to the 3A's—Age, Ability and Aptitude of the student
- Promote eagerness among learners to achieve cumulative learning and for teachers' to maximize skills in enhancing effective teaching
- Mobilizes teamwork and promotes sense of security
- Mastery in the subject matter.

CLASSIFICATION

1. Inspirational methods: Main activity on the part of the teacher, e.g. Simulation and Microteaching.
2. Expository methods: Cognitive emphasis is high, while student activity and experience is low, e.g. Lecture method.
3. Natural learning method: Learning takes place in a natural way, e.g. Field trips.
4. Individualized methods: Main emphasis is for each learner to learn at his own pace, e.g. Programed instruction, self-study, case method and computer oriented instruction.
5. Encounter methods: Providing experience through confrontation or through encounter effective for change in basic behavioral patterns and developing new ways of looking at things, e.g. Role play, simulation.
6. Discovery methods: High on all dimensions like learner activity, experience, experimentation by the learner and cognitive understanding, e.g. Problem-solving technique.
7. Group methods, e.g. Group project, classroom teaching, discussions, demonstration.

CHARACTERISTICS

- Imparting knowledge in an efficient manner
- Inculcates desirable values, positive attitudes and habits of work in students
- Create a genuine attachment to work and a desire to do it as efficiently, honestly and thoroughly as possible
- The principles like 'verbalism and memorization' 'activity and project method' has to be assimilated in school practice
- Provides opportunities for students to learn actively and apply the knowledge practically
- Promotes clear thinking and clear expression both in speech and writing
- Trains the learners the techniques of study, methods of acquiring knowledge through personal effort and initiative
- A well-thought-out attempt has to be made to adopt suitable methods of instruction to benefit all categories of students
- Provide opportunity for the students to work in groups and to carry out group projects and activities to enhance group life and cooperative work.

PRINCIPLES

Methods should be suited to:
- The objectives and the content of the course
- The learning requirements
- Based on sound psychological principles
- Teacher's personality and capitalizes on her/his special assets
- Creative and positive in spirit.

DEMONSTRATION METHOD

The demonstration method is of utmost importance in teaching of Nursing. This method is taught by "exhibition and explanation". It is an explanation of a process. It trains, explains the student in the art of careful observation, which is essential for a good nurse.

Purposes

1. To demonstrate experiments or procedures and explain the utility value of equipment in the laboratory and in the ward.
2. To review or revise procedures to meet a special situation.
3. To introduce a new procedure.
4. To teach the patient a procedure or treatment which has to be carried out in the home. eg: Administration of insulin injection to a diabetic patient.
5. To demonstrate a procedure at the bedside or in the ward or in conference room.
6. Demonstration of a procedure in its natural setting has more meaning (e.g. in ward on patients) than when carried out in an artificial environment (e.g. laboratory).

7. To demonstrate different approaches in establishing rapport with patients, so that the most effective nurse-patient relationship will be established.

Essential Characteristics

1. Every step of a well-conducted demonstration should be understandable and exemplary of the best possible procedure, which might be used under the similar circumstances.
2. Allow sufficient time for reflective and critical thinking as the demonstration proceeds
3. Applied principles in demonstration method performed by both the teacher and the student
   a. The student performing demonstration procedure has to understand the entire procedure before practice. This sometimes necessitates review before performance.
   b. All equipment should be assembled and pretested before the demonstration carried out, as it saves time and ensures that the apparatus should be in good state.
   c. Advance knowledge: Demonstrator should possess advance or mastery over the knowledge of the procedure which has to be carried out. Otherwise, the student's attention will not be focused on the procedure, their mind will be distracted by questions relating to the performance why it is being given, what it means, which has to be followed, the student should possess lab manual which describes the procedure in detail. (Objectives, equipments, steps to be carried out before, during and after the procedure, documentation and after care of equipments)
   d. A positive approach should be used, emphasis has to be placed on what to do, rather than what not to do.
   e. All students in the batch should have a good view of demonstration, precautions should be taken to ensure all round comfort.
   f. Running Comments: The teacher incharge should carry out the procedure with running comments, materials used, equipment necessary, processes taking place and anticipated results. However, the commentary should be limited to essential facts. If an actual patient is used in the demonstration, explanatory and comments must be regulated accordingly.
      The teacher will demonstrate the procedure on dummy first, after return demonstration; and later students practice one to one another (General procedures) and specific procedures will be demonstrated by teacher on clients (after expalining the need and obtain consent).
4. The setting for the demonstration should be true to life as possible. Demonstration of a nursing procedure should be done on a live model wherever possible, e.g. If demonstration is carried out on a patient, obtain consent, explain the purpose of the demo, show every possible courtesy and clarify, if the patient is having any doubts related to procedure, then the clinical instructor carry out the demonstration on an individual.
5. Discussion is followed after the demonstration. This affords an opportunity for reemphasis, questioning, recall, evaluation and summary while or reflection immediately promotes long lasting memory for the learner.
6. Mimeographed directions should be distributed before demonstrating a nursing procedure. This saves continuous dictation on the part of the teacher and writing on the part of the student.
7. Prompt practice: As the main purpose of a demonstration is skill training/ hands-on training, the student should be given an opportunity to practice the procedure as soon as possible after the demonstration. Students vary in their ability to learn. The sooner the practice takes place after demonstration, the better the learning.

Advantages

1. Provides an opportunity for "Observational learning".
2. It commands interest by use of concrete illustrations. The student not only can hear the explanation, but also can see the procedure or process. As a result, demonstration method projects a mental image in the students' mind, which fortifies verbal knowledge.
3. The demonstration method has universal appeal because it is understandable to all.
4. The demonstration method is adaptable to both group and individual teaching.
5. Activates several senses, as the more senses used, the better the opportunity for learning.
6. Clarifies the underlying principles by demonstrating the 'why' of a procedure.
7. Correlates "Theory with Practice".

8. Provides an opportunity for teachers to evaluate the student's knowledge of a procedure and to determine whether reteaching is necessary.
9. Points out the student must have knowledge and must be able to apply it immediately.
10. Serves as a strong motivational force for the student.
11. Return demonstration by the student under supervision of the teacher provides an opportunity for well-directed practice before the student will practice the procedure on the ward.
12. Since the teacher is supervising the procedure, the student will have a sense of security while performing the procedure either in lab or in ward.
13. Ensures closer contact with concrete problems
14. Student will have the facility to acquire cognitive, conative and affective skills improvement.
15. Presents Reality situation, learner will have the opportunity to practice the skill before practicing on the client, e.g. the nursing student in first year of professional nursing training will have the opportunity to practice injection technique in the laboratory on dummy and on the class mates under teachers' supervision before practicing on the clients in OPD or ward or injection room under teachers' supervision.
16. Enables the learner to learn step by step the procedure in a systematic way.
17. Learner has to possess active listening, attention, concentration skills while observing the demonstration of procedure.
18. Learner will learn right way of doing complex tasks.
19. Monitoring of the learners is easy for the teacher if the teacher student ratio followed as per INC norms. (1:5 is advised for clinical supervision)

Disadvantages

1. Teacher can supervise less number of students in a single laboratory session.
2. More time consuming as supervision requires systematic approach.
3. If more number of students were allotted against to norms, it will be very difficult for a single teacher to supervise, as it does not allow for individual pace of learning or one on one supervision will become difficult, if the institution follows ideal ratio, teacher can overcome all these difficulties.
4. Expensive in terms of time, personnel and equipment.
5. Feasibility of acquiring competence is difficult, as repeated number of performing and supervising single procedure is impossible in present situations.

Lecture-Demonstration

Its purpose is to point out relationships as they occur during a demonstration. It may be explanation related to functions of the structure or steps of a procedure and principles associated with it.

This method is used extensively in teaching sciences and nursing subjects. It measured factual knowledge only.

The Television Lecture-Demonstration

The lecture-demonstration is the method used most frequently in TV teaching. Because of the nature of the medium in which photography and audio-tape are combined, and because of time limitations, the preparations of TV lecture is similar to classroom.

Scripts have to be prepared and rehearsal, to ensure proper use of time and photography. Television lecture should not be simply a talking lecture; it should make wide use of all kinds of illustrative materials.

LECTURE METHOD

Introduction

The lecture is one of the most well-known, highly effective teaching method, through which some educational purposes are well served. The lecture, when it is adjusted to stimulate and organize thinking, active learning , challenge attitudes and promote problem solving. It is a teaching procedure, as lecturing is a great art. Consisting of clarification and the explanation of facts, principles or relationships, which the teacher wishes the learners to understand. The teacher talks more or less continuously to the class. Group of learners will listen, takes notes of the facts and the ideas worth remembering and work on them over later; usually, the students do not converse with the teacher. Almost, they might ask a few questions, but these are for the sake of clarification and not for the sake of discussions. The most readily recognized and accepted pedagogical choice is lecture.

Definition

"The lecture is essentially a formal exposition, which makes only incidental use of narrative description in setting forth the basic and all inclusive structure of an entire topic".

Purposes

- Stimulates process of thinking among teachers and learners
- Teacher will gain teaching skills and learn how to attack a problem in a systematic way
- Expertise teaching skills are necessary to make teaching effective and facilitate learning, to teach varied subjects for a larger group of students, lecture method is ideal
- Good teacher with efficient teaching skills and vast subject knowledge is always beneficial for the students as those teachers will be role models for the learners throughout their life time. A good teacher is an asset for an organization
- A lesson taught by an effective teacher always beneficial than several hours of independence studying or unlimited group discussions
- A teacher opens a topic in a field of study, draw attention to a group of students to its' vital elements, extract the essential, bring students abreast of development in the forefront of Research
- The lecture should illuminate, supplement and reinforce the topic being studied, the teacher has to do vast review of the content and thoroughly prepare about a specific topic in advance, formulate a lesson plan and plans the method of teaching quite ahead of time. The lecture should not be a mere representation of exactly what is in the text books nor assigned reading, nor it should be completely unrelated to the subject topic. The teacher should be very careful while teaching to the group of students by whatever method of teaching they adopt
- Teacher will illustrate with suitable examples from other related sources, out of their professional experience, as it enhances students' thinking and understanding the subject effectively and promotes long lasting learning with a factual basis with relevant concepts, practices the same principles wherever it is applicable
- A well prepared lecture will be more beneficial for the students to have organized knowledge in an integrating fashion as the student uses cross references, correlates lecture material with other resources
- Teacher will be exemplify the techniques of analysis in a field of study by using scientific principles
- The teacher can introduce an organizing content in presentation, involves the student with appropriate teaching learning activities, make the students in arriving at the generalizations and conclusions
- Teacher creates interest and enthusiasm in the subject, promotes respect in students' mind for the ideas, worthwhileness of intellectual values through their mode of presentation and instructional materials.

The Ingredients of an Effective Lecture

The art and skill of choosing, balancing and blending all ingredients develop with practice and critique. Some ingredients that demand balance to make a lecture effective.

1. Questions

a. Questions activate learning, promotes thinking and learner interaction
b. Review lecture outline for opportunities to ask and to create some clearly stated questions in advance
c. There are many different methods lecturers can use questioning

Early in the lecture

- Assign listening questions: by giving a specific question to geographical regions of the room-all quadrants, rows or some other means of creating groups. Assign each region a different question. These questions can be a basis for paired or small group discussion at the end of the lecture or ask for a few individual responses when concluding lecture.
- Create cluster questions (groups of questions designed to help learners to understand the topic): that are sequenced in progressing simple to complex, elucidate different aspects of a topic or develop some other organizer appropriate to the topic. Have learners participate in questioning, each learner to write a pertinent

question on a 3 × 3.5 inch card during the first half of the lecture period. Collect and redistribute the cards to groups of learners. Ask each group to respond.

- Present examination-style questions at intervals during the lecture: A multiple-choice format can stimulate discussion when learners defend different choices as the correct answer. This may provide an opportunity to clarify the circumstances in which certain choices would be appropriate.
- True–false or alternative response questions: offer opportunities to correct common errors and misconceptions. When asked about a patient care situation, questions such as "What's wrong with this picture?" give learners an opportunity to apply judgment and use information.
- Give a brief mastery quiz at intervals during the lectures or at its conclusion: Learners required to write the answers. Answering questions immediately after learning facilitates retention.
- Have learners produce a minute paper at the conclusion of the lecture. Pose a question such as "What stood out as most important in today's lecture?" or "What ideas from today's lecture are still unclear?" and allow the learners 1 minute to write the answers. Ask for a sample of oral responses. Offer feedback to learners' answers. Questions give the opportunity for learners to practice with the information and receive corrective or validating feedback.
- Coaching: is the signature pedagogy of nursing questions and feedback in the classroom setting parallel the coaching process in the clinical setting. Conclude the lecture by posing a question for further consideration. The learners' "last memory of lecture is of the questions you urged them to explore further" this approach promotes ongoing curiosity.

2. Learner Preparation

Successful students use lectures as organizers to gain greater meaning from reading assignments.

3. Note Taking

The lecturer can facilitate learning by creating handout materials and guiding learners in their note taking.

- Encourage learners to focus on listening to and thinking about what they are hearing rather than writing.
- Facilitate listening and thinking by providing a handout that contains a skeletal outline of the lecture (not a complete manuscript) that includes the key points with spaces for learners to write). Speak at a pace that allows for writing of important points. For difficult spellings or other useful information, display the information visually or provide the information as a handout. Call attention to points that learners should write. Talk in 7 to 10 minute segments, pause and ask preplanned, rhetorical questions. Ask learners to record their answers in their notes. Pause two or three times to allow learners to consolidate notes and develop questions, Facial expressions and gestures.

Declare a note taking moratorium. Have learners to listen to 15 to 20 minutes of lecture without taking notes. At the end, instruct them to spend 5 minutes recording all they can recall. Then, ask learners to form small discussion groups in which they reconstruct the lecture conceptually with supporting data. Provide a question period during which the learners ask you to resolve questions that arise. At intervals, instruct learners to work in pairs to organize their notes and discuss key points. Instruct learners to close their notebooks for a few minutes at the end of the lecture period and outline or diagram as much as they can remember.

4. Structure

Organization is key to effective lecturing. The lecturer can demonstrate how to organize and use formation. The lecturer facilitates learning by introducing the lecture outline and continually referring to it to help learners create their own internal organization of the information, giving organizers initially and during a lecture contributed more to learning than some other behaviors usually associated with effective lecturing.

The concept of immediacy, which includes eye contact, vocal variation, facial expressions and movement around the classroom. Organization of material and learning of details, was strongly related to performance on tests of the material. Although immediacy and interesting tangents can facilitate connection with learners, these ingredients clearly must be used judiciously. Body language that conveys enthusiasm for the topic and interest in learners facilitates learning, but can also be distracting if exaggerated. Pay attention to learners' responses to your body language and consider the size of the room when communicating with facial expressions and gestures Humor, examples and anecdotes can facilitate learning, but choose carefully and plan to clarify the connection to the topic. Story telling has gained momentum among pedagogies in nursing education . "Stories allow the listener to seek an experience of being alive in them and find clues to answers within themselves". Telling stories as a lecturer and eliciting and encouraging learners to tell their stories contributes to learning (applicable for only certain nursing subject). However, artful and effective use of the technique requires the lecturer's expertise in guiding reflection and illuminating connections. The recommended structure for a lecture begins with a top-down description of main ideas followed by a bottom-up construction of details. To facilitate mastery in new terms, meaningfully "introduce a new idea only after it's born" by stating the term "only after giving an example of the notion that it stands for" .

5. Technology and Visual Aids

Technology and visual representations can aid in the delivery of an effective lecture but cannot substitute for lack of other essential ingredients. Although slides and computer based presentation programs lend a more polished appearance, at times seeing the lecturer construct relationships on a chalkboard or white board has a greater effect. Remember that the visuals are used most effectively to clarify or emphasize information.

Computer-based presentation programs have become extremely popular. If used thoughtfully, such programs can provide an outline for both the learners and the lecturer and can create useful note-taking handouts. However, positive attitude, self-efficacy and motivation will increase when learners receiving lectures. When using Powerpoint, be aware that the use of animation and sound effects can distract learners. Ensure that choice of technological aids is contributing to learning and is neither distracting nor monotonous.

If the class strength is more, the teacher may use microphone to make his/her lecture to be clear to the entire group.

6. Preparation of the Lecture

The goal of lecturing is communication and it is more effective, if it is prepared before hand. The objectives of the course, as well as the immediate objectives of the lecture should be kept clearly in mind. The teacher should know exactly what points she/he has to list, in what order and with what emphasis. The teacher should have a scheme for each lecture in mind, not simply as a set number of pages to be read over, but visualized as a well-articulated structure of thought. The lecture should have a central theme carried to completion in each delivery. The lecture should contain a sequence of ideas kept relatively simple with headings and sub-headings. There should be a definite limitation on the number of sections in which the main topic is decided; too many topics may hide the main topic from view. Time distribution is needed to the various subtopics to make sure that the essential topics are covered. Lecture should contain an introduction to help to establish rapport with the class, to relate each lecture to the preceding one etc., The introduction may be a preview of the main topic to be covered. This helps the new inexperienced teacher through the first few difficult moments of her/his lecture. Introduction can serve as a means of getting the class started promptly. The lecture should be written in outline form, the amount of detail would vary with the teacher's experience in lecturing and her/his knowledge of the subject. Some literal statements of all critical points may be written on the lecture plan for the teacher to read. If illustrative materials are to be used, they should be prepared and tested before the lecture.

Advantages and Disadvantages

Advantages	Disadvantages
Apparent saving of time and resources	Keeps the student in a passive situation
Presence of the teacher	Does not facilitate learning 'How to solve the problems
Covers a large group of students	Offers hardly any possibility of checking learning progress
Gives a feeling of security	Does not allow for individual pace of learning, Low receptivity

Technique

If the lecture is viewed, as a means of presenting information and a method of effective learning, it requires the teacher not only to talk, but also to work with the students. The teacher establishes the contact with the students quickly and places her/his delivery to the capacity of the students to follow lecture, making allowances for note taking and anticipates the sections in her/his lecture that students find difficult to comprehend.

The teacher will make sure that the important points in her/his class are made clear before advancing to the next point. The teacher will use illustrations and interject questions to help, to clarify points before students become too fatigued from the strain of intense listening. A lecture is teacher-centered, the expert teacher will compensate for the restriction of students' verbal expression by sensing how their students are responding in taught to what is being said. The lecturer should conducts internals for clarification of thought, assimilation of ideas.

Guides helpful to the teacher in using the Lecture Method
1. Rapport—Teacher has to establish rapport with her/his students. It will be done:
   i. Through an exchange with students in a conversational tone about some event at the school, this will help to foster a sense of ease and give the impression of personal interest.
   ii. By beginning the lecture with a review of previous lectures, tying them in with the present one.
   iii. To merge the students into a learning group, the questions will be directed to students in various parts of the room
2. Voice—The lecture should be presented in a clear, natural tone of voice.
   The teacher should speak to the students, not at them, nor above or below them. The teacher can use her/his voice for emphasis in her/his lecture by pausing at appropriate points to let her/his words sink in and to let the echoes of her/his voice subside. In a lecture – the rate of ideas is the critical element.
   Keep the students alert and get across their ideas; talk twice, fast, repeat often, even speak indistinctly, by keeping students alert.
3. Gestures—Whatever gestures the lecturer uses should be in a natural part of the total expression of what she/he is communicating. The teacher's actions should blend with speech, they should be spontaneous and animated and a part of the natural style of the individual.
4. Eye contact—The teacher should address the students with their eyes as well as with voice. The eyes have a unique power to transmit the mood of the teacher to the student. If the teacher is alert, eager, enthusiastic, the eyes convey this to the student, who usually adopts a similar attitude.
5. Lecture outline and student's notes—The lecture should be prepared and delivered in several blocks or units, each unit should present not more than fifteen minutes. As each unit is completed, it should be briefly summarized or punctuated with discussion for a short period of time. Lecture should present from written notes, but should not be read. Salient points marked on the outline which has to be delivered slowly and emphatically so that students can copy them if they wish to do so; the connecting arguments should be remembered and delivered in a conversational tone, leaving time and opportunity to unusual interest in any one of them. The lecture should conclude before the end of the period, leaving time to tie up loose threads, review essential points, ask questions or get comments from students.
   The lecture should be delivered on the assumption that the students have completed the reading assignments and are prepared for the lecture. This means that the teacher will have their entire course prepared before beginning their lecture and that she/he will give advance notice to students in each lecture.

The When-to-lecutre Checklist
The When-to-Lecture Checklist identifies goals the lecture can achieve effectively.

The check list:
- Is this information that learners cannot learn on their own?
- Is this information difficult to understand and in need of organization to make it clear and reasonable for learners to grasp?
- Do you need maximum economy and efficiency in presenting a large amount of information to a large number of learners simultaneously?
- Do you want to provide a framework or overview for subsequent learning such as reading assignments or small group activities?
- Do you have information that is unavailable elsewhere?
- Do you want to provide a synthesis of information from various sources?
- Do you want to use your enthusiasm, experience and examples to stimulate interest in the topic?
- Is your purpose to establish broad outlines of a body of material?
- Do you want to set guidelines for independent study?

- Is your purpose to model intellectual attitudes that you hope to encourage in your learners?
- Do you want to encourage learners' interest in a topic?
- Do you want to set a moral culture for discussions?
- Do you want to clarify complex, detailed or abstract information?

How to Improve Lectures

The lecturer can improve lecture performance by incorporating learner feedback, learner performance results, reflection and peer feedback. (Contracting with the peer to make a highly focused observation by looking for evidence of effectiveness previously agreed on between the teacher being observed and the peer who is observing.) Reflect on your actions during the lecture. What worked? What did not work? What will you do differently next time? Identified being open to reflection as one of the themes in learning to lecture. Other themes included attending to learning, reading class situations, unlearning teacher preparation and challenging assumptions of conventional pedagogy. Emphasize the importance of assessing and responding to the learners during the lecture, also known as "reflecting-in-action". Address fears that arise with the challenge of trying something new. Consider the feedback from learners and their performance on measures of the knowledge you have presented to them in the lecture format. Retain as much objectivity as possible when reviewing learner evaluation data. Examine your practice in light of constructive criticism, but also remember that in some simplified definitions, learning equals change. Most people naturally resist change and some learners resist changing their cognitive structures and experiencing new teaching methods. Low ratings on evaluations may reflect this resistance. Strive to improve without becoming defensive or defeated. Critically examine, validate and then act on the feedback you receive. When you can, take advantage of the opportunity to learn from masters, watch and listen to great lecturers and riveting public speakers. Do not take copious notes; instead enjoy the experience and at the conclusion of the presentation, make a few notes about which techniques had the greatest effect on you.

AVOID

- Speaking during powerPoint show, do not display and read the points without further elaboration or examples
- Cramming as much information as possible into each visual or frequently acknowledging, "I know you, can't see this, but. . ."
- Reading from a manuscript
- Reading extensively from a text or other book
- Distributing lecture in a word-for-word manuscript
- Using a PowerPoint handout with 12 slides per page
- Displaying a cartoon or other visual while talking about something else
- Letting visuals speak for themselves. Point out key features or relevance to the topic
- Letting the available technology drive your approach, instead of the subject and learners
- Racing through the last part of lecture where you have placed all the great examples and action implications
- Using a monotone voice and extensive pauses

Ingredients of an Effective Lecture

Ingredient	Lecturer Actions
Before structure	• Make a well-organized plan that contributes to connections of previous learning and experience with new learning, but do not reduce all learning to taxonomies. • Create an outline and notes • Plan a clear introduction, body and conclusion. Plan to tie the conclusion to the introduction (e.g. how we accomplished the learning objectives and outcomes)
Anticipatory reflection	• Plan the time frame and allow for interaction. Learners place high value on appropriate pace • Plan to be student-centered and personal, not to showcase your skills-including skills in using technology

- Anticipate learners' experiences and reactions and plan accordingly
- Consider worst-case scenarios, such as technology failure and plan a tactic
- Look at your lecture outline—select points at which you will ask learners to give information and examples rather than giving the information yourself. Learners place high value on organization and relevance.

Subject-centering

- What organization best communicates the nature of the subject? Examples – to generalizations? Comparisons? Chronological or cause/effect sequence?

During introduction

- Introduce the topic by stating a clear purpose and learning outcome for the session
- Introduce yourself with a connection to the topic at hand
- Provide a framework for the topic and a structure for the information
- Present your outline. Refer back to it at intervals. Display it for yourself and your learners on a white board or chalkboard, flip chart pages, overhead transparency or computer-based display, as a handout or in any visible form
- Orient learners to handout materials

Connection

- Interact with early arrivals
- Maintain eye contact and include all learners
- Check that learners can hear you
- Avoid hiding behind the podium. Walk around
- Make the content a shared experience between you and the learners. If using someone else's plan or notes, make it your own. Blend in examples from the group of learners
- Use analogies, metaphors, smile and examples that are meaningful to the particular learners
- Repeat key points in different ways
- Use pertinent quotes to illustrate points and make information memorable
- Construct bridges to previous learning
- Relate to learners' goals and interests to stimulate motivation and attention
- Continuously weave relationships between concepts, principles, facts, generalizations and examples
- Keep emphasizing the relevance of key points ("what" followed by the "why")
- Alert learners to key points
- Display your enthusiasm for the topic, your comfort with it and your knowledge of it
- Be alert to learners' responses to presentation. Reflect-in-action and modify the approach if necessary, including asking learners what might work better

Questions

- Ask early (avoid setting a passive learning environment) and often
- Apply the 10-second wait-time rule. Give learners time to process and respond to your questions. Assess their readiness to continue or need for pauses. Pauses show a thoughtful approach and capture attention
- Ask, do not tell

Interaction

- Serve the purpose of interaction: to give the students practice in using the lecture information and an opportunity to receive feedback
- Vary the approach at least every 15 to 20 minutes. Research findings show that 15 to 20 minutes is the maximum time for effective listening eg: instruct learners or pairs of learners to summarize, ask for examples or require learners to apply what you have presented
- Survey the group. Ask for a show of hands—Agree? Disagree? Example of. . .? Ask for a comment to support the position
- Construct activities that require the learners to do something relevant with the information

	• Ensure that your directions for group or paired activity are clear. If several steps are involved, interrupt the activity to give instruction for each step. This helps to pace the activity and keep learners on task
	• Introduce brief, focused periods of learner presentation/response, such as debates, reaction panels, role plays and simulations
	• Ask the group to identify any unresolved issues from the previous (or earlier) session and facilitate brainstorming to resolve these issues
	• Be judicious in asking learners to recite their answers and conclusions to group or paired activity. Group or paired work that is well-structured, appropriately focused and timed facilitates learning without learners reciting all of their processes and conclusions for the whole group. It is useful to elicit a sample response or two to a specific question.
Management	• Address disruptive behavior or lateness
	• Troubleshoot the learning environment by controlling the long-winded, encouraging the reticent, introducing controversy and managing other problems that interfere with learning.
Demonstration	• Demonstrate organizing information, comparing and contrasting concepts on characteristics, building evidence to support assertions, selecting relevant information and other cognitive skills that learners must master to use the information you are presenting
	• How you expect learners to use the information (e.g. What does a nurse do with this content?)
	• Visual aids and technologies
	• Make a diagram that displays the concepts or instruct individual learners, pairs or group of learners to construct such a diagram as an activity
	• Use many resources available, related to effective design and use visual aids and learning technologies
	• Consider some of the technologies that can be used to display student responses to questions, such as those that tally responses to questions or identify the first person to respond.
After reflection	• Make some notes immediately about what you think worked well and what did not. Did you leave out something important? Have you thought of a better response to a learner's question? What contributed to your effectiveness or lack there of? What will you do differently next time?
Critique	• Invite the critique of a colleague. Give specific directions to your colleague in advance (e.g. "Please give me some feedback on the interactive window I'll use right after presenting the first patient."). Ask your colleague to focus on specific aspects, but welcome feedback on other aspects
Measurement	• Evaluate learners' achievement of the objectives of lecture. In continuing education settings, lengthy written post-tests may not be practical or desirable, but devise some method, even a few multiple choice questions for group response, to assess learning
	• If at all possible, devise a method to at least sample whether and how learners have put this learning into action in their practice.
Continued quest	• Plan to incorporate the results of your own reflection, critique and measurement into future lectures—whether on this topic or on others
	• Continue your quest for your own learning on this topic—use your own experience, the experiences of others and research evidence.

Frequent Criticisms/Limitations

1. **Time consuming:** The lecture should supplement the book by adding to or clarifying its contents. It should not be a repetition of the book, it should not waste the time by explaining self-explanatory information.
2. **Provides little student activity:** The teacher prepares, organizes and present the lecture and the student sits, listens and takes notes. If the teacher is carefully planned and skillfully presented, the student will be thinking with the teacher. The student will be taking part through mental activity, which means listening, thinking, reasoning and judging therefore she/he is engaging in a learning activity.
3. **The Teacher requires mastery over the subject and special teaching skills:** The teacher should have sufficient knowledge and skill, she/he should be a master of subject matter before a lecture can be successful. The essential factors i.e., personality, voice, poise, vocabulary are necessary for the teacher to deliver the lecture method.
4. **The Teacher is not readily analyzed and summarized by the student:** The teacher plans lecture carefully, organizing it under subheadings and then delivering it slowly, stating the major points with emphasis, the student will be able to take good notes. Beginning students who are not accustomed to the lecture method at first may need some instruction and help on note-taking. If the teacher will pause frequently, asking for questions or comments on points on which they are not clear, students should be able to follow the lecture easily and to take satisfactory notes.
5. **The Lecture is sometimes poorly adapted to the perceptive ability of students:** If the teacher had used the lecture method properly, she/he would have been alert to the needs of the students, evaluated their progress throughout the term by means of tests and quiz and used similar methods to ascertain whether they understood the subject. Unless the teacher is in close touch with the students and is sensitive to their reactions and aware of their responses, she/he cannot possibly use the lecture method with success.
6. **The Lecture is likely to become a sustained dictation exercise:** Poor lecturing was the reading or the dictation of the lecture or the textbook.

   Lecture-Conference groups offer student's learning experiences, which the lecture itself cannot provide. It supplements the lecture by digging into details, providing exercises of application by follow-up individual learning. It offers opportunity to direct individual students, assist the slow learner or the superior learner or the learner with special interests. It gives the student a chance to respond to learning to a much greater degree than possible with just a lecture. Care must be taken to coordinate carefully both the lecture and the conference groups. This requires that the lecture and the conference groups work as a team performing their separate roles in relation to a purpose and planning together and maintaining contact through personal attendance when possible otherwise frequent joint meetings are required. A common course outline may be required.
7. **Lecture is certainly efficient:** the amount of information that can be transmitted is limited only by the speed at which the lecturer can talk. However, information can flow much more rapidly than the learner can receive it, causing much of the information to miss its destination.
8. Educators become obsessed with "covering the material" but might be better served by focusing on what can be left out and learned in a different way, if at all. Today's information-rich practice environment requires nurses to know where and how to obtain information and how to organize it in a useful fashion. Teaching methods that model how to select and organize information, contribute to this learning.
9. It is important to model caring, judgment and use of knowledge rather than simply overwhelming learners with categories of facts.
10. Although lecture delivers content efficiently, an effective lecture requires significant preparation time. The educator must integrate several resources and examples and investigate the learners' familiarity and connections with the topic.
11. The educator must develop delivery skills to maintain the learners' attention and motivation. The lecture method lacks opportunities for individual feedback to learners, connection with a variety of learning styles, active learning and independent learning. However, the educator can overcome some of these difficulties by introducing interactive windows (short discussions and problem-solving exercises) that positively influence recall and learning. Lecture facilitates learning for some, but alternative approaches

are more effective for others. With creative thought, the educator can modify lectures to address various learning styles.

12. Psychomotor and affective learning obviously require more than one-way communication from the teacher. Learners must see demonstrations, practice actively and receive feedback to master these skills. Learners must also practice high-level cognitive skills such as synthesis and evaluation. Although a lecturer might demonstrate synthesis and evaluation, the learner is unlikely to master these skills without active practice.

13. "Classroom teaching in nursing is in trouble," which is evidenced by instructors presenting endless taxonomies, failing to integrate other disciplines and relevant clinical experiences, lacking evidence based literature searches, promulgating confusion about critical thinking and subscribing to the view of teaching as entertainment. The lecture method does not deserve the blame for all of these troubles, but a wellplanned lecture that is blended with interactive windows can counteract some of them.

Conclusion

The lecture can facilitate learning effectively. By reframing the lecture from strictly one-way communication in ways that engage learners and force them to interact with the subject matter, the lecture can support the learning process. The lecture deserves respect from the lecturer. Respect the lecture by choosing it for the purposes it serves best, incorporating approaches designed to overcome the limitations of one-way communication, stimulating active learning and critical thought, and reflecting critically on your lecturing with a view toward improving.

USE OF CLICKERS IN NURSING EDUCATION

In Nursing educational institutions over the last few years, students' strength is becoming larger > 60, maintaining student's attention by the teacher is becoming difficult and more complicated in the classroom , as students are preoccupied with many other distracters deviating the group from learning. In the above conditions, to facilitate learning and engage the students in active listening, to foster critical thinking skills and to provide meaningful feedback, use of clickers will keep the students involved and allow the faculty to 'Run a class like a game show'. The teacher uses a computer with a projector to interact with the students who will use the clickers to make selections. The response systems are of four types:

1. Audience response system (ARS)
2. Personal response system (PRS)
3. Student response system (SRS)
4. Plain Clickers – as a tool

The response system and its components: Computer, projector, base or receiver, key pad, software.

Most systems use wireless technology to transmit the selection from the keypad to the receiver. Browser-based software allows one to connect through internet protocol address with students laptops or personal digital assistance (PDA).

Steps

- Contact Audio – Visual or information services has to find out from the school authority whether ARS is available in class rooms, if so, find out which class room has the facility
- ARS has to be compatible with PDAs
- Implement ARS in a selected class room
- If no facility, keep a convincing proposal through the proper channel i.e., head of the institutions to the authorities for implementation of ARS in big lecture halls
- Provide training for teaching faculty the usage of clickers in their lectures, give the opportunity for them to practice before going to the class room setting.

ARS work

Students are given clickers when they enter the class or they can use their personal clickers by using response software. The faculty member will project the questions on the video screen and asks the students to select an answer. The students will use the clickers to select their responses, which are transmitted automatically; answers are tabulated by selection and can be immediately projected to the class. Some response systems work in collaboration with powerpoint, text books or course learning management systems, e.g. Web CT or Black Board (electronic), interactive, question and answer sessions or an electronic game show.

Advantages:
- Students are not fearful about providing an incorrect answer. They are encouraged to think through the question and select their response anonymously
- Easy to respond
- Less time taking
- Encourages active learning
  - Engage the students by quizzing them on the content in their assigned readings
  - Pretest the class
  - Question and answer session as a review mechanism
  - Engage the students through case studies
  - Promotes further discussion in the class room
  - Interactive classroom encourages students to come to class prepared
  - Teacher can pose questions in a challenging, thought provoking/ Critical thinking or stimulating way
  - Teacher has to create best practices in students viz., creating an interactive environment, becoming active members in the class room, encouraging cooperation among each other, whereby they can interact, consult, work with each other in pairs or in small groups to discuss their solutions/answers with rationale for the questions raised and Teacher provides prompt feed back related to the level of understanding of students and encourages healthy competition
  - Students can quickly assess their level of understanding of concepts, content covered in the assigned reading or knowledge of a specific subject
  - Provide students with frequent indicators of both individual and class learning progress, and can encourage positive effects of self assessment and healthy competition
  - Clickers has the ability to capture the data to facilitate course revisions as well as formative and summative evaluation of a specific course or a particular lecture.

LABORATORY METHOD

The word "laboratory" was applied originally to 'the workroom of the chemist, a place devoted to the experimental study of natural science–Webster Dictinary

Laboratory procedure is considered as planned learning activity dealing with original or raw 'data' in the solution of problems.

It is a procedure involving first hand experience:
1. With primary source materials or facts derives from investigation or experimentation in the solution of a problem, the answering of some questions.
2. Through which the student can acquire psychomotor skills.

Values

For the student:
- To experience a learning situation at first hand
- To use the problem-solving approach to the solution of real problems
- To translate theory into practice
- To develop, to test and apply principles and to learn methods of procedure, with greater reliance on their own power and with greater freedom from restrictions which group work often imposes on the student

For the Teacher:
- To observe the student in action, to assess her/his worth, correct student's mistakes and to guide her/him in promising direction through a penetrating question or two at the time, the teacher can discover whether the student knows 'the why' of what she/he is doing or is trying to follow instructions without comprehending them

- A little encouragement or special help at the right moment may enkindle or intensify interest and provide the basis for independent accomplishment in the future.

Technique

Steps:

1. The Introductory Phase

Involves the establishment of objectives and a plan of work. The planning for a laboratory period (objectives and/or plan of work) may be done in advance by the teacher or cooperatively by the teacher and the students by means of class discussion.

Teacher's Preparation

- To solve a problem
- To understand a process
- To develop a skill
- The selection of a general plan of work and to provide for correlation of the laboratory aspect of the course with the class work
- Teacher advance preparation is necessary to ensure that the proper materials and equipment will be available for the laboratory work
- The teacher can give whatever instructions may be necessary for the students to proceed without wasting time
- Teacher preparation consists of thinking over what the students will be doing i.e., the verbal preliminary instructions that they will require, the difficulties that they are likely to encounter and some of the questions by which the quality of their work can be appraised and their learning experience improved.

Student's Preparation

- Orientation and motivation achieved through proper instructions and guidance
- When instructions are short, they may be given verbally, but when long procedures are involved or complex equipment must be handled, instructions should be in writing
- The teacher who stands at the student's elbow and prompts at every step, achieves the same effect
- Laboratory procedures should be prepared in a manual, state the problem to be solved or the procedure to be followed, fill in the necessary background and a general mode of procedure and leave it to the student to formulate a precise plan of investigation, setting up the plan and reaching their own conclusions.

2. The Work Period

The individual student or groups of students do their particular work under the supervision of the teacher. The laboratory procedure presumes skills on the part of the teacher, emphasis will be more on the organization and the exposition of knowledge. The emphasis is on the ability to guide a student creatively in the accomplishment of tasks, without depriving of the chance to do her/his own work and without allowing her/him to commit serious mistakes.

Teacher should have the right proportion of reserve and readiness in advancing suggestions when necessary, He/she must be able to gauge the student's abilities, to know at what point to offer help and when to withhold it.

The length of the laboratory period is determined by the nature of the problems and the objectives.

The activities should be adapted to the type of work to be done. Students may work individually or in small teams within a large group, e.g. A clinical conference may be used to bring students to study the common problems encountered by the individual students in their nursing care of patients. Adequate records should be kept so that student's progress can be checked and wastage of time prevented. Provisions should be made for individual differences. For the students who will complete their tasks more quickly than others, they can be given additional assignments that will help them to deepen their knowledge or they may be released to work on some related learning areas in which they are especially interested.

3. Culminating Activities
When the laboratory work has been completed, the class should meet together for discussion of common problems.
* For organization of findings
* For the presentation of the results of individual or group problem-solving activities.

Types of Activities to be utilized in the Laboratory Procedure
a. Review of the plan for solving the problem(s).
b. Reports by students on data gathered or other findings.
c. Presentation of illustration materials or special contributions by students working on special problems.
d. Organization of findings and summarization and conclusions by the group.
   The findings and the conclusions may be exhibited and scored or rated by members of the class or by competent judges outside the class.
e. Exhibits of various projects may be set up and explained by their student sponsors.
f. Tests may be used to measure achievement of students.

Laboratory Method in Nursing Education

The laboratory method will be used:
a. In the classroom, in courses that employ problem-solving activities, in which students gather first-hand information.
b. In a laboratory, e.g. Nutrition or Nursing arts settings.
c. In the clinical setting, e.g. Hospital and Community health settings.
   Professional nursing practice requires relevant knowledge, understanding and the ability to apply knowledge in nursing actions. Nursing skills can be learned only through first-hand experience in the clinical laboratory under careful supervision.

Rationale for Clinical Learning Experience

Nursing is a series of arts and science which gives direct continuing personal assistance to individuals who require assistance because of their personal inabilities in self-care, resulting from a situation of personal health. Science is knowledge, art is the purposeful application of knowledge. Nursing is a practice discipline, so knowledge must be emphasized in the learning of an art. The student nurse must learn to become a nurse scientist and a practitioner of the art of nursing. She/he must require the empirical (The knowledge of experience and theoretical) knowledge of thought. The empirical knowledge consists of her/his observation (small part) and in large part the recorded or imparted observation of others.

Theoretical knowledge is comprised of conclusions and ideas based on experience i.e., systematically organised. One obtains knowledge by observation, study, thought and by experience. To learn professional nursing, the student must have the opportunities to gain knowledge through study and experience, to apply knowledge in the life setting and to acquire the attitudes, appreciation of ideals and skills needed to practice the art of nursing.

The nursing curriculum provides through
   i. Class work (Theoretical)
   ii. Clinical learning experiences (Practical)
   Class work and clinical teaching experiences are planned as an integral part of the course, each one supplementing and enhancing the knowledge and the art of nursing. To develop beginning skills in nursing, time practice and continued study are required to become expert in any art.

Teacher Preparation

Objectives should be behaviorally defined so that the proper learning experiences can be identified and evaluated, e.g. objectives for clinical practice is to develop the ability to meet a basic need of a patient, namely, to move and maintain desirable position and to have adequate rest and sleep.

Selection of Learning Experiences

To attain the stated objectives, learning experiences will be selected.

Learning must progress from the simple to complex, to obtain this, the learning experiences should be selected in a sequential practice, it should go more broadly and more deeply than the previous one.

New learning practice requires the student to give more attention because of new element, it serves adequately as a basis for effective learning. This is important for the student in gaining understanding, because it means that concepts and principles are brought in again and again, but each time in a new and more complex illustration so that the student continually has to think through the way in which these concepts or principles help to explain or analyze the situation.

By this type of learning, the student acquires clinical knowledge, skill and particularly clinical or practical judgment. To differentiate from important to unimportant, both in theory and practice comes only with knowledge, experience and with growth of imagination. The cultivation of the powers of each individual student lies in development of skills and the education, training of the individual to know themselves and to know how to use their powers.

To select the right learning experience to meet the clinical objectives and the learning needs of each student, the instructor must

i. Have a Mastery of Nursing knowledge in the area she/he is teaching.

ii. Know the patients – Their state of health, nursing needs, so that she/he can select those patients who will meet the learning needs of each student.

iii. Have rapport with the nursing service personnel, for selection of learning experiences and to have guidance.

Clinical case assignments are made

- To provide the student with opportunity to learn to collect information about their patient
- To assess the clinical condition of patient
- To determine the patient's nursing need
- To make a nursing care plan
- To implement, evaluate and modify the plan as needed
- To learn the importance and the techniques of establishing effective nurse-patient relationships, relationships with other personnel involved in the patient's care and relationships with the patient's family
- To establish continuity of patient care.

Team Assignment is used as learning experience, understanding and having awareness of the learning needs of each student by the instructor or head nurses and the team leader and the members of the team to which the student is assigned are very important. The length of time that a certain patient is assigned to a student depends on the objectives and the achievements of the student. This will vary with each student. The length of an assignment with a clinical situation will vary accordingly to the situation and the learning objectives. The student must have time to get to know their patients, have continuity in their assignments, write nursing care plans, evaluate and modify them to meet patient's unique needs.

Student's Preparation

1. Attaining the background knowledge which she/he will bring to the clinical situation.
   i. The general foundational knowledge, e.g. Humanities, Behavioral Sciences (Psychology and Sociology), Natural sciences, Nutrition, etc.
   ii. Nursing knowledge gained in the classroom, e.g. the theoretical aspects of nursing, correlated with nursing procedures learned in the nursing laboratory.
2. Actual preparation for the clinical assignments themselves, which will help each student to set objectives and high standards of practice for themselves so that she /he will have the means of judging her/his own performance and determine how well she/he is doing.

The Working Period

The working period is the teacher-supervised, learner work period of the laboratory procedure.

Teacher Guidance

The teacher needs very special skills for the implementation of working period. The teacher should respect each student as a person with her/his own inherent dignity and rights, she/he should relate to their students as a friend in that she/he is there to help and to guide the learner. Therefore, teacher should not be antagonistic, authoritarian or thwarting in her/his relationships with their students. Teacher will support their students, reassuring them whenever necessary. An affirmative nod of the head, an encouraging remark, a smile or even simply the presence of the instructor will be sufficient to give her/his support that she/he needs. The instructor will help each student to put information together in their practice of nursing. The teacher has to see that the student has the proper kind of guidance in the new behavior that she/he is seeking to learn, a type of guidance which prevents undue trial and error and waste of time and permits the student to learn through their own efforts, recognizing that all individuals make mistakes and can learn from them. The student learns best when given responsibility as well as opportunity to practice nursing actions.

The Nursing Care Plan

It is used to provide a guide to patient care.

It is a tool, which when properly implemented, helps nurse to provide more complete, unified and continuing professional nursing care.

Content of the nursing care plan should include an analysis of the present needs of the patients; the responsibilities assigned to nurses; suggestions which will helpful in dealing with emotional reactions of the patient; should be useful for better nursing care of the patient.

Students have to learn to prepare written cumulative nursing care plans, implement, evaluate and modify the care to meet each patient's needs.

Clinical Conferences

Small group conferences of students (6 to 12) during the clinical experience period, provide excellent learning opportunity for students. These may be conducted on a topic related to patient care. Whenever a conference is planned around a patient, first obtain consent from the patient. The purpose of conference should be explained to the patient in advance to obtain patient's cooperation. The comfort of the patient should be considered i.e., physical, mental and general welfare of the patient. All conference should use problem approach, the clinical conferences should be conducted in an informal, permissive atmosphere, so that students will feel free to ask questions about their problems. Reading reference should be included in the outline. Teachers will supervise the clinical conference.

Evaluation: Evaluation in the clinical setting done in two phases.

- Firstly daily evaluation of the student as she/he progresses in a course
- Second phase-done by culminating activity. It is the evaluation at the end of the course and is made to determine whether the student has acquired the knowledge, the skills, the attitudes and the appreciations necessary for her/him to be promoted to the next course. Evaluation of clinical practice begins with the behavioral definition of the objectives set up by the faculty
- Behavioral definitions can be used as a basis for setting up specific criteria for areas of expected competence and for rating the level of competence of each course. This helps to make the evaluation more objective and provides both the student and the instructors a more valid record of growth
- It provides common criteria and thereby prevents each teacher from using her/his own individual criteria.
- These criteria and rating levels of performance should be communicated to the student, so that she/he can use them for the evaluation of her/his own performance
- Objectives methods, e.g. Records, checklists should be used to gather data on the performance of the student
- Conferences with each student should be held frequently in which the student should be encouraged to evaluate herself and her performance as well as having the teacher's evaluation
- The notes that the teacher makes concerning the student practice should be made available to the student and discussed with her/him at frequent intervals, so that she/he may compare her/his own evaluation with that of her/his teacher's evaluation

- A final record, which summarizes the typical behavior of the student, substantiated with anecdotes, should be prepared and placed in his/her permanent file. It should be discussed with the student encouraging her/him to write any reaction on the record if she/he wishes to do so
- The final record should be kept confidential.

Guide to effective use of the Laboratory Procedure in the Clinical Studies

1. Every human being is a person who has the right to be respected because of his personal worth and dignity as a human being. Therefore, the teacher should show respect for the student, patient, the doctor and all other persons encountered in the clinical setting.
2. Every nursing student is an individual, she/he has her/his own needs, interests and abilities. The teacher should consider individual differences when planning and supervising nursing students.
3. Every student should be helped to establish realistic and worthwhile goals for both her/his class work and her/his clinical learning experiences.
4. The teacher should assess and help the student to assess her/his knowledge in relation to the particular setting, supplement and reinforce it through clinical teaching and through the student's own efforts in reading and study.
5. Selection of learning experiences should be selected in relation to the knowledge and skills of each student and flow along a continuous from the simple to the complex.
6. The teacher should adopt her/his instruction and supervision to the capacities and needs of each student.
7. The teacher should familiarize the student with the situation and to reassure her/him in functioning in it.
8. Every nursing student, regardless of her/his educational level, is at times stressed, anxious and insecure. The teacher should relate to each student as a friend and be there to help and guide her/him.
9. Every student desires to grow personally and professionally during her/his clinical education. The teacher, through discussion and conferences should show interest in each student and in her/his progress towards and achievement of attaining her/his goals.
10. The teacher should encourage each student to act independently when warranted but should be available when the student needs her/him.
    Clinical experience must be well planned and well supervised.

ROLE PLAY

Definitions

'An educational technique in which people spontaneously act out problems of human relations and analyze the enactment with the help of the other role players and observers'.

'Role Playing is a discussion technique that makes it possible to get maximum participation of a group through acting out', e.g. some problem or idea under discussion. Role Playing, sociodrama and psychodrama are closely related, and the term role-playing and sociodrama frequently are used interchangeably.

'The spontaneous acting out of roles in the context of human relations situations'.

Types

Role play is of 2 types: 1. Sociodrama 2. Psychodrama, both sociodrama and psychodrama require not only players, but also an audience, who help the players to interpret their roles.

Sociodrama

It deals with the interaction of people with other individuals or groups, eg. Mother, Nurse, Leader etc. It always involves situations of more than one person and deals with problems that a majority of the group face in executing their roles.

Psychodrama

Practiced in a group setting, mainly concerned with the unique needs and problems of a particular individual. It should not be attempted except under the guidance of a trained therapist.

Audience identification which he/she acts out in roles critical observation, brought about much greater learning than passive watching.

Thirty minutes is long enough for the actual role playing and the discussion.

Values/Advantages

1. The actor really tries to feel the part of the character he is portraying and puts himself in that person's situation. The audience, by being assigned actors to watch, gets some kind of emotional involvement.
2. It is enjoyed by people who do it.
3. It does need equipment/articles/makeup based on the theme selected.
4. It is a method to involve a group through participation.
5. It can be used to:
   a. Arouse interest in a problem.
   b. Make a problem seem real to a group and thus the solution seem attainable.
   c. Help a person to understand the point of view of the other person.
   d. Train in leadership skills.
6. It can bring out data about human behavior and human relations which are not made available by more traditional methods.
7. In role playing, the student not only hears about a problem or tells about it, he lives through it by acting it out. He experiences it emotionally and then uses this experience to produce and test insights into the problem and generalizations about ways of dealing with it.
8. Individuals may develop new skills for dealing with problems in human relations.
9. Role playing allows the group to get case material, can be tailored to fit the specific need and situation of the particular group that is using it.
10. It allows many attitudes and feelings that fundamentally affect group process, but usually are left unexpressed and subjective, to be brought before the group for review.
11. It can be used to illustrate and objectify many of the causal and the dynamic factors in group process that frequently are ignored.
12. It is a way of presenting problems related to human relations, the students can experiment with behavior, make mistakes and try new skills without hurts that experimentation in real-life situations may involve. In this environment, the learner can try out new behavior not in the presence of judges, but of co-learners.

Applicable for students

1. Develop communication skills, leadership, interviewing skills, social interaction and obtain constructive feedback from peers, e.g. learning how to put another case, how to listen, how to lead a discussion, how to be a member of team responsible for patient care.
2. Develop sensitivity to another's feelings by having the opportunity to put oneself in another's place, by noting that there is a difference between what a person says and what a person does and develop empathy and understanding, e.g. noting how gestures, facial expressions, tone of voice, assuming role of another, the actor gets feeling tone and responds emotionally to role and develops insight into another's feelings.
3. Develop skill in group problem-solving, e.g. the group works as a whole to develop the problem of concern to the group. To develop the situation, to identify critical issues and to have mutual agreement.
4. Develop ability to observe and analyze situations, e.g. Discussion following role-playing provides the opportunity to identify critical issues, to suggest alternatives for dealing with a situation and to appraise the actor's concept of role.
5. Practice selected behaviors in a real life situation without the stress of making a mistake. A person is more apt to permit true feelings to be expressed when it is safe to do so, e.g. the student is exposed to reacting to and having others react to their point of view, strengths and weaknesses–with dramatic impact retained and working with others in a similar situation.

Applicable for teacher

In the teaching-learning situation, it provides for the teacher with the opportunity to:

a. Note the individual student's needs by observing and analyzing his/her needs in a simulated real life situation.

b. Assist the student in meeting his/her own needs by either giving her or encouraging group members to give her on the spot suggestions.

c. Encourage independent thinking and action by stepping aside or giving indirect guidance, for emphasis is on the students helping themselves.

Disadvantages

1. Role Playing is a means, not an end.
2. It requires expert guidance and leadership.
3. Sometimes participants may feel threatened.
4. Used as an education technique, not as a therapeutic one. Strongly dependent on student's imagination.
5. Time consuming in developing group readiness, should not be used when pressure of time is there.
6. Limited only by the teacher's ingenuity and realistic use.

Points to remember while conducting Role Playing

1. There should never be one answer to a situation presented.
2. The time of the play should be brief.
3. Enough time should be allowed for discussion and analysis of the situation.
4. Evaluation concerns the teacher and the participants through discussion or follow-up as to specific individual behavior or sequential of group actions.

Steps

I. Select a problem/Theme for role-playing
   a. The group leader, who recognizes a problem that can be used effectively and suggests it to the group. (OR)
   b. The group can list problems on the blackboard and decide which problem they want to workout. The problem selected should be one:
   - For which there is not a clear 'Yes' or 'No' answer
   - Which is of real concern to the majority of the group
   - On which the group has indicated either by vote or general consensus that they want to focus attention.

II. Set up the role playing scene
   a. The group should come to a clear agreement on the chief objectives to be realized in role playing.
   b. The group working together with the leader decides:
   - Specification of characters that are involved
   - The attitudes and personalities of the characters
   - The setting of the story
   - The point on which the story should begin.
   c. The leader may brief the players on the situation, which they have decided to portray. The leader may arbitrarily assign individuals to take the various roles or members may volunteer to play the different roles.
   d. The player's lines are never fixed but for just what the player thinks his character would say in a given situation.

III. Getting underway in Role Playing
   a. The role takers usually go out of the room and are given a few minutes to 'warm up' or to get the feeling of the roles they are about to play. Specific names, other than their own, should be used to help them to get into their roles.
   b. The role players should attempt to express the attitudes which the group has assigned to the various characters as well as to achieve the goals decided upon.
   c. The story grows out of the natural reactions of the characters enacted in the role-playing.

IV. The Part the Group Plays
   Those members not involved in the actual role playing act as observers. They may be assigned to watch particular role player or to look for important clues, which come out of role playing.

V. Cutting the Role Playing

The leader may cut at point where enough action has already occurred to provide a basis for discussion.

VI. After the Role Playing is Cut

a. Get immediate reaction of the role players. How they felt in their roles and how they responded to other responses in the scene.

b. Use in the discussion the role name of each person so that the player will not feel he is being evaluated.

c. When role players succeed in really projecting themselves into the roles assigned them, they usually give during the discussion valuable insights into the problem and provide additional material for discussion.

VII. The Audience Observers

The comments of the audience observers constitute the heart of the role playing as a discussion technique.

a. How did the group think the role was handled?

b. What were the good points of the action ?

c. What were the poor points or omissions ?

VIII. The Role Playing Scene: might be played by different people so that there might be a comparison of the behavior of different people.

IX. Cautions to be taken while Role Playing

a. Use role play only when it will be useful; not just for the sake of doing it.

b. Be careful about the interpersonal relationship within the group.

c. If there is a popular role, give it to a person with enough status in the group to carry it successfully. If necessary the leader might play it to spare the feelings of others.

d. Avoid un-covering deep-seated personal problems, which require professional help.

X. Summarize

a. The leader sums up with the group the chief points or principles which have come out in the role playing and the comments of the observers which follow.

b. The comments on the specific problems should be related back to the more general problem under consideration.

Process

1. Need: Develops within group, concerns all members
2. Role Play: Explained as a method. Geared to level and readiness of the group
3. Problem: Controversy and Conflict. Probe different view points
4. Purpose: All members identify objectives
5. Situation: Specific attitudes and motivations delineated
6. Casting Roles: Ask for volunteers. Provide atmosphere which allows for volunteering or choosing actors. Do not use own names. Recorder may be chosen to note various aspects of the presentation
7. Briefing and Warming up: Cast members may be excused to develop own role or review problems. Rest of the group discuss possible situation. Situation may be presented in the form of a script to present a frame of reference
8. Method: Players: One group represents
   - Reverse Roles
   - Alternate group substitute roles.
9. Audience Participation: Certain members identify with — a) Actors b) Group asked to look for critical issues
10. Stopping: Cut when purpose is achieved
11. Discussion and Analysis: Actors discuss own performance first. Group discusses scene. Teacher encourages discussion, but keeps in background
12. Evaluation: Observe whether the purpose is achieved or not.

SOCIODRAMA

Sociodrama, is the unrehearsed acting out of a problem or situation confronting a group. Spontaneous drama and discussion are natural outlets for tension, natural methods of disseminating views and of informing one self. Teachers can use sociodrama at all levels. Several members of the group enact a scene in the presence of the whole group. The scene may deal with real problem of human relation within the class or with any material being studied which permit different interpretations.

1. Sociodrama improves skill in the democratic process.
2. Communication is speeded.
3. Individuals gain greater insight into their own beliefs, tensions, honest convictions and prejudices.
4. Understanding of others' results.
5. Real attitudes and values are revealed.
6. The analysis of difficulties in group thinking is enhanced.

The audience is invited to participate and make suggestions both during the scene and after spontaneous action is essential. The actors should have a brief period together for planning, the general setting, line of development and views to be expressed. Following the scene is thought by many to be most valuable part of this technique.

Process

a. Demonstrating a Sociodrama for a New Group:
   1. Select a simple, illustrative situation that will be fun, meaningful and theme oriented.
   2. Select a volunteer cast.
   3. Arrange the scene, using a few simple props, if necessary.
   4. Inform the castes about the scene and what to be done.
   5. Leader will introduce all the actors.
   6. Develop and enact the scene. As it progress the director may secretly suggest to one of the cast, a problem which will encourage argument or discussion.
   7. Encourage audience participation by stopping the scene from time to time to get new ideas.
   8. Try out new ideas. The actors may be asked to try out suggested ideas of members of the audience and asked to replace members of the cast for that purpose.
   9. Reverse roles, to increase the opportunity and variety of participation.
   10. Discuss the scene after it is concluded. The director asks questions regarding the subject of the scene, the problems presented and the solutions suggested.
   11. Limit the drama for 10 to 15 minutes.

b. Performing in a Real Life Situation
   1. Select a scene, which is related more directly to the kinds of problem, situation this group has encountered.
   2. Decide roles. The director may ask the audience to help in selecting the roles and indicating how they should be played.

PROGRAMD INSTRUCTION

Programed instruction or programed learning is a learning in which the student works from the known to unknown, from the familiar to unfamiliar. It is planned to control the student's responses and to provide a feedback to the student in a pattern designed to accomplish maximum transfer of learning. Attempts were made since Socrates' period toward a systematic involvement of self-activity on the part of the learner in the learning process. But, today, the teaching machine focusing so much attention clearly and specifically on the value of student self-activity and on the importance of reinforcement in the learning process.

Programed instruction is self-sufficient. It is very well planned and organized that when once it is programd, it takes care of itself and leads the learner for successful learning without the intervention of the teacher. Programed Instruction is an instructional technique designed to suit the changing learning situations.

Definitions

"A kind of learning in which a 'program' takes the place of a tutor for the student, and leads him through a set of frames of specified behaviors designed and sequenced to make it more probable that he will behave in a given desired way"—*Kochhar, SK 1992*

"A process of arranging material to be learned in a series of small steps designed to lead a learner through self-instruction from what he knows to the unknown of new and more complex knowledge and principles".

" Programed Instruction is a planned sequence of experiences, leading to proficiency in terms of stimulus response relationship"
– James E Espich and Bill Williams

History

- The Programed Instruction emerged out of experimental researches on operant conditioning, it incorporates the principles of reinforcement to effect behavioral changes in successive approximation to the desired goal. The total behavior is broken into meaningful operants, which are chained together to form the whole
- Programed Instruction offers possibility of providing a conceptual framework, which allows for the planning and organization of learning courses with a view to realizing specific, operationally defined objectives or performance levels.

Socrates is the first programer who developed a program in geometry recorded by Plato in the dialogue menu.

'Gita' is the first programed text in the world. It has all the ingredients of programming, e.g. initial behavior, small steps, immediate knowledge and self-evaluation by the learner are present. Here the instruction has been designed most systematically and psychologically.

Programed Instruction has emerged as a complete system of education and training due to the continuous contribution of psychologists from time-to-time.

EL Thorndike (1874 to 1949) in his 'law of effect' used Programed Instruction which presents immediate reinforcement for the learner's correct response.

Sydney L Pressey developed Programed Instruction of testing items i.e., multiple choice items.
During the first world war, *HB English* invented a device which has all the ingredients of programming to help trained soldiers squeeze a rifle trigger.

BF Skinner, (in middle of fifties) developed a theory of learning i.e., Operant Conditioning, in which the behavior of the learner is shaped in successive approximation to the desired goal.

Characteristics

A learning program is carefully ordered and organized sequence of material to assure the best possible learning conditions for a student. It uses the principles of reinforcement.

1. Assumptions stated clearly in writing: A program builder has to make certain assumptions about the student to whom his program is directed.
   a. Program builder reads at a particular level of competence.
   b. He should have a command of vocabulary i.e., consistent with the language of the program.
   c. Students' background in the subject matter.
   A specific subject should be put down explicitly in writing before the program maker begins to arrange his learning material.
2. Explicitly stated Objectives: The program designer must determine the goals or objectives of the learning program i.e., the defining of knowledge, skills, attitudes that the student is expected to acquire through completion of the program. All the objectives should be defined in Operational, Observable, Measurable terms in order to facilitate the construction of the program and its subsequent evaluation.
3. Logical Sequence of Small Steps: Subject matter, broken down into fragments of information, is arranged in an orderly sequence of growing difficulty so that the student may progress steadily from one point in the

program to the next. It will help in the logical, deliberate development of the learning material, simplify the acquisition of knowledge, it also tends to reduce the number of student errors.

4. Active Responding: Programed Instruction requires interaction between the student and the program to prevent passiveness of the program. Active involvement of the learner in teaching-learning program.
5. Immediate Feedback of Information: As soon as a student makes each response, the program informs him of his correctness or incorrectness. The more rapidly this check or feedback follows his responses, the more effective becomes reinforcement.
6. Individual Rate: The student learns the subject matter, in view of the rate of learning needed review, repetition and additional materials will be stressed.
7. Constant Evaluation: From examining the student responses to the items, he can obtain an approximation of the program's success.

   The teacher gathers objective data upon which to improve the program by assessing or observing the number of errors.

   To assess the student's progress, allows the program builder to plan other learning experiences of a meaningful and helpful kind.

Principles

1. Objectives Specification
a. The programer should specify the objectives of the program in behavioral terms
b. The programer identifies the terminal behavior, which the learner would be able to show at the completion of the program
c. The programer further specifies the conditions under which the terminal behavior is to be manifested and states explicitly any restrictions to be imposed
d. The standard of judging the acceptable performance is mentioned in definite terms.

2. Empirical Testing
The programer after writing the initial draft of the program tries it out in three phases.
a. Individual try-out: The first draft of the program is tested on an individual in face-to-face testing. The reactions of the individual are recorded for each frame.
b. Small Group try-out: The program is tested on 5 to 10 representative students of the class for whom it is developed.
c. Field try-out: After modification on the observations of small group, it is administered in actual classroom conditions.

3. Self-Pacing
In programed Instruction, the learner decides the rate at which he/she progresses through the program. He/she adjusts the pace of work to his/her own abilities and motivation level. He/she is not forced to work with the speed of other students of the class. The principle of self-pacing incorporates the concept of individual differences in teaching-learning.

4. Principle of Active Responding
A response must be made by the learner and induces sustained activity. The learner remains busy and active when he works on a program. A good program requires a thorough understanding of the previous frames before moving to the next frames. Active responding on the part of the learner means learner involvement in the learning process is active.

5. Student Testing
The teacher can regularly assess the progress of students. He/she can find out the weaknesses of students' progress and can modify the weak portion of program in the light of the students' performance. The student can also continually evaluate the performance on the program.

Comparison of Programed Instruction & Traditional Method

Programed Instruction	Traditional Method
It makes practical use of teaching principles.	The principles will difficult to apply in crowded classroom
It is an individualized technique, self-pacing is provided.	Group technique.
Immediate feedback is given to the learner.	Vague and not well defined objectives.
Specifically defined objectives.	Subject matter is not organized.
Subject matter is well-organized in increasing difficult order.	Student remain quite/passive when confronted with material.
Student is forced to participate actively by continually.	and there is no assurance that teacher is assimilating the
making responses.	information.
The unit will be presented in small frames with	Matter is not divided into frames.
meaningful information.	This cannot be accomplished with same precision that is
A program is developed empirically through	achieved in programed instruction.
series of try-outs on typical students.	

Dynamics

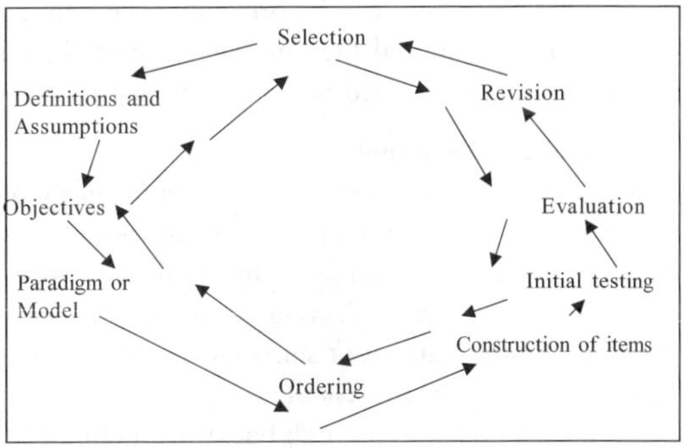

1. The selection of the subject to be programed requires, an assumption by the program builder about the learner who will use the program.
2. The programer lists the objectives of the materials to be programed. These factors then influence the programer's choice of a paradigm for the arrangement of items.
3. Construct the items in accord with established learning techniques.
4. Short sequences after their completion they can be tested and revised on an initial basis.
5. After exposure to a larger number of students, the sequences can be analyzed for errors and shortcomings. The sequences can be evaluated for effectiveness in terms of how the student learns from them and this information can be used for revision of the programs. Two-directional development of programed matter with each step functioning as a spring-board for the next one and as a reexamination of what has happened before using it.

Comparison between Teaching Machine and Programed Text

Teaching Machine	Programed Text
1. There is a greater control of the learner's behavior, because the program can be locked inside.	1. There is no control. The student can skip ahead without answering a frame by merely turning a page. Programed text is not cheat proof.
2. Mechanical control in the machine can assure that only one frame is presented at a time.	2. There is no control regarding presentation of frames.
3. The student must respond to the frame before proceeding to the next frame.	3. The student may not respond to the frame proceeding to the next as there is no check.
4. The machine covers the students' answer with a shield which prevents the student from changing it.	4. The student can change his response when he likes to change it.
5. Machine maintains an accurate record of responses by the learner on the answer tape which is locked inside.	5. A reliable record of responses by the learner cannot always be had.
6. Objective data for research on learning process can be collected.	6. Objective data cannot be collected.
7. 'Pinball effect' in young children which increases interest and motivation of the learners.	7. Students feel boredom after working sometime on a programed text.
8. Pinball effect is important in maintaining motivation of older students working on long programs.	8. Long programs create monotony.
9. Logistically, machine program in terms of cost and quantity of paper is cheap.	9. Programs are comparatively costly. Great amount of paper is needed to develop programed instructional material.
10. Teaching machine can employ reusable microfilm and can store long programs in a small space.	

Types

Programming is planning and presenting instructional material. In planning and presentation we follow the principles of programming. There are compulsory and optional principles of programming. Programers differ in their use of the optional principles so their programs also differ in their style.

1. Adjunct programming

Sidney L Pressy of Ohio university, America, developed adjunct programming. He named it as ' Adjunct Auto Instruction'. A large step text followed by test items. The information may run to pages. After reading the information, the learner answers a series of questions. Each answer is checked with correct answer given at the end. If the learner is wrong, then he is told which page (and line) he should read to get the correct answer.

The questions need not necessarily cover all the points dealt within the passage read. The questions are meant to clarify the points and clear the misconceptions. They help the learner to determine whether or not, he has mastered the content, whether he needs to revise the topic or needs any additional help from the teacher.

Adjunct programes can be prepared relatively easily and quickly. We can make use of textbooks, select passage from them and then prepare a series of questions to clarify and emphasize the key points in the passage. This type is used best in the industrial context.

2. Mathetics programming

Used in industrial training field, 'Mathetics' is a Greek word, means 'the process of learning'; 'to mathetics' means pertaining to learning. *Gilbert* developed this type. He developed an instructional model involving 3 stages to learn or to teach the behavioral structures. These stages are Demonstrate, Prompt and Release.

In chain learning, the learner learns or does a series of small pieces of information or event when learnt becomes the stimulus for or starts the next piece of information, the second event starts the third event and so on the learning goes in a chain.

To present material through backward fading of a chain. First the criteria response is demonstrated. Then through backward fading the sequence is presented 'Retrogressively'. Prompts are given and finally the complex chain is released. The response made acts as the prompt to get the immediately succeeding response.

In mathetics program, the step size is as big as is required. The number of steps are as few as possible. The learner responds by writing down the answer or performing the task. Task completion is the reinforcement given.

3. Computer assisted instruction

To impart formal and informal education at all levels and in all the areas.

Computer Aided Instruction facilitates instant access to information with infinite patience, accuracy and provides opportunity for systematically organised maximum learning for all learners. It provides complete individualizing instruction.

Computer Aided Instruction mechanizes human brain and human beings are converted into machines.

Types

a. Logo: This system was developed by Feurzeing and Papart at MIT Logo is a simple programming language, which can be taught to children. The program provides instruction, which can be used to produce pictures on an oscilloscope or make a little mechanical robot. The children who learn logo make up their own programs to draw flowers or faces or generate designs on the screen.

b. Stimulation: The computer in programs enable the student to mount an experiment in symbolic form.

c. Controlled Learning: It indicates both drill and practice. Drill and practice program is supplementary to the regular curriculum taught by the classroom teacher. The classroom may also introduce the basic concepts. The students, later on, review and practice fundamental skills on an individualized basis at instructional terminals. The computer provides immediate feedback to individual learners simultaneously as they work through a set of exercises. The record of individual student's performance is furnished to the teacher for evaluation.

Role of Teacher
A powerful tool for the teacher in the instructional process.
* The teacher will be liberated from his routine work
* The Computer Aided Instruction can complete accurately and rapidly huge data.

Experts needed in Computer Aided Instruction
1. Computer Engineer
2. Lesson Writer
3. System Operator

4. Linear or extrinsic programming

Prof. BF Skinner is the exponent of this type of programming. He was concerned with the shaping and conditioning of behavior. As per Skinner, a creature can be guided to a desired behavior by means of a series of carefully structured small steps on the condition that each correct step is immediately reinforced by some kind of favourable experience or reward. The process of rewarding the correct response to a stimulus renders the response highly probable in the sense that it will be repeated in future.

The frame contains two sets, out of which some keyword is missing. After reading the answer, the student writes the answer. The moment he makes a response, he is given the desired answer. The desired response is very often a confirmation of the student's response. Each student is taken through many stimulus response steps.

Example: Just as the moon is a satellite of the Earth, the Earth is also a _________ of the Sun, since it _____________ the Sun (Satellite, Circles.)

Steps
a. Information is presented in small steps.
b. The learner responds actively at each step.
c. Immediate knowledge of results is given.
d. Self-pacing by the student is possible.
   It is known as linear because each learner takes the same path through the instruction.
   Progresses from frame one to frame two, three, etc., in an unalterable, preplanned sequence.

$$1 —— 2 —— 3 —— 4 —— 5$$
sequence.

This program does not provide for branching for able or slow learners.

This program is also called Extrinsic because a learner has no choice of his own in following the path or sequence.

It is best suited in subject areas where facts and information can be properly sequenced.

Limitations
1. Lack of Motivation: Learning becomes dull, monotonous as a good deal of time is taken to teach a few and simple points. Steps are small materials, lack challenge and interest for children, particularly the gifted ones.
2. Serial Order Learning: Learning is acquired in a serial order. But in actual life situation, learning may not be serial.
3. No Freedom of Choice: The learner has no choice of his own to respond. Creative imagination and judgmental ability of the learner to respond are inhibited. Learners do not contribute towards a discovery of answers but follow a rigid line prescribed by the writer.
4. Tendency to Guess: The learner finds out the clue as to what is to be filled in the blank and key terms are guessed.
5. Used in Limited Areas: Where the subject matter can be properly sequenced. For example, Science, Maths and Vocabulary development in languages.

5. Branching or Intrinsic style:

The frames are not kept before the students in a numerical sequence. The student's answer determines which frame he has to see next.

In this system, the student is given a problem and a number of answers, out of these one answer is correct. When a student selects an answer, he is directed to a specific frame. This frame shows him if his answer is wrong and why it is wrong. Then the frame takes him to the first question so that the answer may be given again or it will direct him to a sub-programe and will help him to get the basic knowledge for answering the question. Depending on the answers he gives, the student may branch ahead, may branch 'backward' and secure further explanation or move ahead to the next step. Whatever may be the case, the student has to give a correct answer to the question and until he gives the correct answer, he cannot proceed to the next frame, e.g. Licensure exam for Health professionals in USA/Canada.

Limitations
1. Guessing: The learner may give the correct response without understanding the subject matter of the frame.
2. Difficulty in Praising Branches: Infinite branching cannot be provided. It cannot cater to the needs of all individuals because it is very difficult to find out the total number of branches for every individual.
3. Diagnostics may not suit the needs of individual learners.
4. Branching style cannot be used below fifth class.
5. The cost of preparation is high, Audio-visual equipment needed is very costly.
6. There is no guarantee that the pupil has learned everything the program is intended to teach.
7. The program is unable to control the student.
8. It is written primarily for diagnostic purposes so that the student can be provided with specific remedial material needed as he/she selects responses.

Advantages of Programed Instruction
1. Student is kept Active and Alert: He gets good exercise in using new words, concepts and relationships; lack of attention is at once detected. Even when student commits a mistake he does not have to wait for long to know it. He can work according to his own schedule. If due to illness or any other reason, he cannot attend school for some days or months, he can start from where he left when he comes back.
2. The teacher gets relieved of doing ordinary Jobs and she/he can play the important role like guide, counselor, motivator and organizer. The teacher can become a model for the students and avoid becoming the administrator of simple learning tasks that can be better handled by programed materials.
3. Social and emotional problems can be eliminated.
4. The problems of discipline have been automatically solved by the use of self-instructional material.
5. A well-programed self-instructional device is tailored to cater to the needs of individual students of the class.
6. Programed instruction makes learning interesting.
7. Every student can work at his own pace.
8. Programed instruction is useful in memorization of facts, nomenclature, procedures and mastering of simple facts, concepts formation and learning of principles.
9. Programed instruction is useful in situations where the human instructions are not available.
10. Can improve the communication potential of conventional textbooks.
11. Intellectual and some motor skills will be taught more efficiently, e.g. Foreign language, spelling-bee contest.
12. The discernment of the logic of various disciplines and inspiring students to creative thinking and judgement.
13. Programed instruction is a great trust in the direction of individualized instruction. A well-programed self-instructional device is tailored to cater to the needs of individual students of the class.
14. Scoring is done, item by item, diagnostically thus reducing the necessity of testing and allowing the Teacher to determine the exact problems of each learner. Knowing the trouble spots, the teacher can correct them by a modification of the program. The teacher can give classroom explanation if the error is common or he may arrange individual conferences on specific points.
15. The learner is challenged by his own capabilities. The novelty of learning by a device provides extra motivation to the learner. Continued success on a program augments this motivation.

16. The student is immediately reinforced for correction of his response and this reinforcement sustains the motivation of the students.
17. More complex of the concepts will be known.
18. Programed instruction is useful in memorization of facts nomenclature, procedures and mastering of simple facts, concept for motion and principles of learning.

Steps in Program Writing

1. Preparation
- The teacher should be thoroughly familiar with the topic and limit the area to be dealt
- The teacher should see that the topic is suitable for the program
- Preparation of a content outline-It will help him to cover all the material to be taught
- Behavioral objectives should be stated in terms of instructional goals in operational, observable, measurable terms to facilitate the construction of the program and its subsequent evaluation
- Goals further analyzed, finally decided the components of goals are explained by component behavior
- Constructing a test for entering behavior and for terminal behavior criterion.

2. Program writing
- The content outline and analysis of behavioral objectives leads to the terminal behavior through a series of instructional devices
    - The presentation of material in frames
    - Stimulus and stimulus context
    - The cues for evoking responses
    - The response evoked by stimuli
    - Enrichment of material.
- Ensuring the response of the student: Overt behavior is essential for learning technical terms
- The complete record of student's written responses should be utilized later for revising the program
- Conformation or correction of students responses: When the student knows that his response is correct, he obtains confirmation; where it is incorrect, he receives correction
- Using prompts to guide student responses: Prompts are cues provided in the program frame to guide the student to make responses correctly
- Providing careful sequencing of the frames: It will depend on two factors
    - The description and analysis of behaviors to be taught through the programs
    - The conditions necessary for the learning required by the various tasks.

3. Try out and Revision
When the first draft is ready, it should be tried out on several persons and reedited. The original frames should be typed and their response given on the back page. It should be given to a small group of students. The students make use of the typed content (index cards) and turn to the reverse side of the cards for confirmation. It has to be seen where the mistakes are being committed. This will facilitate revision of the frames later. These programed materials are experimentally tried out in classes, items that are frequently missed are changed. The original draft is edited once again. Tried out further and final revision is prepared.

Application of programed instruction in education
1. For Regular Instruction: The teacher can use programed material regular instruction in any subject in which the programed material is available. The teacher may use it in conjunction with methods., e.g. Textbooks, TV films, Lectures, Discussion. Programed instruction can be used to teach a selected unit in a course or entire course of a subject.
2. Enrichment of Curriculum.
3. Remedial Instruction: It can reduce the percentage of failure in maths and science. Applied right from pre-primary school to university education.
4. Industrial Application: Programed Instruction is used in industry because:
    a. Lack of qualified instructor and lack of sufficient time to the instructor.
    b. Assembling employees into classes is a problem
    c. Employees work in shifts

    d. Employees work in a scattered location

    e. Heavy costs of staff and maintaining of the training center

    Each employee is supplied sufficient self-instructional material which he can use individually at any time and any place. Thus, it is possible to trained employees in many skills at local plants without sending them to training centers

5. The use of programed instruction has been introduced successfully in army, navy and air force
6. Correspondence Courses: Successful medium of educating the masses as well as those who want to continue their education
7. To improve Agricultural practices for Agriculturists, the programed material is prepared
8. To improve sanitary habits of public
9. Non-formal education
10. Used in banks to train cashiers
11. Modification of deviant behavior
12. Vocational training and psychotherapy training
13. Programed Instruction for exceptional, handicapped children
14. Can be used to enrich the curriculum to cater to the needs of gifted children.

Problems of application
1. The problem of quantity and quality
2. Shortage of good teachers in the country
3. Lack of good programers
4. Resistance
5. Lack of funds and facilities

INDIVIDUALIZED INSTRUCTION

Definitions

'The tailoring of instruction to the particular needs and abilities of the learner'.

'It takes place if learners are working alone at their own pace'.

'It is a system of instruction in which any or all of the following factors are adopted to the needs of the each individual student. The factors are – Pace, medium of presentation, study style, context and evaluation technique'.

'An arrangement that makes it possible at all times for each student to be engaged in learning those things that are most appropriate for himself as an individuals'.

'An instructional system is individualized when the characteristics of each learner plays a major part in the selection of objectives, materials, procedures and time; how to achieve the objectives are based on the individual learner'.

Meaning

'Individualization which effects the release of human potential has long been an important function of classroom teacher'.

'The teacher works on a personal, one-to-one basis with each student. It is a tutorial system which is normally followed in teacher-pupil relationship'.

Objectives

1. Maximize potentialities.
2. Universalization.
3. Facilitation of new schemes.
4. Implementation of life – long education.

Characteristics

1. Specification of Instructional Objectives: The objectives should be defined in operational terms—i.e., behavioral changes can be observed and measured in an objective way.
2. The initial behavior of the learner is measured prior to his entrance into a given instructional sequence.
3. Individual prescription: The instruction is tailored according to the needs, capabilities and interests of individual learners.
4. Learner selected objectives.
5. Active responding: The learner actively participates in the learning process by making frequent observable responses or manipulation of materials employed in the instructional sequence.
6. Explicit Contingencies: Reward or reinforcement are systematically arranged to follow precisely defined behaviors of the learners.
7. Immediate Feedback: The learner is immediately informed of the result of his performance on a task. This motivates the learner for further learning and sustains his interest in the learning task.
8. Frequent Feedback: Frequent feedback is arranged to maximize opportunities for the learner to assess the adequacy of his performance.
9. Successive Approximation: Arranging for each step in an instructional sequence require an achievable increment in the learner's performance towards the desired outcome of the sequence. The learner is led to the terminal behavior step by step.
10. Self-pacing: Learner controls his progress through an instructional sequence himself.
11. Mastery Criterion: Requiring a high level performance of the outcome specified for a given step in an instructional sequence as a condition for progress to the next step in the sequence.
12. Use of Proctors: Providing repeated testing, immediate scoring, tutoring and a marked enhancement of the personal social aspect of the educational process by using students who have already mastered a step in an instructional sequence to monitor, prompt and praise the performance of students at work on that step.
13. Critical Information written.
14. Multimedia presentation.

Methods

1. Programed Instruction
2. Teaching Machine
3. Computer-assisted Instruction
4. Personalized-system of Instruction
5. Learner-controlled Instruction

Problems in implementation of Individualized Instruction

1. Reluctance on the part of teacher community to modify old practices to accommodate the social and economic need of the society. The resistance may be altered through continuous persuasion.
2. The educational planners fail to anticipate the problems which the administrators and teachers encounter in introducing an innovation.
3. Absence of problem-solving effectiveness in their day-to-day affairs.
4. It requires the use of multimedia techniques to impart instruction due to budgeting problem.

Tentative suggestions to implement Individualized Instruction

1. The teacher must observe and listen to his students with increased ease and concern.
2. Achieve openness in classroom relationship.
3. The teacher should recognize and accept different ways of responding according to individualized need and style.
4. The teacher should encourage questioning, probing and responding in ways that lead learners to assume responsibility.
5. The learners should be encouraged to discover and exercise his own resources to find out the solutions of problems.
6. The teacher can use the techniques of placing learners in different roles.

7. The teacher should endeavor to achieve free and constructive communication with learners.
8. Teacher should clear the way, by whatever means for stretching learner's mind and abilities in creative, self-fulfilling attempt.

DISCUSSION METHOD

Introduction

Discussion occurs when a group with group orientation purposefully interacts orally for enlightenment or policy determination. If the aim is enlightenment, members systematically define, analyze and exchange information. When the end is problem solving, members systematically define, analyze, evaluate possible solutions and attempt to agree upon a high quality decision to which all or the majority will be committed.

A group of 3 to 15 members, can be formed and some kind of organization is formed. If the group is large i.e., more than 12, it inhibits the group members ability to communicate with everyone else in the group.

Interaction: Group members must be able to communicate freely and openly with all the other members of the group. Groups will develop norms about discussion and group members will develop roles which will affect the group's interaction.

Goals: A group must have a common purpose or goal and they must work together to achieve that goal. The goal brings the group together and holds it together without conflict and tension.

Definitions

'Group discussion is a cooperative, problem-solving activity which seeks a consensus regarding the solution of a problem.'

'Three or more participants who have an agreed topic to discuss and share their view in all the aspects and submits/presents their view in the form of report to bigger gathering.'

Salient Features

1. Discussion involves a group.
2. Discussion is oral.
3. Discussion involves interaction.
4. Discussion is purposeful — Members will have a clear, specific purpose which brings them together on a particular occasion. A committee or conference group meets to solve concrete problems.
5. Discussion proceeds systematically from the question or problem toward increased understanding or decision.
6. Discussion should proceed with the classification of a limited question.
7. Systematic forward movement that leadership becomes a vital contribution.
8. Members must accept group orientation. Defining the problem and its wording. Analysis of the nature of the problem and its components. Exchange of information, which leads to a contribution to increase understanding on the part of each participant or listener. The teacher by necessity must guide the contributions in a predetermined direction so that students will be exposed to certain subject matter.

   In the problem solving discussion, the group wishes to find a solution that will be left for every one in the group to which all or most will be committed. During discussion members are searching and inquiring. They have to make up their minds about best solution.

Activities to be carried out during group discussion

- Identification of Group leader to lead the group of participants to discuss about a specific topic and one member will record all the discussions in a sequential order
- Identification of problem/issue–Discussion focused towards group orientation, while the debates persuade the group towards its proposal
- Operationally Defining the Problem
- Discussion is cooperative when the participants speak informally and conversationally while the debate is a competition between debater and advocates: It talks for equal amounts or alternating time against a proposal, analyzing the views related to problem based on their detailed knowledge exposure or experiences or specific observations

- Suggested alternatives
- Weighing of alternatives
- Deciding the solution of problem in innovative way or coming to conclusion related to issue/problem
- Ending the session with general agreement or conclusion about a specific problem of discussion.

Types of Discussion

1. Closed group Discussion

   These are private or non-public. Most committee meetings are held as closed group discussions. Only members of the committee are present in the room and they are the only participants in the discussion. The talk is addressed to members held for the purpose of enlightenment or decision making.

   Closed group discussions will be held in different kinds of situations.

   a. Study Group: Members meet together to study some subject of common interest. Students in a classroom use this type of discussion.

   b. Work shop: A group of people with common interest will be gathered on specific days, the common theme will be discussed, the sub-themes will be carried out in different sessions. At the end all the groups will present their reports in general. The workshop starts with inauguration, ends with valedictory. All participants will be given Certificates of participation.

   c. Staff meeting: The head of institution formulates the agenda and call for faculty meeting. In the meeting all the points in the agenda is discussed, views are shared and recorded.

   d. Briefing sessions: Here information is needed by a group whose members are ready to undertake a common task.

   e. Round Table: Here the participants with a common problem, talk together around a table, for a purpose of learning from each other.

2. Public Discussion, e.g. Panel discussion, Dialogue, Symposium and Forum.

3. Discussion techniques for small groups

   A small group is one in which, face-to-face relationship among participants and an opportunity for each member to actively participate in discussion

   a. The Individual conference
   b. The informal class group discussion
   c. The seminar
   d. The clinical conference
   e. Role play
   f. Case analysis.

4. Discussion techniques for large groups

   a. Multiple discussion groups
   b. Symposium
   c. Panel.

Small Group Discussions

The Individual Conference

It is 'conversation with a purpose' simply as an interview.

Purpose

To obtain facts or to give information. As a teaching tool, the conference primarily provides an opportunity to discuss the students' problems privately. The purpose of conference in teaching is guidance.

Principles

- Attitude of the teacher towards the student – teacher relationship, her/his conception of its value, i.e., attitude
- Continued professional guidance
- Friendly attitude of concern for the self-development of the student and the solution of the problem
- To give aid to the student
- The teacher needs to comprehend, associate or integrate the knowledge she/he has received
- When student explains her/his problem to the teacher focusing on 'why'.

Skills needed
- Observation
- Use of setting
- Establishment of rapport
- Meeting resistance
- Recognizing ambivalent feelings
- Use of questioning
- Establishment of authority
- Silence as a skilled procedure.

a. Skill in Observation: Implies the use of senses, mainly seeing and hearing. The learner may verbalize her/his feeling and attitudes, more can be gained by the teacher who carefully notices the facial expressions, the manner of speaking may indicate the learner's state or feelings. The observer must be aware of subject phenomena i.e., learners own background, attitudes or experiences.

The interview or conference with the student should take place in a friendly, private atmosphere.

Rapport must be established between teacher and the learner.

Acceptance of herself/himself, putting emphasis on the dignity of the person over the exaltation of the personality.

The teacher must be sensitive to the student's resistance.

The learner may have very ambivalent feelings. He/she is face to face with the teacher, he/she knows that he/she needs help, and yet he/she may not want to disclose his/her shortcomings. He/she is aware of the need for guidance.

The teacher has the skill, to act subtly by proper timing and expression of help being given. If handled correctly, the student even may feel that she/he has solved the problem by herself/himself. A distinction must be made between authority and learner.

The teacher may use authoritative approach, she/he bases her/his suggestions, criticisms or comments on existing norms or knowledge.

b. Silence: The teacher may listen quietly to the student's views without expressing comment or passing judgement.

Individual conference used in nursing course to clarify class material, to supplement instructions, to explain answers to questions of individual students which do not concern the entire class.

It is used as a means of assisting the individual who is having difficulties in keeping up with the class or the student with the potentiality of advancing ahead of the group as a whole.

Individual conference is successful clinical teaching, assisting the student to understand the relationship between class content of courses and the application to problems of nursing practice and patient care.

The Supervisory Conference

The instructor has the opportunity to learn the student's interests, the progress or lack of progress in relation to the student's concept of past experience. Outlining the conference and making the appointment with the instructor is the student's responsibility. It will help him/her to think and realize his/her needs – his/her areas of strengths and weakness. The teacher will assure the student of her/his willingness to serve as a resource person to guide her in planning and in problem-solving and in his/her progress. To gain the student's respect and confidence, the instructor needs to be an expert practitioner herself/himself. By the use of interview type questions, the instructor guides the progress of the conference and keeps it focused in the problem area. She he presents intellectual challenges to the student and stimulates motivation. Constructive criticism will be done in evaluating learning procedure. Good rapport, friendliness is essential. Questioning should be skillful in order to aid the student in discussing the problem that he/she had.

Seminar
- It uses Problem-Solving approach
- To give students, the opportunity to participate in methods of scientific analysis and research procedures

- The teacher should help the student to select, formulate and organize the most significant student problems or topics, suggest available sources of information and allow sufficient time to gather the information by following outlines of proposed seminar, teacher guides the students in selection of appropriate/suitable Audio Visual Aids to present the topic comprehensively
- Students are expected to do considerable library research, if feasible obtain primary source data and analyse or critically evaluated and conclusions reached under the direction of the teacher
- As the seminar progresses, the students will assume increased responsibilities for preparing and presenting the topic for group by having the discussion
- Group has to be 10 to 15 students, duration of seminar will be 1 to 2 hours.

Symposium

To investigate the problem from several points of view. Symposium consists of a set of program of prepared speeches followed by audience discussion.

Several people present speeches representing different approaches to the same problem. These form the basis for the general group participation. Each individual may be given separate topic or taken together, they represent a broad consideration of the topic. A series of related papers are presented.

Technique

Success depends on the personnel involved and the degree of preparation.
- The teacher should plan the program ahead of time
- The teacher and members should know the objectives of the symposium and the breadth of the topic to be discussed
- The teacher or student may function as chairman, she/he will introduce the topic and speakers to the audience
- To have unity and proper sequence, the chairman may give transitional statements between speeches. Then, she/he gives a brief summary at the close of all the speeches and opens the discussion to the audience
- She/he directs questions to the various members of the group, trying to give all individuals an equal opportunity.

Disadvantages
- Lack of time
- Inadequate opportunity for all the students to participate actively
- Time is limited to 15 to 20 minutes
- Audience participation is limited.

Panel Discussion

This method, originated by Prof. Hasy A. Overstreet.

Panel is "a discussion in which a few persons carry on a conversation in front of an audience", when the group is too large to work effectively through the usual round-table procedure.

Purpose: To reproduce the features for the benefit of a larger group. It is a socialized group conversation in which different points of view are presented.

When handled intelligently and creatively, the panel stimulates thought and discussion and clarifies thinking. Because several people engage in a free exchange of opinions, the panel influences the audience to an open-minded attitude and respect for the opinion of others. The quick exchange of facts, opinions and plans tends to develop more critical attitude, and better judgment. It can be helpful to stimulate discussion, encouraging thinking and developing group opinion.

Technique

The members of the Panel include:
- The chairman
- The audience.

  The panel consists of 4 to 8 members seated in a semicircle facing the audience.

The members of the panel should be quick thinkers and facile talkers, represents different points of view.

The members should be prepared by knowing the limits of the topic to be discussed and the regulations which guide the discussion.

The chairman should be selected carefully, as much of the success of the panel will depend on her/his leadership. She/he should be a person with wide mental flexibility who has a sense of fair play and is able to determine the relevance of remarks as they are made. Chairman must keep the discussion to the subject and see that all members of the panel have an equal opportunity to express their views.

She/he should act as a neutral referee.

The chairman begins the panel discussion by exploring the whole proceeding. First, the members of the panel are introduced by name and background of experience. The topic is announced and the limits of the discussion are stated. The chairman may start the procedure rolling by making a comment or two or by directing a question to a particular person. After that she keeps the conversation to the topic, encourages expression of the difference of opinion and organizes the discussion with occasional summaries. A general summary before discussion is opened to the audience.

The panel discussion should provide a natural setting in which the audience will have the opportunity to ask questions, evaluate replies and make constructive contributions.

Questions from the audience may be directed to certain speakers.

Workshop

A group of individuals who work together towards the solution of problems in a given subject field during a specific period of time. Sessions are organized under sub-themes. Interested participants will form as a group for the session and discuss in detail for a given period of time, the group leader will present the report in general meeting. Participants will have the opportunity to present the paper during the sessions.

Values of Group Discussion

- Creates analytic and critical abilities, creativity, encourages the student to think for herself/himself
- To develop critical habits of study
- To interpret problems of the past, throw light on the problems of the present and to gain insight into ways for shaping the future
- Keeps him to advance in creative thought by his own efforts, to make progress as a result of the responses of him and others to the stimulus of questions and volunteered expression
- It enables the student to enrich his/her own participation
- It gives the student an opportunity to learn how to adjust to social situations
- The student acquires new knowledge from discussion and develops the ability to reexamine and analyze her/his own reasons and contributions in the light of ideas presented by others
- Self-activity is increased as student is participating
- Group benefits as there is a pooling of ideas and harmonizing of attitudes in the solution of a common problem
- Cooperation in highest sense is developed, since open-mindedness, respect for the other person's opinions and concern for the effective group discussion
- Increased knowledge, intellectual abilities, skills, interests, changes in attitudes and values, better personal and social adjustment, increased cooperation.

Essentials of good group discussion

1. Clear formulation of realistic goals.
2. A permissive atmosphere conductive to full participation. Planning in terms of time and resources available.
3. Work on specific problems rather than broad general problem area.
4. Participation by each group member.
5. Physical conditions so that each member seen and heard.
6. Opportunity for members to get acquainted.

7. Scoring Maximum Results from Group Discussion
   - Prepare for discussion.
   - Come to the discussion with questions in mind.
   - Speak freely
   - Listen thoughtfully to others
   - Be brief, do not monopolize the discussion
   - Strike while the idea is hot, don't wait for the leader to reorganize before speaking
   - Don't let the discussion get away from you
   - Indulge in friendly disagreement
   - Give credit to others by acknowledging their contributions
   - Interaction is important
   - Group discussion depends upon sharing of ideas, knowledge and experiences. It is based on varied factors like good leadership
     - Clear identification of the problem to be discussed or the goal has to be reached
     - Preparation by the leaders and the participants
     - Active participation by all members of the group
     - Accurate information.

TEAM TEACHING

Definitions

"A method of coordinated classroom teaching which involves a team of teachers working together with a single group of students".

"An arrangement whereby 2 or more teachers, with or without teaching aides cooperatively plan, instruct, and evaluate one or more class groups in an appropriate instructional space and given length of time so as to take advantage of the special competencies of the team members".

"An instructional situation where 2 or more teachers possessing complementary teaching skills, cooperatively plan and implement the instruction for a single group of students using flexible scheduling and grouping techniques to meet the particular instruction"–*Carlo Oslon*

"A type of instructional organization, involving teaching personnel and the students assigned to them, in which 2 or more teachers are given responsibility, working together for all or a significant part of the instruction of the same group of students"–*Shaplin and Olds*

"tTeaching team is a systematic arrangement with a leader and assistants and with an optimum use of technology cooperatively instruct a group of students, varying the size of the purpose of instruction and spending staff time and energy in ways that will make the best use of their respective competencies"–*David W Beggs*

"A form of organization in which individual teachers decide from pool resources, interests and expertise in order to devise and implement a scheme of work suitable to the needs of their learners and the facilities of their school"–*David Warwick*

Characteristics

1. A form of instructional organization.
2. A group of teachers decides to take action. It is not imposed upon them. The cooperating members fully understanding it, they are enthusiastic about it and have to be prepared to give the time and energy to make it work.
3. Resources are pooled for the benefit of all concerned. Resources include factors, e.g. Specialization in interests, knowledge, skills, experience, time-table, departmental equipment, facilities and free time for meetings.
4. Team teaching centers on the needs of the learners.

Objectives

1. To utilize the better talents and interests of the teachers.
2. To increase grouping and scheduling flexibility. Team Teaching provides flexibility in the grouping of children according to their interests and aptitudes in the subject.
3. To improve the quality of instruction.

Principles

1. **Size and Composition:** It should be appropriate in terms of learning experiences and purposes of the group.
2. **Time factor:** Time should be allotted keeping into consideration the importance of the subjects. In team teaching arrangement a fairly fluid time-table is essential.
3. **Learning Environment:** It should be provided by making arrangement of laboratory, good library, workshops, listening and viewing rooms.
4. **Duties assigned to teachers should be appropriate:** The duties should be assigned on the basis of interest, qualification and personality characteristics of individual member. Selection of members of team should be made very carefully.
5. **Level of instruction:** The level of team teaching must be appropriate to each learner within the group. The initial behavior of the learners should be properly assessed.
6. **Supervision:** The extent of supervision of the group's activities depend on the purpose of the group.

Advantages

1. **Ensures economical use of resources:** Time and energy are saved by team teaching in maintaining discipline in the class.
2. **Ensures interested and enthusiastic teaching:** While planning, the teachers consider their own skills and divide the classroom teaching accordingly.
3. **Deploys teachers to methods and areas of their expertise:** Teachers can concentrate on those areas for which they expressed preference or have specialized knowledge. Their time and energies can be used more economically and effectively.
4. Makes teaching experience centered.
5. Provides a framework within which subject integration is possible. Team teaching places the needs of children above the needs of the subjects.
6. **Makes teaching learner-centered:** Pupil's needs and reactions decide the direction and scope of the syllabus.
7. Provides opportunities for staff cooperation.
8. Takes students out of the classroom into the real world.
9. Helps in smooth sailing from the elementary level to the high school level and then to the college level
   - Common understanding among students and teachers, which fosters mutual trust and cooperation and creates the most suitable atmosphere for learning and teaching.
   - Team teaching provides experimental framework in which all or most of the current reforms can be incorporated and integrated.
10. **Opportunity for free discussion:** Team teaching gives an opportunity for free expression to all the students of the team. Team teaching stimulates thought and discussion among teachers who are jointly responsible for a group of children. Professional behavior is likely to develop best where there is a strong sense of involvement and responsibility.
11. **Development of human relations:** Team teaching provides this opportunity and trains the students in human relations essential for social adjustment.
12. Development of the professional status of the teacher.
13. **Exposure of group to more specialists:** The students get opportunities to be benefited by the special knowledge of various teachers constituting the team.
14. **Breakthrough from a rigidly compartmentalized school organization:** Team teaching makes more flexible use of staff, equipment and the school building.

15. Evaluation: The teachers can evaluate the teaching of one another and can give suggestions to improve it. Students become more aware of teaching style, their own approach and more disposed to examine alternative approaches.
16. Quality of Instruction: Definitely improved in team teaching organization.

Limitations

1. Lack of cooperation among the teachers: They hesitate to cooperate for the organization of successful Team teaching
2. Team teaching necessitates delegation of power and responsibilities: The administrators do not want to delegate their powers to any other agency
3. Disregard to the dynamics of small group
4. Traditional conservative attitude: They fail to adapt themselves to the new situations and find it more troublesome
5. Lack of accommodation
6. High-cost.

SIMULATED TEACHING

Definition

'Role-playing in which the process of teaching is displayed artificially and an effort is made to practice some important skills of communication through this technique. The pupil-teacher and the students simulate the particular role of a person or actual life situation. The whole program becomes a training in Role perception and Role Playing".

Meaning

Simulation is the basis of sensitivity training, sociodrama, role-playing and psychodrama. It is not actual teaching. Certain underlying skills to teaching can be modified, described and practised like any other skill. It is assumed that through role perception, the psychological appreciation of the classroom problems will grow and develop in the student. Teacher is a basis for handling the problems in the class.

Principles

1. Players take on roles which are representatives of the real world and then make decisions in response to their assessment of the setting in which they find themselves.
2. The experiences simulated are consequences which relate to their decisions and their general performance.
3. 'Monitor' the results of their actions are brought to reflect upon the relationship between their own decisions and the resultant consequences.

Application of Simulation in Teacher Training

Crrruikshank (1968) has developed a teacher training system which includes:
- The participant is introduced into the situation (i.e., if he is a new teacher in a school)
- The participant is provided with information and opportunities to solve the problems (for beginning teacher)
- The participant is exposed to a variety of potential solutions to a particular problem
- The participant is given the opportunity of observing the results of his chosen line of action
- The participant is introduced to the situation by film strips
- The participant is also given the materials, e.g. the rules, regulations, curriculum handbook and records, to familiarize to the topic
- The participant is presented with role-playing situations, written and responds to incident as a response sheet
- The participant then identifies the factors influencing the problem, locates the relevant information, suggests appropriate alternative course of action, communicates and implements a decision
- Small group discussions

Simulators
- It is deliberately designed to omit certain parts of the real operational situations
- Simulators are designed for procedures like
  - For adjusting electronic representation of motor skills
  - Identification of targets
  - Emergence signals
  - Conceptual tasks involving reasoning
  - Team functions.

The Procedure of Simulation

1. Selecting the Role Players: A small group of 4 or 5 student teachers is selected. They are assigned different letters in an alphabetic order. The role assignments are rotated within the group to give chance to everyone. Every member of the group gets an opportunity to be the actor and the observer
2. Selecting and Discussing Skills: The skills to be practiced are discussed and the topics that fit in the skill are suggested. One topic each is selected by the group members for exercise
3. Planning: It has to be decided who starts the conversation, who will top the interaction and when
4. Deciding the Procedure of Evaluation: How to record the interaction and how to present it to actor, has to be decided so that a proper feedback on his performance could be given
5. Provided Practical Lesson: The role players should be provided reinforcements on their performance to give them training for playing their part well.

Activities in Simulation

Role-Playing: The role, false or actual is performed in an artificial environment. This may give the pupil, an understanding of a situation or relationship among real life participants of a social process. He will gain some perceptions of the actions, attitudes and insight of persons or situations.

Socio-drama: It seeks to utilize role-playing as a means of finding out the solution to a problem situation assigned to the role-players. The problem may be false or based on real life situation and the actor is required to find out an acceptable solution of the situation.

Gaming: The situations involve outcomes affected by decisions made by one or more decisions. It is designed in a manner which enables chance to affect the outcome.

Advantages of Simulation in Teacher–Education

1. Simulation establishes a setting where theory and practice can be combined.
2. Simulation requires the teacher to be active participants in the process.
3. No risk is involved. The decisions are made and carried out without physical or psychological harm to children or school as a result of practice-teaching.
4. Controlled teaching assignments are possible. Student, teachers obtain experiences which are realistic and thus they become critical.
5. Simulation is a teaching device that motivates and involves students. It changes teacher behavior. Introduces novelty in the whole learning process. Level of freshness and novelty is maintained throughout the learning session.
6. Students are not expected to identify the group time and follow it. Every student is expected to have experiences, which are different from the usual laboratory type experiences common to all.
7. Stimulates the students for the acquisition of purposeful activities and they feel keenly interested in role-playing, socio-drama and gaming activities.
8. Removal of student-teacher polarization
   Simulations are self-monitoring. Participants recognize their aim progress by various feedback methods. Students are involved in decision-making. They observe their own evaluation of these consequences which influence their future actions.
9. Personal tensions in the teaching situation are likely to be reduced by the process of self-monitoring.

10. The teacher's role may be as interpreter of the simulation and as a guide, but he/she does not have to pose as an expert or as a judge.
11. Simulation as a universal behavioral mode.
12. Gains related to relevance and learning.
13. Decision-making skills into action. It develops various skills in children in increasing difficulty order.
14. Role awareness – The individual when he plays the role of others becomes conscious of that role.
15. An interdisciplinary view – It provides an integrated view as well as a vehicle for free interdisciplinary communication.
16. Dynamic framework.
17. Bridging the gap to reality – Simulation works to bridge the gap between unreal and real. Students enact real situation and learning becomes more interesting and lively than purely theoretical.
18. Gestalt communication – It is holistic in nature. It permits the learner a greater flexibility in addressing facets of complexity.

Values

- Enables the learner to learn directly from experience
- Promotes high level of critical thinking
- Develops in the students an understanding of the decision-making process
- Enables the individual to empathise with the real-life situation
- Provides feedback to the learners on the consequences of actions and decisions made
- Motivates the students by making real life situations exciting and interesting
- Enables teachers and learners to assess the realism of the situation by uncovering misconceptions.

Limitations

1. Simulation cannot be made in all subjects of the curriculum.
2. Simulation cannot be conveniently used in case of small children because mechanism is too difficult for them to follow.
3. It requires a lot of preparation on the part of teachers, very few teachers are prepared to take up the extra work which is required to make use of the technique as a success.
4. Learning is a serious activity which is highly individualized and needs concentration on the part of the learner. Simulation reduces the seriousness of learning.
5. Minimum of feedback sequence to choose.
6. Time-consuming.
7. Difficulty in using analytic approach.
8. Need for many simulators.

MICROTEACHING

Introduction

A training procedure aimed at simplifying the complexities of the regular teaching process. The trainee is engaged in a scaled-down teaching situation. Scaled down in terms of class size (small group 4-6 learners), length of class time (5 to 10 minutes), teaching tasks (practicing and mastering of a specific teaching skill, e.g. lecturing, questioning or leading a discussion) and strategy, flexibility, instructional decision-making, alternative use of specific curriculum, instructional materials and classroom management.

Definitions

"A scaled down teaching encounter in class size and class time. The number of students is from 5-10, and the duration of period ranges from 5-20 minutes"–*Allen, 1966*

"A device which provides the novice and experienced teacher alike new opportunities to improve teaching, it is a real teaching scaled down in time and size of the class, 1-5 students for 5-20 minutes"–*David B Young*

"A teacher education technique which allows teacher to apply clearly defined teaching skills to carefully prepared lessons in planned series of 5-10 minutes encounters with a small group of real students often with an opportunity to observe the results on video tape"–*Buch MB, 1968*

"Use of cloud-circuit television to give immediate feedback of a trainee teachers' performance in a simplified environment"–*Urwin, 1970*

"A teacher training procedure which reduces the teaching situation to simpler and more controlled encounter achieved by limiting the practice teaching to a specific skill and reducing teaching time and class-size"–*Clift and others,1976*

Microteaching is a scaled down sample of teaching. The complex act of teaching is broken down onto simple components. Only one particular skill is attempted and developed during Microteaching session. The teaching act is scaled down in terms of the content of the lesson, duration of the lesson and size of the class. A student-teacher teaches a short lesson of 5 to 8 minutes to a small group of learners (5 to 8). The lesson is self-contained and a single concept is taken up in the lesson. At the end of the lesson, the learners in the class leave and the teacher trainee discusses with the supervisor. Then the teacher-trainee is given time to think about the discussion and modify his lesson and plan accordingly. The process can be repeated till desirable skill is developed. The success depends on the teach-reteach cycle, which can be completed in about 30 minutes.

Meaning

The short lesson is recorded on an audio or video tape recorder and the trainee gets to hear and see himself immediately after the lesson. The learners who attend the lesson are asked to fill in rating questionnaires evaluating specific aspects of the lesson. The trainees self-analyses of the lesson based on the authentic feedback from the tape together with the pupil's reaction and a supervisor's analysis and suggestions, assists the trainee in restructuring the lesson which he/she then immediately re-teaches to a new group of learners added by improvement when he/she teaches again. The microteaching sequence is practiced usually in a microteaching laboratory in a teacher-training institution or an inservice training program in regular schools.

Characteristics

1. *Micro-element:* Microteaching reduces the complexity of the teaching situation in terms of:
   a. Number of students to be taught.
   b. Duration of lesson.
   c. Subject matter to be taught to enable the trainee to concentrate on a particular teaching skill at a time. One should master the components of the task of teaching before he/she attempts to perform effectively the complicated task of teaching at macro-level.
   d. The number of instructional objectives and the content is kept low.
   e. It reduces the teaching skill and size of the topic, it is focused on micro-events.
   f. It is highly individualized training device to prepare effective teachers and provides feedback for trainees' performance.
   g. Microanalysis of the teaching process consists of analyzing the minute details of teaching.
2. *Teaching skills and teaching strategies:*
   a. Pre-instructional skills
      • These include writing of instructional objectives
      • Sequencing and organizing knowledge to be presented in order to achieve specific objectives
      • Appropriate content
      • Proper organization
      • Selection of proper audio-visual aids
   b. Instructional skills
      • Skills of introducing a lesson
      • Skills of explaining and illustrating
      • Reinforcement
      • Probing questions

- Reinforcing pupil participation
- Diagnosing learners' difficulties

c. Post-instructional skills
  - Skills of writing test items
  - Interpreting pupil's performance in a test
  - Planning remedial measures

It enables the trainees to develop these skills and perfect them in such a way as to master the teaching strategies.

d. Feedback: Several reliable and authentic sources are used to provide feedback: oral feedback by the supervisor, observation schedules filled in by the peer group participating in the micro lesson, audio and videotape recording.

3. *Safe Practice ground:* Teaching is performed under simulated conditions with a small group, the trainee is on a safe practice ground.
4. *The Teaching Models:* The trainee gets many opportunities to study the desired pattern of behavior through demonstration given by the supervisor or a tape guides, the trainee can develop his own style.
5. *The Research Laboratory:* According to Allen and Rayan, the following areas of research seems to make the most effective use of the microteaching settings:
   - To optimize the procedures and sequences in the microteaching situation
   - Research in modeling and supervising techniques
   - Task analysis of teaching act
   - Investigation of the relationship between teaching behavior and students performances
   - Aptitude treatment interaction studies, to provide optimal training procedures for teachers with different abilities, interests and backgrounds

Principles

1. Enforcement: Feedback, re-teaching makes teaching perfect.
2. Practice and drill: Teaching is a complex skill which needs constant drill and practice. It affords practice in each small task or skill and thereby the pupil teacher gain mastery.
3. Continuity: Microteaching is a continuous process: teaching-feedback–re-teaching-feedback till perfection is attained.
4. Microscopic supervision: Supervisor has an observation schedule which he fills up while supervising and makes assessment at a rating scale. The supervisor sees through the lesson all important points, paying full attention to one point at a time.

Strategy

- Supervisor has to conduct orientation training for teacher trainees on each teaching skill by model presentation followed with discussion about the presentation
- Supervisor has to prepare time-schedule of micro lesson for each teacher trainee
- Delivery of lesson under controlled conditions by the pupil-teacher
- Supervision of the lesson by the supervisor
- Videotapes of the lesson to be televised at closed circuit television
- Discussion about the presentation/feedback from pupil supervisor and supervisor in-charge
- Preparation of the lesson after the feedback
- Re-teaching of the same lesson to another small group of the students by the pupil teacher.
- Again discussion with the supervisor and feedback.

Five 'R's in Microteaching

- Recording
- Reviewing
- Responding
- Refining
- Re-doing

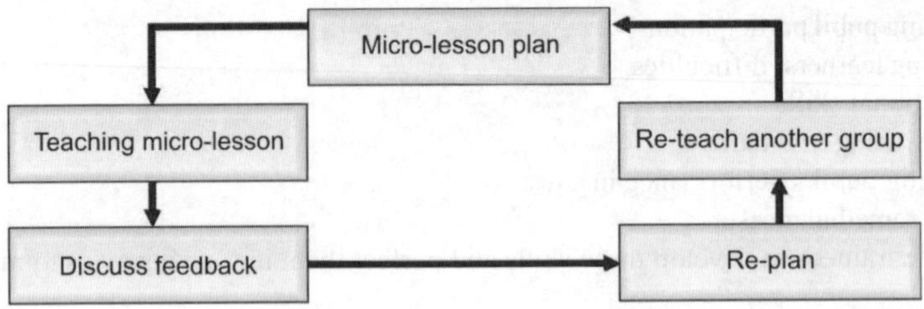

Fig. 5.1: Microteaching cycle

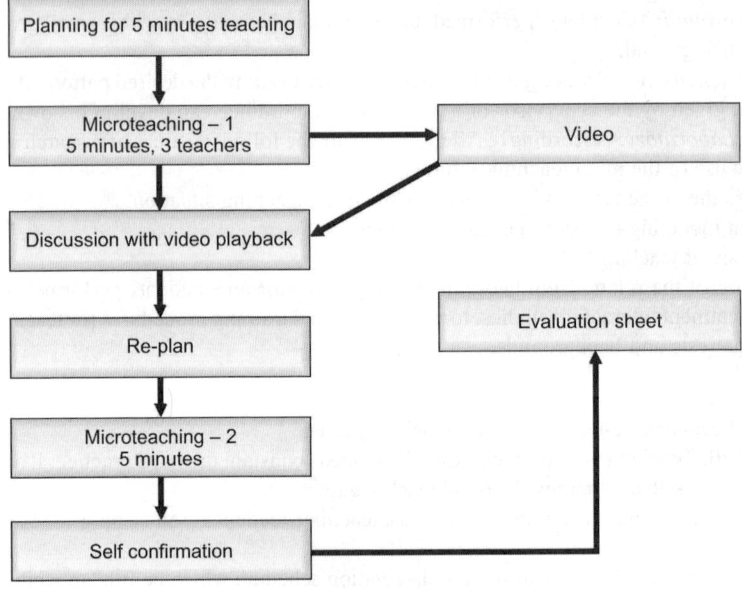

Fig. 5.2: Microteaching flow chart

Need

To ensure the desired skills are actually acquired by the teacher trainee. Supervised teaching and learning practice are more useful after the student teacher goes through the microteaching cycle.

Teaching is a complex task involving a number of teaching activities (overt teaching behavior) and covert teaching activities come into play.

Overt behavior–Observable, measurable and recordable behavior.

Covert behavior–They bring about a change in opinions and beliefs.

Often covert behavior leads to overt behavior.

Desirable microteaching behaviors which constitute teaching skills, e.g. Standing still, thinking, framing a question, facing the students, listening, looking around for a response.

Recalling the names of students, Calling the students by name, Pausing to think.

Different teaching skills are not exclusive to each other. It is better to identify some observable skills and then desire means to quantify them.

Microteaching is all about demonstrating, quantifying and improving such teaching skills.

Stanford model listed the general teaching skills involved in Microteaching

- Stimulus variation
- Closure
- Nonverbal clues
- Set induction
- Silence
- Reinforcement of student participation

- Fluency in questioning
- Divergent questions
- Illustrating and use of examples
- Planned repetition move

- Probing questions
- Recognizing attending behavior
- Lecturing skills
- Completeness of communication.

Passi et al listed teaching skills as follows
- Writing instructional objectives
- Fluency and questioning
- Explaining
- Stimulus variation
- Reinforcement of learning
- Using a chalk board
- Recognizing attending behavior.

- Introducing a lesson
- Probing questions
- Illustrative with examples
- Silence and nonverbal cues
- Increasing participation
- Achieving closure

Procedures adopted in Microteaching

Microteaching is integrated with student teaching program
- Lecture method
- Diagnostic lessons

- Demonstration lesson
- Micro lessons for practice.

Apparatus needed in Microteaching

Microteaching can be conducted with or without closed circuit television
- Video on camera with a zoom lens
- Two monitors
- Two clocks
- 100 yards of wire

- Videotape recorders
- Recording tapes
- Dozen lamps
- Switch gear.

Objectives

1. To enable the teacher trainees to learn and assimilate new teaching skills under controlled conditions.
2. To enable the teacher trainee to gain confidence in teaching and mastering a number of teaching skills on a small group of learners.
3. To utilize the academic potential of teacher-trainee for providing much needed feedback.
4. To give the teacher trainees training in the component skills of teaching at the pre service level.
5. To gain maximum advantage with little time, money and material.

Steps

1. Defining the skill: A particular skill is defined to student teachers in terms of specific teaching behaviors, and the objectives such behaviors aim at achieving.
2. Demonstrating the lesson: The teacher educator can give a demonstration lesson using the particular skill.
3. Planning the lesson: The student teacher prepares a lesson plan based on the pre decided model on a suitable topic relating to the particular skill which he proposes to practice.
4. Teaching the Micro lesson.
5. Discussion on the lesson delivered: The lesson delivered by the trainee is followed by discussion to provide him feedback. Peers who participated in the lesson as learners, peer observers or the supervisor can provide the necessary feedback. Feedback can also be provided by audiotape or video tape recorder. The student teacher observes and analyses his lesson with the help of the supervisor.
6. Replanning the lesson: In the light of the feedback and supervisor's comments, the student teacher replans the same lesson or a different lesson in order to use the skill more effectively.
7. Reteaching the lesson: The revised lesson is retaught to a different but comparable group of learners.
8. Rediscussion or re-feedback: The lesson is again observed or audiotaped or videotaped. Observations are noted. Feedback is again provided on the re-taught lesson.
9. Repeating the cycle: The teach-reteach cycle is repeated till the desired level of skill is achieved. The supervisor is to enable the teacher trainee to perfect his performance in the particular teaching skill.

Phases

1. Knowledge acquisition phase
   - Observation of analysis
   - Discussion of the demonstrated skill.
2. Skill acquisition phase
   - Preparation of the micro lesson involving the skill
   - Practicing the skill while teaching.
3. Transfer phase
   - Evaluating performance leading to feedback
   - Replan, reteach and transfer of skill to actual class teaching in macro sessions.

Role of Supervisor

- Supervisor will help the teacher trainee to develop component skills of teaching to both the theory underlying skills and the practical conditions of the classroom
- Provides continuous consultation and helps the teacher trainee skills learnt in microteaching setting to the actual classroom
- Demonstrates the teaching skill which has to be developed in the teacher trainee
- Prepares a special schedule of microteaching lessons in the practicing schools
- Supervises the lesson and discusses with the pupil-teacher in a group of other pupil-teacher
- Evaluates the trainee's class and fills the rating questionnaire schedule and gives feedback
- Supervisor should act as a role model for teacher trainees.

Comparison between Traditional teaching and Microteaching

	Traditional teaching		Microteaching
1.	Objectives are not specified in behavioral terms.	1.	Objectives are specified in behavioral terms
2.	Class consists 50 to 100 student teachers	2.	Consists of 5 to 10 students
3.	Teaching becomes complex and threatening	3.	Relatively simple and nonthreatening
4.	Feedback is not immediately provided	4.	Immediate feedback is provided
5.	The role of supervisor is vague and is not helpful to improve teaching	5.	The role of supervisor is specific and well defined to improve teaching
6.	Pattern of classroom interaction cannot be objectively studied	6.	Objectively studied
7.	School teacher practices whole complex teaching behavior	7.	Student teacher practices only one skill selected for practice
8.	Time duration is 45 to 60 minutes.	8.	Time duration is 5 to 10 minutes.

Advantages

1. Superior performance.
2. Real teaching: The teacher and learners work together in a practice situation.
3. Accomplishment of specific tasks: Tasks are the practice of instructional skills, the practice of techniques of teaching, the mastery of certain curricular materials or the demonstration of the teaching method.
4. Increased control of practice.
5. Expansion of the normal knowledge of results or feedback dimension in teaching.
6. Helps in solving some of the problems involved in student teaching practice: As microteaching focuses upon specific teaching skills, it enables the supervisor and the learner to approach the job in the spirit of mastering the teaching model. The appraisal of the student teaching becomes more objective because he himself is involved in the appraisal of his micro lesson.
7. Effective in modifying teaching behavior.
8. Helps in developing important teaching skills: Microteaching was effective in developing the skills of questioning, reinforcement, silence and nonverbal cues, illustration and use of example.
9. Effective technique for transfer of general teaching competence to classroom teaching.
10. Provides a good prelude to a macro lesson: It helps in building confidence step-by-step, provides continuous reinforcement to the teacher trainees performance and improves his/her teaching behavior. A good micro lesson prepares the way for a good macro-lesson.

11. Different feedback forms: As oral feedback by the supervise by the peer group audio and videotape recording provide accurate and powerful feedback.
12. Provides safe practice ground.
13. Provides many opportunities to trainee to study the desired patterns of behavior.
14. Lessens the complexities of the normal classroom teaching by 'scaled down teaching'.
15. Individualizes teacher training
16. Facilitates the combination of a number of devices.
17. Facilitates the development of teaching skills., e.g. Reinforcement, Probing questions.
18. It is a teaching in a relatively simple (only one skill is selected practice) and non threatening (because the number of students is hardly 5 to 10).
19. The student teacher can easily focus his attention on clearly defined aspects of the behavior.
20. Provision for much fuller and more objective feedback to the trainee than in other teacher training procedures.
21. Immediate evaluation and additional trails will be done.
22. The student teacher can concentrate on some specific aspects of teaching-learning.
23. The microteaching sequence proves most effective when one or two teaching skills are selected for emphasis.
24. Patterns of classroom interaction and communication between the teacher and the students can be objectively and easily studied.
25. The objectives of microteaching are specified in terms of behavioral outcomes.
26. Individual micro-lessons are observed by other teachers and improvements can be suggested by them by observing video recording.
27. It is more manageable than classroom teaching as number of persons involved is less and duration of time is also less.
28. Observable, demonstrable and quantifiable skills are used.
29. It operates in a healthy environment where only the fellow teachers and colleagues are available.
30. It enables the student teacher to view and hear her/his own performance and thus enable him/her to make self-criticism.
31. Senior teachers can guide the junior teachers in a practical manner where improvement of skills can occur by identifying their strengths and weaknesses.
32. Subsequent cycles of microteaching results in critical analysis and improvement in teaching skills.

Limitations

- It is only a simulated technique with less number of persons over a short period of time
- It is expensive to procure and to maintain video recording equipment just for microteaching
- Limited to lecturing
- Conducted under controlled environment where different audio-visual resources, etc. are provided
- Real life situations are quite different
- It does not apply to skills like decision-making, Preparation of audio-visual resources, Maintaining student records, etc.
- Minimum of feedback sequence to choose from, the feedback provided by a simulation is not total but only the most likely feedback
- Time consuming
- Difficulty in using analytic approach
- Need for many simulators since instruction is individualized
- Scope is narrow
- Requires more skill.

ASSIGNMENT METHOD

It is generally advocated for teaching different subjects to learners in the higher classes. The syllabus is split up into significant units or topics. Each unit or topic, in its turn is subdivided into learning assignments for learners. The learners are usually required to prepare the assignments in writing. Written assignments help in organization of knowledge, assimilation of facts and better preparation for examinations.

Types
1. Preparatory assignment: Used for circulation purposes. The learners can be prepared for the work, which is to follow on the next day. After this preliminary pilot work, the teacher can lead the class with ease and understanding.
2. The study assignments: Learners carry on the study individually or in a group. The assignments can vary with the individuals, 'each according to his need' and 'each according to his capacity'. The assignment can range from a page or paragraph assignment to a topic, problem, project, exercise, report, unit, chapter, and experiment. The teacher guides the learners in their problems.
3. The revisional assignments: It is given for
   a. Providing drill to the work done by the students.
   b. Checking their retention and reproduction of facts, incidents, etc. of the topic.
   c. For checking the understanding of the topic.
   These assignments worked out in advance keeping in view the specific objectives of the subject matter being tested.
4. The remedial assignments: These assignments are devised in the light of pupil's reactions to the preparatory assignments, study assignments, revisional assignments.
   The purpose of these assignments is to remove weak points and clear misunderstandings.
5. Common assignments: Every member of the class works. These assignments are useful for basic learning of all the students in general.
6. Small group assignments: Tailored to the needs, interests and abilities of each small group in the class. Thus, in a heterogeneous class, a basic assignments will be given to the slow learner and the same assignments, in an enriched form will be given to the intelligent students.
7. Individual assignments: Is different and distinct for each pupil. It is designed in accordance with each pupil's achievement, level, interest, abilities, aptitudes and need. It solves educational problems created by differences in a large group of students.

Criteria of a good assignment
1. Definite, clear and interesting.
2. Sufficiently challenging to stimulate pupil's interest in it.
3. Significantly related to the topic of which it forms a part.
4. Lead learners to meaningful complete learning experiences.
5. Appeal to the pupil's curiosity or his/her desire to achieve a well established interest.
6. It should not be too, big i.e., not to take more than a week to prepare it.
7. It should not take more than two class periods to discuss it in broad outlines.
8. It should be flexible enough to meet the different range of interests and abilities represented in the group.

Procedure
The syllabus of the subject for a particular class, may be divided into suitable units and then, a tentative plan for preparatory study assignments has to be chalked out.
1. Preparation for the assignments: Efforts should be made for developing the pupil's interest in writing the assignments. Broad heading under which assignments has to be written should be outlined. The necessary information, which would help the learners in working out the assignments, should be given. The work can be completed in one period.
2. Writing the assignment: The pupil may write assignments at home or in the class. If they write the assignment in the class under the supervision of the teacher, they should be allowed the facilities to review books and ask questions whenever necessary. This work may take more than one class period.
3. Selection of pairs of pupil for mutual correction: The pupil may be given a variety of probable errors, which may occur in the subject to help them in their correction work. Common errors may be omission of vital facts, wrong statement of facts, statement of irrelevant facts, failure to bring out casual relationships, errors in language and spelling, etc. the pupil may be asked to point out all those.

4. Peer Review: The group of learners may be asked to correct their assignments by peer review or within the class exchange of assignments.
5. Correction of sample assignment scripts: It is done by the teacher and preparation of common list of errors.
6. Discussion of the list in a correction class: The common errors committed by the pupil should be discussed in a correction class to prevent their recurrence.

Advantages

1. It is a kind of activity method, the learners learn through their own activity as self-study and writing.
2. The assignment gives the pupil guidance in an expert way, prevents failure for the arousal of interest and ensures success.
3. Assignment places the greatest emphasis on individual pupil work. Thus the learners learn to be on their own.
4. Through written assignments, the learners get training in the organization of facts which is very useful.
5. An assignment enables the teacher to know the interests of learners in a particular subject area. He/she is also able to discover the specific abilities of the individual pupil, which may be developed and used for their own good.
6. Assignments provide the best possible mindset, which is prerequisite for effective learning.
7. It makes learning an exciting experience for learners.
8. The teacher can foresee the difficulties, which the students may have to face in the learning of a topic. He/she can guide the learners by intelligently putting thought provoking questions in his assignments. Guidance provided to read or to study a topic will prepare the learners to face the difficulties boldly.
9. The method helps both teaching and learning processes. The experience gained through the assignments will help in remedial teaching and learning.
10. The method is suitable for the learners of different ability levels–gifted, average and slow.

Limitations

1. Time Consuming even though it is brainstorming for the learners.
2. Lack of Resources for broad review related to topic.
3. Internet availability and accessibility is limited to students or expensive for browsing the information.
4. The learner has to develop skills in preparing and incorporating the content in topic.

PROBLEM SOLVING METHOD

To train the minds of the learners by confronting them with real problems and giving them the opportunity and freedom to solve them. The major purpose of the problem is to afford training to the learners in thinking, in solving the problems mentally. Problem solving approach is meaningful, developmental, sequential, based on the discovery of generalizations. It involves the thought process that results from doubt, proplexity or a problem. The approach leads to the formulation of generalizations that are useful in future situation involving the solution of problems. It is an important contribution to learning.

Steps

1. Discovering, considering, discussing, selecting and stating the specific problem or question.
2. Collecting, organizing, comparing and judging significant information in the light of the defined problem.
3. Exploring the problem and framing some possible solutions.
4. Drawing preliminary conclusions for further exploration and study.
5. Evaluating findings and establishing a conclusion.
6. Considering the summarization with the possibility of further study.

Essential Qualities of a Problem

1. It should be in line with the need and interests of a particular group of learners.
2. The problem should be valuable and timely.
3. It should impart functional and rich learning.

4. The learners should feel that the problem is their own. The teacher can motivate the learners in a manner to make the learners think out, the problem under study by themselves.
5. Learners should identify the problem and its means of execution to avoid wastage of time.
6. Conclusions and generalizations once found, has to be stated very clearly so that these can be further used in the solution of new problems.

Major Approaches

- Inductive
- Deductive
- Analytic
- Synthetic.

Inductive Approach

Here the child is enabled to arrive at the general conclusion, establish laws or formulate generalizations through the observation of particular facts and concrete examples. After a number of concrete cases are understood the student can successfully attempt the generalization, e.g. in a grammar lesson, the teacher while teaching 'noun' may give examples and then, help the learners to frame a sentence by listing the noun.

Merits
1. It is easy to understand a grammatical or mathematical principle establishes through a number of simple examples. The doubts, about, how and why of a formula are clarified in the very beginning.
2. It is a logical method.
3. It gives the opportunity of active participation to the students in the discovery of a formula.
4. It is based on actual observation, thinking and experimentation.
5. It reduces dependence on memorization and homework.
6. When a new rule has to be taught, inductive approach is the best.
7. It gives freedom from doubt and helps in understanding.

Drawbacks
1. It contains the process of discovering the formula with the help of a sufficient number of cases, but 'what next' is not provided in it. The discovery of a formula does not complete the study of the topic. A lot of supplementary work and practice is needed to fix the topic in the mind of the learner.
2. Inductive reasoning is not absolutely conclusive. 3 or 4 cases are picked up to generalize an observation. Therefore the process establishes a certain degree of probability which can, of course, be increased and made more valid by increasing the number of cases.
3. It is likely to be laborious and time consuming.
4. At the advanced stage, it is not so useful as some of the unnecessary details and explanations may become dull and boring.

Deductive Approach

The learner proceeds from general to particular, abstract to concrete and formula to example.

The preconstructed formula is explained to the students and they are asked to solve the problem with the help of that formula. The formula or definition is accepted by the learner as a well-established truth.

The teacher announces the relevant formula or definition.

The students accept the general statement or the rules and the formula without challenging regardless of whether they are correct or incorrect in harmony with outer reality, the approach is authoritative and developmental.

Merits
1. The method is short and time-saving. The books and teachers thus have some preference for it.
2. It glorifies memory, as the students have to memorize a considerable number of formulae and definitions.
3. During practice and revision stage, deductive method is adequate and advantageous.
4. It combines with the inductive method to remove the incompleteness and inadequacy of the later.
5. It enhances speed and efficiency in solving problems.

Drawbacks

1. It is very difficult for a beginner to understand an abstract formula, if it is not preceded by a number of concrete instances.
2. Pure deductive work requires a formula for every type of problem and an extensive use of this method will demand the blind memorization of a large number of formulae. It will thus cause an unnecessary and heavy burden on the brain.
3. Memory is more important than understanding and intelligence.
4. If the pupil forgets the memorized formula which is very likely in cramming, he cannot recollect and reconstruct the formula easily.
5. The students cannot become active learners.
6. It is not suitable for the development of thinking, reasoning and discovery.

Inductive and Deductive approaches aim at establishing the validity of the thought process. Deduction can only give formal validity because the rule is taken for granted. This may be misleading if the general statement is wrong. It is only induction which tests the material validity i.e., whether the application of deduction is actually real or not. Thus induction must supplement deduction to complete the thought process. Induction is to be forerunner or predecessor of deductive. The deductive will give a good follow-up, if the understanding is earlier obtained through induction. The loss of time, due to the slow speed of induction, can be covered up through quick and timesaving process of deduction. Deduction serve as complement of induction. Induction leaves the learner at a point where he cannot stop. The after work has to be completed by deduction.

Deduction is a process suitable for a final statement and induction is most suited for the exploration of new fields. Probability in induction is raised to certainty in deduction.

The modern teaching always starts with induction, leads to deduction, where the knowledge learnt is verified and then ends in induction, where the knowledge is applied to further examples.

Analytic Approach

Analytic means the breaking up of the problem in hand so that it ultimately gets connected with something obvious or already known to us. It is the process of unfolding of the problem or conducting its operation to know its hidden aspects. We start with, what we have to find out. Then we think of further steps and possibilities which may connect the unknown with known and lead us to find out the desired result.

Thorndike says that all the highest performance of the mind is analysis.

Merits

1. It is logical method, leaves no doubts and convinces the learner.
2. It is a suitable method for understanding and discovery.
3. The steps, in its procedure are developed in a general manner. Each step has its reasons and justification.
4. The student is throughout subjected with questions and thus increases the power at every step.

Drawbacks

1. It is a lengthy method.
2. Difficult to acquire efficiency and speed with this method.
3. It may not be applicable to all the topics equally well.

Synthetic Approach

We proceed from known to unknown. Synthesis is to place together things that are apart. It begins from something already known and connects it with the unknown part of the statement. It begins with the data available or known and connects them with the unknown. It is the process of putting together known bits of information to reach the point where unknown information becomes obvious and true.

Both are independent. The teacher can help for the analytic form of the solution and synthetic work left to the learners.

Merits

1. Problem solving constitutes a realistic method for presenting the type of experience that the pupil will face throughout his career. It gives him/her a fine chance to think, to judge and evaluate, to compare and select

which is best. Whenever a specific question has to be answered, the facts have to be marshalled and directed toward solution. The individual is challenged to bring to bear all his information and experience in such a problem, which arouses his/her interest and awakens his/her curiosity.

2. The problem furnishes a natural objective. He/she can easily see its significance and works for its solution.
3. This method provides for logical way of thinking in the learners. The pupil can see the necessity and sequence of following each step systematically.
4. The problem enables the pupil to utilize what he/she knows and focuses this knowledge upon the unknown. He/she learns to attack fresh problems with the knowledge at his/her command.
5. The problem can be adjusted to groups as well as individuals. It thus promotes adaptation without sacrificing the social values that arise from cooperative understanding.
6. The method develops initiative and responsibility. The pupil appreciates that the process is not a task which is assigned, but an inevitable requirement of the situation.
7. The traits of open-mindedness and tolerance develop as the children see many sides to a problem and listen to many points of view. The horizon of thinking is widened. They learn to think critically and independently and they learn to struggle for solutions of selected problems.
8. Good and cordial relations between the teacher and pupil are established and promoted.
   The pupil feels free from arbitrarily imposed tasks of the teacher. He/she learns to appreciate the guidance of the teacher. Thus, a foundation is laid for good and happy relations between teachers and taught, which is indispensable for the success of the teaching learning process.
9. The problem can be adjusted according to the needs. It can be a small unit or a long-term assignment.

Limitations

1. This method will become monotonous if used too frequently. So, it can be used as one of the procedures and not as the sole method.
2. The pupil can start over estimating themselves. Problem solving in the classroom means solution of simple problem. It is just an exercise to give training to the learners. But there is a danger. The solution of simple problems may easily lead the pupil to think that he/she has acquired a technique i.e., applicable to complex social problem as well as to classroom exercises.
3. There is a danger that the problems may be selected which may be trivial, untimely or problems that generate more feeling and emotion than thought. This danger can be avoided, if the teacher is very cautious in selecting the problem.
4. The method may easily become a seminar method i.e., too advanced for learners. Very capable teachers are required to avoid dissatisfaction and discouragement on the part of the learners.

Synthesis	Analysis
The learner is just like a man being led blindfolded to the desired goal	It is lengthy method, needs the help of synthesis for the removal of this defect. If it is not followed by stimulus, it will not be useful
——	Synthesis is the complement of analysis, they always go together
——	Analysis leads to synthesis and synthesis makes purposes of analysis clear and complete
It helps to retain the knowledge in memory	It helps to understand
Forms the follow-up work	It forms the beginning

PROCESS RECORDING/INTERPERSONAL RELATIONS RECORDINGS/PATIENT-NURSE INTERACTION INTERVIEWS

Introduction

It is a tool used in "Teaching, Counseling and in Psychiatry field". The art of effective communication is a dynamic process. Nursing students are continually attempting to cope with the wide range of human interactions and have an opportunity to observe and provide care for person's with varied stressors and exposed to wide range of experiences. Often they are faced with conflicts which arise within the interpersonal process. How effectively they can cope with these conflicts will depends on a large measure on "The factor of Readiness".

Nurse has to use effective use of interpersonal communication techniques according to their intellectual level, maturity of judgment and capacity for adaptability. The importance of the therapeutic nurse-patient relationship, the emotional support required by patients, the identification and the understanding of patient's emotional and physical needs and the methods of assisting patients to work out solutions to their health related problems are being recognized. Process recording is being utilized as a tool to help them in assisting nursing students to acquire understanding of and to establish competence in IPR.

Definition

"A verbatim account of a visit for purposes of bringing out the interplay between the nurse and the patient in relation to the objectives of the visit"–Walker

"An exact written report of the conversation between the nurse and the patient during the time they were together and a record of the nurse's feelings about what was going on at the time and as far as possible, how the patient said what he did"–Hudson

Purposes

- Used as a data collecting instrument for
    - A teaching tool
    - A self-evaluation tool
    - A therapeutic tool—Patients can be helped more efficaciously by a nurse who has knowledge of the dynamics of human behavior and skill in using their own behavior, as a therapeutic tool
    - Communication tool
    - helpful tool in learning about IPR and gaining competence in related skills
- Brown and Fowler described many folded functions of a nurse
    - Observer/Spectator
    - Participant
    - Introspectionist
- Evaluates the effectiveness of their own communication and assessing the communication skills of others
- Able to assess their own strengths and weaknesses in IPR, which becomes the base for the assimilation of new knowledge and skills.

Elements of Communication studied through Process Recording

- Conversational skills
- Structured Interviewing skills
- Verbal and nonverbal cues to the patient's needs
- Skill in meeting the patient's needs
- Awareness of their own behavior
- Assessment of their own strengths and weaknesses (introspection, analysis, synthesis skills) in communicating and meeting the felt needs of the client
- To develop self-control of behavior
- Promotes the nurse-patient interaction
- Skills in verbal communication, responding to the needs of client by Interaction
- Generic experiences for student's own growth with their own efforts.

Technique

1. Preparing the student for process recording
    a. The teacher assists the student to formulate the objectives in behavioral terms regarding "Nurse-Patient Interaction"
    b. Discuss with the student the objectives of process recording as a teaching and learning tool and the teachers' expectations in terms of progress and scheduled time to accomplish the desired goals.
    c. Teacher has to teach the student to learn the process of documentation in writing a process record.

2. Recording nurse-patient interaction
a. The "exact verbatim report of the Patient-Nurse conversation", "the student's conscious feelings", "their interpretation of the patient's feelings" and "analysis for meanings and clues to patient's needs" has to be recorded.
b. The instructor's and the student's evaluation of the total process record experience to be effective teaching and learning instrument, the necessary conditions needed are:
   - A minimum of 2 people
   - The confidentiality of the interview has to be reassured (The student also must be impressed with the importance of keeping the interview material confidential)
   - All verbal interaction has to be documented
   - Notations on thoughts, feelings and actions that the student experiences during interaction
   - Notations on the nonverbal communication of the patient
   - Notation of the interaction done as soon as possible after the interaction occurs, noting the time lapse between actual recording interaction.

3. Evaluating the nurse-patient interaction
a. After the interaction data collected by the student has to be documented, the student has to possess the knowledge of subject during the learning experience.
b. Analysis of data is time consuming.
c. During the process of analyzing the recordings, the objectives of the learning experience should be kept clearly in focus.
d. The teacher must discuss with the student before allotting the process recording. Each student is an individual and will relate to each patient in their own unique way. The individuality of the student must be respected.
e. The teacher helps the student to explore the reason for nurse-patient interaction.
f. Student needs guidance in analysis of process recording as per pre plan, a theme has to be identified to conclude generalization, a summary, abstraction, characteristic of an event consisting of many details, the student has to pay attention while documenting as these behaviors indicate an individual client's mood, thought or action.
g. Themes abstracted from the process recording facilitates comparison of one interaction situation with another, thus providing a frame of reference for interpretation of what has taken place during the interaction and what prognosis is being made over a period of time. The process of theme abstraction involves identifying cues from the patient's verbal and nonverbal communication or from the nurse's response to the interaction, analyzing the significance of these cues and then formulating a theme that summarizes the patient's behavioral response. Once the theme has been formulated, the nurse should seek consensual validation of her conclusions. The teacher's function in this phase of learning is to provide the consensual validation for the student's conclusions or if she/he does not agree with the student, to repeat the theme abstraction process together with the student describing, analyzing and formulating another theme. As the student's skill increases she/he may assume greater responsibility for independent analysis of both the patient's communication and her/his own. Thus, self-evaluation is an integral part of process recording analysis.
h. It provides the teacher with an accurate account of the student's clinical learning experience.
i. It makes it possible for the teacher to utilize interaction situations post facto in helping the student to learn communication skills. This eliminates the necessity of he/she being present during the interaction, as this is frequently anxiety provoking for the student.
j. The instructor has to use the technique correctly.
k. Time consuming.

Form
   1. Goals for working with assigned patient.
   2. Important factors in patient's personality development (from history).
   3. Somatic therapies and medications used for patient (past and present).
   4. Date of each recording.

5. Amount of time, which you spent with the patient.
6. Describe briefly the setting or situation previous to conversation.

Format in process recording

Conversation between Student-Nurse and Patient	Student's comments	Instructor's comments
		Signature

7. Identify the patient's needs as represented by behavior.
8. Identify mental mechanisms that you think the patient is using and give examples.
9. After completion of this assignment, comment on how well you were able to meet the goals which you set up for working with assigned patient.
10. Evaluate the process record as a learning experience for the student at the end of the assignment.

PROJECT METHOD

Definitions

"A project is a problematic act carried to completion in its natural setting"–*Stevenson*

"A whole-hearted, purposeful activity proceeding in a social environment"–*Dr Kilpartrick*

"A project is a bit of real life that has been imparted into the school", in project method, "learning by living, this life has spontaneity, purpose, significance, interest and freedom"–*Ballard*

"The strong desire to achieve a certain end provides intense stimulus and increases the interest of the child in, what he is doing".

"Any unit of purposeful experience in which the dominating purpose is an inner urge that fixes the aim or objective of the action and guides its process to completion".

To be a project, the learning activity must be:
1. Problem oriented in nature.
2. Aimed at a definite, attainable objective and measurable goal.
3. Purposeful, natural and life like in its procedure to attain the goal.
4. Directed and planned by the student by himself.
5. Practical in nature with emphasis on a single, complete unit of purposeful activity, resulting in a concrete achievement. The undertaking must be complete in itself.
6. True creative thinking, true mental activity are essential.

Characteristics of a Good Project Method

1. The method aims at teaching the child to get the best out of life.
2. An attempt to use experience – the trust and best master–whose lessons are unforgettable.
3. Project method gives an opportunity for self-expression and for relating the self to the community.
4. The experiments of the project method has to reset the whole curriculum and break all barriers of subject matter.
5. The project method proposes the whole sequence of activities involved in a complete undertaking. Children has to develop their knowledge by trying out theories into practical solution of problems in the course of which they would come to appreciate the principles involved. Fresh knowledge is acquired only as a result of the felt needs of the learners.
6. A project can be a large unit of appreciational learning or of attitude development, that increases motor skills and technical knowledge.
7. A project is a play activity and children engaged in carrying out of activities.

8. The project method is a complete surrender to the child's point of view. It seeks to offer the pupil complete freedom of choice of the problem to be solved, as well as the means to be employed.
9. In the project method the procedure of the school is liable to be determined by the technique of workshop, because the child learns much better from his own activity than from constant instruction.
10. Establishes a positive relation with life.
11. The project method lends itself naturally to group work.
12. It is a large unit plan of teaching. A project is a learning unit of appreciable length, difficulty and learning value.
13. The method seeks to have individuals see and understand life in its unity.

Types of Projects

A. Dr. Kilpatrick has suggested 4 types.
1. Producer type: Projects in which learners are getting to do something like participating in workshops or game activities, conducts exhibition, planning to execute a model of a circulation for Anatomy lab, etc.
2. Consumer type: Projects in which learners are getting the experience and are enjoying eg: participating in cultural activities, extra cultural activities and in games and sports.
3. Problem type: Project in which a solution to a problem, is worked out, e.g. drugs and solutions calculations in basic principles of nursing and practice.
4. Drill type: An activity once performed, is repeated to acquire greater skill, e.g. swimming or singing. Project method involves all types of mental and manipulative activities.

B. Based on purposes and the objectives by which the learning activities are unified and shaped.
1. Projects calling for the production of some physical or material product, e.g. innovation of chemicals useful for Home activities to maintain cleanliness.
2. Learning project, acquisition of some ability, e.g. learning of Injection technique.
3. Intellectual or problem projects, e.g. narrating some experience in the form of mental activity like writing poem, stories, songs, drama or novel, etc.

Essentials of Good Project

1. The project should stress present and future values and experiences that supplement and extend rather than duplicate learning.
2. The project must have a bearing on varied subjects and the knowledge acquired through it may be applicable in a variety of ways.
3. The project should be timely, challenging and feasible.

Organizing a Project

1. The teacher must review the subject content, analyze the felt need of learner and demand needs of the respective university and carefully provide individualized guidance in selection of the project with their own efforts. The teacher will act as facilitator, counselor for the student during problem selection, synapsis preparation and viva presentation.
   Teacher has to see projects are educative and according to the capability/Strengths/ability of the learner and based on their speciality requirement and at the need of hour (like societal felt needs), sometimes it may arise in the classroom teaching or discussion.
2. Whole-heartedness acceptance of the project, almost every learner has to be secured, if the teacher wants to ensure its success.
3. Organized planning is essential before hand. It may be in the form of drawing or list of steps to be followed, materials to be used, a Audio-visual aids to be prepared or other specific indications of what has to be done.
4. The project is an activity oriented to meet certain purposes.
5. To avoid interruptions and delays later, sufficient preparation could be done before executing the project.
6. During the execution of the project, the teacher should carefully supervise the learners in manipulative skills to save time and prevent waste of materials and to guard against accidents or unecessary/subjective problems and recurrent failures.

7. The relation between chalked out plans and the developing project has to be constantly monitored. Spot modification not advisable, but, if there are any, these should be noted and the reasons explained for future guidance.

8. To maintain standards, ethically approvable and qualitative one, teacher has to take careful steps or precautions, whereby learners' learning capacity will be maximized and helpful in future, evaluation of the project has to be done both by the learners (self-evaluation, peer evaluation) and by the teacher (Concurrent and Final Evaluation, viz. Open Viva, theory exam at the end of an academic year). Teacher also may face certain problems when they want to maintain the standards and improve students' capacities, she/he is implementing specific steps, certain times hard decisions has to be made which may result into strained interpersonal relationship, communication gaps may result, so teacher has to handle the situation very carefully, as it is very sensitive to deal, counseling skills may be necessary to implement activities into action, in order to build the future of fraternity in general and the learner in specific.

9. Learner has to possess skills in self-assessment, Observation skills, Interaction and listening skills, insight, the value of information/knowledge in subject matter, inquisitiveness, interest in improvement, self motivation skills and positive approach/optimism attitudes.

10. Teacher has to facilitate or provide conducive environment to organize the project method successfully.

11. Teacher can promote interest among learners to communicate research findings of project by publishing project results through articles in journals (National and International).

12. In Project method based on intellectual skills, aptitude, attitude, interest of learner the instructional objectives and activities, mode of teaching, assignments will be allotted. But teacher always put efforts in successful completion of project by individual student at the maximum and meets University specifications. Overall teacher will act as "Moderator" and monitors the learners' activities to maximize the learners' abilities.

Merits

1. The psychological laws of learning will be utilized in teaching learning process
   a. Law of readiness
   b. Law of exercise
   c. Law of effect
   d. Psychological concept of maturation.

2. Follows naturalism principle, i.e. the learner will have the liberty in selecting the problem of his/her interest in his/her speciality which university enrolled, (requirements and availability of Research Guide interest, broad review of related literature in area of interest).

3. Derives social values.

4. Training will be given in social adjustments.

5. Maintains learner's honesty, qualitative nature.

6. Trains for a democratic, individualistic, independent way of life.

7. Learning through problem solving.

8. Student and the Teacher grow in a positive direction.
   a. The student stimulated by and encourages in his/her exploration of varied materials, which ultimately approach other areas of learning in a similar manner.
   b. The teacher will grow in her/his understanding of learner's creative developments.

9. Confers on school work.

10. Promotes sense of reality.

11. Intrinsic standard of evaluation set up.

12. Satisfaction of completing the whole task.

13. Economical: The children take more interest and learn in the shortest possible time. Atmosphere of freedom is conducive to learning. Leaner will pick-up knowledge without strain.

14. Upholds the dignity of labour.

15. Qualities like self-reliance, resourcefulness and responsibility among the learners will be enhanced.

16. Ideal for the subjects like Science, Handicraft, Geography, Dramatic work and Literature.

Limitations

1. Learning haphazard and incidental.
2. The role of communication subordinated to the glorification of active learning.
3. The practical difficulties of covering a syllabus rule out the project method as the basis of teaching in most schools.
4. Time-consuming and limited by availability and cost of materials.
5. Most valuable among learners of lesser academic ability, as it provides an opportunity for the practical enthusiasm.
6. Leave gaps in the learner's knowledge.
7. May be too ambitious and beyond the learner's capacity.
8. For success in schools run on the basis of this method, the requisite conditions more in the way of buildings and equipment, more ability, zeal and preparation on the part of teachers, more science and a higher art in the work itself than needed in other schools. The employment of this method will call for more highly qualified teachers and a more generous staffing ratio.
9. Opportunities for correlation with the academic subjects are extremely limited.
10. The method of organizing instruction is unsystematized and upsets the regular timetable work.
11. Difficulty to ensure any kind of systematic progress in instruction.
12. A complete reorganization of the school is needed for new teacher.
13. The resultant education emphasizes relationships in breadth not in depth.
14. Too ambitious.
15. Learner may ignore maxim "the simple to complex".
16. Among learners the critical powers outrun their executive skill, hence their criticism of the products of their work may inhibit them from taking fresh projects.
17. Time bound projects introduce artificiality and may require more than necessary help.
18. Projects may be adopted or abandoned at will.
19. It is not easy to formulate projects having a satisfactory degree of width and comprehensiveness at a later stage of education.
20. The project approach often results in an incomplete mastery of the tools of learning which are essential means to learner's education later.

Teacher's Role

The teacher has got mature experience, deeper and broader knowledge. learners need suggestions and guidance at every step. The teacher has to save the learners from faltering and floundering. So the teacher has to skillfully guide in the selection of topic for project method. The teacher suggests help when it is required. Teacher possess good prompter. The relations of the teacher to the learners are to be much closer and informal than it is an ordinary classroom teaching. He/she performs their role like a friend with rich or vast and mature experience. She/he is a director, her psychological knowledge must be thorough and scientific.

The teacher must be a keen observer and a true sympathizer. She/he should be able to win the goodwill of the learners so that they will not feel discouraged. She/he is a storehouse of information and knowledge so that she/he may anticipate the difficulties before-hand and suggest remedies as and when necessary. Teacher should command respect of the learners so that the learners might look to her for help, guidance, solace and affection.

- The project method is based on correlated teaching
- The teachcer has to guide the execution of the project that the maximum number of subjects concerned are learnt by the learners, gaps are properly filled
- Teacher has to see that complete and integrated knowledge is given. Experiences and contributions of the group should provide increase knowledge in the particular context
- The teacher has to spare enough time for the success of this method. Only a devoted and enthusiastic teacher can make a success of the project method, not the discouraged, time-serving and bell-watchers

CASE STUDY

Nursing Care Study

Case study is a comprehensive study of an individual. The medical case study centers about the patient, his disease and the related medical treatment. The Nursing case study centers around the patient, his problems, his needs and the nursing care he/she receives. The emphasis is on the patient and his/her needs during illness and recovery and the nurse's method of meeting these needs.

The doctor studies the patient for the purpose of diagnosis and treatment, while nurses' study the disease for the purpose of deciding intelligently the best type of nursing care to be given. To do this she/he needs to know not only the techniques of nursing care, but also disease condition in detail.

Nursing care study place emphasis on the actual nursing care of the patient. It is a case study in which there is a comprehensive study made of the individual patient to bring about a fuller understanding of the needed nursing care, to improve the nursing care given to the patient and to prepare the patient to return to his community not only cured of his present illness but also fortified with knowledge and ability to improve and maintain good health standards for himself, his family and his community.

Values

1. Provides an opportunity for the student to solve nursing problems.
2. Stimulates the student to meet her/his problems by critical and reflective thinking. The student learns the scientific method of study or approach to a problem and how to apply this method to her/his problems.
3. Emphasizes the fact that the patient is an individual personality and not just so many procedures or symptoms.
4. Accentuates the health and the social aspects of Nursing. The student comes to realize what an important opportunity and vital responsibility and she/he has, as a teacher of health in the home, the hospital and the community.
5. Points out the relationship and the cooperation of the various agencies interested in the patient's problems and welfare such as social service and public health nursing.
6. Acquaints the students with professional literature which has special bearing on nursing problems.
7. Helps to establish in the student's mind a definite syndrome of various diseases. This enables her/him to record actual case given to the patient, as well as the study of theoretical treatment of the disease.
8. Helps the student to integrate all knowledge of the various subjects.
9. Contributes to the building up of a specific body of knowledge in Nursing Science.
10. Helps to improve the general nursing care of the patient.

Limitations

1. Too often it has been used as an end in itself, instead of as a means to an end; this is to help the student to understand more fully the needed nursing care. If too many nursing care studies are demanded, the student does not have time to do a thorough study.
2. The type of study selected also limits its usefulness. If the new student attempts to study a complicated nursing care, it probably will be poor learning experience for her as well as discouraging one. She cannot do a good case study because she does not have sufficient background to solve the problems encountered.
3. Time factor—If the student is to make a good nursing care study, she/he must be given sufficient time to study her/his patient as she/he cares for him. Good nursing care studies require time.

Principles

- The student should make her/his nursing care study on patient for whose nursing care, she/he is responsible
- The selection of the patient for the student's nursing care study has to be done cooperatively by the clinical instructor and the nursing student
- The first consideration of the student in the development of her/his nursing care study will be the nursing care of the patient
- She/he has to study the patient's social status, cultural background, economic level, hobbies and special interests, for an understanding, these factors will contribute to the patient's welfare

- She/he has to study the medical aspects of the patient's condition as this knowledge is needed for her/him to give intelligent nursing care.

The first part of the study should be concerned with the confirmation and facts about the patient, his/her disease condition, social and personal history and how this knowledge is applied in the nursing care of the patient.

The second part of the nursing study takes in the responsibilities and the activities with which the nursing student will be concerned in giving complete nursing care to the patient.

The nursing care study serves as an excellent medium to help the student to develop the skills and techniques needed to function well in the nursing team.

In nursing care plan, which can be used as a part of the nursing care study has two major divisions:

1. Prescribed medical orders, treatments and medicines
2. The nursing care given to the patient: The nursing care should include the supportive and therapeutic care given to the patient
3. Through the nursing care study emphasis should be on the individual need of the patient and how these are met.
4. Through conferences the student can be helped to express her/his understanding of the patients need for teaching and the manner in which the student helped to meet them, including the problems.
5. The nursing care study serves as an excellent means for the student to demonstrate her/his nursing skill, scientific knowledge, sociologic and psychological insight into the problems of the patient and skill in interpersonal relations with the patient as a nurse.

Advantages
1. It provides for individual difference of the students, self-expression in writing.
2. It provides experience in organizing and writing a paper in a scientific manner.
3. It provides a source of material for future uses.

Limitations
1. It leaves no opportunity once the study is completed, to branch out and incorporate new ideas.
2. It requires a great deal of time to rewrite into an acceptable form.

Oral Nursing Care Study

It is presented by one or more students in the form of a verbal report to the clinical instructor or to a group of students.

Advantages
1. It provides an opportunity for the instructor to direct a student's thinking into new channels and to correct errors of information.
2. It serves as a basis for a better personal understanding and relationship between the instructor and the student.
3. It is time saving. It does not require lengthy recopying of notes into acceptable form.
4. It offers an opportunity for public speaking experience.
5. If discussion is invited after presentation the case becomes cooperative and all benefit from the study. This is a source of motivation to the student because she shares the benefits of her/his study with other students.

Limitations
1. It does not offer an opportunity for writing and other creative expression, since only notes are used for presentation.
2. It leaves no record which may be kept for future reference.

WORKSHOP

Definition

"A meeting during which experienced people in response positions come together with experts and consultants to find solutions to problems that have cropped up in the course of their work and that they have had difficulty in dealing with on their own. Participants themselves select the objectives they wish to reach and help in choosing the problems for group work".

"A systematic approach to deal in detail about educational problems by means of a short meeting".

A mini workshop: "A short workshop lasting for 3 or 4 days".

Principles

- Allowing the participant to prepare and select the objectives to be reached, will increase the participant's motivation.
- Giving the participant an active role will make teaching more effective
- Providing the participant with regular opportunities to see the progress he/she is making will increase his/her learning speed and improve the quality of the knowledge and skills he/she acquire
- Person's attitude towards other people
- To learn better human relations
- Every individual has worth and has a contribution to make to the common good
- The most crucial learning at any given time has to do with the individual's current problems
- Cooperation is a technique and as a way of life which is superior to competition, is primary factor to be allowed

Feature

Complete active involvement by each participant, the central theme of attendance is to work and to learn from practical experience.

Purposes

1. To put teachers in situations that will break down the barriers between them, so that they can more readily communicate.
2. To give teachers an opportunity for personal growth through accepting and working towards a goal held in common with others.
3. To give teachers an opportunity to work on the problems that are of direct, current concern to them.
4. To place teachers in a position of responsibility for their own learning.
5. To give teachers experience in a cooperative understanding.
6. Teachers will learn new methods and techniques which they can use in their own classrooms.
7. Teachers will have the opportunity in collaboration with others, to produce materials that will be useful in their teaching.
8. Teacher will be put in a situation where they will evaluate their own efforts.
9. To give the teachers an opportunity to improve their own morale.

Methods used to organize workshop

Group discussion

Participants will have the chance to discuss and solve the problems of greatest interest to them. Each member can find something in the experience of others that has a bearing on the questions of most interest to him will make his work more meaningful.

Plenary sessions

Organizers and participants responsible to find solutions to the problems selected. Participants may act as group leaders or rapporteurs.

Procedure

- Select the 'theme' of the workshop
- Identify the resource personnel and obtain consent
- Organizing team will prepare Budget plan, Venue fixation and accommodation facility arrangement for the participants has to be taken care (Choose the place, where participants can stay comfortably attend total activities) in advance.

- Confirm the date of workshop, it should not coincide public holidays, professional commitments of political meetings. At least one working day will precede the opening of the workshop
- Print brochure (pamphlet/hand chart) specifying the aims, registration fee, activities specifying sub themes with specifying session name, speaker, program specified
- Select homogeneous participants (2 months before day of workshop, 45 days before confirmation of participants is needed)
- Written confirmation detailing the specified conditions
- Committee of sponsors, assistant organisers, volunteers has to be formulated
- National language is working language
- Documentation of activities in workshop is required budget for equipment, checklist, publicity has to be planned
- Inform press
- Coordination of activities
- Preliminary introductory session, orientation towards workshop's theme and objectives, program specification.
- Formation of groups
- Assignment, clarifying sessions, practical exercises, group presentation, preview of next working day, individual consultation and evaluation.

Outcomes of Workshop

- Widening of specified knowledge, profession and personal growth; social interactions, friendships team spirit and human relations, etc. will be benefitted, activities held in workshop also one has to plan in advance.

QUESTIONING

Introduction

Questioning is a very ancient method of teaching used by Socrates, who actually invented it. Questioning is used by almost every faculty in all the fields in the classroom and there is a need for all instructors to improve their questioning techniques. The key to successful questioning is asking questions at an appropriate cognitive level that stimulates a response. Questioning is the educative activity, it is the first stimuli to the mental life of the child and it remains throughout the life.

Teaching is constant expansion of knowledge , development of educational material and the way to verify this development is by questioning the student. Questions will be asked in a class, on a newly taught topic, teacher has to be positive and creative, aimed at enhancing the knowledge and understanding levels of learner, sharpening their alertness to its implication and exposing problems which they can help to solve. Incorporating good questioning procedures into classes requires planning and forethought. Create an atmosphere in which students feel fairly relaxed and free to ask and answer questions.

Levels

To organize the purpose of questions, 'Bloom's taxonomy (1956)' described six levels of "educational objectives". In each level requires a response which uses a different kind of thought process. Based on this, questions can be framed, which will stimulate higher order of thinking activities among students.

Motivation to learn can increase insight deeper to the problem, the instructors uses questions to guide students' thought processes in a specific direction and guide the students' to improve thinking on a subject, the teachers extend their knowledge, encourage learners to think logically and deepening their understanding of a subject.

Functions

- To measure achievement and skills of students
- To determine what extent the student has prepared and mastered the essential facts in a class or assignment
- To test the student's understanding of facts
- To secure grades for purposes of record

- To stimulate and direct thought
- Promotes new viewpoints
- Understanding of cause and effect
- By judicious use of questions, teacher can help their students to develop an attitude of critical inquiry, analysis, comparisons and evaluation
- To ensure the organization of content, interpretation of materials and experiences gain the unity by the appropriate use of questions, the teacher can determine whether the student is acquiring the right interpretation, as it promotes deeper insight
- To make generalization and organize material correctly
- To facilitate interpretation and evaluation of information
- A wise, critical, inquiring attitude helps the student to function effectively in the society
- Every activity requires choosing of issues and in making decisions
- To make a final judgment, the individual must read, study, compare and evaluate
- Teacher will construct questions which give the student experience and practice in judging a situation which is extremely valuable
- Provides immediate feedback on the progress to both learners and educators
- To discover interests and abilities of students: Questions can lead to knowledge of special interests and abilities of the student soon recognizes and appreciates the teacher's sincere interest, regard and shows her/his gratitude by warmth and friendliness
- To promote the development of critical thinking
- To facilitate adaptability to new situations, make competent decisions in clinical areas
- To develop attitudes and appreciations
- Questions can stimulate thoughts, habits and skills, followed by development of affective reactions, e.g. attitudes, ideals, appreciations
- Well formed questions, properly directed and asked, can condition the student toward likes and dislikes (ethical values) appreciation or indifference
- To obtain individual or class attention: When a class grows restless or tired, often a pointed question will arouse interest and challenges attention.

Purposes

- To arouse interest
- To draw students to activity
- An opportunity to participate and share the responsibility for learning activities
- For grading the students
- To assess the student's abilities, interest and needs
- To challenge students to expand their knowledge base and develop new ideas and creativity
- To find out each individual's work preparation
- To expose the difficulties in preparing items in Questionnairre.

Types of Questions

a. Memory or act questions—The student required to recall readily available answers, which read previously or discussed or mentioned in some way or other.
b. Thought questions—Student has to create or form an answer from the general knowledge she/he has about a particular subject.

Characteristics of the effective question:
- Based on the objectives, mastery over the subject matter, teacher will formulate questions
- Questions could be within the range of the student's experiences and university syllabus knowledge; otherwise, the student will not understand the questions and will only guess the answer
- Questions should present a challenge which stimulates an educative response in keeping pace with the objectives

- Questions which require comparison, evaluation and thinking are preferable to the simple recall type
- Questions has to contain only one idea, many faceted question will confuses the student, who usually answers one phase and forgets the remainder, then he/she may loose marks, as she/he did not answer one part of multi faceted question.

Questions to be avoided:
- Leading questions—Suggest the answer often require only a 'yes'/ 'No' reply
- Catch questions—The guessing of a puzzle or trick does not explain relationships or require any thinking and therefore does not encourage learning
- Discussion question—The student does not know what points to include in the answer.

Questions should be well worded:
- Clear and concise
- Intelligible
- Grammatically correct and express in good English
- Question should not be ambiguous; the central idea should be clearly conveyed from the teacher to the student
- The question should not suggest the answer
- Question should require an extended answer
- Question should not be stated in textbook phraseology.

Technique of Questioning

Technique is the way or manner in which the questioning has to be carried out, it is an art that requires practice, development and should be directly related to the objectives to be achieved. The teacher needs poise and self-confidence to use the technique of questioning skillfully, otherwise the clarity and rapidity of thought before the class is impossible.

- Address the questions to the class in general: Before directing it to a particular student the question should be asked for the entire group in order to secure the entire class attention and to create interest, thought, to all members of the class, all student can form an answer in anticipation of being called on; if one student is initially addressed, the remainder of the class relaxes, assumed that they will not have to think of an answer
- Distribute questions as evenly as possible to all students—So that everyone gets a chance, reduces the mechanical routine, Prevents wasting class time, trying to get an answer out of a student who doesn't have one to give, all for the sake of a grade. Students should be called on, according to their needs and abilities
- The teacher will check her/his class roll from time to time to see that all have been called on.
  - Allow sufficient time for formulation of an answer
  - The student must be given time to think, but not allowed so much time that her/his mind wanders off to something else; give a pause after posing a question to permit time for a thoughtful response.
  - Ask questions in a natural, interested, conversational tone, to create confidence, If the teacher uses an 'of-course-you-can-answer-this' attitude, (it may be presumption) the student will make an attempt, even though she may know only a part of the answer.
  - Students should be given as much credit for answering as possible, insist upon accurate, complete and intelligible answers
  - Organize questions around sequences, leads to the development of a particular understanding, idea, appreciation or ideal. This prevents fragmentary and unrelated questioning and unifies the work of the course
  - Ask questions to the inattentive student, to arouse students, prevent inattention and thereby avoid discipline problems
  - Vary your pace of delivery, lower order questions can be asked quickly and higher order questions should be asked slowly. Give sufficient time for the students to recall and answer the question
  - Prompt learners: by presenting the question in a another way if the student is unable to answer, give some hint where the learner can pick up and recall the content, so that he/she will be able to develop an answer

- Encourage the students, to expand the answer by probing; if needed additional information has to be given, by other students for better response
- Call on others, motivate the non participants (who seem to be active listeners, but reluctant to participate) to participate in discussions
- Create a trusting learning environment, where incorrect responses/unconventional responses are welcomed and explored, to encourage all persons in the group
- Ensure simple questions, the questions has to be simple, fluent and clear to the students
- Positive question, the questions of the session is asked in a positive manner.
- Waiting time, a waiting time of 3 to 5 seconds is needed, if learner is not responding for the question.
- Question should not be repeated, if the students know that a question will be repeated, they may not be attentive for the first time.
- Natural question: Questions should be asked in a natural, interesting and conversational manner. Create confidence by asking questions to the student.

Dynamics of Effective Questioning

Questioning is used as a teaching tool, according to Perrott (1982) an effective questioning strategy depends on the mastery of the following specific instructional techniques.

1. Phrasing of question: Ambiguous and confusing questions should be avoided. Clear, simple, fluent words has to be used in effective questioning.
2. Delivery of question: Faculties call the attention of the learner to the content of question before limiting the potential target population for response; questions should be framed to maximize learner participation. Address the question in general rather than a single student.
3. Wait time: The interval between the end of the question and the request for a response. The wait time will allow the learners to think through the question, compose an answer and respond, personal anxiety will be reduced and facilitates to tolerate the silence.
4. Listening technique
   Listening strategies will:
   - Reinforce the learner response behavior
   - Enhance participation
   - Contribute to successful use of questioning as an instructional tool
   - Watch for nonverbal signals indicating learners' desire to respond to or ask a question
   - Focus on the learner who is speaking and pay attention to what is said
   - Maintain eye contact with the learner and use other nonverbal signals to indicate attentiveness.
   - Ask for necessary classification when response is concluded
   - Evaluate the response only after it is complete.
5. Dealing with inadequate responses:
   - Faculty should be diplomatic in dealing with inadequate responses
   - Effective faculty response to incorrect answers helps the learners to redirect their thinking to the correct answer
   - Personal attacking, e.g. sarcasm, reprimand, accusation can be avoided.
6. Feedback: Feedback is a two-way process with information exchanged between the faculty and the student regarding levels of understanding and performance. The faculty's response to a students' answer is very important. A nod, a smile or a comment can encourage the student to respond in a positive way
7. Faculty behavior: The social and emotional milieu of the learning situation will be effected by faculty's verbal and nonverbal behavior, e.g. tone of voice, eye contact, movement, gestures, facial expressions, nodding, etc. are the signals of approval which can motivate the student.

Teacher reaction to student questions and responses

Success of the class depends greatly on the attitude and the response of the teacher towards learners

1. Encourage students for active participation to increase their participation.
2. Questions should be significant: Avoid sidetrack, trivial and ambiguous questions.

3. Courtesy: Both the teacher and student should be courteous in asking and answering questions.
   In the eagerness to speak, students sometimes break in on each other or several will try to answer at once.
   The teacher should be courteous in recognizing or passing over a student who wishes to answer.
4. Grant the student the right to disagree: Real thinking promotes opinion. The student ought to be encouraged
   to think for themselves and to form their own opinion.
5. The teacher should admit that he/she doesn't know an answer.
   If an answer is not known, admit it by saying, 'I will find out' or ' I will look it up and let you know'.
6. Rarely assist the student in her/his answers: Let the student work out her/his own contribution without
   prompting to prevent confusion and interruption of student's thinking.
7. Never pump answers from students: Allow sufficient time to think and answer. If an answer is not forth
   coming, go on to another student; pumping never produces answers, it only wastes time.

"Microcomputers in the classroom" is a hand-on course for educators wishing an overall orientation to microcomputers. Their operation, software and rudimentary concepts of programming. This course is offered 3 to 4 times per year, students from all disciplines are eligible.

Computers for teacher's activities at the university level
- Availability of technical support
- To meet the needs of students, teachers and administrators
- To assist with operational programs
- To maintain high standards for professional development and practice
- To nurture appropriate interest in research
- To increase knowledge about teaching and learning process
- Action oriented research
- Training and support activities
- Professionals should get involved in planning for collecting and interpreting data to aid in decisions in their schools
- Resources of the colleges and universities, training and support offered to teachers through colleges should take the advantage of the special resources available there
- Microcomputers are used throughout the university in many different ways
  - Information systems
  - Process control
  - Laboratory equipment
  - Specialized graphics etc.
- Students should have the opportunity to learn about current and future uses of microcomputers
- Exploration of microcomputers applications opens doorways onto the entire world of computing
- To give appropriate attention to matters of learning and teaching.

Computers in Nursing

Computer influence every sphere of human activity and bring many changes in education, health care, scientific research, Medical transcription and in social sciences. In Developed countries, computers have become part of every man's life, whereas in India, it is limited to certain fields. Usage of computers in health care system will save the time, economises energy and help the nurses to provide quality nursing care and saves time.

Uses

In clinical practice
- Admission and transfer system allows nurses to obtain basic biographical information about the clients before they arrive to the ward/unit
- When a discharge or transfer is entered in the computer, all the appropriate departments will be notified, e.g. Pharmacy, Dietary, House keeping, Census and Client's location in the unit, etc. everything will be readily available thus it saves the time of the nurses

- Nursing documentation: Computer typing is very legible. Nursing process, care plan, implementation of activities, nursing notes and discharge plans can be computerized. It can be stored in a format determined by the institution. Through computers drug calculations, flow rates can be done more accurately and easily. Multiple program choices can be chosen for application of nursing theories in implementation of nursing care activities. Communicate Physicians orders, monitor clients' values and also receive lab test results and patients' information to the respective wards but maintains invasion of privacy.

In Nursing Education

Computer assisted instruction programs are very useful in self-paced learning. Learners will interact with computer (as it takes the role of teacher):
- Drill and Practice
- Most common and least complex method
- A learner is presented with a series of questions or problems about materials, e.g. drug dosage calculations, IV drip rate calculations, terminology
- Writing up of textbooks; collection of education materials
- Library maintenance
- Tutorial programs
- Display new material
- Tutorial information
- Feedback
  - Simulations, the real life situations will be presented to assist learners in problem solving and decision making skills in a safe environment
  - Interactive video instruction (IAV) can provide learners with true-to-life simulation
  - Video pictures, graphics can be incorporated in the design of software.

Nursing Research
- Review literature or search for related articles, e.g. Internet, Med line, search line
- Tool for data collection
- Dissemination of findings and results
- Tabulations or statistical analysis and description of tables
- Preparation of research reports, project report.

Nursing Administration
- Computerized patients classification system can be used to assign nursing staff based on how severely ill the clients are:
  - Clients are classified on the basis of their abilities or need for nursing care
  - Computerized inventory system keeps track of supplies received and disbursed
  - Client billing system
- Diagnosis or reports
- General computer application software, e.g. word processing, electronic spread sheets, data based management sheets
- Budget planning
- Maintenance of individual records
- Calculation of number of nurses required on each unit (Nurses with clients ratio).

PUPPET SHOW

Puppet show is one type of dramatic expression. It always plays an integral part in the lives of people regardless of their background, it serves as a substitute for real experiences, as a reconstruction of experiences and as a way of interpreting social, political or religious beliefs. It is a flexible media seen. It can be adapted to any subject and depends on the proposed purposes and the desired result.

Purposes

It develops:
- Effective listening and looking skills
- Improves group cooperation
- Enhances feeling of security and confidence
- Maintains self-control
- Understand the subject content.

It promotes:
- Creative ability
- Developmental learning in language and in the fine arts
- Experimentation in the use of language, rhythm
- Self-expression.

Types

1. Finger Puppet
2. Hand puppet
3. Rod Puppet
4. Marionettes.

Procedure of Puppet Show

The puppets should be selected according to the level of audience. If we are presenting a show in a rural area, the puppet selected should be made with the local available material.

Precautions to be taken while doing puppet show

- Selection of puppets
- Synchronization i.e., voice and action
- Way of presentation.

Advantages

- Creates interests
- Gives the knowledge in a brief period
- Effective method
- Motivates students
- Easy to carry and operate.

Disadvantages

- Needs group cooperation, coordination
- Required skills in preparation and supply
- Skills in presentation.

EDUCATIONAL FIELD TRIPS

Introduction

The world is your classroom. Learning can-and-should happen everywhere. Field trips have been a part of education for thousands of years, but despite challenges, a carefully planned and integrated field trip offers tremendous learning potential for all students, but ensuring that field trip is a productive learning experience for students takes planning. The use of educational field trips has long been a major part of the education programming for both youth and adults. An educational field trip can be an integral part of the instructional program, designed around specific educational objectives. Field trips helps to find opportunities on topics you're teaching, in your county or within a given distance from your school suggests related lesson plans and classroom resources. Planning is critical to a successful trip. Good planning must precede field trips, real or virtual. Remember it is the journey, not just the destination that provides the learning experience. A field trip should be designed so participants can easily make connections between the focus of the field trip and the concepts they are learning in the rest of the educational program, Ensure field trip compliments the curriculum by meeting specific expectations.

Definition
"Any teaching and learning excursion outside of the classroom".

Types
- Physical Field Trip, e.g. School playground, outdoor education centers, Botanical parks, science center, museum, zoo, grocery store, fire station, veterinary clinics, agricultural operations and natural resource operations
- Digital and Virtual Field Trip: Virtual field trip collection is a wonderful way to teach and learn about the outside world. For example, travel to museums and even outer space.

Purposes
- To make a connection between reality and theory—Hands-on
- Can be used as an introduction to a unit or a culminating activity
- To provide an authentic learning experience
- Exciting, students eager to meet and interact with others in outer areas, memorable life experience
- They can experience all five senses i.e., see, touch, feel, smell and taste
- Students remember the field trips because they learn new by using different methodology
- A valuable tool in the extension agent's educational toolbox
- Provides participants with first hand experience related to the topic or concept being discussed in the program
- Provide unique opportunities for learning that are not available within the four walls of a classroom.

Problems in arranging Field Trips
- Funding limitations
- Time constraints
- Increased liability concerns many education professionals at requests for field trips
- Risk for sexual indulgence, e.g. if teenagers are going chances to get attracted with opposite sex.

Preparation for Field Trip
- Have a sound pedagogical reason for the field trip. Students should be prepared for learning outdoors, because of the pre-trip activities you have done. Parents should be informed of where you are going and what mode of transportation and of the number of adults per student that will be along. Visit the site in advance and find any possible danger areas. Warn students about these areas. When you arrive at the site, remind the students of the dangers and how they have to handle. Is your trip a chance for the students to have free exploration? or do you want them in activities the whole time? Plan according to the particular group you have. You must use your own judgment, always have the students in small groups, either for their explorations together or for their activities. Set the functional groups so there is at least one responsible sort of student in each group
- Discuss with total group the organization of the program, specific objectives, activities to be carried out, categorize the activities and prioritize the activities, inform your expectations and expected student behavior and role performance and responsibilities
- Prefer to have activities for the students to carry out at different places at the site. If there are six small groups, try to have six activities and to run each activity. The students rotate through the activities. This means that each activity should take the same amount of time. If one activity takes much less time than the others, you can have the students sketch or write or measure a good learning activity that extends the action they are involved in
- Field trips are only slightly more hazardous than the classroom. In other words, with proper planning, they are not very dangerous at all. The keys to safety are: Anticipation, planning and adequate supervision.

Planning and Organizing a Successful Field Trip

A. Pre-Trip Stage

1. The administration component:

- Involve all the steps taken by the field trip organizer to arrange the logistics of the field trip
- Securing permission from appropriate administration, organizing transportation to and from the field trip location, contacting the field trip location to verify the schedule and activities and obtaining signed permission slips from parents/guardians of youth attending the field trip. Determine your destination and write your objectives for the visit
- Consult your administration and gain approval. Every school is different concerning approvals and there might be blackout dates and other items that you need to consider
- Determine transportation rules and decide on the mode of transportation
- College/School principal has to obtain permission from the authorities where the field trip was planned
- Planned and effectively organized, Check for school/board policy on field trips, Student to supervisor ratios, Fund raising, Involve the students from the Plan of action as much as possible, Involve school principal and vice-principal (Authorities) and Management (Private sector)
- Although the activities of the administration component are important, if organizers only focus on logistics, a major segment of the pre-trip stage is missing and field trips may not be educationally successful
- Prepare a checklist to ensure that all tasks are completed (e.g. booking facilities and transportation, parental notifications, medical forms, supervision, safety precautions, emergency information) and have the school administrator sign the checklist once completed
- Be sure to visit the site ahead of time, in order to plan for safety, resources and resource personnel facility
- Plan on route activities to enrich their experience during the field trip
- Provide parents with rationalization for the field trip and trip itinerary.

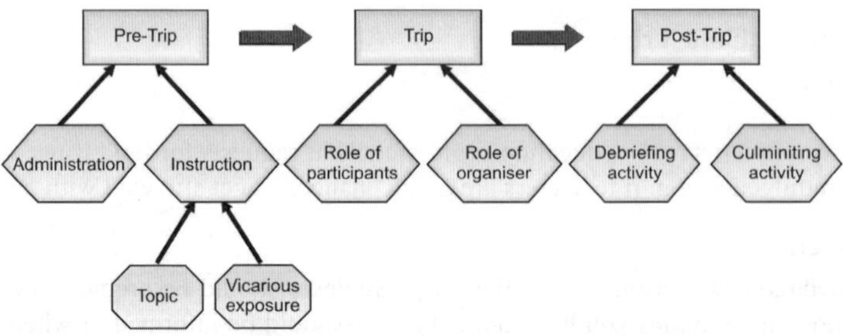

Fig. 5.3: Field Trip Planning Model

2. The instruction component:

- The pre-trip stage is critical in preparing participants for the experience. Participants, especially youth, often have high levels of anxiety when going on a field trip. Anxiety levels can be especially high for field trips to novel, unfamiliar settings. Often a field trip is the first experience a person has with a particular location. When individuals experience high levels of anxiety, learning cannot take place. To reduce anxiety, field trip organizers need to make participants feel comfortable and safe at the location of the field trip just as they would in a typical classroom
- Provide participants with vicarious exposure to the field trip site as part of pre-trip instruction. Vicarious exposure could involve the field trip organizer showing participants photographs, drawings or a videotape of the site to be visited. This can occur at a meeting prior to the field trip or materials may be sent to participants prior to the event. Another option would be to post important field trip information on the Internet so that participants can visit a website prior to the experience. Items such as the location of toilet facilities, rooms and basic features of the site should be identified. If participants will be at the field trip site during a meal time, such arrangements should also be discussed. Studies in science education have shown time and again that providing participants with vicarious exposure prior to a field trip significantly reduces individual anxiety and increases overall trip effectiveness

- Pass out permission slips and an information sheet for students including due dates for money and signed forms and the cost and details of your trip. You can also ask for chaperones at this time
- Collect money and keep a careful accounting. Make sure to follow all school rules concerning the collection of money
- Remind students as the due date nears and call parents if you are not getting enough chaperones
- Create student groups. Remember that many destinations will have rules concerning student-chaperone ratios so check these out early. Also spend some time determining your groups. Do not allow students to just choose their own groups because this is a recipe for disaster. Further, try to remember student personalities. Make sure to take it easy on the chaperones, e.g. do not put the most trying students together in one group if it can be at all avoided
- Create a lesson for students to complete in conjunction with the field trip.
- Work sheet with questions to answer while at the destination, an essay that they must complete upon return or some other activity. Check with your field trip location because they might have ready-made lesson plans that you can use
- Create a contingency plan in case things go wrong, e.g. what if the students are finished one hour before the buses are set to return?
- On field trip day, get to school early. Make sure you have all required forms and attendance sheets ready to go. If you need to get lunches from the cafeteria, make sure you have these also. Be prepared to orient your chaperones concerning your expectations, their groups and the class assignment. Let your students know your expectations and then go and have fun
- Debrief concerning the field trip the next day after your return. Talk about the group impressions and what students learned. You can use this to further their learning and also to decide if you will go on that particular field trip again in future years

Review Guidelines for safety and behavior rules and expectations with youth
- There are many potential liability situations that can occur on a field trip, it is ultimate responsibility to ensure that the following safety guidelines are meet concerning safety and behavior while outside the classroom
- Set behavioral expectations for the field trip and describe and discuss them with the students prior to departure
- Have students create their own code of behavior with teacher involvement and veto power
- If junior students are mature enough to be responsible and accountable for their own behavior, have them sign a written code of conduct; therefore, creating a behavioral contract
- Introduce the idea of team work to enable students to live to the written code of conduct
- Describe the consequences for not behaving properly prior to embarking on the trip
- Provide parents with behavioral expectations and ask them to ensure that the students know and understand the code of conduct and the consequences
- Ensure that the student/supervision ratio meets board/school standards
- Eliminate all the safety concerns identified in the school/board policy
- Use board approved transportation
- Create passenger manifest and file with appropriate school personnel. Also, take along passenger manifest to check that everyone is accounted for
- Implement a buddy with students as an additional safety precaution
- Ensure that safety gear and first aid equipment are readily available and in plain view
- Permission slip letters to parents/guardians of youth participants
- To increase the educational effectiveness of field trips, pre-trip instruction should also focus on the content topics and concepts that participants will be investigating during the field trip. It is important for field trip organizers to give participants verbal clues regarding what to look for during their activities. Pre-trip instruction makes it easier for participants to focus on the educational goals of the trip. As part of pre-trip lessons, organizers should demonstrate the use of any equipment and explain in detail any activities that will be occurring during the field trip

- During field trips, learning activities involving groups of 2 to 3 individuals are most effective. These groups should be assigned during the pre-trip stage. Specific roles of each group member during activities (such as observer, recorder, graphic artist) should also be explained in advance.

B. Trip Stage

1. The role of the participants

- It is accomplished by establishing a field trip agenda and sharing this agenda and field trip objectives with the participants. A suggested agenda for a field trip starts with a brief amount of free time for individuals to explore the field trip site on their own. This open exploration may not be appropriate in all locations. For example, individuals could not roam freely inside an equipment manufacturing plant. They could however, have free time to view items in the visitor area or lobby prior to the guided tour. This exploration time allows participants to get comfortable with their surroundings. Once the basic curiosity of the facility is satisfied, learners are better able to focus their attention on the content topics to be learned
- A whole-group guided tour: During the tour, the organizer or tour leader can point out specific items that relate to the educational goals of the trip. This also provides an opportunity for participants to ask any questions they may have developed during their exploration time

  A small group learning activity: Working in pre-assigned groups of 2-3 participants can complete an activity such as a short worksheet. The worksheet should be designed in a manner that is challenging to learners yet not frustrating. The worksheet should clearly relate to the educational goals of the field trip.

2. The role of the organizer

It is also an important consideration during the trip stage. Although monitoring and management of the experience is important, monitoring participant learning is also a major organizer responsibility. Throughout the field trip, the organizer should be actively engaged in teaching activities. However, on field trips the organizer should utilize different teaching approaches than those used in traditional classroom settings. Organizers should interact with participants to help answer questions they might have. Organizers should also initiate discussion with small groups of participants by asking them questions. During field trips, organizers should function more as facilitators or guides rather than directors. By playing an active rather than a passive role during the field trip, organizers can increase student interest and learning.

C. Post-Trip Stage

1. Debriefing activity: During the debriefing session, participants should be encouraged to share and discuss their experiences during the field trip, e.g. sharing and discussing data or results of assigned small group activities as well as sharing feelings about specific aspects of the trip or overall impressions. Participants should also be given an opportunity to identify and discuss problems encountered during the field trip.
2. Culminating activity: This activity should give participants an opportunity to apply the content knowledge they gained during the field trip. Culminating activities should help learners tie together content they covered in regular educational program sessions and content learned during the field trip. They can be whole group or small group experiences. Both the debriefing and culminating activity should occur as soon after the trip as possible. Planning and organizing a successful field trip can be a great deal of work for the organizer. However, by following the simple steps in each of the pre-trip, trip and post-trip stages, participants can greatly benefit from your labor. Also when a well developed field trip plan is presented to administrators, many of their concerns are usually addressed. Field trips should be an integral part of extension programming. If faculty properly plan and execute educational field trips everyone can benefit from the experience.

How does field trip support the curriculum?

Before you request permission to take the trip, take the time to identify the following instructional elements in a document you can share with colleagues and with your students: Curriculum materials or guides that have been developed by staff members from the site you will visit.

- Learning outcomes for the trip
- Standard course of study alignment
- Essential concepts underlying the content and structure of the trip
- Key vocabulary that will be a part of the trip.

Preparing students

This phase of any field trip is perhaps the most demanding and time consuming, but is crucial to the success of the experience for everyone. The following suggestions will make a difference in your next field trip:

- *Introduce the trip as a part of a lesson*—Lesson plans that have been designed around a visit While you may not find a lesson that exactly suits your needs

- *Stimulate student's interest for the trip*—Use artifacts from previous trips to this site such as photos, brochures or videos. Consider inviting students who previously participated on this field trip as guest speakers to talk about their experience. This is especially useful for overnight trips to distant places, where students will want to know what to expect

- *Discuss your expectations for learning and behavior*—Students may have certain expectations of their trip based on previous trips taken with other teachers or organizations. Prepare them mentally for the experience by reviewing as *schedule of activities or itinerary.* Explain what and how they will learn and what tools they will use. Do not assume that students possess the observation and exploration skills necessary to conduct the activities you or someone else has designed. It suggests having students practice these skills in the classroom by describing common objects to one another, such as a clothes pin, a paper clip, or a paintbrush. If the result of the field trip is a product such as a multimedia presentation, report, or dramatization, consider giving students a rubric before the trip to guide their exploration. And remind students of the consequences of inappropriate behavior during the trip.

- *Prepare students with a twenty-four hour "staging period"*—Remind students to get a good night's rest and to eat a nutritious breakfast prior to departure. Ask students to mentally prepare themselves for the experience by thinking about how their behavior at school might not be appropriate in public spaces. Remind them to dress appropriately, which means taking into consideration the weather and the venue. Like behavior, clothing that passes the school's dress code may not be appropriate in another location.

- *Develop a schedule of activities or itinerary*—Review this with students and ask them to agree to follow this schedule. You can ask them to sign the itinerary as they would a learning contract.

- *Create a packing checklist for overnight travel*—For overnight travel, create a packing checklist for boys and one for girls. Most students tend to over pack, which can be disastrous if you are traveling long distances. If students are paired to share rooms, encourage them to decide who will bring electric appliances that can be shared.

Preparing others

- *Obtain prior approval from your school or school system*—Though you may have standing permission from your administration, there may be other events that require students to be present on that day. Check your school's calendar before you schedule your trip.

- *Obtain parental permissions*—Your school may have a standard form for permissions. Remember to carefully describe why the field trip is important and how it relates to the curriculum. Consider using the permission form as a recruiting tool for chaperones.

- *Complete medical permission forms*—You may have to create your own medical permission form which includes all information related to student health, and parental permission for medical treatment in the case of an emergency.

- *Fundraising just say no*—Educators are kind-hearted individuals who want to ensure equal access to educational opportunities for everyone. If the trip includes costs to individual students, consider other options for funding aside from fund-raising activities. It is most likely that students have already participated in numerous fund-raising activities and, depending on their age, door-to-door sales may not be a safe option. Consider asking parents to fund the trip or make a tax-deductible donation to the school to make the trip possible.

- *Prepare chaperones for their role*—Send a letter or hold a meeting with chaperones prior to the trip to establish agreement of chaperone role and responsibility. Do not take for granted that adults will intuitively know their role. Review your expectations of how they will assist you to ensure student learning and safety.

- *Hold a meeting with bus driver(s)*—Whether you are using your school system's buses or traveling with a private bus company, make sure to introduce yourself as the lead teacher to all drivers. Thank them in advance for helping you to make the trip run smoothly. Make sure they know where you are going and that they have a copy of the itinerary which should have departure and arrival times for all activities.

Preparing teacher by themselves

- *Conduct a pre-visit to scout the site*—Do you know where the bathrooms and toilets are located? Are there any possible distractions nearby like a music store or bakery? What spaces are available for students to take notes, make sketches, or take pictures or video? Can you obtain a map of the visit to share with students in advance? What can you discern about crowd control within the visit space?
- *Develop a participant checklist*—Develop a system for accounting for everyone on the trip, including chaperones. This may be a checklist with everyone's name that you can check off as you depart for various stages of the trip. You might also consider assigning a number to each participant and conduct a "count off" before leaving.
- *Check the weather in advance*—Check weather conditions of your destination prior to the trip so that you can prepare yourself and your participants accordingly. Check for current weather information for your destination.
- *Reconfirm travel and accommodations*—If you are planning overnight travel, hotel bookings, tickets and so on just prior to departure.

For students

- Hard surface like a clipboard for note-taking or sketching container (zip-lock bag, grocery bag, etc.) for collecting artifacts, Recording device like pens, pencils, markers and paper; handheld devices; laptops; cameras, video cameras or digital cameras and a tape recorder students might bring some money for purchasing accessories to use in class presentations. You might encourage students to purchase postcards which can better capture sites of interest and allow students to focus their attention to the site itself. Carefully monitor students in gift shops and stores since some students may spend too much time shopping rather than exploring
- For young students and overnight trips, equip students with a small note card containing the lodging contact information and/or cell phone number of lead teacher/chaperone.

For teachers

Container for class supplies, a first-aid kit and a container to protect student prescribed medications along with prescription form.

A "Hot File"—A plastic or large envelope to transport the following important documents:
1. Emergency contact information for your school and school system
2. List of students who must take medication during the trip
3. For travel out of state or foreign travel, copies of insurance documents
4. Checklist of all students and chaperones in attendance
5. Extra cash for emergency situations
6. Contact information of site contact(s) i.e., name, phone number, role and office location on site.
7. Trip itinerary

Cell phone for emergency calls and wrong turns.

Student identifiers. To easily spot your students in a crowded space, think about how you will identify them with a quick glance.

Consider inviting another faculty member along who might take this trip in the future. They can shadow you while also serving as a chaperone.

Pros of Field Trips

- They are a way to reinforce and expand on concepts taught in class
- They offer students another method to learn concepts and are especially good for the many tactile/kinesthetic students in your classroom
- They allow for a shared reference that can be referred to later as you are teaching new concepts
- They allow you and your students a different format in which to get to know each other and bond.

Cons of Field Trips

- You have to plan ahead above and beyond your normal lessons

- You will need to complete and collect paperwork from your students
- You need to keep your students organized and well-disciplined. Your field trip might turn out to be a disappointment.

CLINICAL TEACHING

Introduction

Nursing education is a practice discipline, the students will learn the subject matter by doing the things and practices the skills. Nursing is a science, as it is based on systematic body of knowledge and principles of education. It also implies as an art, as it requires professional skills especially based upon humanitarian approach and behavioral sciences background. Clinical Teaching is performed by a faculty within a curriculum i.e., planned and offered in a response to professional, societal, educational expectations and demands, using available resources, e.g. Human, intellectual, physical and financial etc. the context of curriculum. Nursing education is having more emphasis on skill development based upon two aspects i.e., Theory of Nursing and Nursing Practice. Clinical teaching include skills, e.g. Identifying Knowledge gaps, finding and utilizing new information and initiating or managing change, team work and collaboration skills in working with interdisciplinary team. Teachers can provide appropriate activities that will facilitate clinical learning activities, provides real life experiences and opportunities for transfer of knowledge to practical situations. Clinical teaching is an expensive enterprise. "Clinical" means involving direct observation of the patient. The central activity of the teacher in the clinical setting is Clinical Teaching. The teacher's role in the clinical setting is competent guidance. The teacher guides, supports, stimulates and facilitates learning by designing appropriate activities in appropriate settings and allows the student to experience that learning.

Old nursing curriculum contained only a few hours of teaching and many hours of clinical practice. Through the intervening years, the amount of nursing knowledge has grown exponentially and the time allowed to learning by doing has contracted steadily. The clinical experiences for nursing students will be provided in the places where the actual clients are being cared for. Since the practice involves human life and handling real life situation, it is essential, such training and experiences should be supported by good clinical teaching. In clinical practice, the theoretical knowledge and skills learned receive repeated testing. The student has the challenge of putting this knowledge and skills gains in real life situation to make them practitioners in nursing. To bridge the gap between classroom and clinical instruction is, to expose the student to a series of laboratory stimulation in real settings. Clinical experience requires the presence of a clinical instructor to guide, reinforce and correct behavior.

In the nursing curriculum to correlate the subject matter learned in ideal situation (e.g. lab and classroom) to real situation, the clinical instructor organizes the clinical experiences. The student nurse learns the bedside nursing from senior nurses in real field situation.

In classroom teaching there is possibility for careful demonstration of procedures, the ideal equipment will be collected well in advance and sufficient time was permitted for developing skills based on theory underlying sound practice under close, strict supervision.

After learning in ideal situation, the student will practice the procedure (by implementing care to the clients) in real situation utilizing available facilities.

Clinical instruction is directly concerned with teaching students about the care of clients.

Clinical Skill

Nurses need to develop and utilize specific clinical skills to practice their professional activities in clinical settings (Community & Hospital) to fulfil the needs (Felt and Demand) of clients and their families in specific and community in general and to maintain standards of living e.g. Rapport building, Empathetic communication, Paraphrasing, Skills in Counseling, Communication, Interaction, Interpersonal skills, Reflective Practice skills etc.

Clinical Experiences

The nursing care activities performed by the students for the care of clients as a part of educational program. Learning is an active, personal process. The student is the one who experiences the learning. Teacher is plan and provide appropriate activities that will facilitate learning.

Clinical experiences are classified into three types.

1. Laboratory experiences: Students will learn the skills in laboratory situation on dummy or doll under strict supervision under guidance of clinical experts in specific field, the experience will be selected according to the needs of students and the requirements of the curriculum.
2. Supervised nursing care practice: Students after practiced in the ideal situation i.e., lab, they will practice nursing care procedures in the real field under expert's supervision. *Nursing care experience* will be *planned, allotted, guided* and *supervised.* The nursing care experiences will be provided for the students in each subject area. The students should practice compulsory clinical experiences.
3. Interneeship: After acquiring knowledge and practice in all areas, according to the needs, requirements and interest of the students, the faculty allow the students to practice skills, the teacher will act as an coordinator of the program.

Purposes

- To prepare nursing students for professional practice
- Independent learning activities learnt first in the simulation laboratory and then in clinical practice
- Creating and maintaining a climate of mutual trust and respect that supports learning and student growth
- Faculty must respect the learners and trust their motivation and commitment to the profession they seek to enter
- Provide opportunities for real life experiences and transfer of knowledge to independent learning activities to real life and practical situations
- Facilitate learning based on educational theories, learner development, knowledge and socialization
- Participates in clinical design with evaluation of program outcomes
- To provide individualized care in a systematic, holistic approach
- To develop high technical competent skills
- To practice various procedures
- To collect and analyze the data
- To conduct research
- To maintain high standard of nursing practice
- To become independent enough to practice nursing
- To develop cognitive, conative, affective and psychomotor skills
- The students will develop the techniques related to observation
- To meet the needs of client
- To improve standards of nursing practice
- To develop various methods in delivering care
- To identify the problems of clients
- To learn and implement nursing care during various diagnostic procedures
- To learn various skills in giving health education techniques to the clients and significant others
- To help in integration of theoretical knowledge into practice
- To develop communication skills
- To maintain interpersonal relationships and inter-institutional relationship
- To develop proficiency and efficiency in carrying out various nursing procedures
- To assist physician in carrying out therapeutic procedures
- To learn managerial skills
- To become professionally active member
- To encounter reality in the practice of nursing, synthesis learning, practice activities described in the course objectives
- The outcomes of clinical practice are: Critical Thinking, Decision Making, Psychomotor skills (Clinical reasoning and problem solving), Interpersonal skills, Organizational skills and Cultural competence.

Essentials for Good Clinical Instruction

The clinical instructor has to select a clinical area, where the clients require good nursing care and also it should provide chance for the students to practice high standards of nursing care practice.

The clinical instructor and the head nurse should consider the needs of students to develop the individuals at a higher level of functioning.

They select the area where opportunities are available for the instructor to teach and the students to learn according to the requirements set by the institution.

Identify the nursing personnel (head nurse and staff nurse) who are interested in attending and sharing the discussion in nursing care conferences, nursing rounds and other sessions where clinical conditions were discussed.

Competent teacher should be available. The head nurse and instructor should cooperate with one another to plan and to provide improved nursing care practice.

Conducive environment is essential.

Functions of the Clinical Instructor

- Set the objectives, standards for practice
- Develop evaluation tools
- Obtain permission of the institute
- Prepare master rotation plan and clinical rotation plan
- Set up the clinical area in an ideal manner
- Keeps ready equipment in working condition to provide nursing care
- Plans and directs the instructional program activities within one clinical area
- Directs and supervises the students in providing client's care
- Assists in patient care
- Demonstrates nursing procedures on patients and ask the students to return demonstrate procedures to develop skill and confidence
- Develops an understanding of research for better patient care
- Analyses the difficulties and guiding the students accordingly
- Maintains high standards of patient care
- Encourages, motivate and inspire students
- Supervises and evaluate the performance of students
- Maintains strict discipline
- Maintains students' records, e.g. duty rosters, individual assignments, evaluation tools, clinical teachings and performance of students
- Conducts individual conferences with the students to solve any problems arose and to meet their professional and personal needs
- Attends the lectures which was arranged for students and make arrangements for presentation of the topic, e.g. bringing clients keeping ready overhead projectors etc.
- Supervises assignments like ward teaching class, case study, health talks
- Participates in faculty conferences
- Focusses attention of the students upon the medical and nursing problems of the clients to whom they are assigned
- Helps the students to develop ability to adjust general plans of care to the needs of individual patients
- Assists the students in preparing teaching plans
- Demonstrates skillfully the nursing procedures of special importance on the particular area
- Guide the students in acquisition of new skills
- Directs the students in their use of library resources for writing and preparing clinical assignments of students
- Guides the students in conducting nursing research activities
- Develops potentialities of each student.

Qualities of a Clinical Instructor

- Enjoys bedside nursing
- Expert in bedside nursing

- Good communication skills and develops good rapport among the nursing personnel
- Mastery over the methods of delivering the care, advanced knowledge in educational psychology and other advanced areas, e.g. specialties
- Develops confidence, has to be maintained since success in clinical nursing rests upon her/his ability to win the cooperation of doctors, head nurse, staff nurse, other professional colleagues, technicians, the auxiliary staff, ability to work well with other persons
- Possesses adequate theoretical background
- He/she should enjoy in teaching the students in hospital situation
- She/he should be appointed on the basis of outstanding skills
- Ability to implement the knowledge into practice
- Ability to communicate the knowledge to others
- Should have good teaching skills
- Physically active
- Very wholesome, healthy, smiling and pleasing personality
- Neat, nicely dressed (good poise)
- Good conduct
- Empathetic, sympathetic in nature
- Should understand total nursing program
- Should have detailed knowledge about area, in which she was placed
- Should have positive philosophy of life
- She/he must know teaching and evaluating methods
- She/he has to maintain good working relations
- She/he should be responsible for all arrangements of experiences in her clinical area
- She/he has to participate in professional activities
- She/he has to maintain good conducive, democratic environment
- She/he has to maintain freedom of speech
- She/he should have sensitive to others feelings, good judgmental type
- Non-interference
- Sincerity, punctuality, cooperative in nature
- Good team spirit
- Agreeable
- Cheerful
- Pleasant
- Amicable
- Good observer
- Cultured person
- Enthusiastic
- Social and professional responsibility
- Tolerant
- Open-mindedness
- Courageous
- Initiative
- Conscious
- Accurate
- Listener
- Supporter
- Guiding, counseling and evaluating the students
- Sense of fitness
- Interested in professional affairs
- Sense of justice

- Self controlled
- Trust worthy
- High technical, competent spirit
- Mentally alert
- Good discriminating power.

Clinical Teaching Methods

In clinical area, the student nurse will learn technical/clinical skills, by using the principle of "Learning by doing", Purposive/specific clinical skill will be learnt with, application of theoretical knowledge into practice. The student will practice and gain skills based on scientific principles. The teaching methods will improve the clinical knowledge of student and able to practice all procedures systematically to render qualitative care to the client. Varied clinical teaching methods will be used to enrich the student's knowledge in clinical area. Those are:

1. Client family centered approach

Individualized care will be provided in holistic manner, to meet total needs of the client systematically. Here, not only the client will be assisted for therapeutic measures, the family members also will be educated about the illness of the client in detail-causes, clinical manifestations, treatment, rehabilitation measures if any, prevention and their responsibility in taking care of client in meeting the client's needs.

2. Conference

Group Conference

A conference is the act of consulting together, two or more individuals in an formal meeting for the purpose of giving or exchanging ideas. It involves a two-way flow of conversation.

Clinical conferences—The specialist will discuss about a specific clinical diagnosis in detail with suitable audio-visual aids to make the group to understand the subject clear. The participants from the same clinical speciality, who are interested to learn about the specific case and its' management were gathered in a lecture hall, if they have any doubts, clarifications will be made clear by the specialist. The participants were selected based on their interest or requirements as a partial fulfillment of the program or the course.

Staff conference

These types of conferences will be held in teaching institutions eg: faculty meeting and in hospitals, nursing superintendent or Head Nurse or In charge Nurse will conduct conference to all nurses.

The leader of the conference, opens it by briefly stating the purpose and briefly review the objectives of theme of the conference.

Teacher starts the discussion by asking a carefully thought out question or prelude to the conference or making a statement designed to bring out needs, suggestions or problems of various staff members.

The leader should accept each persons' suggestions as worthy of consideration make a note it on a black board or small pad.

Each member should encourage to express their thoughts.

The leader then summarizes the suggestions. A group discussion about the specific theme or topic is usually in order.

The leader ends the conference by stating the next steps and delegating responsibility that may be entailed.

Nursing care conference

Purposes

- To set objectives and criteria for nursing care
- To implement Nursing Process effectively for a client with specific diagnosis
- To portray the nursing problems typically associated with a particular disease in detail and to narrate the related nursing care to meet the specific needs of client
- To learn ways to help clients, identify their needs and solve their own problems
- To suggest approaches to the patient and their families to plan the ways and means to help themselves in getting assistance and obtaining specialist services

- To plan methods for improving care
- To solve problems which interfere with good nursing care
- To evaluate results of nursing activities and plan for better practices

Individual conference
- To get the staff member to take the lead in the conference and in developing the plan for care with the team member by asking judicious questions as necessary
- To help the staff member and feel confidence in their own knowledge and ability
- To see that the staff member learns the process of planning nursing care and understand her responsibility in this
- To make sure that an effective plan for a particular client is developed and evaluation of its progress.

The team leader should recognize when assistance is needed and arrange to meet with the staff member. The purpose of conference is explained and the nurse is asked to come to the meeting and given thought to the kind of help she thinks, she needs.

The team leader will suggest that the staff members be familiar with the patient's record and that she/he has read the literature on the disorder from which the patient is suffering. The nurse spoke with the client and tried to determine his needs, formulate objectives for his case and prioritize the care activities.

The team leader also prepares herself/himself for the conference by becoming familiar with the client and his/her record, she/he too thinks through the client's need and a possible plan for care. This prepares her/him to ask questions designed to stimulate the course of thinking.

Team conference
The professionals, who will held responsible for particular type of clients' (disease conditions or in a specific ward like TRR, ICCU, Post Operative units) usually calls for a team conference, there, the specific disease condition or the common illnesses and its pathogenesis, clinical manifestations, treatment, nursing care will be discussed.

3. Bedside clinic
The Nurse who is presenting case will obtain consent from the client by explaining it's need and vitality; then the group may visit the client or the client may be brought to the conference room during the discussion. This method is of helpful, when some members of the group are unfamiliar with the client's condition or when there are special observations, which need to be mentioned and all group members has to learn, to present the discussion in a more meaningful. In this conference, when the client is to be visited is predetermined. The group knows the purpose of the visit and what to be observed. Frequently the client is engaged in purposeful conversation, the teacher will use this opportunity to demonstrate and to help the client to identify his needs and the assistance can be given to him/her in handling his problems. Client should feel ease; embarrassment of client has to be avoided. Client should know the group and what is expected from him, comfortable environment should be maintained and minimum group members (4 to 6) should be allowed.

4. Nursing rounds
A small group of the staff members, not more than five and a leader or teacher visit, the bedside of clients. Nursing Superintendents, ward sisters will do the rounds in the hospital wards. It helps the nursing members know about all the patients in the wards, their problems and ways of solving. It is an extension of the clinic method.

Procedure
- Students will be informed about timings of nursing rounds in their ward, so that, they will be ready with the clients' report to discuss during rounds
- Students will follow nursing rounds, the clinical instructor or ward supervisor will stop at the bedside of each patient for a brief period to have a short discussion and discuss the most significant nursing diagnosis and the intervention required to resolve the identified problem
- The instructor will instruct the concerned student nurse to inform assessment findings and report nursing care provided to a specific client during rounds

- During Case presentation, the student who is taking care of the patient for a week or so, has to present the case to the total group of the students so that all the students will be aware about total condition related to the case. If any cardinal manifestations are identified, with the clients' permission, they can demonstrate to the total group. The presentation of the background information is followed by additions and suggestions from the group
- Case presentation should be short and relate to only to problem or situation of immediate interest
- The contents to be discussed in nursing rounds are carefully selected, well organized, clearly and interestingly presented, for each client only 3 to 4 minutes have to be spent.

Types
- At the time of giving the transfer report at the change of shift
- Specific time of the day, when rounds are not interfering with general activities of the ward, Head Nurse or senior nurse will make Nursing rounds with all junior staff along with student nurses- to acquaint the staff with all patients in the ward for better understanding of the clients' condition and more specific care needed to achieve the nursing goals, to implement nursing process effectively for each patient.

Advantages
- To demonstrate important clinical manifestation in clients
- To clarify terminology used and studied
- To narrate client's reaction to disease
- To demonstrate nursing Procedures and to discuss clinical findings
- To demonstrate the effects of drugs
- To illustrate skillful nursing care
- To compare methods of meeting the needs
- To illustrate successful improvisation
- Rounds are useful in situations, where assignments are made to provide continuity of care
- Instructional purposes for student nurses
- To learn about disease, pattern of care, treatment
- To acquaint nurses with all patients
- Nursing rounds purpose should be explained to all the students as they are directed towards the improvement of nursing abilities and clinical skills.

The client should always be introduced to the group, encourage question and comments with almost consideration for the feelings of client.

At the completion of nursing rounds all the staff members will meet in the conference for summary and further explanation.

Disadvantages
- Requires very careful planning
- A small group of students, can be taken at a time
- Time consuming

Medical rounds
The Chief Physician or surgeon in charge of the ward with their team of doctors will be making rounds in the clinical wards to assess the condition and prognosis of client with treatment, need for discharge or continuation as in patient, any change of medications, modifications of care etc. during rounds the concerned doctor will be discussing the clients' condition in detail and the observations made during assessment, lab reports, the prognosis made they will discuss further line of management., during rounds nurse incharge also will accompany them to make a note of any instructions to be carried out by nursing team to implement Nursing care activities.

5. Ward-teaching program
The Clinical Instructor will assign the topic well in advance and give the date for ward teaching class for all the students in group posted to the clinical area., the topics are related to the clinical conditions and basic associated clinical field knowledge, when scheduled student will present the topic in teacher presence along with appropriate Audio-visual aids to other group members.

Purposes
- To supplement, to integrate the classroom instruction
- To aid the student to make correct applications of scientific principles basic to the specific nursing activity
- To enable the student to gain a real understanding of individual differences and substitute variations of case and circumstances to tactfully respond and adjust to them by adopting nursing procedure and treatment without violating basic principles
- To inspire the student for self development.

6. Ward class

A class will be conducted based upon current clinical experience of the students for whom the class is planned and for the students at one level of experience, who are having similar experience in a specific department.

7. Ward clinics

- A client is presented to the group, who illustrates typical clinical manifestations and require all nursing care procedures
- Obtain permission from the Physician/Incharge doctor and Incharge Nurse to conduct ward clinic
- Instructor will explain before hand, and obtain consent from the client and explain about the purpose of the clinic
- The students will be able to practice procedures in real situation
- Suitable place has to be selected
- Students should understand the purpose on improving the standards of nursing care and their contributions has to be directed towards at its end.

8. Case method

Case study/case presentation

The student will be given an opportunity to provide nursing care for specific client, after 4 or 5 days of careful study, the student nurse will prepare case study by referring and comparing with the text book with the client's condition, the student presents the case before the group companions in detail, general discussion about the client will be dealt.

Case analysis

A concrete case for analysis and discussion by a group of students under the leadership of the instructor. Sufficient information is presented to the students to make judgment of problem or situation in case.

Case incident technique

A critical incident technique which requires immediate decision and action is taken from a case and presented to the students for their analysis and decision. No background information is given to them regarding details of the incident at the time, it is presented. The instructor will have facts about the case, can be given as requested by the students.

9. Assignments

Types

Patient assignment—The Clinical Instructor after posting the students in clinical area as per clinical rotation, in wards/clinical area will allot the specific client to specific student to render clinical care for a specific period of time.

Work assignment—The Clinical Instructor will list the work to be carried out by the students in general in order to carry out clinical activities by total students posted in the ward like setting up of TPR Tray, Injection Trolly/Cart, Medicine Trolly/Cart, Inventory, care of Sponge bags, Hot water supply, maintainance of equipment, CSSD Supplies etc. Teacher will take precautions when preparing assignments rotation, all the students will get equal opportunity and gain similar experience

Student assignment—For example, in clinical block (at the end of academic year, CON will take permission from clinical authorities and will provide total care of the clients for 24 hours and ward activities in general (2 to 3 specific wards like Medical, Surgical and Post operative wards), students will work under different shifts (like Morning, Afternoon, Evening) under strict clinical supervision., The faculty also work around the clock along with students and monitor the activities of students, provide needed assistance if any, teacher will allot specific team of students a particular patients (Final year student will work as a team leader, under them III year, II year, I year students will be given, the four members will held total responsible for meeting clients' needs, for whom they are responsible . Each student will carry out specific activities under team leader and clinical Instructor supervision)

Special assignment—In clinical area each learner will be assigned special assignment like maintaining Drug Register in the ward, Linen supply, CSSD supplies etc. by the clinical supervisor. The student is responsible for completion of specific assignment.

Functional assignment—The clinical supervisor allot specific function to be carried out by specific student in their clinical posting, e.g. village Mapping, Organization of Health Education Program for focused groups etc., Combination of assignments—To provide holistic care for the patient, combination of clinical activities has to be carried out by the students.

Team assignment—e.g. Clinical experience in Block, assigning the tasks for specific students in organizing field trip

Case method assignment—e.g. In clinical experience teacher will provide opportunity for each student to provide care for clients with specific diagnosis

Objectives
- To give best possible care to the client
- To consider the educational need of the trainee
- To develop good managerial skills.

Principles
Only clinical instructor has to list and allot assignments for each student
- Assignments should be clear, congenial, simple, short, understanding in nature
- Before giving assignments, the instructor has to observe
- The standards and policies of institution and clinical area
- Objectives of curriculum
- Duration of experience
- The individual differences
- Capabilities and (ability of the trainee) weaknesses of trainee
- Background of the trainee
- Personality of the trainee
- Make assignment according to the ability of the student to complete the task efficiently
- Prepare assignments on priority wise
- Assignments are not complete till it is checked
- Assignments should be individualized
- Same nurse has to be assigned a single client for minimum of 5 days, then only it is easy to adjust and understand the disease condition of client; frequent change causes confusion and problems in the ward
- Delegate all duties among trainees
- Anticipate emergencies in the ward and make provisions ready
- Each trainee should have adequate assignments; allow the trainee (some time) for refreshments
- Do not assign same duties for long time
- Let all assignments should be shared by all, teacher has to be responsible to provide each trainee equal experience.

10. Brain storming method

Here the intellectual capacities of trainees will be utilized in solving or suggesting solutions to problems and make the group to become active and answer the problem among them only. The instructor will act as referee and give answers for the unsolved problems, e.g. the counseling of AIDS – in this topic, the expert in the field will make certain opinion regarding AIDS and made the group into 2 or more sections, according to the number of trainees, each trainee will be given one paper to write opinions and will give 3 minutes time and ask the trainees to read the opinion and request whether it falls into high, low, do not know etc. teacher has to give explanation. Then the referee will ask other groups, are they satisfied with that particular explanation, if no, trainee is answering correctly for any problems, then the expert would clarify it. Here the brain of the trainees will be sharpened and the entire class will participate in discussion, the group will become active and enthusiastic.

11. Group discussion:

A cooperative, problem-solving activity which seeks a consensus regarding the solution of a problem.

Values

1. It encourages the student to think for themselves, to develop critical habits of study.
2. To interpret problems of the past, that she/he can throw light on the problems of the present and to gain insight into ways for shaping the future.
3. Helps her/him to advance in creative thought.
4. Enables the student to enrich her/his own conceptions by reacting to those of others.
5. The teacher can observe the student as she/he participates in the class and can plan for individual differences.
6. It gives the student an opportunity to learn how to adjust to Practical situations, to meet needs of clients.
7. Gives an opportunity to cooperate with others in the reflective session like In calculating drug dosage calculation by problem solving.
8. Self-activity will be promoted.
9. Cooperation in its highest sense is developed.
10. It provides conducive social environment by the development of favorable attitudes towards cooperation and responsibility.
11. Leadership skills will be developed.

Guide for discussion teaching

1. All group members should have a common understanding of the goals towards which they are working.
2. Procedures which will best help the group to achieve its goals should be set up by the group itself.
3. Group members have to learn to become maximally effective in the performance of skills relevant to their goals.
4. Possible barriers for effective group action should be considered by the group and plans made to avoid or overcome them.
5. All members of the group should participate in all of the aspects of group functioning.
6. Evaluation procedures will help the group to learn how effectively they are working toward the attainment of their goals.

Outcomes

- Increase knowledge, intellectual abilities, skills, interests and cooperation
- Changes in attitudes and values
- Better personal and social adjustment.

Discussion techniques for small group

- The individual conference
- The informal class group discussion
- The seminar
- The clinical conference
- Role playing
- Case analysis.

Discussion techniques for larger groups

- Multiple discussion groups
- Symposium
- Panel.

12. Demonstration method:

Advantages
- It activates several senses, which increases learning because the more senses used, the better opportunity for learning
- It provides an opportunity for observational learning
- It clarifies the underlying principles by demonstrating the 'why' of a procedure
- It commands interest by use of concrete illustrations
- It correlates theory with practice
- It gives the teacher an opportunity to evaluate student's knowledge of a procedure
- To determine whether re-teaching is necessary
- Used as a stronger motivational force
- Return demonstration under supervision of the teacher provides an opportunity for well-directed practice before the student must use the procedure on the ward
- To demonstrate procedures in the classroom and in the ward (in natural setting)
- To demonstrate experiments and its use
- To teach the patient, a procedure or treatment which he must carry out in home
- To demonstrate different approaches in establishing rapport with patients, so that the most effective nurse-patient relationship may be established.

Essential characteristics
- The demonstrator should understand the entire procedure before attempting to perform for others. This sometimes necessitates review before performance
- All equipment should be assembled and pretested, as it saves time and ensures that the apparatus will be in good working condition
- Advance knowledge of the procedure to be followed in the demonstrations to avoid distraction of student
- A positive approach should be used. Emphasis should be placed on what to do, rather than what not to do
- Demonstrator should accompany the procedure, with reviewing comments relative to procedure and its anticipated result. It should be limited to essential facts
- The setting for demonstration should be true to life as far as possible
- A discussion period should always follow the demonstration
- Mimeographed directions should be distributed before demonstrating a nursing procedure, as it saves continuous dictation on the part of teacher and waiting on the part of the student
- The student should be given opportunity for prompt practice for better learning. student will be given opportunity to do return demonstration/ practices in the lab on doll or dummy or on live object, again he/she will be given an opportunity to practice clinically under strict clinical supervision.

13. Laboratory method:

Planned learning activity dealing with original or raw 'data' in the solution of the problems.

Laboratory method is a procedure involving first hand experience – With primary source materials, through which the student can acquire psychomotor as well as mental skills.

Values
For student
- It gives best opportunity to experience a learning situation at fist hand
- To use the problem-solving approach to the solution of real problems
- To translate theory into practice
- To develop, to test and to apply principles
- To learn methods of procedures
- Initiates group work.

For teacher
Provides the teacher an opportunity:
- To observe the student in action

- To assess her/his worth
- To correct her/his mistakes
- To guide her/him in promising directions
- A little encouragement or special help at the right moment may intensify interest and provide the hopes for independent accomplishment in future.

Technique
- Introductory phase.
Involves establishment of objectives and a plan of work

Teacher preparation:
Discuss objectives or plan of work with the 'students by means of class discussion:
- To solve a problem
- To understand a process
- To develop skill
- To provide for correlation of lab aspect of the course with class work
- To give instructions for the students, to proceed without wasting time
- In thinking over what the students will be doing.

Student preparation:
For orientation and motivation achieved through proper instructions and guidance
- The work period
  Supervised study activity, in which the student is involved in a first-hand experience designed to achieve particular objectives by solving the problem
- Culminating activities
  After the lab work, the class has to meet together for discussion of common problems, for the organization of findings, for the presentation of the results of individual or group problem solving activities.

14. Process recording:
'An exact written report of the conversation between the nurse and the patient during the time they were together' and ' a record of the nurse's feelings about what was going on at the time, and as far as possible, how the patient said what he did'–*Hudson*

Purpose
To assist the students in acquiring, understanding of and competence in interpersonal relationships.

Used as a:
- Teaching tool
- Self-evaluation tool
- Therapeutic tool.

The elements studied in process-recording are:
- Conversational skills
- Skills in interviewing for a specific purpose
- Verbal and non-verbal cues to the patient's needs
- Skill in meeting the patient's needs
- Awareness of behavior in relation to the patient
- Control of behavior as a result of awareness
- Recurrent themes in the nurse-patient interaction
- Skills in verbal intervention
- Interaction patterns

Phases
a. Preparing the student for process recording
  - The teacher must help the student to define clearly the objectives to be accomplished regarding nurse-patient interactions

b. Recording nurse-patient interactions
   Recording of:
   - The exact report of the patient-nurse conversation
   - The student's conscious feelings and her interpretation of the patient's feelings
   - Analysis for meanings and clues to patient's needs
   - The instructor's and the student's evaluations of the total process recording experience.
c. Evaluating the nurse-patient interactions
   - After the interaction, data have been collected by the student, the teacher and student has to analyze the recordings based on objectives
   - Self-evaluation by the student to develop a deeper understanding of her/his own behavior and the effect of her behavior on others
   - Develops keener insight into the behavior of the patient.

15. Health talks:

This method will be used when teaching for clients and their relatives or a mass, either in hospital and in community in a planned way like a planned Health teaching, e.g. educating the mass about health and its aspects. Health talks can be conducted incidentally based on need or requirement of the client. Clinical Instructor has to supervise the students during planned health talk presentation, as a part of clinical assignment or requirement to complete the clinical experience.

16. Problem solving:

To find an immediate solution to a practical problem in an actual setting. Clinical learning activities provide rich sources of realistic practice problems to be solved. Some problems are related to patient and their health needs and some arise from clinical environment. Most clinical problems tend to be complex, unique and ambiguous, nursing process is itself a problem solving approach. Problem solving requires new reasoning methods and problem solving approach. Clinical activities should expose the learners to realistic clinical problems of increased complexity. Clinical Practice requires high level cognitive abilities, e.g. Critical thinking and problem solving abilities, specialized psychomotor and technological skills and a professional value system.

A clinical problem-solving process is defined by Fraser as one in which, a practitioner:
- Elicits relevant and specific information from patients to help distinguish between working diagnoses
- Generates appropriate working diagnoses
- Seeks relevant and discriminating physical signs to help confirm or refute working diagnoses
- Correctly interprets and applies information obtained from all sources about a patient
- Applies knowledge of basic, behavioral and clinical sciences to the identification, management and solution of patients' problems
- Recognizes limits of competence and responds appropriately as a result of their nursing education and experience of working with patients, nurses developed quite an advanced process of clinical problem solving. This observation made us realise that the main aim of training should be to promote this innate clinical problem-solving process.

17. Observation:

It is one of the basic and oldest method to gather clinical data or acquiring information through occurrences that can be observed through senses with or without mechanical devices. It is systematically planned and recorded and checked for their validity and reliability. Planned, methodical watching that involve constraints to improve accuracy. It provides variety and depth of information. Greater accuracy. First hand and sequence of information will be available, all subjects are potential respondents. Two types of observation is used in clinical research 1. Participant observation, e.g. the observer will be part of an interview, 2. Non Participant observation, e.g. observing patient's record and knowing patient's information.

The role of clinical instructor in clinical experience
- Planning and directing the program activities
- Prepare the objectives, clinical assignments to a set of student

- Obtains permission from authorities and respective clients, to demonstrate specific procedures to be carried out
- Supervise the students while they are providing patient care
- Supervise the students to demonstrate/return demonstration of procedure to develop clinical skills and gain the confidence, to practice
- Develop an understanding of research for better patient care
- Analyze the difficulties and guiding the students accordingly
- Maintain high standards of client care
- The clinical instructor will assign list of assignments need to complete like per week one ward teaching class, one health talk, one case presentation – with suitable audio-visual aids, drug book maintenance, lab procedures and normal values and specific clinical assignment to improve clinical performance of the students and standardize it as a requirement or norm. the teacher has to correct it before presentation for which the institution has to follow student and faculty ratio strictly, then only standards will be maintained
- Encourage, motivate and inspire students to supervise and evaluate the performance of students
- Maintain strict discipline
- Keep record of student activities, duty roster, assignments, clinical teaching and performance of students.

Program of Clinical Teaching

After curriculum planning, the administrator, clinical in-charge and clinical instructor sit together and prepare master rotation plan for all years in the curriculum then the clinical incharge and instructor have to prepare clinical rotation plan.

Principles of Master Rotation Plan

- Plan in accordance with curriculum plan for the entire course/program
- Plan in advance for each student in the class
- While planning consider the maxims of teaching
  - Simple to complex
  - Specific to general
  - Synthetic to analytic
  - Concrete to abstract.
- Post students based on their background preparation and availability of guidance extent
- Select areas that can provide expected learning experiences
- Acquaint the clinical staff and clinical supervisor with clinical objectives and rotation plan
- Provide each clinical experience of same duration to all students
- Rotate each student through each learning experience
- Plan for all students to enter and leave the ward at the same time.

Factors to be considered in Planning Clinical Rotation

- Standards, policies, philosophy and objectives of organization
- Curriculum outline
- Requirements laid down in syllabus and course
- Course objectives
- Indian Nursing Council (INC) guidelines
- Nature of clinical facilities available, location of ward
- Teacher-student ratio
- Permission from the authorities and payment of fees
- Formal theory classes
- Facilities, e.g. transport convenience
- Availability of appropriate time to avoid over lapping of students
- Clinical instructors and experts in the field availability (their leave should correlate with students vacation)
- Number of teaching units and wards (bed strength according to specialty/size of the ward)

- Number of staff nurses employed to provide nursing services in the hospital or in the field
- Sectors that are solely dependent on student services during day and night
- Duration of clinical experiences required
- Size of ward
- Select wards depending on the length of learning experience to be provided
- Adhere to rotation plan.

Principles in Planning Clinical Rotation

The clinical rotation must be planned in conformity with:
- The curriculum pattern for courses
- Formal theory classes (Doctors and concerned classes)
- Availability of clinical instructors
- Expert in the field has to give guidance (if no assistant is available, her vacation period has to coincide with the student's vacation)
- Availability of appropriate time to avoid over-lapping of student
- If all the instructors in the clinical area are equally well prepared, clinical rotation and scheduling of classes should be so planned as to equalize the teaching loads
- Seasonal variation has to be followed
- Give weightage for all subjects
- Provide the clinical experience in specific area according to INC rules
- Field practice in public health nursing should be provided
- Strict supervision is necessary so that, whenever students do the mistake or any doubts raised in the area, the teacher will be able to guide the students and clarify their doubts
- Whenever the clinical rotation for one class is being planned, the planner must know the clinical rotation already in effect for other classes in the school
- The scheme for clinical rotation should be planned, well in advance to ensure sound planning. Block rotation should be planned (if it is present in their curriculum).

Preparation for Clinical Experience

- The curriculum coordinator, program incharge, clinical instructor will sit together discuss and formulate the clinical objectives and goals to be achieved according to the nursing standards (INC rules) and needs of the nursing curriculum
- Select the learning experiences, according to:
  - INC guidelines and University guidelines
  - Bed strength
  - Specialty availability
  - Standards and policies of hospital
  - Transport convenience
  - Location of wards
  - Clinical Fees
  - Facilities.
- The clinical instructor has to go to the clinical area, approach hospital Superintendent, Nursing Superintendent, Residential Medical officer seek permission, inform about the duration of experiences, objectives need to be achieved.

Principles for Organizing Clinical Experience

The clinical experience should be organized based on the fulfillment of four criteria:
1. Continuity
   Refers to the vertical organization of major curriculum events.
2. Sequence
   Each successive experience build upon the proceeding one, but go more broadly and deeply in the matters involved. It is a logical order, based on psychology and educational needs and standards of curriculum the student experiences has to be planned.

3. Integration

Refers to the horizontal relationship of the curriculum, to get a unified view and unified behavior in relation to the elements dealt with the courses are so organized that they reinforce one another and point toward general objective, e.g. integration of Nutrition and Psychology to Medical Surgical Nursing.

4. Coordination

Between one area to another area. Theory has to coordinate with practical experience. Integration is possible, when good understanding between teachers to have intermingling of the courses

Factors to be considered by the teachers while posting students in clinical area

- One experience will provide many nursing activities
- Different experiences should be provided to reinforce many activities
- Provide experiences in different situations so that the activity will be reinforced. For example: bed making for post-operative patient
- No gap or exceptions for provision of clinical experiences
- There should be relationship between theory and practice
- Before the clinical experience, major theory has to be covered
- Concurrent evaluation to avoid mistakes and subjectiveness
- Increase complexity of experience, if the student is able to do, e.g. if she is able to do simple task, provide complex opportunity to learn
- Along with theory and practice provide the chances and opportunities for the student, to develop personality also
- Provide experiences continuously, no student should be left alone
- Overcrowding of experiences should be avoided
- Division of students into groups, should be based on supervisory principle (i.e. span of control) depended on
- Alphabetical order
- Registers
- Number of teachers
  - Observation of students
  - Number of students
  - Number of clinical areas to be completed.
- Clinical instructor has to make evaluations, based on the proforma, immediately after completing the experience
- Totality of experiences should be provided, to fulfill the objectives
- Maxims of the teaching has to follow
- Meaningful experiences should be provided
- Theory should proceed along with the lab or coincides with the lab
- Period of experience will be changed according to the curriculum standards and interests of the student
- All procedures have to be observed for each student
- The rotation plan should be flexible, not too rigid
- Arrangements of experiences based on situations, material, equipment
- Before going to any clinical area, the clinical instructor should arrange pre-experience meeting, where she will discuss the objectives, routines, policies, standards of ward assign—ments to be completed, tasks to be fulfilled; evaluation proforma, what activities have to achieve in order to reach the objectives.
- The clinical instructor should involve the staff members in the field, to guide, to teach and to supervise
- Before planning next clinical experience, instructor has to discuss with the student
- Assigning clients depends on:
  - Student's level of knowledge and experience
  - Availability of Faculty
  - Patient's point of view, condition wise and system affected
  - Doctor's wise

- Geographic area
- Needs of patients
- Functional wise.

SELF INSTRUCTIONAL MEDIA

Introduction

Generational changes are rooted in shifts in culture and will be viewed as reflections of changes in society. Generational differences reflect changes in the culture as a whole. Generation is a useful proxy for the socio-cultural environment of different time periods. Instead of making sudden shifts from one generation to the next, changes occur gradually. Authors are beginning to respond to generational changes by shortening textbooks in concern with respective curricular requirements and publishing more material in easy-to-digest tips, where the learner can understand subject easy manner. This trend is likely to continue; young people today, enjoy sitting quietly with a book and reading. Instead, they attempt to multi-tasks, doing homework while surfing the web and exchanging instant messages with friends. Educators can take several steps to teach better this generation, to meet its members on their own ground by breaking lectures into short themes, using video and promoting hands-on learning. However, standards for content and learning will be maintained and also should remain the same and should be fair to everyone. Educators can supplement the material that must be learned. As students feel more entitled, more will demand for better grades by keeping sincere efforts and learn on their own. In Medical and Nursing education, however, allowing students to learn the material in detail is essential, as they are dealing with human lives. Today's students frequently need the purpose and meaning of activities spelled out for them. This is an opportunity, if young people understand the deeper meaning behind a task, they can bring their energy and passion to bear on it.

Information and Communication Technology (ICT)

Medical and Nursing Education resembles evolution in that it rewards by ensuring the survival of the fittest. When taught properly, the fittest of Generation will succeed, engaging in networks, technology transfer, capacity-building, developing teaching materials and sharing experience of their application in teaching, training and research, making knowledge accessible to all; creating new learning environments, ranging from distance education facilities to complete virtual higher education institutions and systems, capable of bridging distances and developing high-quality systems of education, thus serving social and economic advancement and democratization as well as other relevant priorities of society, while ensuring that these virtual education facilities, based on regional, continental or global networks, function in a way that respects cultural and social identities; noting that, in making full use of information and communication technology (ICT) for educational purposes, access to new information and communication technologies and to the production of the corresponding resources adapting ICT to national, regional and local needs and ensuring securing technical, educational, management and institutional systems to sustain it.

Benefits to higher education

- Increase access to instructional resources through the Internet
- Share experiences through technologies
- Increase access to higher education through distance teaching and learning
- Increase flexibility in what to learn, how to learn and when to learn
- Motivate potential learners to engage in higher education.

Learners and teachers has to be engaged in various activities to realize the above benefits

- Train lecturers to improve their competence in using the new technologies in their instructional activities
- Train and assist lecturers in producing teaching and learning resources
- Train lecturers and students in computer literacy
- Acquire adequate facilities so that the identified new technologies can be used as part of the instructional resources in the institutions
- Run sensitization workshops to promote new technologies in higher education.

Purposes of Technology in Teaching

The introduction and use of information technologies in teaching in the schools would serve a dual purpose.

a. For the purposes of acculturation

For acculturation purposes, a learner who is being prepared for technologically oriented world needs to be immersed in technology early. Technology is a new world culture, and like all cultures is best acquired in early by the learners. Orient the thoughts and attitudes of learners through technology, For a learner at any level to seek information through technology the awareness has to be created and a need established. Only then would the individual invest on and utilize technology. The use of the new information technologies have become inevitably for survival. While adults have to adopt with difficulties to the use of new technologies, young individuals can learn and should be given the opportunity to learn easily and naturally by early contacts with these technologies.

b. For more efficient instruction

Technology is about "machines". Machines make work easier, achieve more work in less time. It can therefore be expected that employing technology in teaching would introduce better efficiency in the instructional system. This is achieved by expanding the possible modalities of learning (redundancy) and add some measure of reality to learning (concreteness)

Photography: It provided a means of capturing visual information on paper leading to developments like motion pictures, still pictures, photocopiers etc. Photography has led to further developments in information accessing in education through mass media like the Television. Photography can be improved by using computerised cameras which adjust automatically for light exposure and object distance.

   i. Increases the perceptual scope of the learner (immediacy)

   ii. Motivates the learner by making learning easier more interesting and challenging.

   iii. Provides the teacher with more reflective time for improving instruction.

   Makes record keeping and evaluation easier

Developments in Mass Communication—Mainly the radio and television, had much impact on education, making distance learning possible, telecommunications also produced the telephone systems and satellite systems which have turned the world into an open learning classroom. A combination of all these technologies have resulted in limitless opportunities for the educational system.

The **Development of computers** is capable of processing information from all other systems once the information is digitised. The computer combines all the advantages of the other information technologies, processes information at high speeds, generates new information and converts information from one encoding system to another. It support the teaching/learning process. Each learner works at his or her own pace and on individual basis. Used in combination with any of the other technologies computer provides limitless possibilities in information processing and information generation. In CBL, a structured environment in which computers are used for teaching purposes.

The main implication of the computer for instruction is data processing, its ability to aid the further development of all the other information systems used in education, the main changing agent for the future, most work will be done through computers so the computer as a technology has become an important subject for the educational system In the school system, the computer can serve as subject, as media, and as a tool for creative work. As a subject the student learns about computers. This is computer literacy. It has therefore become important at this age to learn the basic uses of computers, to learn to operate the computer, to learn to use various computer software and to learn to develop computer software for various purposes.

As media, the computer is used for teaching and learning. This is Computer Assisted Instruction (CAI). The knowledge of computers and programed instruction are used to produce computer programs that teach. It becomes possible to tailor instruction to individual needs. Learners can advance at their own pace or use the programs at school or their homes. Teachers can utilise packaged lessons or produce their own courseware. CAI adds a lot of flexibility to learning systems.

Computer-assisted instruction (CAI) is being used with increasing frequency by educators to supplement traditional classroom instruction. Instructional challenges create a strong need for an effective teaching and learning tool to enhance the traditional classroom experience. The advent of multimedia CAI offers educators a means for addressing these instructional problems.

Multimedia CAI is an integrated form of CAI that combines two or more components into an electronic learning environment, including text, audio narration, photographic images, graphics, video, animation, and 3D visualization. This combined format makes information management faster, more efficient, more extensive, and in some cases, may enable activities that could not be performed any other way.

As a tool for creative work, the learner uses the computer to advance her/his ideas, trying out new methods or projects and experimenting with and creating new concepts. In this format to use the computer also serves as a problem solving tool, calculating, manipulating and analysing data.

The **telecommunication process** includes teleconference, telephone teaching, telewriting.

- Developments in **motion picture** production culminating in the video-tape and videodisk (laser disk) which in combination with the computer, provides interactive video systems
- Interactive **audio systems**
- The white board (**electronic board**)
- Finally the computer and computer software

Advantages in combination with other technologies:

- High speed processing of information
- The ability to adapt to various input formats and encoding systems
- High capacity for information processing and storage
- Convenient information packaging formats (compact discs etc.)
- Relatively easy manipulation techniques
- Relatively low cost of the technology
- Adaptability to user conditions and modes.

Simulation teaching: using a computer to represent the operation of a system in a real-life situation

Internet: Through digital telecommunication networks Internet explores information super highway which almost instantly offers users unlimited research and information opportunities in various specialised fields.

Closed circuit television: which provides teaching and information only to identified learners linked to the circuit by means of a cable. .Such a teaching system permits a simultaneous presentation of a subject to a large number of clients. This technique may prove efficient when combined with verbal and non-verbal supports and if it makes room for learner's participation.

Satellite-assisted teaching: The use of communication satellites, transmission systems enables learners in large areas to benefit from teaching offered in a remote location. Distance teaching becomes the most efficient means of teaching far-flung clients according to their specific needs in terms of time and place. Instructional programs and information can be accessed at a distance by radio wares, microwaves, tele-systems etc.

The Library as a Resource: A guide to teaching and learning in higher education is incomplete without any reference to libraries and library resources. The library should be the hub of teaching and learning in higher education. It provides a wide variety of teaching and learning resources including the new terminologies which actually are refinement of some traditional learning and teaching resources. The book here used in its widest sense will continue to be the main instrument of teaching and learning. There may be CD-ROMs and microforms but these were first in book forms before being transferred into electronic media. Books are cheaper to use and easier to come by. Books, computers, microforms and the like will complement each other and help to bring fresh insight into the traditional teaching and learning resources. Tertiary institution's libraries will increasingly become multimedia based. This is why they are now called library resource centres, instructional resource centre, etc. The library will be the umbrella site for all learning and teaching resources in the tertiary institutions, the library will provide opportunities for teaching staff and students skills required for the effective use of books and other learning resources.

Printed materials are of two types 1. Reference books are those consulted for specific pieces of information. The references and reading lists given by lecturers provide the extra reading that leads to a mastering of the subject. Periodical and journal articles further complement books and provide up to date information especially in the fields of science and technology, 2. Non-reference books are of two types – a) Textbooks are used by teachers and students in the pursuit of a course of study. The content is presented in understanding way for the learners, Index will be helpful to search related material. b) Supportive or complementary books elaborate on text books and enable teachers and students to have a broader perspective of the topic.

Non-printed resources: These are made up of audio-visual software and hardware – sound of all types, particularly useful for teaching languages, music and drama, visual resources which concretize learning, reducing the problems of over verbalization and a combination of the visual and aural video cassettes; film slides with their attendant gadgets for use. Students and teachers should be taught how to operate and use these gadgets in various teaching and learning situations. The availability of these materials will encourage self investigation and reduce dependence on the lecturers. All teachers should be encouraged to produce audio-video resources in their subject areas.

Bibliographic sources: Bibliographic citations and compilation in all subject areas will be helpful to gather the content which is needed.

The library catalogue: The library catalogue is a tool for unlocking the treasures of the library. The components of the book and their various uses. Students should be encouraged to read various disciplines so that they can have a better perspective of life and knowledge. A proper use of library resources will produce robust students who are self-reliant and creative, who are able to weight one opinion against the other thus arriving at their own judicious conclusions.

E-learning: Acronyms like CBT, CBL (Computer-Based Training/Learninng), IBT (Internet-Based Training) or WBT (*Web-Based Training*) have been used as synonyms to e-learning. It is naturally suited to *distance learning* and flexible learning, but can also be used in conjunction with face-to-face teaching, in which case the term *Blended learning* is commonly used. The "e" should be interpreted to mean exciting, energetic, enthusiastic, emotional, extended, excellent and educational in addition to "electronic". It comprises all forms of electronically supported learning and teaching, which aim to effect the construction of knowledge with reference to individual experience, practice and knowledge of the learner. E-learning is essentially the computer and network enabled transfer of skills and knowledge. E-learning applications and processes include Web-based learning, computer-based learning, virtual classrooms and digital collaboration. Content is delivered via the Internet, intranet/extranet, audio or video tape, satellite TV, and CD-ROM. It can be self paced or instructor led and includes media in the form of text, image, animation, streaming video and audio.

Assessing learning in a **CBT** usually comes in the form of multiple choice questions or other assessments that can be easily scored by a computer such as drag-and-drop, radial button, simulation or other interactive means. Assessments are easily scored and recorded via online software, providing immediate end-user feedback and completion status. Users are often able to print completion records in the form of certificates.

Computer-supported collaborative learning (CSCL)—is one of the most promising innovations to improve teaching and learning with the help of modern information and communication technology, the concept of collaborative or group learning whereby instructional methods are designed to encourage or require students to work together on learning tasks has existed much longer.

Virtual Learning Environment (**VLE**)—In higher education especially, the increasing tendency is to create a VLE (which is sometimes combined with a Management Information System *(MIS)* to create a Managed Learning Environment) in which all aspects of a course are handled through a consistent user interface standard throughout the institution.

A *learning management system* (LMS) is software for delivering, tracking and managing training/education

Advantages of e-learning
- Improved performance of students was observed in e-learning than traditional teaching method
- Increased access to everyone in the globe and as as Web-based training becomes a standard

- Accommodates the three distinct learning styles of auditory learners, visual learners and kinesthetic learners
- Convenience and flexibility to learners, self-pacing, for slow or quick learners reduces stress and increases satisfaction, individualized instruction and the learning sessions are available 24 hours x 7 days
- To develop digital literacy skills required in their discipline
- Reduce overall training time, Spread training out over extended periods of time, increases retention
- Participate in class activities when convenient (not tied to class meeting times)
- Access public content such as webcasts or other course content
- Access courses from a variety of locations
- students are able to acquire knowledge and skills through methods that are much more conducive to individual learning preferences
- easily distributed to a wide audience at a relatively low cost once the development is completed
- Provides educational web sites such as those offering learning scenarios, worksheets and interactive exercises for group of learners in a specific program
- Inclusive of a maximum number of participants with a maximum range of learning styles, preferences, and needs
- Consistent delivery of content, Expert knowledge is communicated, Proof of completion and certification, essential elements of training initiatives, can be automated
- On-demand availability enables students to complete training conveniently at off-hours or from home
- Interactivity engages users, pushing them rather than pulling them through training
- Confidence that refresher or quick reference materials are available reduces burden of responsibility of mastery.

Disadvantages of e-learning

a. To the Trainer or Organization:

- Up-front investment is larger due to development costs
- Technology issues that play a factor include whether the existing technology infrastructure can accomplish the training goals, whether additional tech expenditures can be justified and whether compatibility of all software and hardware can be achieved
- Inappropriate content some times
- Cultural acceptance is an issue in organizations where student demographics and psychographics may predispose them against using computers at all, let alone for e-learning.

b. To the Learner:

- Technology issues of the learners are most commonly technophobia and unavailability of required technologies
- Portability of training has become a strength of e-learning with the proliferation of network linking points, notebook computers, PDAs, and mobile phones, but still does not rival that of printed workbooks or reference material
- Reduced social and cultural interaction can be a drawback. The impersonality, suppression of communication mechanisms such as body language and elimination of peer-to-peer learning that are part of this potential disadvantage are lessening with advances in communications technologies.

Web-based Learning: These are vehicles for distance education characterized by the use of computers and the internet will deliver course work. It is the newest trend in distance education, supported by web based course management and delivery programs eg: web CT/ Black board allows the instructors to display their course content to students via a secure web site.

" The use of the world wide web (WWW) to create entire or partial courses, curriculum content, which is available to the students online".

Web based learning activities can serve as an effective medium that can expand learning options that cannot be replicated in the traditional class room. Primary characteristic of web based learning environment is whether they are synchronous, asynchronous or a hybrid of two.

Synchronous learning environment involve the learner and other learners or instructors being online and communicating at the same time. For example: online chat rooms, In video class room/ computer conference systems,white boards etc. Asynchronous learning environment, takes place over elapsed periods of time. Web/CT/Black board environment in which students log on, view and read postings and submit assignments. It allows the students to access and down load course materials and afford several advantages over their synchronous counter parts, since they do not require students to be online at the same time , helps them to perform their work at their own pace to post comments, complete assignments. It overcome the barriers like transportation, weather, child care and employment issues etc.

WEB conferencing software tools: For example, shared white boards, document sharing, presentations, instant polling, text and side bar chat that allow for most activities found in a traditional face-to-face class room, as well as interactive television distance education courses with modifications for online, mostly synchronous activities with audio and video delivered over the *WWW.students* and instructors have a camea and microphone on their computers thus hybrid technology has implications for teaching clinical skills in web based learning environment.

Interactive video disk (IVD) program: A series of video clips were shown to the students, that depicted Nurse and Client interaction in a counseling environment. After watching the clip stored on the IVD with a computer, the students were asked a question on how the nurse proceed in the situation portrayed on IVD. Based on each student's response, another video clip would be played that showed what happened to the characters, based on that decision, two different IVD programs were used, a sense of competence in the knowledge is achieved, e.g. Child Assessment Psychopathology, Counseling for the child abuse or Substance Abuse etc., can be taught.

Satellite broadcasts of classes: Students at the location could see and hear the classroom at the broadcast location. ITV where students at both locations could see and hear each other and the WWW where student would receive mainly text based course content over the internet, often using a web based distance education software program, e.g. Web CT/Black board

Web interface: It allows students to conceptualize different cases from a range of Theoretical approaches. The web site allows users to listen to and read case intakes, listen to segments of a clinical interview link to different theory web sites and participate in a theories, case conceptualization discussion forums, by using this site, students can send conceptualization of different cases to the other students or an instructor. After submitting their response, students can review how a specialist representing the same set of expert resources responded to these questions.

Values

- Web based learning activities can serve as an effective facilitative medium that can expand learning options that cannot be replicated in the traditional class room
- As an additional to class room teaching, web based learning environment is helpful in teaching clinical skills. students will enjoy in participating in a web based learning environment. So blended/hybrid/multimodal method of combining face to face and web based learning environments are essential, e.g. the teacher can use web base learning, to demonstrate nursing procedures and in nutrition practicals, food preparations, recipes with calories specifications etc. can be demonstrated
- Guide and to develop the best practices for educators
- Instructors will discover new and better way of providing clinical skills
- Focus on outcomes rather than process
- Formulate educational policy and maintain accreditation standards
- Change from behavioral to cognitive approach, i.e. enriches knowledge associated skills, reflect the cognitive, affective, experiential components of learning to the attainment of the programs' specific goals
- Lower cost, as it reduces the number of faculty and their salaries
- Revision of curriculums is easy
- Studies compliance, safety, challenge, social justice, new thinking and consolidation

- Enhances emotional capacity
- Creates a safe learning environment that facilitates risk taking and examining one's way of thinking
- Critically examine their knowledge and world views
- Promotes new way of thinking and excitement.

Limitation

In teaching clinical Sciences, it is less effective than face to face instruction, to teach practice skills online and unable to socialize students to the profession in a web based learning environment with a focus of human interaction and hands on training and teaching of practice oriented skills, relationship building , clinical skills based clinical courses are incompatible within administrative, community or policy development practice.

More Examples for Self Instructional Media

- Experiential Learning
- Independent Study
- Interactive Instruction
- Self reading case materials
- Reviewing expert responses
- Web based environment for file sharing & digital portfolio assessment
- Text based chat rooms.

QUESTIONS

- Advantages of nursing care study(2 M, RGUHS, Feb, 2010).
- Advantages of Patient Assignment (5 M, NTRUHS, June, 2010).
- Assignments (5 M, RGUHS, Sept, 2009).
- Attitude scale (2 M, RGUHS, Aug 2010).
- Barriers of an effective group discussion (2 M, RGUHS, Feb, 2010).
- Bed side clinic (5 M, NTRUHS, June, 2009 and Feb, 2010 and 5 M, NIMS, Dec, 2009).
- Case method (5 M, RGUHS, Feb, 2010, 2 M, RGUHS, Aug, 2009).
- Case method in teaching (5 M, NIMS, May, 2008).
- Characteristics of a good demonstration (5 M, RGUHS, Aug, 2010).
- Characteristics of good assignment (5 M, MGRUHS, Dec, 2006; Oct, 2007; Feb, 2009; 2 M, RGUHS, Feb, 2010).
- Clinical assignment (5 M, MGRUHS, Feb, 2009).
- Clinical teaching (5 M, MGRUHS, Aug, 2007).
- Computer assisted learning (5 M, RGUHS, Sept, 2009; Aug, 2010).
- Define teaching. Enlist the various methods of teaching. Discuss in detail any two methods with advantages and disadvantages of each(10 M, RGUHS, Aug, 2010).
- Demonstration Method (4 +4 M, NTRUHS, Dec, 2007 and 5 M, RGUHS, Sept, 2009).
- Describe any four methods of class room teaching (10 M, MGRUHS, Aug, 2008).
- Describe clinical methods of teaching with suitable examples (15 M, Baba Farid UHS, 2010).
- Describe clinical teaching methods (8 M, Feb. 2008 and 10 M, Rajasthan UHS, March, 2010).
- Describe different methods of class room teaching (6 M, NIMS, May, 2007).
- Describe the advantages and disadvantages of Lecture Method (5 M, NIMS, May, 2007).
- Difference between bedside clinic—Nursing rounds (5 M, MGU, Oct, 2007).
- Differences between programmed instruction—Microteaching (5 M, MGU, Oct, 2007) .
- Differences between role play—Brainstorming (5 M, MGU, Dec, 2008).
- Differentiate between seminar—Symposium (5 M, MGU, Dec, 2008).
- Differentiate between seminar and symposium (5 M, RGUHS, Feb, 2010).
- Discuss the problem solving Approach or Method of Teaching in detail with suitable example (15 M, RGUHS, May, 2009, M.Sc. N and 5 M, MGRUHS, Feb, 2009).

- Discuss the various advantages and disadvantages of demonstration method(5 M, NTRUHS, June, 2010).
- "Discussion" is one of the Teaching Methods in Nursing Education; List the Different Methods of Discussion (5M), Explain any two methods in detail (10 M, MGRUHS, Feb, 2009).
- Enumerate the methods of teaching, Explain in detail about clinical teaching (5+10 M, NTRUHS, Nov.2010).
- Enumerate the various methods of teaching, Explain in detail about Lecture Method (15 M, RGUHS, May, 2010).
- Explain Simulation as a teaching Method in Nursing Education (5 M, Baba Farid UHS, 2008 and 5 M, RGUHS, Feb, 2010).
- Explain the advantages of Micro teaching (10 M, NIMS, May, 2008).
- Explain the various methods of assessing the skill of a nursing student and elaborate any one method (15 M, NTRUHS, June, 2010).
- Explain various methods used in Clinical Teaching? What are the Functions and Responsibilities of Clinical Supervisor (15 M, RGUHS, April 2009 and 10 M).
- Field Trips (5 M, MGRUHS, Aug, 2007 and 5 M, RGUHS, April, 2008, M.Sc. N).
- How does the knowledge of different modes of teaching help you as a nurse educator" illustrate (15 M, RGUHS, May, 2009).
- "How does the knowledge of different modes of teaching help you as a nurse educator" illustrate (15 M, RGUHS, Oct, 2009).
- How many members are present in Panel Discussion and how are they seated? (2 M, MGRUHS, Feb, 2009).
- Importance of assignment (2 M, RGUHS, Aug, 2010).
- Individual conference (5 M, RGUHS, Aug, 2010 and 5 M, RGUHS, Feb, 2010).
- Laboratory Method of teaching (5 M, NTRUHS, June, 2009).
- Lecture Method (5 M, Rajasthan UHS, Jaipur, Feb, 2008 and 5 M, MGU, Nov, 2009 and Dec, 2008).
- List down the purposes of Assignment(2 M, MGRUHS, Feb, 2009 and 10 M, RGUHS, April, 2009).
- List the Different Teaching Methods? (5M), Write about "Field Trip" as a method of teaching for a group of students (9M) Baba Farid UHS, 2009).
- List the four Clinical Teaching Methods (2 M, MGRUHS, Feb, 2010).
- List the group methods of teaching. How will you conduct a seminar on AIDS for a group of 2nd year B.Sc Nursing Students? (10 M, RGUHS, Aug, 2010).
- List the methods of teaching. Explain any one method of teaching. (10 M, NTRUHS, June, 2009).
- Mention the various methods of teaching and explain any two(7 M, NTRUHS, July, 2008).
- Microteaching (5 M, Baba Farid UHS, 2009 and 5 M, Rajasthan UHS, March, 2010 and Feb, 2008 and 5 M, MGU, Nov, 2009 and 15 M, NIMS, Sept, 2010 and Oct, 2009).
- Nursing Care Studies (5 M, MGRUHS, Aug, 2007).
- Nursing clinics, Ward Management (4 +4 M, NTRUHS, Dec, 2007).
- Nursing Rounds (5 M, NTRUHS, June, 2010; 5 M, MGU, Dec, 2006).
- Panel discussion (2 M, RGUHS, Aug, 2009, Feb, 2010).
- Problem Solving (5 M, NIMS, Sept, 2010).
- Process recording (5 M, NTRUHS, June 2009; 2 M, RGUHS, Aug, 2010; 5 M, NIMS, May, 2010).
- Professional teacher (5 M, NIMS, Oct, 2009).
- Project method (2 M, RGUHS, Aug, 2010 and (5 M, MGU, Dec, 2006).
- Puppets (2 M, RGUHS, Feb, 2010).
- Questioning technique (5 M, RGUHS, Aug, 2010; 5 M, MGU, Dec, 2008).
- Role of a group leader in group discussion (5 M, RGUHS, Aug, 2010).
- Role Play (5 M, NTRUHS, Nov.2010).
- Self instructional module (5 M, MGU, Oct, 2007).
- Simulation (5 M, NTRUHS, Feb, 2010).
- Symposium (5 M, NTRUHS, June, 2010; 5 M, MGRUHS, Feb, 2009).
- Teaching Learning Principles (15 M, NIMS, Oct, 2008).
- Team Nursing (5 M, NTRUHS, July, 2008).
- Technique of questioning (2 M, RGUHS, Feb, 2010).

- Three principles of assignment (3 M, MGU, Dec, 2008; Oct, 2007) .
- Three principles of Teaching (5 M, MGU, Dec, 2006).
- Use of computers in Nursing (5 M, RGUHS, Aug, 2010).
- Uses of Microteaching (2 M, RGUHS, Feb, 2010).
- What are the advantages of computer aided learning in the present context (10 M, NIMS, May, 2008).
- What are the Incentives the teacher use to encourage students?(2 M, MGRUHS, Feb, 2009**).**
- What are three Methods that are commonly used in Teaching with cases (2 M, MGRUHS, Feb, 2009**).**
- Workshop (5 M, RGUHS, Sept, 2009).
- Write a demonstration plan to a first year B.Sc. (N) 20 students on Oral care (12 M, NTRUHS, June, 2010).
- Write any four purposes of Lecture Method (2 M, MGRUHS, Feb, 2009**).**
- Write the Steps in developing a Project?(2 M, MGRUHS, Feb, 2009**).**
- You are appointed as a clinical Instructor, what factors you will consider while preparing clinical facilities for students (8 M, NIMS, Oct, 2009).

Inservice Education

INTRODUCTION

Education is a tool for improving life and is one of the most important needs for the well-being of any society. Learning continues throughout life and is called 'lifelong learning'. Learning is about improving one's knowledge, skills and attitudes to make life easier, fuller, longer and more enjoyable. Learning has a practical purpose. It helps us to cope with the changing world socially, economically, culturally, physically and spiritually. Learning provides us with practical tools to improve the quality of life or to change it. Our efforts, to educate ourselves should not stop after the completion of basic training program. Continuing education gives us opportunities to engage in lifelong learning. Continuing education is provided through non-formal, formal as well as informal education. Through continuing education, we can organize appropriate learning activities. These programs aim at equipping learners with essential knowledge, attitudes, values and skills to enable them to improve the quality of life as individuals and as members of Nursing community. Therefore, education is a powerful instrument of social progress without which neither an individual nor a nation can attain professional growth. The training of human life continues in various forms in each period. An individual needs training throughout his life by adapting improved technologies and to gain new knowledge and skills. Nowadays, the education spending is not expenditure; it is a human capital investment. Nursing is regarded as a problem solving procedure i.e. based on Knowledge of the Sciences and is developed through testing Nursing practices in specific situations. The quality of life refers to the level of well being of a community and the degree of satisfaction in meeting the basic needs. It helps employees to acquire or upgrade their vocational skills, to enable them to apply in their daily lives, to conduct income-generating activities. Such skills may help them to change their vocation, improve their current career prospects. Income Generating Programs can initiate income-generating activities. People become more independent and flexible in how they earn money.

DEFINITIONS

"A planned learning experience provided by the employing agency to enhance their employees' Professional Knowledge and skills, to follow new technology specifically related to job; Inservice training is an applied education".

"The broad concept of all education, above the level of basic nursing programs, offered in hospitals or institutions for their employees".

"A program of instruction or training provided by an agency or institution for its employees. The program is held in the parental institution or out side agency and is intended to increase the skills and competence of the employees in a specific area, Inservice education may be a part of any program of staff development".

"Inservice education includes all the experiences that teachers acquire after they start their professional activity in job"—*Hite & Howey, 1977*

"Identifying the needs and expectations of participants before the program start, meeting their identified expectations and needs during these programs and providing various opportunities to their involvement to the various levels of Inservice programs"—*Ozen, 1995*

AIMS

- To enable individuals to be successful in their professions
- To develop professionalism - to make their adaptation to the changes and novel situations in their professional life and to improve their required performances in order to meet the student's needs
- To investigate behavior and programmatic changes that improve the quality of instruction within the school
- Provides the opportunity to learn information or techniques that have the potential to improve job performance, which is a powerful motivator to the staff
- To improve work performance of the professionals
- The needs of students, the community needs and demands can be identified, training needs can be determined and relevant training programs can be designed
- To develop quality in education and to increase the effectiveness of teachers
- To achieve the required knowledge, skill and attitude
- When the objectives, supported with appropriate methods and activities, The success of the program will be enhanced
- To help the participants to become Productive, should focus on entrepreneurial skills, to upgrade the standard of living and to improve the quality of life of individuals, families and communities
- To improve employee's knowledge through upgrading the services rendered with scientific principles
- To discover potentialities, to alert personnel in working environment
- To keep in face in changing society to meet the employee's needs
- Acquisition of new knowledge related to technological advancement
- Improvement in performance of professional activities by developing specific skills required for practice
- It improves the staff members to get chances for promotion
- To develop right concept of client care
- To maintain high standards of nursing
- To observe and bring change in staff behavior
- It reduces mechanical action to a minimum and promotes economy, safety and efficiency of personnel in their work situation
- It reduces turnover and absenteeism
- Effective production will be observed through their work performance.

Components

1. **Orientation skill training program**—It introduces a new employee to the basic aspects of her/his job. In hospital field, if any new nurses are appointed, first the supervisor has to discuss with them—Their job chart, standing orders, policies of institution, objectives and it's fulfillment, procedures has to be carried out. If she/he is well oriented to her/his working situation, he/she will be getting adjusted to the new environment very easily and performs the work effectively. Orientation skill training has to be given for development of knowledge and skills (cognitive, conative, affective domains). In community field, orientation training camps will be organised to school teachers, village leaders, AWW, MPHW and HV by the Public Health Nurse about the concept of health and illness, etiological factors for disease, identification of case, prevention and treatment in order to reach Health For All. In Nursing Educational Institutions, the administrator has to conduct Orientation training programs and introduce the new employees about the Organizational Policies, objectives and its fulfillment related to training programs, the job responsibilities, line of authority etc. so that they can perform their job effectively.

2. **Continuing education**—The activities which contribute to the development of three domains and leadership, management for the nurses. These skills are very helpful as the nurse is expected to function with the help of auxillary personnel in her/his working condition. Her/his competence is very much needed.
   Types:
   - Centralized Inservice training—In nursing service department, one department will held responsibility for improvement of knowledge, skills, practice of their nursing staff. They will devote full time for Inservice education program and its activities.

- Decentralized Inservice education—This is planned for staff members who work together, giving care for clients with similar conditions and share common nursing goals. Programs are planned around the special relevant interests of the employees, e.g. TRR, ICCU units.
- Combined or coordinated Inservice education approach—There will be a central nursing Inservice education department consists of nurse in each division, who held leadership responsibility for staff development activities, whose time is devoted fully for teaching-learning situations. They plan, conduct, evaluate the program and further plan their programs basing on the need arises.

3. **Management skills and leadership training**—For the administrators and the senior professionals, for the persons who possess higher qualifications, who is having the chances for promotion and the supervisors, the authorities will give Inservice training to obtain management skill and leadership skills in order to supervise the institution to achieve the targets by reaching goals and preparing the persons to solve their problems and to meet their needs and to have conducive environment to improve their work performance.

4. **Staff development program**—To meet the educational needs of nursing students and to meet the curricular requirements, there must be provision for regular staff development programs.

"Staff development is directed toward expanding to the fullest, all the potentials of an individual, so he/she can provide better patient care".

"A process that assists individuals in an agency or organization in attaining new skills and knowledge, gaining increasing levels of competence and growing professionally. Various resources outside the agency employing the individuals may be used".

Whenever teachers are asked to behave in a different way they must change:
- what they know—Awareness, knowing about
- what they believe—Attitudes, feelings about
- what they can do—Skills, knowing how
- what they actually do—Performance, putting their knowledge, attitudes and skills to work in the classroom. (Harris, 1989; Ryan, 1987; Oldroyd & Hall, 1991)

Components:
- Orientation programs
- Inservice education—Faculty development programs
- Continuing education using self—Instructional media
- Attending short—Term courses, workshops, seminars and presentation of scientific papers.

5. **Individual Interest Promotion Programs (IIPs)**—Health Administrators will provide opportunities for individuals to learn about and appreciate their social, cultural, spiritual, health, physical and artistic interests. The aim is to promote leisure activities, life improvement and personal development. The program activities can be categorized into various types: hobbies, cultural activities, self-reliance, sports and activities for personal development. To be more specific, these activities may include reading and writing poetry, painting, making speeches, studying local law, participating in politics (organizing local elections), using computers, taking photographs, traditional dance, swimming, religious meditation or flower arrangement. Learners can choose the activities that they are interested in.

6. **Future Oriented Programs (FOPs)**—Health Professionals will provide members of community with opportunities to acquire new skills, knowledge and techniques. With these, they are more able to adapt themselves and their organizations to ongoing social and technological change. To prepare learners for the future activities.

Methods of delivering Inservice education—Forum; Ward teaching; Discussion; Laboratory; Conferences; Seminars; Workshops; Field trips etc.

Principles
- In the workplaces, support the idea of enlarging of knowledge and technical efficiency
- Inservice training is integration of life-long learning and self-development concepts, training of Staff to be taken into periodic intervals
- It is correlated to education-productivity and the professional progress
- Inservice training activities are shown continuity
- Inservice training objectives determine to the kind of education, which is given to staff.

Nature

Different criteria/ factors are used in determining the kind of Inservice education. It can be categorized according to the person's ability, work place of staff, organization's personnel requirements, training organization, place of training, the stage of trained staff inservice, attributes, tasks of trained staff; In implementation phase - executive training, development training, field training and internship training are the phases. There are two methods of training in application location: on the job and off the job training. In professional knowledge, it is primarily necessary to measure the knowledge. According to the measurement results or need of the group or technological advancement, Inservice training groups has to be set. Training programs should be prepared as focused groups. Academics could contribute in determining the training program about the structure and content. Therefore, the regulatory authority is able to contact the universities, institutions and resource persons to arrange the workshops with the participation of participants from varied institutes.

Stages in Inservice Education Program-Systems Approach (Fig. 6.1)

1. Analysis—viz., Analyze needs, goals, priorities, resources, constraints and alternate delivery systems, Determine scope and sequence of training program (by task and job analysis).

Use a needs assessment process. Training programs are developed to meet the felt and demand needs; needs should be arrived at systematically by identifying discrepancies between current conditions or outcomes and desired conditions or outcomes. Thus, when inservice training programs are being designed, analysis involves to gather the information about discrepancies and to use that information to make decisions about priorities (determining identified needs should have priority). The

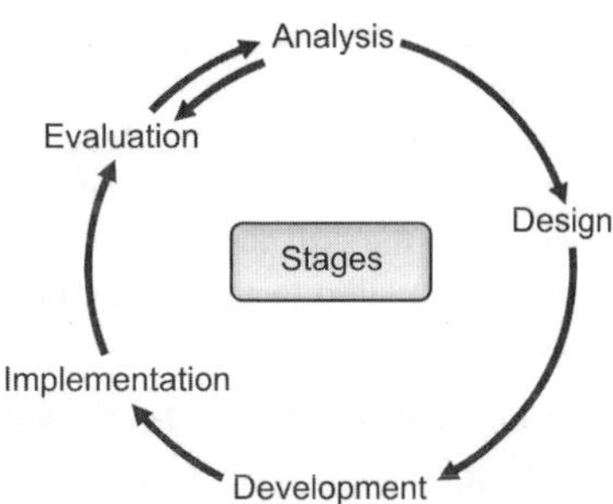

Fig. 6.1: Stages in inservice education program

determined priorities must have the goals for the inservice training effort. Training needs are often derived from a job analysis or from a comparison of the present performance of a person with the performance desired of them. There are many ways to collect information about needs. The inservice training designer must know which method is appropriate and what questions to ask. When needs and goals have been identified, inservice education planners need to identify parameters of the needs: resources, constraints and alternate delivery systems. Finally, there is a need to restate original needs and goals as performance objectives which are sufficiently specific and detailed to show progress on goals.

2. Design – viz., Determine training approach, develop learning objectives, performance measures and training program specifications

The overall curriculum is outlined and the foundation for the construction of the training program is developed. The components that make up the foundation all derive from the information and data gathered during the analysis phase, Some skills are best taught in the classroom; some in the lab; some through simulation etc. The nature of the task to be learned will suggest the setting in which it should be taught and evaluated. Plans are made for various sized group activities and needed teacher guides are noted.

Learning objectives should derive directly from the results of the task analysis and should be stated in terms of observable behaviors. it ensures training will meet actual training needs and that the results of training are measurable, In development of test items to measure the achievement of the learning objectives. Using the clues provided by the action word in the objective (e.g. construct, recall, list, classify), the appropriate test items can be devised, e.g. To measure a trainee's ability to recall information, a completion item would be appropriate. A performance test item, on the other hand, would be appropriate to measure a trainee's ability to construct something. Once developed, test items are used to form pretests, progress tests and posttests. Pretests allow to confirm that trainees are ready to enter the program or to identify that they need remediation or that their skills are such that they can be accelerated through or exempt from the program. Post-tests provide a basis for assessing whether a trainee has completed the program successfully. The results of this phase, sequenced objectives and a test item bank also provide the basis for the development of another foundation product: a preliminary curriculum (or course) outline (or plan). Outline provides the instructional objectives that materialize during the development phase.

3. Development – Viz. Develop Curriculum Guide, Lesson plan, Supportive media and Politest/Revise materials

The analysis and design phases explain what will be taught: what tasks trainees need to learn to perform and what learning elements (e.g. steps, knowledge, skills, safety) are involved in those tasks. The next phase development deals with how those tasks and supporting content will be taught: learning activities, training materials and instructional methods will lead trainees to mastery of the required skills and knowledge. The documents that outline the results of these development decisions are the unit plan and the lesson plan. Because this is a systems approach, each phase builds upon the work of the previous phase(s). Thus, the curriculum outline grows out of the analysis and design phases and then guides the development of unit plans, and the unit plans guide the development of lesson plans. The curriculum outline provides the base of the instructional program, unit plans add substance to the curriculum and lesson plans provide the specific detail. Likewise, the objectives, which were developed on the basis of task analysis reflect the preferred training setting (e.g. knowledge, simulation, actual performance). This information, in turn, suggests what activities would be appropriate, what materials are needed and what methods should be employed. If the objective states that the trainee needs to perform a manipulative skill, e.g. Methods, materials and activities should facilitate and support skill development. Teacher might demonstrate the skill in class (or show a videotaped or filmed demonstration) and provide trainees with a handout that lists the steps and safety requirements involved in performing the skill and once the trainees have seen the skill performed and read about the steps involved, they could be required to participate in an activity involving practice of the skill, perhaps in a guided laboratory experience.

4. Implementation—viz. Implement training plan, Conduct training, Formative evaluation and Document training results

Implementing the plans to use. This assumes the presence of trained instructors, access to the needed facilities and equipment and the availability of trainees who possess the prerequisite (entry-level) knowledge and skills to succeed in the planned program. Each instructor is responsible for preparing and constructing instruction on the basis of the established (and approved) plans. A normal part of instruction is record keeping or documenting what occurs in the training process.

5. Evaluation—viz. Conduct summative evaluation, Analyze collected information and Initiate corrective actions

Evaluation of trainee progress and achievement. Program evaluation is a culminating experience. However, evaluation is also an inherent part of all phases of the process; it is continual. The results of evaluation feed back into the beginning of the process analysis is to provide a basis for planning future program modifications or additions; in other words, the systems approach is a circular process. The continual evaluation carry out is 'formative process' of evaluation. One must ensure through evaluation that teacher has to identify the right tasks and analyze them accurately and completely. For the analysis phase, verification can serve evaluation function.

Inservice Education Coordinator

"Under the general supervision, The Director of Nursing, is responsible for patient care related staff development activities including needs assessment, planning, implementation, coordination and evaluation; presents and/or coordinates inservice training programs for patient care staff and other staff relating to patient care needs is responsible for the orientation/monitoring of all new employees. Performs other duties as assigned".

Functions

- Assesses ongoing nursing staff development needs for the organization and for individuals within the organization
- Develops and implements group and individualized staff development plans
- Develops inservice programs including course design and training materials
- Develops community/in-house resources which can be used to meet staff development needs
- Develops in-house materials and audio-visual tapes which can be used to meet identified needs
- Acts as a presenter for educational programs; accesses films, tapes, books for staff review
- Prepares inservice training budget recommendations; reviews and approves the purchase of professional journals and literature for nursing staff

- Develops and presents (or coordinates) inservice programs for non-patient care staff in areas related to patient care and safety
- Maintains and updates inservice training records for professional staff
- Provides orientation to all newly hired employees regarding patient care practices and the philosophy of patient care practiced by the facility
- Provides remedial training programs for employees lacking basic job knowledge and skills to operate audio-visual equipment
- Coordinates the facility's Infection Control program
- Is responsible for complying with the Medical Device Reporting Act; serves as co-chairperson of the facility's Safety Program; monitors OSHA compliance; maintains employee health files
- Responsible for coordinating state mandated fire/disaster drills. Also conducts monthly survey on resident's skin integrity and advises unit nurses on intervention strategies
- Knowledge and Abilities: Thorough knowledge of General Nursing, Geriatric, infection control and psychiatric nursing principles and practices; ability to use basic computer skills; knowledge of adult education techniques; knowledge of therapeutic and team techniques
- Develop individualized and group (staff development) programs; ability to conduct large and small group training programs; ability to operate audiovisual equipment; ability to relate well to other staff and residents; ability to evaluate training programs and budget training needs
- To work more productively and teach according to times necessities, teachers who take the responsibility of the brought-up qualified needed man-power globally, should be trained and become sufficient in their jobs. When employees think education is always important, the teachers are the important members of the process of education who are responsible for growing the society and the individuals, directing the society and the quality of any educational system cannot be better than the quality of its teachers
- The teachers should develop themselves all the time and become efficient professional teacher
- Since teachers are the individuals who take part in the process directly, it is important to elicit their opinions about the issue. Inservice training programs should be reconstructed taking the expectations and needs of the teachers into consideration.

Planning and Organization of Inservice education program or Staff Education Program in clinical settings

- The complexity of the Inservice organization will depend on the size of the hospital and on the individual hospital philosophy and the kind of service it renders
- The hospital administration supports the need for nursing Inservice education. Certainly, the Director of Nursing service and her/his immediate assistants do much to stimulate a successful program. These are the people who, by their example, become the ideals for other staff
- The size of the hospitals may determine the type of Inservice system. There may be one person at the organizational level of Assistant Director of Nursing, who functions as Coordinator of all Inservice efforts, Whoever has the responsibility for conducting the program must be given the time to function in this capacity
- The larger hospitals may find it necessary to appoint instructors for each service, with all working under the direction of the overall coordinator. Other hospitals may have no formal program; rather, leave the responsibility for Inservice to incharge nurse or various groups within the staff organization
- Orientation duties may be assigned to certain line supervisors or head nurses and other on-the-job training parceled out to capable staff nurses. orientation of all newly employed staff; committee participation to formulate nursing policies and procedures; career counselling; programming field visits etc.
- The Inservice coordinator must work closely with supervisors and head nurses in planning and executing worthwhile programs on their divisions. She/he should be the resource person for obtaining essential media, either from within the institution or from outside agencies
- The Inservice department very likely would be responsible for the nursing library and other audiovisual facilities owned by the hospital

- It should be an unwritten understanding that all staff members will attend continuing education programs. The institution will decide whether or not attendance is mandatory or that employees will be paid for attending on off-duty time
- Inservice instructor should have background B.Sc. (N) or Senior Diploma holder with principles of education helps
- Creative thinking is a more valuable asset for the instructor. The responsibility for teaching may be a part-time one assigned to a head nurse or other graduate. Whoever does it must be relieved of other duties when necessary
- An advisory committee, with representatives from all services and various staff levels, is helpful in determining the overall Inservice plan
- Staff - development programs planned by the employees generate greater interest and enthusiasm. Rotating the chairmanship of this committee gives individuals training in leadership. Participating in the presentation of programs enhances teaching experiences and helps develop speaking abilities. Although all of the four phases of staff development are equally important, one part may be more in need of revision than another. This can be determined through a staff committee evaluating the methods and outcomes, possibly using a questionnaire and suggestions
- When new staff were recruited, the inservice educator or In charge Nurse of the ward has to plan for orientation training and special training on skills development specific to the particular department is essential. Based on the required skill development the duration of training will be varied. Individually planned orientation is more beneficial to all concerned
- Some orientation must be based on the needs of the individual, with the starting point a review of previous experience. A skill-inventory list may be helpful
- The new employee needs time to review the job description of other workers on the staff as well, so that his own position and responsibilities are clear. When the specific needs of the new employee have been determined, the orientation to the job position can be made
- When refresher nurses are involved, additional time must be allowed and broadened subject areas must be covered
- All staff development programs must ultimately lead to improvement of patient care through more effective use of employee potential
- The types of programs to be presented may include Problem-solving sessions; Procedure book revisions; Operation and use of equipment; Role-playing for teaching patients and solving employee conflicts; Conferences to discuss and plan; nursing care for specific types of patients; coordination with members of other disciplines to discuss continuing patient care and outcomes of treatment; discharge-planning and public health follow-up; Conferences within the staff and other departments and with other facilities, determining standards of patient care. Other methods for presenting continuing education in the hospital setting might be: Daily morning reports; Tours of other departments, hospitals, manufacturing plants; current library facilities accessible to all, with reference books available for loan; reference library on nursing, use of programd instruction; various presentations involving units; Clinics; Audio-visual media; Seminars; Workshops; Group meetings; Telephone information service etc.
- There are many sources of financial aid for continuing education programs. Every effort should be made to permit personnel to participate in outside programs, with special consideration being given to time arrangement. Educational institutions now grant on duty leave of study permitting teachers time for advanced study
- The final phase of staff development involves leadership training or management development of personnel to assume responsible positions such as team leader, head nurse or supervisor. Well prepared leaders cannot fail to set the pace and simulate the rest of the staff to increased productivity. Inservice education is a vital part of the total hospital nursing program, all phases of the program for staff development will contribute greatly to the improvement of nursing care.

Model of Inservice Education Program

The model works by using three levels of learning experiences to build a base of new and improved knowledge and skills accompanied by attitudinal change. From this strengthened knowledge base, it should result an improved standard of patient care and increased job satisfaction for nurses (Fig. 6.2).

General programs—Short courses are organized. Course topics are relevant to all nurses regardless of practice area. Topics like Nursing Process, Intravenous Therapy, Clinical Assessment of nursing students, Stress Management, Assertiveness training, Communication, Ethics and Patient Education etc.

Each course runs over a three to four week period, consisting of sessions held for two hours once a week, during work time. Each nurse is notified well in advance so that roster arrangements can be made with the charge nurse. Some courses have been conducted in the evenings for the benefit of night staff. The Course period will be considered as On Duty only.

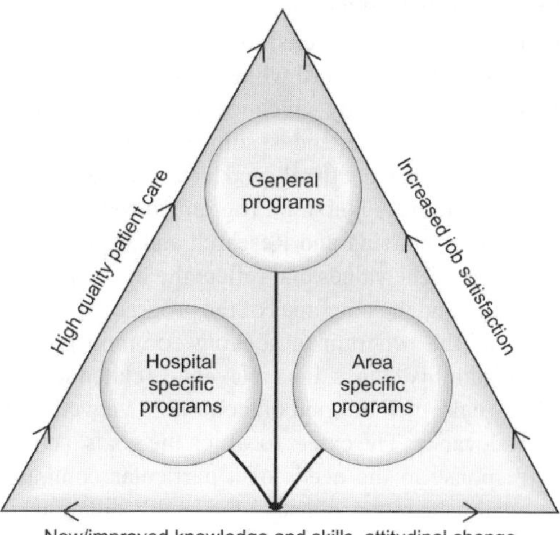

Fig. 6.2: Benefits of inservice training program

Hospital specific programs—Hospital specific programs are held on a regular basis in a central area. They may take the form of a film or videotape followed by discussion, demonstration of equipment or a formal lecture. Each session is of 45 minutes duration and is usually repeated once. Subjects covered by these programs are specific to the individual hospital i.e., general, paediatric or obstetric. Staff are encouraged to request programs on issues of interest or concern. Head Nurses, Nursing Supervisors, Nursing Superintendents also provide information on areas of need acts as resource persons.

Conducting an Inservice Education Program in Nursing Educational Institutions

The Principal or the Nursing Administrator will organize faculty development programs, Staff development programs, Leadership training programs to enhance the knowledge in relevant fields for specific group of teaching faculty. For newly appointed staff, Orientation training programs will be conducted to orient them policies, objectives, responsibilities in the organization and to update the faculty in relevant fields with technological advancements, inservice training programs through work shops, seminars, conferences, demonstrations, discussions will be organized. The report will be written and maintained in a register, the title of the program, the number of participants, duration, discussions in brief, the resource persons, organizational committee, representatives and their experiences will be recorded.

Evaluation of Inservice Training Program

"The systematic assessment of the operation and/or outcomes of a program, compared to a set of explicit or implicit standards as a means of contributing to the improvement of the program or policy."

Nursing as a response to the health care needs of an individual or to the community and of the Nation. Nursing Profession has the opportunity to observe gather information on and how the individual or the community as a basis for assessing the health needs of an individual, the validity of the program goals as related to the essential components of Nursing and to the health care needs of the situation (individual, community and country).

The evaluation procedure involves gathering objective evidence that is representative of the program and analysis of the evidence in relation to the criteria to ascertain the state of development of the program. The evaluation report gives the result of the analysis in a manner that establishes the validity of the findings and the credibility of the evaluation as a whole. The information provided in the evaluation report is of value to the teaching staff in decision making in relation to the problems arising during this program.

Selection of Criteria

Criteria should be selected to be of assistance in answering the questions posed by evaluation. The qualities or Values deemed worthwhile change and evolve as society's views on what is valuable change. For this reason, the criteria by which we judge anything reflect the prevailing values of the times, which in disciplines allied to Science depend to some extent on the current state of knowledge. Therefore it seems reasonable to select values that are timely and have worldwide appeal, not only in Nursing, but in the wider domains of Health and Education. A Nursing Program consists of a number of related parts – Curriculum, Teaching of Nursing, Practice of Nursing and Research and Administration functioning together to achieve the common goals or objectives. The values that reflect the development of a program are thought to be: the relevance of the goals, activities and the outcomes of the program to the particular community or country. The relatedness of different parts of the program in seeking common goals and in discovering the means to achieve them and the accountability comes, thus relevance, relatedness and accountability of the program in assuming responsibility of its goals, methods and outcomes are viewed as the critical attributes or criteria of program development.

1. Relevance: The extent to which the goals, activities and outcomes of the nursing educational program are a response to the needs of a particular community or country. Ideally a nursing educational program is established in response to the health situation and to the needs for health and nursing services at a point in time and in relation to the attitudes of that particular community or country towards the health goals, e.g. prevailing knowledge, values, plans and innovations. The goals and purposes of the program are related to the function of graduates will perform, which is, in turn, related to the health problems of the country and the type of care and services that these problems demand. The extent to which the program is responding to the needs of community, indicators of which may be economic, educational, political etc., may be said to be indicative of the degree of relevance program. The relevance is low when the goals and purposes of the program are not influenced by the changing the needs for nursing and for health services. The criterion of relevance is of concern with respect to the content of the program, the methods of teaching and to the relationship of teacher between teacher and the student will in general fit the expectations and values of the community and be appropriate, In particular to the type of students recruited into the program. Relevancy in teaching is usually related to the teaching staff's understanding of the culture of the community and of the learning modes of the people. The degree of relevance of a program to the community and country will over time, influence its' rate of growth, resources and viability.

2. Relatedness: The extent to which the parts of the Nursing program (Curriculum, teaching of nursing, Nursing Practice, Nursing Research and Administration) which influence each other in developing program goals and in shaping their achievement. The way the teaching staff practices nursing will influence the way they teach the nursing, it influences overall curriculum planning and all aspects of curriculum administration and over all how the institution may behave as a whole and a closer association between means and ends. Increased unification of this nature, where teachers, students and administrators will all together functioning toward common goals is suggestive of a high degree of relatedness. If the parts of these works differently in their own way of direction, suggests low degree of relatedness. In a Nursing Education Program the teachers will select the clinical situations where the students will get an opportunity to work effectively along with the clinical specialists as a part of the team.

3. Accountability: The extent to which the program teaches the student nurse that the primary responsibility in nursing is to that patient. Similarly in teaching the primary responsibility is the student. Assessment is the core function of Nursing, responding to the patient is a major consideration in assessing the development of a nursing program. In addition to the goals and purposes of the course, the types of Nursing course and the way in which the nursing taught, the nature of supporting and related courses and the preparation and experience of teachers all contribute to the study of accountability in a nursing program, i.e. how the student learns to develop nursing action as a response to the particular patient. In health services, nursing predominates therefore more nurses are required than other professionals in health care settings. For this reason nursing has to sustain a great deal of strain and is subjected to greater pressures for change from the public, from other health care professionals and more over within the nursing profession itself. In these circumstances nurses must be accountable for shaping of the young professionals and their path in nursing in the building of new health care services, hence the understanding of nursing is essential. Educational

institutions as the forerunners of change can demonstrate accountability in guiding the evolution of nursing and nursing services. Accountability in the teaching of nursing demands that the teacher assist the student to focus on the patient and to perceive the situation, including the therapeutic regime, the procedures, the clinical settings and the time is a feature of the process of Nursing.

The criteria of relevance, relatedness and accountability when applied to an educational program assist in describing the development of that program and form the basis of evaluation process.

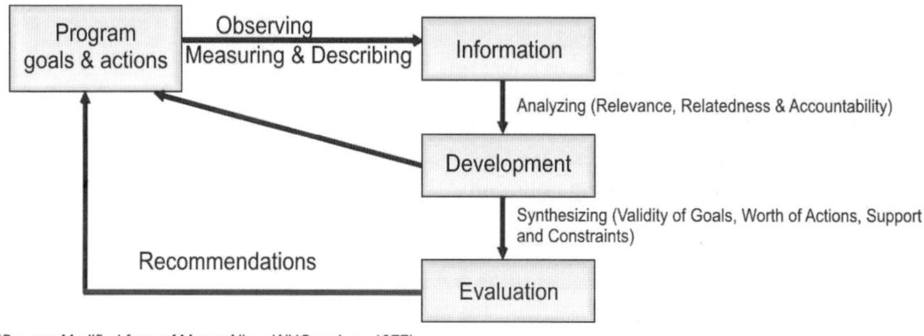

(Source: Modified form of Moyra Allen, WHO series - 1977)

Fig. 6.3: Model of evaluation process

Figure explains the process of evaluation. First the evaluator observes, measures, describes the program goals and actions collects the information to provide a data base for analysis. The criteria provide the structure of analysis and the results, conclusions, inferences indicate the development of the program, it provides the information base for monitoring the program so that the direction of goals and activities may be changed and the accumulated information provides a feed forward into the program plans. This process describes the every day monitoring and shaping of the nursing program by the persons involved. Periodically a more formal type of evaluation may be carried out for the purposes of accreditation, research, examination by the parent institution or at request of teaching faculty. The information development is scrutinized and synthesized in relation to the questions that the evaluation seeks to answer. This phase usually leads to a series of recommendations for the purpose of directing the future development of the nursing program.

An evaluation is directed toward gathering information on the various parts of the system so that one may have greater understanding of its dynamics. This knowledge increases the predictability of outcomes and the probability of the success when modification or changes are being considered.

CONTINUING NURSING EDUCATION

Introduction

Continuing Nursing Education (CNE) is a modern imperative, it must be future-oriented, geared to the facing new situations and the making of new responses appropriate for these situations. New knowledge is emerging rapidly in the Physical, Biological, Behavioral and Medical Sciences, which constitute the foundation of nursing. Problems in nursing must be solved by rational effort based upon systematic inquiry. Continuing nursing education programs should be developed by nurses and conducted within nursing or in general education system in cooperation with the nurses.

Definitions

"It includes the experiences after initial training which help health care personnel to maintain and to improve existing knowledge and skills and to acquire new competences relevant to the performance of their responsibilities. Appropriate continuing education should reflect community needs related to health and lead to planned improvement in the health of the community".

"All the learning activities that occurs after an individual has completed his basic education"—*Cooper*

"Education which builds on previous education"—*Shannon*

"Continuing education in nursing consists of systematic learning experiences designed to enhance the knowledge & skills of nurses."

Continuing professional education activities have more specific content applicable to the individual Nurses' immediate goals, are generally of shorter duration, sponsored by college, universities, health agencies, professional organizations and conducted in a variety of settings".

Features
- Unified approach
- Relationship with other systems
- Comprehensiveness
- Accessibility for all health professionals
- Integration with the management process
- Analysis of needs as a basis for learning continuity
- Internally coordinated
- Relevance in planning
- Credibility and economics
- Appropriateness in implementation.

Need
- To ensure safe and effective nursing care, nurses need to keep abreast with interest, knowledge and technical advances
- Should cater the services to meet the needs of population
- Development of nurses will occur by updating their knowledge and skills to prepare them for specialization
- For career advancement
- Professional roles are altered as new knowledge and technologies emerge and to meet the societal needs present and in future
- To develop competent Nurse practitioners
- To acquire specialized skills and to meet technologic adjuncts
- To meet the professional forces or challenges like changing function of the nurse, an increasing trend toward specialization, shortage of specialized nurses, variation in the nature and difficulties in formal education preparation and the mobility of the nurse population.
- Clinical specialists are needed for direct patient care, for teaching and consultative roles to help the students and staff nurses to reach higher levels of competency
- Nurses with research aptitudes and preparation are needed
- Nurses in administrative positions need to increase their understanding of the administrative process
- To design effective methods of maximizing the contribution of individual's efforts to provide nursing services to patients
- Nursing requires a high degree of skill, knowledge, competence and educational preparation to function effectively
- The demand for specialized nursing service is increasing more rapidly
- Planned programs are needed to increase nurse's competence as practitioners
- Need for additional preparation for the positions nurses already holding or to prepare themselves for other positions
- It provides opportunities for educational growth compatible with the realities of both work situation and the home responsibilities
- In the world, scientific advancement, technologic innovations, social change are occurring rapidly and new patterns of health care changes in the role expectations of all health care personnel are emerging to meet these needs and demands, qualified nurses are essential
- To maintain role as bedside nurse and to assume supervisory, administrative role and to perform delegated functions, to specialize and to generalize practice, continuing nursing education is essential
- CNE is needed for the nurses who wish to shape their own destiny must be aware of the forces at work, which will affect their future roles

- To provide and prepare faculty who see continuing nursing education as a personal responsibility as well as professional and university responsibility
- To provide a variety of continuing nursing education opportunities of high quality to nurses in both education and service changes.

Functions

- To meet the health needs and public expectations
- To develop the practicing abilities of the nurse
- For recruitment purposes
- To recognize gaps in nurse's knowledge levels
- To test ability and skills and to choose further advancement in studies
- To improve the communication between the participants, faculty, community and health sector
- To test the participant's ability to do formal academic studies
- To shape or support university educational policies and practices
- To ensure the quality of education
- To grant budget for extension studies
- To maintain academic standards
- To meet educational requirements.

Philosophy

Continuing Nursing Education encompasses various aspects of life and is not limited to professional education. Continuing Nursing Education is concerned with the development of the nurse as a person, a practitioner and a citizen. These are closely interrelated, but each must be considered in identifying philosophy of education.

Nurse's philosophy of life, nursing, education and belief etc. will influence the philosophy of continuing nursing education. If focuses on individual learner. Philosophy is thought of relating to basic beliefs. Actions are guided by one's beliefs, how one teaches relates to his beliefs about learning and education. Philosophy provides a direction for action, it is useful to think through one's personal philosophy. The educator has to think through his personal values and beliefs. One's personal philosophy of education is expressed, not by what he says he believes, but by what he does, what one believes about learning, the rights of the individual and the needs of society all are reflected in one's approach to teaching, this is Philosophy in action.

Philosophy is based on values and social change. The thoughtful teacher recognises that one's philosophy of education is always an emerging one, rather than a static one. Learning must be a continuous process throughout the life span, not limited to formal courses of study. Facts are more meaningful and more readily learned when there is an opportunity for immediate application. The aims and methods of formal education are shifting, to solve the problems of communication, continuity, coordination in providing patient care.

Nursing is based on knowledge of the physical and psychological functioning of man within his environment, expanding the knowledge related to manand and his dynamic, proliferating fields of operation is of concern. To sharpen the judgment and an increased understanding of ideas and values as they shape personal and social goals. To maintain worth, dignity of the individual, compassion, care and nurture in their professional role. To shape personal and social goals by acquiring more knowledge, sharpening the judgment and an increased understanding of ideas and values. To develop basic nursing abilities and new dimensions of adjustment to a changing society, provides liberation of the individual for maximum personal growth.

Elements

The philosophies of continuing nursing education recognises

1. Learner as a person, as a nurse and as a citizen

Thus continuing nursing education is seen as a totality, a sound philosophy of education recognises all three aspects of lifelong learning.

- Diversity is a part of learning process and contributes to the development of the individual so the teacher has to make the learner to involve in nursing and non-nursing courses, e.g. Music, dance or participating in extra-curricular activities like NCC, NSS. It discourages provincialism among nurses, benefits by learning with persons from other walks of life

- The learner in his/her life plays many different roles, e.g. adult, family member, learner, friend etc. for every aspect of life, there are some continuing education elements
- It aims as self-directed learning.

2. Teacher/Nurse educator

- He/She has to accept the concept of life long learning and his/her responsibility to encourage nurses to recognize the value of participating in different types of educational activities
- Educator must be aware of sources of information about related continuing education activities. e.g. Self directed individual study, inservice programs, formal basic courses and Academic studies etc.
- Teacher's task is to help the student how to learn, how to approach situations with an open, inquiring attitude, how to interpret what he observes and how to examine the system of values which gives meaning to his life as adult, can learn effectively, gathers many facts, make inferences, takes action and evaluates the effectiveness of his action by testing theories, ideas and to face an uncertain and changing future
- The teacher must help the learner to discover new approaches and potential developments in the field
- Teacher should act as a role model, friend, guide and philosopher
- The teacher is a dispenser of wisdom and knowledge, guide in the learning process, assisting wherever appropriate, encourages the activities that promotes individual thought
- The skillful teacher has to aware of the difference in learning what is already known and encouraging exploration in those areas yet to be discovered
- Creative teaching is essential. The effective teacher takes advantage of the assets, which the learner brings with him. A warm, helping, trusting relationship creates conducive environment for learning
- Teacher has to show interest and concern for every member of his/her class
- He/she is able to instill in his/her students a sense of their own adequacy and the feeling of confidence on themselves, which are necessary for the learning process
- The continuing nursing educator has to play multiple roles like:
  - Guide and counselor to the learner
  - An arranger and organizer of learning experiences
  - Motivator and an encourager of students
  - Evaluator of programs
  - Involving resources/experts for teaching the students
  - Producing instructional materials
  - Select and evaluate materials prepared by others
  - Administrative role (planning, directing, budgeting and evaluation)
  - Public relations role to change the image of nursing and in recognizing the contributions and potentials of nurses.

3. Educational preparation

- Master's degree in his/her area of nursing expertise or with a doctorate in adult education
- Credentials with more publications
- Writing and organizing skills
- A continuing learner
- Clinical expertisedness
- Depth of nursing knowledge and skills in its application
- Interest in the subject, enthusiasm in teaching
- Skills in working with adult learners
- Adequate knowledge about teaching skills and methods of teaching
- Broad base knowledge.

4. Competencies and other characteristics

- Concern for people
- Flexibility
- Sensitive to group response

- Willingness to travel
- Detailed advance preparation and organization for teaching
- Resourcefulness
- Determination
- Self-confidence
- A sense of humour
- Broader outlook
- A zest for life
- An innate curiosity
- Love of adventure
- Desire to search the unknown
- Interest in self-development and in others development.

5. The faculty administrator
- Teaching is part of his/her responsibility
- He/She should possess a high degree of administrative skill
- He/She will be able to assess the various abilities/talents of different faculty members and utilizes their resources at the time of need
- Helps the faculty members to strengthen their teaching skills
- Provides conducive environment for faculty members and learners to promote personal and professional development
- Gives adequate orientation, creating opportunities on the job which contributes faculty growth
- Encourages supplemental education and creativity
- Facilitates the faculty members to explore new concepts, develops imaginative approaches to help the nurses to meet their learning needs
- Fosters the expansion of learner's talent
- Maintains balance between the routine and other interesting activities, helps the learners to realize and accept their broad responsibilities
- Faculty members must accept responsibility for helping the institution to meet its goals and must learn how to work with colleagues to bring about desired changes
- He/She should make the faculty members to support and abide the institutional policies by familiarizing them
- Adequate administrative support permits the maximum use of faculty time for their effective performance
- The effective administrator is prepared to meet the unexpected
- He/She must guard against the interference of his/her own needs with benefit of the program
- Supports his/her faculty and accepts responsibility, encourages team spirit, working with other members
- Appreciates the person's contribution.

6. Motivation of the learner
- To accept personal responsibility for their own continued learning, motivation of the learner is essential.
- To arouse new areas of interest among the learner and involve them in planning, designing the learning activities
- Internal motivation i.e., the personal needs desire to learn is more effective than external incentives like certificates, grades and credits etc.
- Expanded learning opportunities for nurses which required their work experience and need to be motivated
- The truly motivated person will learn without external requirements being placed upon him/her
- He/She learns actively, as her/his thirst for the knowledge, as self motivated
- For the motivated learner, difficulties encountered in the process are seen as challenges, not as obstacles.

7. Involvement of the learner in the learning process
Learner has to participate in the learning process. Learning depends upon the student himself/herself. Learning can be done only by the learner. It depends upon the effort put forth by the learner.

8. Organized learning experiences

Teacher is involved more directly in program planning and in the conduct of courses and deciding which educational experiences and the activities are most suitable for specific group of learners, in certain aspects, teacher will include learner's views while organizing the learning experiences.

9. The needs of society

Quality of life and needs of society influences the learning needs of the nurses. The critical issues facing society can be met by a concerned, well informed citizen, who are willing to devote thought, time and energy to their solution. Citizens are vitally concerned and actively involved in seeking solutions to the problems faced by that society. Adequate preparation for participation approach is essential for continuing nursing education.

10. Universalisation is necessary for continuing nursing education

11. The leisure

The individual has to learn how to use leisure time constructively, participate in more educational activities or specific skill development.

12. Liberal education

Future nursing practice will place heavy demand on all health professional's efforts, human practice requires practitioners with the insight, understanding and attitudes which can be fulfilled through liberal education.

13. Inter-professional continuing education

It is imperative for the future; educational programs now include course content open to all those in various health fields. Nurses have to accept and participate interdisciplinary continuing education. It requires input from all professional groups for whom it is intended.

Principles of CNE

- Provision for school and nursing faculty involvement in planning and teaching the continuing nursing education (CNE) courses tend to maintain high educational standards for the program
- An adequate staff is essential for planning, implementing and evaluating a program which is based on learning needs and which has an impact on the quality of nursing care provided
- Responsibility of the Director of Continuing Nursing Education are:
  - Determination of learning needs of the nurse population
  - Development and implementation of a program to meet these needs
  - Evaluation of results
- Staff services are required with sufficient number with adequate talents to implement the planned program:
  - Advisory
  - Secretarial
  - Administrative
  - Supportive(additional supportive services may required periodically)
  - Assistance with:
    - I. Research
    - II. Publicity
    - III. Questionnaire
    - IV. Evaluation tools
    - V. Data analysis
    - VI. Computer programming.
- An advisory committee has to be appointed, which includes:
  - Faculty members from a variety of areas of nursing practice
  - Directors of hospital nursing services
  - Representatives from the state licensing authority, health department and voluntary agencies
  - Extended care facilities
  - Hospital association
  - Medical and allied health professionals

- Regional medical program
- Other agencies involved in the delivery of health care in the community.
- The community may serve as a liaison between the school of nursing and the health community and fulfill communication and public relations function for the university
- Continuing nursing education program may be decentralized (i.e. faculty of an academic department would initiate, plan, implement and evaluate its own program of continuing education) or centralized (a separate department or extension division is responsible for the continuing nursing education program of the entire university)

Decentralization is characterized by programming within each academic department, faculty involved in consultation and surveys with the public interested in their subject field were most knowledgeable about the needs for continuing nursing education.

Centralization is characterized by a separate department or extension division:
- Financial support is by either university grants or self-supporting
- Faculty may be assigned to continuing education as a regular part of the normal teaching load, but for periods they will get extra remuneration or non-university faculty may hired on a contract basis to teach specific courses.

Planning

A successful continuing nursing education program is the result of careful and detailed planning.

Aspects of continuing nursing education planning:
- Broad planning has to be done by institution andagencies responsible for continuing nursing education
- Specific planning has to be done by individuals for their own continuing education
- Planning is essential to:
  - Meet the nursing needs
  - Use available resources
  - Meet needs at all levels i.e., local, state, regional, national and international
  - Avoid duplication and fragmentation of efforts
  - Keep at a minimum, any gaps in meeting the continuing education needs of nurses
  - The selection of teaching faculty may depend upon the availability of the person and his expertisedness or teaching ability. The content of the program is designed around faculty knowledge and learning needs of the participants
  - In interdisciplinary approach requires representation of all the groups involved; determination of common and compatible goals for successful programming
  - Planning is an ongoing process, the rapid technologic advances and proliferation of knowledge demands continuous planning to meet ever changing learning needs.

Planning Process

1. Establishing goals with the purpose or philosophy of the organization: Purpose gives direction in planning. It identifies the reason for existence. Purpose are based on the learning needs and societal needs; so it has to be reviewed from time to time and restated as appropriate.

   Planning formula

   It provides a framework for program planning
   - What has to be done?
     - Understand clearly what your unit is expected to do in relation to the work assigned to it
     - Break the unit work into separate jobs in terms of man power, material and money you have at your disposal
     - Think each job responsibilities.
   - Why it is necessary?
     - Alternate methods which are necessary to meet the goals.
   - How it has to be done?
     - Look for better ways of doing it in terms of the utilization of men, materials, equipments and money.

- Where it has to be done?
  - Study the flow of work, availability of material and equipment best suited to do the job.
- When it has to be done?
  - Time schedule for the maximum utilization of time, money, material.
- Who should do the job?
  - Determine what skills are needed to do the job successfully; select or train the individuals best suited for the job.

2. Establishing goals and objectives:
   - Planning moves toward goals which are significant and realistic, which can be attained. Goals serve to stimulate and direct action and should be reachable.
   - An objective is specific, it is a desired end or accomplishment to be sought

   Objectives
   - To assist the nurse in identifying and meeting current learning needs and those needs generated by changing professional practice
   - To encourage the nurse to identify and influence societal changes which have implications for nursing and to modify practice accordingly
   - To promote the development of leadership potential of the nurse
   - To identify nursing problems and in seeking solutions to them
   - To develop varied teaching methods for extending nursing knowledge and competency
   - To disseminate new information from varied channels
   - To assist the nurse educator in increasing teaching effectiveness
   - To facilitate a return to practice
   - To assess the health needs of nurses, hospitals and community to plan, implement and evaluate educational programs in hospitals and health facilities
   - To seek opportunity for and collaborate with other health disciplines to effect improvement in the delivery of health care systems.

3. Determining needs and priorities (the course of action required to meet the specific objective):
   Assessment of needs will be done by survey, through mailed questionnaires, interview (formal and informal discussions) with participants (feedback) and check list, After assessing the needs prioritization of needs has to be done.

4. Assess the available resources for establishing the program:
   Careful assessment of ways and means to meet the established program goals. Faculty, finances and facilities may be seen as the major resources required for a continuing nursing education program.
   A broad survey of the major resources are necessary to the total continuing nursing education program and a more detailed assessment for any specific course or activity. Planning involves deciding upon the resources necessary to the activity and then determining the availability.
   Adequate financial support, appropriate faculty, facilities with easy accessibility space and necessary equipment required to conduct offering.

5. Plan the budget appropriate for the program:
   Separate budget is required for each specific activity and each individual offering is expected to be self-supporting. Budget requires ascertaining all the anticipated costs of the offering.
   The fee is on the basis of the cost involved and the expected enrollment sometimes budget for inservice training or continuing education programs will be sanctioned by government, university grants or fee collected from participants. The coordinators has to write the proposal after the problem has been identified and the substantiating data collected, guidelines has to be studied and to be followed in writing the proposal.

   Writing the proposal
   The proposal should be written with carefulness clear, concise familiar terms which include enough detail so that reviewers have a thorough understanding of what the project intends to accomplish.

Format for proposal preparation:

a. Cover sheet includes
- Name of project
- Summary of project (optional, one paragraph)
- Name of funding source to which proposal is directed
- Name and address of institution submitting project
- Name of principal initiator and others involved in proposal preparation
- Date of submission.

b. Proposal abstract (optional)

c. Proposal narrative
- Statement of objectives
  - Description of the nature of problem
  - Documentation of existence problem with appropriate data
  - Description of the existing efforts to solve problem or create opportunity
  - Define target group
  - State goals of project.
- Procedure
  - Description of phases or sequences of procedures
  - Description of work performed at each stage and duration
  - Show how work will be organised
  - Personnel handling each component of work.
- Facilities required
- Resources that will be identified and utilized
- Evaluation procedures.

d. Budget narrative

Explain each budgetary item
- Criteria and data used to make estimates
- Breakdown of budgetary materials where appropriate.

e. Appendices
- Statement outlining details of institution requesting funds
- Vitae of personnel involved
- Supporting statements from proposed clientele
- Supporting statements from cooperating individuals or agencies.

Sample format for budget

Project title

Project period from ……………... to ………………..

Personnel services:
- List all position titles
- Percent of time on the project
- Funds needed to cover emergencies.
- Give the annual rates
- Projected increases in the salaries

Supplies and expenses:
- Office supplies
- Duplicating services
- Instructional material
- Telephone
- Reference body and publications
- Printing of forms.

Equipment:
- Office equipment

- Duplicating equipment
- Cost of maintenance agreement
- Audiovisual equipment
- Purchased or rented.

Travel
- Number of trips
- Place of trip
- By whom
- Cost per trip

Space needs and monthly rental
Other costs
- Insurance
- Miscellaneous

Trainee costs:
- Subsistence
- Travel
- Salary or stipends
- Space for classes

Sample proposal abstract
- Proposal title
- Submitted by
- Problem
- Objectives
- Procedures
- Timetables
- Budget total

6. Organization

Programming of professional courses in nursing is a joint responsibility of a Director of continuing Nursing Education and a Dean of School of Nursing. The formal channels of communication make possible the optional use of the nursing faculty to explore the needs of continuing nursing education, to set priorities, to plan courses and to teach them. University faculty may be assigned to continuing education in nursing as a part of the regular teaching load or an extra compensation basis. The opportunity for faculty involvement is highly desirable and provision of advisory committee at the operational level is needed (Also see Figs 6.4 to 6.7).

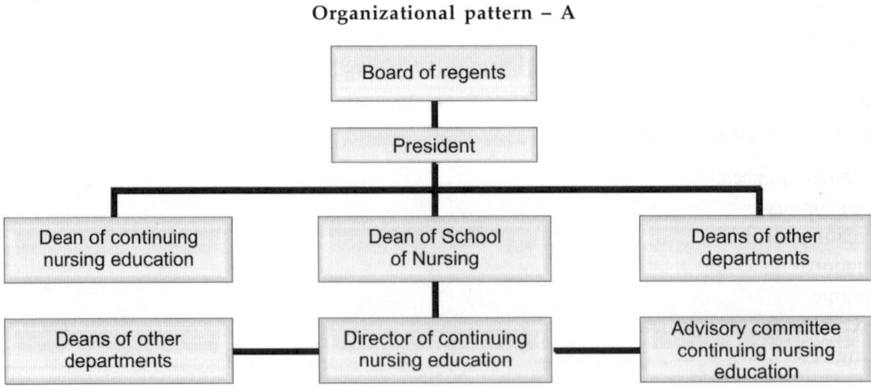

Fig. 6.4: Organizational chart of continuing nursing education showing joint responsibility

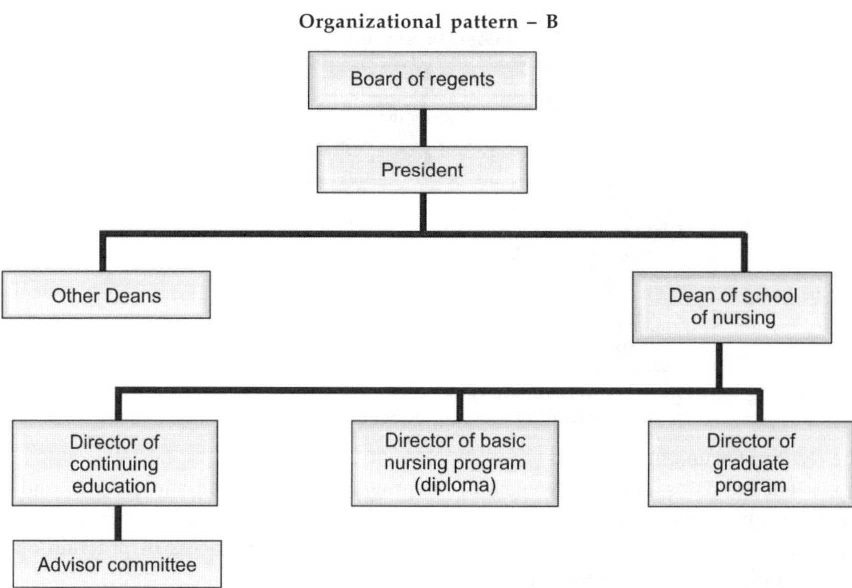

Fig. 6.5: Organizational chart of continuing education in nursing showing decentralized responsibility for the continuing nursing education program at a departmental level.

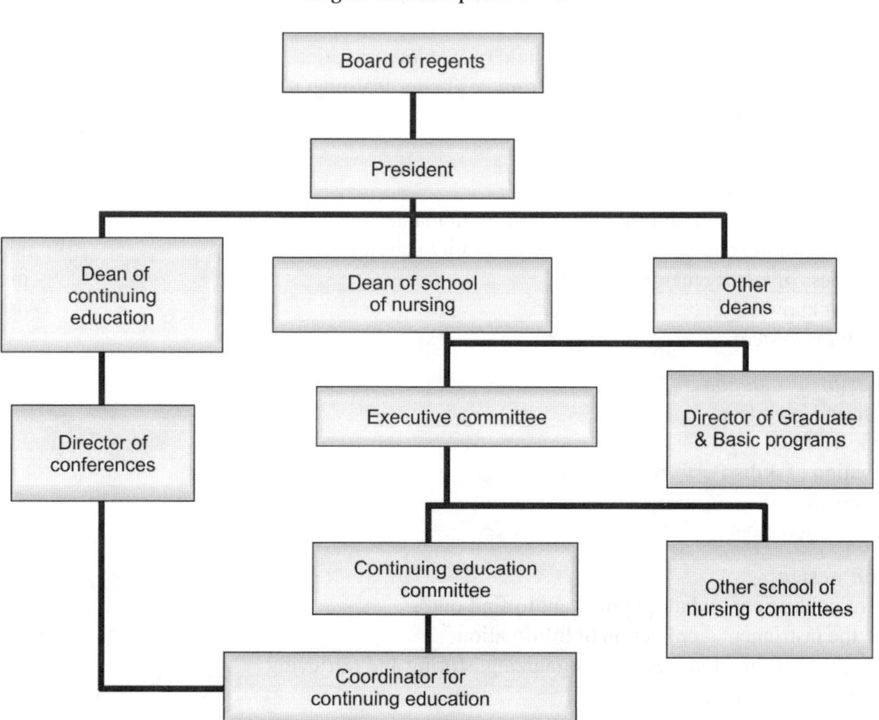

Fig. 6.6: Organizational chart showing joint responsibility for the continuing nursing education program on a committee level.

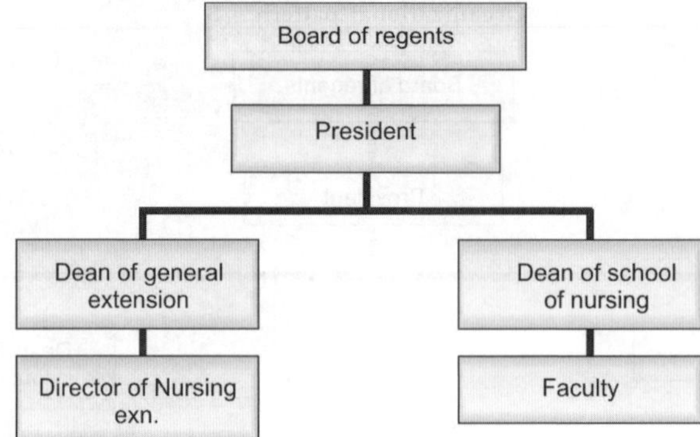

Fig. 6.7: Organizational chart showing centralized responsibility for the continuing nursing education program.

Evaluate the results at stated intervals

Evaluation is needed to assess the effectiveness of the program or the progress in order to find out to what extent pre-set goals have been achieved evaluations should be done at different stages of the program e.g. Preparatory stage; Implementation stage; the impact of programs; the process of program operation, the management systems, efforts and performance evaluation.

Purposes of evaluation
- To identify the areas which require greater attention in terms of participation of trainees, academic activities and management (at planning stage)
- To identify bottlenecks in various activities carried out during the operation of the program (implementation stage)
- To assess the applicability of training in field or in actual situation
- Qualitative improvement in instruction promotes better learning, determines future changes and needs
- For quality control or qualitative improvement

What to evaluate?
Evaluation should cover
- The professional growth and satisfaction of participants
- The outcome of the course and the whole program / activity / task
- Effectiveness of faculty members
- Transfer of knowledge
- Effect on the system

Procedures for evaluation
- Pre-test and post-test
- Attitude tests
- Observation of skills/Performance Evaluation
- Questionnaire
- Audio or video tapes

Evaluation design
- Focus of evaluation – what do you want to find out?
- Devise the instrument – collection of information
- Organize the information – coding, organizing, storing and retrieving
- Analyze the information
- Report the findings
- Reassessing the goals
- Updating, modifying the plan periodically based on needs
- Evaluate the design for validity, reliability, credibility, timeliness and pervasiveness

QUESTIONS

- Continuing Nursing Education (5 M, NTRUHS, June, 2009 & 5 M, RGUHS, Oct, 2006).
- Define Continuing Education in Nursing, Discuss the need of CNE (10 M, NIMS, May, 2010).
- Define Continuing Nursing Education? Design and Prepare a Plan of Continuing Nursing Education for the Health Care Workers of a Primary Health Centre? (15 M, RGUHS, May, 2010).
- Define Inservice Education, What are the components of Inservice Education, Prepare an Orientation Program for 6 days to orient 25 newly recruited ward sisters in a 500 bedded hospital (2+2+8 M, NIMS, May, 2007).
- Define in-service education. As a nursing superintendent how will you organize in service education in a hospital nursing service? (15 M, NTRUHS, Nov, 2010).
- Define Validity, What are Types of Validity (2 + 5 M, MGRUHS, May, 2010).
- Describe types of reliability (5 M, MGRUHS, May, 2008).
- Inservice Education (4 M, NTRUHS, Dec, 2007 & 4 M, RGUHS, 2009).
- Plan a budget for Continuing Nursing Education Program for the clinical Instructors for a period of one week (12 M, NIMS, Sept, 2010).
- Staff development program (10 M, RGUHS, M.Sc.(N), 2006 & 5 M, RGUHS, Aug, 2010).
- What do you understand by the term "Inservice Education". Plan a week inservice education training program for operation theatre nurses in your hospital (15 M, NIMS, October, 2009).
- Write the importance and need for Continuing Education in Nursing (15 M, NIMS, Oct, 2008).
- Write the scope of Inservice Education Program, Plan an Inservice education program on disaster management for staff Nurses at 250 bedded hospital (3M+7 M, NIMS, May, 2008).

Audio-Visual Aids (Instructional Media)

INTRODUCTION

Audio-visual material must be seen in their relationship to teaching and to the learning process as a whole, until teacher understands the relationship between audio-visual material and teaching-learning process, he cannot be expected to make intelligent or fruitful utilization of the techniques, which offer lot of assistance in day today activities of teaching.

'Audio-visual aids', 'audio-visual materials', 'audio-visual media', 'communication technology', 'educational Media or instructional media' and 'learning resources', 'educational technology' and 'instructional technology' are broadly meant the same. Audio-visual aids are both complimentary and supplementary in nature for teaching. The most appropriate teaching aids are ones that can best convey the "messages" to the learners. Several factors are influencing in selection and utilization of audio-visual aids eg: Sound, Motion, Color, Abilities or background of learners, presentation and explanation etc.

The nursing profession which requires mastery of underlying scientific skills, intelligent attitudes and appreciations must necessarily aim for the highest quality of education for its students. Instruction can be enriched tremendously through the use of Audio-visual material. The contribution which these devices can make to specific areas of study is therefore well worth the thoughtful attention of all nurse educators.

Definitions

"An instructional device in which the message can be heard as well as seen".

"Aids that are used by a teacher in teaching learning situations for effective communication".

Concept

Audio-visual aids are sensitive tools used in teaching and as avenues for learning. These are planned educational materials that appeal to the senses of the people and quickens learning, facilitates for clear understanding.

A Chinese Proverb: 'If I hear, I forget, If I see, I remember, If I do, I know' says the importance of sensory perception in teaching and learning situation.

When we see it with our eyes we remember it for a longer time and when we perform an activity with our own hands, we understand its process. This is because of the fact that the more the senses are stimulated and involved the more will be the learning and retention among learners.

- By Seeing-87%, Hearing-07%, Odour-03%, Touch-02%, Taste-01% individual will grasp.
- Audio-visual aids enhances clarity in communication. Provides diversity in method of teaching. Increases the forcefulness of the subject being learned or taught. Serves in the instructional role in order to supplement and enrich the teacher's own learning. The student will be able to get direct experience of a real life situation or indirect sensory experience or symbolic experiences will be used.

Meaning

The sensory objects or images which initiates or stimulate and reinforce learning. It helps the process of learning i.e., motivation, classification and stimulation. Audio-visual aids are multisensory materials which motivates, classifies and stimulates the individuals. It makes dynamic learning experience more concrete, realistic, clarity, establish, co-relate and coordinate accurate concepts, interpretations, appreciation and enables him to make learning effective, interesting, inspirational, meaningful and vivid. It provides significant gains in informational learning, retention, recall, thinking and reasoning, activity interest, imagination, better assimilation and personal growth and development.

Need of Educational Communication Media

- Audio-visual aids as a means of communication—Words are wonderful, they are easily produced, reproduced, stored and transported. But the overuse or excessive use of words can result in serious problems, chiefly, the problem of verbalism (using or adopting many words or phrases). "Without considering what they mean and forgetting." Contribute to the growth or clear understanding, increase vocabulary development
- Complement verbal instruction: Teaching will help in reducing verbalism. They help in giving clear concepts and thus help to bring accuracy in learning. They enable the students to learn faster, remember for longer duration, gain more accurate information, understand the concepts with adequate meaning. Thus learning becomes more meaningful, enjoyable and effective.
- Simply words whether written or spoken by a teacher cannot and will not provide the required information. It has to be supplemented by audio-visual aids, e.g. Visual aids–Charts, posters are helpful in clear understanding of concept, listening to language will make it more clear for e.g. Demonstration of CPR technique or any nursing procedures by audio-visual aids will supplement and enrich clear understanding of concepts in clear way, e.g. listening to audio cassette, video cassette are essential. Cartoon films are also a very useful medium for developing writing skills. We can show these films and ask the children or learners, to write about them. With the use of these audio-visual aids classroom teaching can be converted into a very joyful learning experience
- Audio-visual aids provide significant gains in informational learning, retention, recall, thinking, reasoning, activity, interest, imagination, better assimilation and personal growth and development. The aids are the stimuli for learning 'why', 'how', 'when' and 'where'. The 'hard to understand principles' are usually made clear by the intelligent use of skillfully designed instructional aids. Develop continuity of thought
- Recall pre-requisites—Use media to help students to recall what they learned in the last class, so that new material can be attached to and built upon it
- It promote memorization, stir imagination, thinking process and reasoning power, call for creativity and inventiveness and reinforce the learners
- Enhances transfer of information—Pictures enhance retention. Instructional media help students visualize a lesson and transfer abstract concepts into concrete, easier to remember objects
- Increase the meaningfulness of abstract concepts by stimulating correct thinking. The use of audio-visual aids also helps in better retention of the content, e.g. Teacher has to provide a number of opportunities for listening, speaking, seeing, smelling and touching things and objects. This will give the students first hand experiences. Educational experiences that involve the learner physically and that give concrete examples are retained longer than abstract experiences such as listening to a lecture
- Saves energy and time—In this age of knowledge explosion, teacher want to explain the students a number of things in a very short time. A good deal of energy and time of both the teachers and students can be saved on account of the use of audio-visual aids as most of the concepts and phenomena may be easily clarified, understood and assimilated through their use. The use of audio-visual aids can be very helpful in this. A well-developed language program supported by suitable, relevant and effective aids provides a number of enriching experiences. These ultimately lead to the development of language skills in the learner
- Realistic—The use of audio-visual aids provides reality to the learning situation
- Vividness—Audio-visual aids give vividness to the learning situation
- The aim of teaching with technological media is 'clearing the channel between the learner and the things that are worth learning'. The basic assumption underlying audio-visual aids is that learning (clear understanding) stems from sense experience
- Encourages healthy classroom interaction–audio-visual aids, through their wide variety of stimuli, provision of active participation of the students, and vicarious experiences encourage healthy classroom interaction for the effective realization of teaching-learning objectives

- Reaching remote areas—It can serve as an open window through which the student can view the world and its phenomena by bringing remote events into the classroom. Audio-visual aids like radio and television help in providing opportunities for education to people living in remote areas
- Promotion of scientific temper—In place of listening to facts, students observe demonstrations and phenomena and thus cultivate the scientific temper
- Development of higher faculties—Verbalism promotes memorization. Use of audio-visual aids stirs the imagination, thinking process, reasoning power of the students and calls for creativity and innovation as well as other higher mental activities on the part of the students, thus helps the development of higher faculties among students
- Reinforcement—Audio-visual aids prove effective reinforces by increasing the probability of re-occurrence of the responses associated with them and thus render valuable help in the teaching-learning process
- Positive transfer of learning and training—Use of audio visual aids helps in the learning of concepts, principles and solving the real problems of life by making possible the appropriate positive transfer of learning and training received in classroom
- Positive environment for creative discipline—A balanced, rational and scientific use of audio-visual aids develops motivation, attracts the attention and interests of the students and provides a variety of creative outlets for the utilization of their tremendous energy and thus keeps them busy in classroom work. In this way, the overall classroom environment becomes conducive to creative discipline
- Catering to individual differences—There are wide individual differences among learners. Some are ear-oriented; some can be helped through visual demonstrations, while others learn better by doing, The use of a variety of audiovisual aids helps in meeting the needs of different types of students
- Audio-visual aids or technological media are additional devices that help the teacher to clarify, establish, co-relate and co-ordinate accurate concepts, interpretations and appreciations enable him/her to make learning more concrete, effective, interesting, inspirational, meaningful and vivid. They help in completing the triangular process of learning viz., motivation-clarification-stimulation
- Clear images—Clear images are formed when we see, hear, touch, taste and smell, as our experiences are direct, concrete and more or less permanent. Learning through the senses becomes most natural and consequently lie easiest Present objectives to the learners-Hand out or project the day's learning objectives. Sensory experiences of all kinds contribute to strengthen and enrich the learners' perception.
- Vicarious experience—It is beyond doubt that the first-hand experience is the best type of educative experience. Provision of active participation of the students and vicarious experiences encourage healthy interaction for the effective realization of teaching-learning objective. They direct, dramatize the experiences. Offer a variety of experiences which stimulate the senses and promote self activity among learners
- Audio-visual aids provide rich perceptual experiences which are the basis of learning
- Variety—Audio-visual aids give variety and provide different tools in the hands of the teacher
- Freedom—Facilitate freedom among learners, increases retention as they stimulate response of whole organization to the situation in which learning takes place. When audio-visual aids are employed, there is great scope for children to move about, talk, laugh and give their comments. Under such an atmosphere the students work because they like to work and not because the teacher wants them to work
- Present new content—Not only can media help make new content more memorable, media can also help deliver new content (a text, movie or video)
- Support learning through examples and visual elaboration—One of the biggest advantages of media is to bring the world into the classroom when it is not possible to take the student into the world
- Opportunities to handle and manipulate—Many visual aids offer opportunities to students to handle and manipulate things
- Based on maxims or principles of teaching—Use of audio-visual aids enables the teacher to follow the maxims of teaching "concrete to abstract', 'known to unknown' and 'learning by doing'
- Helpful in attracting attention—Attention is essential in any process of teaching and learning. Audio-visual aids help the teacher in providing a proper environment for capturing as well as sustaining the attention and interest of the students in the classroom work, e.g. A picture on the screen, a question on the board, etc. serve to get the student's attention.

- Helpful in fixing up new learning—Gained in terms of learning needs to be fixed up in the minds of audio-visual aids help the learners in achieving this objective by providing several and stimuli to the learners
- Elicit student response-Present information to students and pose questions to them, getting them involved in answering the questions
- Provide feedback-Media can be used to provide feedback relating to a test or class exercise.
- Assess performance-Media is an excellent way to pose assessment questions for the class to answer or students can submit mediated presentations as classroom projects
- Provide adequate learning experiences. Audio-visual aids will supplement the teacher's words or thoughts
- Promotes real life experience
- People generally remember:
  - Ten percent of what they READ
  - Twenty percent of what they HEAR
  - Thirty percent of what they SEE
  - Fifty percent of what they HEAR AND SEE
  - Seventy percent of what they SAY
  - Ninety percent of what they SAY as they do a thing.
- Good motivators: Teaching aids are good motivators. They help to make the students work with more interest and zeal as well as to become more attentive and supplement the teaching
- Improve and make teaching effective
- Enable the audience to look, listen and learn provides first hand experience
- Make learning interesting and profitable
- Quicken the phase of learning
- Economize teacher's effort
- Foster/develop the knowledge
- Overcome possible hurdles during the act of teaching
- Bring expected behavioral change among the learners
- Stimulate curiosity
- Provide concrete experience or direct contact with reality or serves as a source of information and life likeness in the teaching-learning situation
- Provide a basis for more effective perceptual and conceptual learning
- Make personal involvement of the student in active learning and meet individual needs of the learners
- Provide an opportunity for situational type of learning, e.g. field trips
- Facilitate and advance the process of applying what is learned to realistic performance and to the life situation
- Add zest, interest and vitality to any training situation, provides integrated experience
- They give variety to classroom techniques, provides change in the atmosphere of the classroom and allow some freedom from the formal instruction or traditional type
- Spread of education as a mass scale-It will provide opportunity for promoting adult education
- Multi-sensory approach—The students will get opportunity to handle, touch, feel, operate, manipulate the audio-visual aid. It gives added appeal because it satisfies temporarily at least the natural desire for mastery and ownership
- Facilitate change in attitude
- Audio-visual aids educate learners for life, promotes international understanding
- Increase the concreteness, clarity, effectiveness of the ideas and skills being transferred
- The teacher has to organize his teaching material in a systematic order to impress the ideas more clear in the mind
- Visualize and make teaching more real acts as an antidote to the disease of verbal instruction
- Stimulate thinking and motivate action
- Change attitude or point of view of learners
- Stimulate self-activity on the part of the learner by which it offers reality of experience

- When audio-visual aids properly used can make a significant contribution to learning, reinforcing the role of text books, oral instructions and practicing exercises
- To present objectives to the learners, e.g. The teacher can prepare a hand out to project the objectives to the class
- To present the new content in a memorable way
- Supports learning through examples and visual elaboration, e.g. The teacher can quote examples by showing diagrams and pictures to make the students to understand in a better way
- The teacher can give the information on content in points by projecting audio-visual aids and encourage the students by posing questions and get the response and feedback from them
- Teacher can assess the performance or understanding level of students about the subject with the help of questioning by audio-visual aids.

Drawbacks in using Audio-Visual Aids

- These are not essential for all instructional programs
- These are helpful for teaching, but aids will not substitute teachers and books
- Possible risks of 'Spectatorism 'instead of 'attitude of thoughtful enquiry'
- It requires more time for planning and preparing
- Tempts the teachers to narrow down the subject
- Audio-visual aids are not ends, but means

Problems in using Teaching Aids

- Apathy of the teachers—Teaching with words alone is very tedious, wasteful and ineffective
- Ineffectiveness of the aids—Preparation, presentation, application and discussion are necessary whenever teacher is using aids for teaching
- Certain features will fail in effective usage of audio-visual aids
- Absence of proper planning
- Lethargy of the teacher
- Without proper preparation
- Correct presentation and appropriate application and discussion.
- No proper follow-up work
- Financial hurdles—The lack of finances and suitable planned programs, is not enabling them to do their best
- Absence of electricity, when it is needed—Most of the Projectors, Radio and TV cannot work without power
- Lack of facilities for training—Teacher education institutions/colleges or specialized agencies should make special provision for pre-service and in-service training of teachers and workers in the use of these aids
- Language difficulty—Most of the available educational films are in English, These films should be dubbed in the local languages and production of films originally in local languages should be encouraged and promoted
- Not catering to local needs, if aids are selected improperly by not considering sociological, psychological and pedagogical factors, its' effectiveness will be reduced
- Indifference of students—The judicious use of aids arouses interest but when used without a definite purpose but simply for a show, they lose their significance and importance
- Improper selection of audio-visual aids—Teaching aids or media are not selected according to the classroom needs

Classification of Audio-Visual Aids—I

1. Auditory aids, e.g. radio, recordings, mike, phonograms, megaphone, microphone, gramophone, record player producing sound but no pictures.
2. Visual aids

a. Non-projected /Unprojected Visual aids e.g. i) Three-dimensional materials-specimens, models, globe, mock–ups, objects, puppets, ii) Display boards, e.g. black board, white board, bulletin board, flannel board, magnetic board, peg board, iii) Graphic aids, e.g. cartoons, charts, pictures, flannel graphs, boards, cartoons, maps, photographs, flashcards, illustrations, posters, printed materials and diagrams
   b. Projected aids, e.g. epidioscope, slide projector, overhead projector, film projector, sound or silent films, film strips, slide projectors
3. Audio-visual aids-producing sound and motion pictures, e.g. television, video
4. Aid through activity, e.g. field trips, preparation of models, collection of material and exhibition, computer assisted instruction, demonstration, dramatics, experimentation, programd instruction, teaching machines
5. Traditional media, e.g. puppets, dramas, folksongs and folkdance.

Classification of Audio-Visual Aids—II

1. Visual aids
   a. Projected aids, e.g. Films, Filmstrips, Opaque Projector, Overhead Projector, Slide Projector.
   b. Non-projected aids
      i. Graphic aids, e.g. Cartoons, Charts, Comics, Diagrams, Flashcards, Graphs, Maps, Photographs, Pictures, Posters, Printed materials, Globe, Flip books, Illustrated books, Models, Specimens, Text Books, Silent Motion Pictures
      ii. Display boards, e.g. Blackboard, Bulletin board, Flannel board, Magnetic board, PEG board
      iii. 3-D aids, e.g. Diagrams, Models, Mock-ups, Objects, Puppets, Specimen, Exhibit.
2. Audio aids, e.g. Radio, Recordings (tape, disco) and Television, Video tapes, Language laboratories, Sound distribution systems, Public Addressing System
3. Audio-visual Aids, e.g. Television, Video films, Video Compact Disks, Cartoon films, Motion Pictures, Computers
4. Activity aids, e.g. Computer assisted instructions, Demonstrations, Dramatics, Experimentation, Field trips, Programd instruction and Teaching Machines.

Classification of Audio-Visual Aids—III

- Big media, e.g. Computer, VCR and TV
- Little media, e.g. Radio, Filmstrips, Graphic AIDS, Audio Cassettes, etc.

Classification of Audio-Visual Aids—IV

1. Visual Aids
a. Non-projected aids, e.g. Pictures or Illustrations, Photographs, Flash Cards or Strips, Posters, Charts, Diagrams, Maps, Graphs, Comic Strips or Comic Books, Exhibits
b. Projected Aids, e.g. Motion Pictures, Films 8 mm, 16 mm, Slides, Films, Film strips, Transparencies for Overhead Projectors
c. Three Dimentional Aids, e.g. Models, Objects, Specimens, Mock-ups, Puppets, Mobiles and Planatoriums
d. Display Boards, e.g. Black Boards, Bulletin Board, Peg Board and Flannel Board
e. New media—TVS, Video Recordings, Computers, Language Laboratory.

2. Audio Aids
a. Radios, Recordings–Tapes, Discs, Gramphone,
b. Audio Visual Kits, Displays and Exhibitions, Programd Learning kits
c. Audio-visual Equipment, e.g. Motion Picture Projectors–16 mm, 8 mm–Reel Type, 8 mm–film loop or cartridge film projectors Slide Projectors–Manual and Automatic. Film-Strip Projectors. OHP, Tape Recorders (Casette, Disc type), Opaque Projectors, Epidiascopes/Opaque Projector, Video Recordings, Television

Classification of Audio-Visual Aids—V

- Hardware Teaching Aids, e.g. Computer, Epidiascope, Magic Lantern, Motion Pictures, OHP, Radio, Slide and film Projectors, Tape Recorders, Teaching machines and Television
- Software Approach-Software approach is characterized by task analysis, writing precise objectives, selection

of appropriate learning strategies, immediate reinforcement of responses and constant evaluation. Newspapers, books, magazines, educational games, flash cards may also form part of software. Uses the principles of psychology for building in the learner a complex repertoire of knowledge modifying his/ her behaviour

The diagram shows how Edgar Dale's "Cone of Experience" (1969)—Organized learning experiences according to the degree of concreteness each possesses (Fig. 7.1). At the bottom is hands-on-experience, e.g. Experimentation, Projects, Field trips. As you ascend the cone, concrete experience begins to drop out, with stimuli becoming more abstract; the stimuli require more skill on the part of the learners to interpret the messages they carry. For certain types of learning (such as changing attitudes or teaching motor skills), experiences at the bottom of the cone are more appropriate than those at the top. Learning experiences at the bottom of the cone tend to hold student attention longer and involve active student participation. Media at the top of the cone are said to be more passive but are suitable for transmitting large amounts of information quickly, which is best depends upon your purposes and circumstances. While the web is becoming popular for distributing other types of mediated messages, it is not always practical, and other types of media are more appropriate.

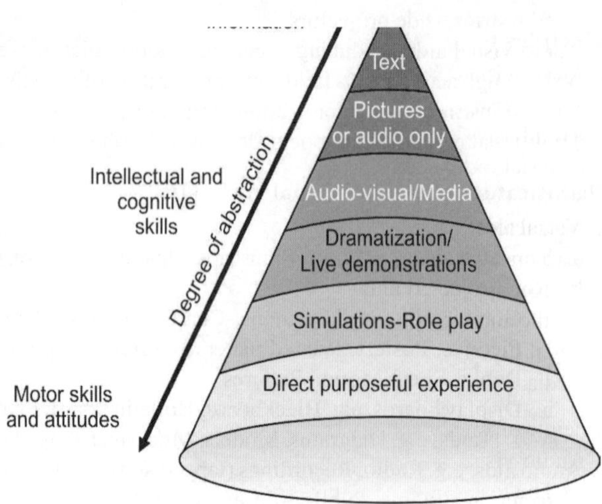

Fig. 7.1: Dale's cone of experience

Characteristics of good Teaching Aids

Teaching aids should be

- Clear, clean, interesting and in good condition
- A suitable size based on number of audience, i.e. it must be large enough (bold) for the whole class or small for group work
- Adequate, accurate, giving up-to-date information
- Must be relevant to the topic being discussed
- It must not be over-crowded with details
- Illustrate the specific point being taught
- Realistic in terms of the learners' ability to interprete aids
- Related to learner's experience
- Meaningful
- Purposeful
- Accurate in every aspect
- Simple
- Cheap/Inexpensive
- Improvised
- Easily portable
- According to mental level of the students
- Motivates the learners.

Sources of Audio-Visual Aids

"A source of supply or support available means"

- Government

- Educational institutions
- Professional organization
- Non-government organization
- National and international voluntary organizations
- Commercial producers of educational material.

Principles to be followed for the effective use of Audio-Visual Aids
- Audio-visual materials should function as an integral part of the educational program
- Audio-visual aids should be centralized, under specialized direction and leadership in educational program
- An advisory committee should be appointed to assist in the selection and coordination of audio-visual material for different subject content
- Audio-visual educational program should be flexible
- Instructors have to help the students how to select and Present/use audio-visual aids for a group of learners
- Budget appropriations should be appropriately made by subject teacher or curriculum committee regularly for the audio-visual educational program
- Legal aspects should be considered in the production and the utilization of educational communication media.

Principle of Selection
- Audio-visual aids should suit
  - The teaching objective
  - Unique characteristics of the special group of learners
  - The age level
  - Grade level etc
- Specific educational value and stimulate interest and motivation
- True representatives of the real things
- Help in the realization of desired learning objective.

Principle of Preparation
- Locally available material has to be used in selection of audio-visual aids
- Students should be associated in preparation of audio-visual aids
- Teacher should receive training and experience in preparation of audio-visual aids, so that she/he can guide the student effectively in selecting and preparing educational media.

Principle of Physical Control
Arrangement of aids safely to facilitate their access to and use by the teachers.

Principle of Proper Presentation
- Teacher has to carefully visualize the use of teaching aid before their actual presentation
- They should fully acquaint themselves with use and manipulation of the aids to be shown in the classroom
- Adequate handling of aid to prevent damaging
- Display properly so that all the students are able to see it and observe it to derive maximum benefit out of it
- Avoid distraction of all kinds so that students will pay fully attention for the presentation.

Principle of Response
The teacher should guide the students to respond actively to the audio-visual stimuli so that they derive the maximum benefit in learning.

Principle of Evaluation
Continuous evaluation of audio-visual material—Based on realization of desired accompanying techniques in the light of realization of desired objective.

Factors Influencing in Selection of Audio-Visual Aids

Audio-visual aids are designed to clarify and speed up instruction but they cannot take the place of the instructor—a basic principle to bear in mind when employing audio-visual aids is that a few audio-video aids utilized well will have better instructional results.

Audio-visual aids will be used either single or in combination depend upon

a. The objectives of training program/the teaching objective i.e., the type of behaviour change you want to bring in learner or to change the attitudes of the learner or to gain certain skills
b. The nature of subject matter being taught
c. The nature of audience
   - Number, e.g. small group-flash card, large group-movies
   - Age
   - Educational level
   - Socio-economic status
   - Interest
   - Experience
   - Knowledge of the subject
   - Intelligence levels/maturity level of learners.
d. Cost effectiveness
e. The teacher's familiarity with originality and skill in selection, preparation and use of aids.
f. Teaching aids must be used with skill and understanding.
g. The availability, functioning or working condition of aids.
h. Knowledge of resources and availability of facilities
i. Appropriateness i.e., is it relevant to the topic being discussed.

Criteria for selecting Audio-Visual Aid

The teacher has to put the following questions to his/her mind before selecting any audio-visual aid for teaching activity:

- Do the materials give a true picture of the idea they present?
- Do they contribute meaningful content to the topic under study?
- Is the material appropriate for the learners? (Age, Intellectual levels and Experience)
- Is the physical condition of the materials satisfactory?
- Do they make learners better thinkers with a critical mind?
- Do they tend to improve human relations?
- Is the material worth with the time and efforts involved?

If the teacher finds satisfactory, then only he/she has to choose the material for using in teaching-learning process.

Guides for Selecting and Preparing an Audio-Visual Aid

- Aid must be easy to see and to understand
- Simple and direct
- Easy to handle and transport
- Emphasize the key point
- Good working condition
- Time and place
- Group/Audience
- Please the senses
- Accurate and Correct
- Represent the things that are common
- Conveys upto date ideas
- Encourage the viewers to eye your ideas

- The message/content to be conveyed should be written, brief, clear, easy, attract the vision of others
- Letters should be neat, clear, easy to hold, visible, simple words, leave the space between letters, give gap between word to word
- Avoid over-writing, overcrowding, clumsiness in writing, give space between lines
- By seeing the visual aid, the learner should get interest, positive attitude, clear to understand and uses its knowledge effectively and adequately in his learning process
- Select the colors, which are natural of related items, appealing, attractive, clear and visible, appropriate to the pictures.

The Effective Use of Audio-Visual Aids

a. Planning
- Know clearly the objectives of the presentation
- Plan well in advance
- Anticipate the problem and avoid them
- Anticipate the size of the audience, the aids should be visible, audible for entire group of audience
- Ample number of aids (different types) has to be planned, plan to use a variety of colorful visual aids as they help change in phase of presentation and keep the audience hold and develop interest, enthusiasm, creativeness among the group of audience
- Plan in advance to keep ready audio-visual aids, and present them appropriately at the time of presentation.

b. Preparation
- Select a convenient and comfortable meeting place, seating arrangements must be suited to the specific purpose
- Anticipate the need for special effects like well ventilation/total lighting or darkness, based on the selected aid at the right time
- Make sure that all equipments are in good working order, before starting the meeting
- Rehearsing or previewing is required, to avoid delays or gap in presentation and to have smooth presentation
- Arrange the audio-visual aids in sequence and have them within easy reach
- Keep aids out of sight until actually required for use, to catch attention of viewers.

c. Presentation
- Motivate the audience and stress the key points they should observe during the presentation
- Present aids at the right moment and in proper sequence
- Display only one aid at a time
- Remove all unrelated materials
- Stand beside the aid, not in front of it
- Speak facing the audience and not the side, never pose back to the audience to maintain interest among the group.

d. Evaluation
- At the end, evaluate by providing the discussion and application to discover and dispel misunderstandings, if any
- Undertake follow-up studies and observe results.

DESCRIPTION OF VISUAL AIDS

'One picture is worth than a thousand words'.
Visual aids includes—Projected aids and Non-projected aids.

Non-Projected Aids
Printed Aids and Materials
Material in printed version, e.g. Books, Booklets, Flip Books, News Papers, Pamphlets, Handouts, etc. used to educate the general public or community in general and individuals in specific.

Photographs

- Exact visual recordings of things which will occur in real life situation
- It may be white and black or colored or mounted or unmounted photographic prints
- It may be used
  a. In personal teaching situations
  b. As display type visuals in exhibitions or bulletin boards
  c. Projected with an opaque projector which is suited to teach illiterates
- For effective teaching, a photograph must
  a. Tell a story
  b. Illustrate only one point, give accurate results
  c. Have plain and simple background
  d. Shows the main subject prominently
  e. Shows action, emotion and useful for easy understanding.

Illustrations

Non-photographic reconstructions of reality, e.g. drawing, paintings, sketching, etc.

Blackboard

The most commonly available aid in the classroom situation is the blackboard. It is helpful in meetings and in group discussions. Blackboard can be prepared with a piece of plywood about 30" × 40" square or rectangular in shape. Paint the plywood with blackboard paint. To carry from one place to other place, blackboard can be made in two pieces and hinge it in the middle. Have a small strip of wood attaches to the inside of the fold so it can be slid across the board after it is opened and make the board firm. While conducting meetings of discussions, write the topic for discussion on the board. Illustrate the points on the board.

Uses

- Used in conducting literacy classes
- Opportunity for creativity
- It makes group instruction more concrete and understandable
- If it is used properly, it can set standards of neatness, accuracy and speed
- It can restore the attention of the group
- For jotting down spontaneous thoughts, time saving
- To work out formulaes like drugs and solutions, biochemistry equations, etc.
- For listing topics
- Many vague statements can be clarified by writing words, graphs, drawings, pictures or sketches, outlines, diagrams, directions, summaries, maps, etc. They can be used again and again, as they can be easily cleaned with a duster
- Initiates aural, visual sensations, helps in learning
- It can be a means of motivation and interest
- It can be used for recording the progress and status
- It provides many educational opportunities in all curricular and co-curricular activities, e.g. we can present:
- The Facts, Principles, Processes, Procedures, making Assignments, assign Individual Responsibilities, Writing Questions, Problems, Sources and References, Summaries, Outlines, Directions
- Practicing individual drill or creative work, graphic demonstrations, Screen for still pictures, projections, symbolic representations, Review the total lesson, Announcements, Closely supervised student activities, etc.
- To state questions, to cite examples of work desired, to pose problems and to list sources for study
- To illustrate forms of charting and to provide opportunity for nursing students to practice charting
- Abstract statements can be clarified in the exposition stage and a summary containing the salient features can be given at the recapitulatory stage
- It provides lot of scope for creative and decorative work
- The teacher can erase writings and drawings and start a fresh
- Inexpensive and no electricity is required.

Rules in using Blackboard/ You can improve your chalkboard skill

Board should be kept clean always and uniform strokes with eraser can be made to clean the board.

Write the letters and drawings should be in large or bold in size, legible, so that all learners can be able to see it.

- Avoid spelling mistakes
- Writing should be in straight line
- Develop one point at time
- Do not talk as you write
- Face the group after writing and continue the discussion
- Extreme lower corner of blackboard should not be used, as, total members cannot see
- Do not fill the board, only salient features have to be written and remove the unwanted information
- Do not use abbreviations.
- While writing on the board, the teacher should ensure that the class is attentive
- Use colored chalks if necessary, e.g. To draw the diagrams and different parts can be drawn by using different colors like anatomy diagrams
- Do not stand in front of the board, stand to one side so that learners may see what and how you are writing.
- Use a pointer, if necessary.
- You may prepare a diagram, a figure, etc. in advance to save time. It may also be very motivating for the children in creating reading readiness
- Practice using the blackboard repeatedly until you gain the skill.

Limitations while using Chalkboard
- No illustrate moving parts
- It own't convey sound
- Limited for small group of audience
- Prone for chalk dust allergy

Types
1. The ordinary chalkboard held by an easel: A portable and adjustable blackboard put on a wooden easel can be taken out of the classroom while taking the class in open, useful for teaching of art subjects in small class.
2. The roller type chalkboard with a mat surface: Made of thick canvas wrapped on a roller.
3. The magnetic board: Teachers can make three-dimensional demonstration with objects on a vertical surface. Small magnets are used to hold suitable objects fixed wherever they are put on this vertical surface. Board is made up of steel on which magnets can be fixed. The creative impulse is aroused among the students while they use it as an exercise.
4. Black ceramic unbreakable board: It will be framed with aluminum or teak wood frame as per the requirement, useful for chalk piece writing.
5. Black or green glass chalkboard: It will be framed with teak wood and available black or green color, useful for chalk piece writing.
6. Lobby stand board: It is useful in lobby. Alphabets and figures are changeable. It will be lightweight and easy to carry. Stand height will be 6 feet.
7. Exhibition board: It can be folded and expanded easily. Both side useable. It will come with two panel, three panel and four panel. Papers and pamphlets can be fixed with push pin.
8. Double side stand board: One side white board for marker writing and another side blackboard for chalk piece writing. It is fixed on wheel stand. It can be moved from one place to another place easily.
9. Reception board: Gold color powder coated aluminium frame. Golden letters can be fixed on this board.
10. Tariff board: Useful for price list, reception, welcome to delegates and wedding.
11. Paging board: One side with marker pen writing and one side letters interchangeable. It is useful at public places to receive the VIP's.

12. Pressing graph perforated board: It can be used vertically, horizontally in any place like educational institution, administrative office.
13. Write and wipe off white board: Marker pen can be used for writing and it can be erased easily with duster or ordinary clothes or brush.
14. Information notice board (open type): It is framed with aluminum frame, notices can be fixed with push pins, available in green, blue and maroon color.

When Using the Whiteboard

- Include a whiteboard plan in your lesson outline that determines which aspects of the lesson will be illustrated on the boardlist of concepts to be learned, timelines, outline for the day's presentation
- Bring plenty of spare markers to class
- Use different colored markers to highlight important aspects of the lesson
- Write neatly and horizontally, making certain your handwriting is large enough for students to read. Board work should be organized so that students will be able to interpret their notes later
- Write on the board in several places (top, bottom, right side, left side). Go to the back of the room to see if you can read what you have written from any location. Be sensitive to obstructions, including the heads of students that may block the lower part of the board
- Give students time to copy what has been written
- Avoid modifying the board while students are copying information
- Talk to the students, not the board. With a little practice, you will find that you can write while you are partially facing the class.

Bulletin Board

It will be used for both informational and educational purposes. It can motivate, supplement and enrich learning, stimulates thought. It employs intrinsic motivation through the medium of interest, curiosity and desire for knowledge. The successful use of this aid depends on the interest it inspires, demands attention and promotes reflective thinking.

It is a simple device placed either indoor or outdoor, kept in a suitable place, it can provide a suitable place for the display of all kinds of creative work of the students.

It is a soft board, that hold papers to be pasted with the help of suitable pins or tags.

Items generally used in bulletin board are:

- Photographs
- Cutout illustrations
- Publications
- Drawings or Art
- Specimens
- Posters
- Newspapers
- Pasting up of announcements, assignments, distinctions, achievements.

Uses

- To communicate the ideas or the information
- To describe the ways of doing a particular item
- To follow-up instructions on things demonstrated and emphasized
- Posting photographs to show local activities
- Local announcements which has to be notified to all
- To motivate the learners with inspiring thoughts
- To present the ideas of many individuals and localities, when the material is gathered from a variety of sources
- To intensify impressions and vitalize instruction
- To add variety to the classroom activity

- To provide information
- To supplement and correlate instruction. It saves time, i.e. material that cannot be presented during the class hours, nevertheless can be on bulletin board.

Principles in the use of the Bulletin Board
- A board for posting notices should be kept separate from those for current events and study
- A suggested plan for placement of bulletin board is to have one near the educational administrator's office, another near the library or studyroom for material in relation to study, third board in conference hall or main halls, 4th one in classroom
- The contents of the boards should be organized around a central theme of content and materials should be dated to ensure that, it does not remain or longer than desired
- The appearance must be neat, orderly and attractive manner
- The material should be changed frequently and systematically to encourage interest
- Notices should be removed as soon as they have fulfilled their purpose
- The contributions should be well-labelled
- Student contributions should be encouraged and placed
- A bulletin board committee should be appointed, they will held responsible to provide material, and for editing the contents and should have the power to place or remove the contents of the bulletin board. Administrator is one among the committee members
- All material should be organised in an attractive manner by dividing the board into sections, each item placed under a suitable section, with proper labeling
- Crowding of display materials has to be avoided
- The learners may be given opportunity or responsibility for collection and display of appropriate material in connection with specific lessons or events
- The bulletin board should be kept a little above the eye level of the average individual.

Types
1. Flannel board/Felt board
2. Magnetic board
3. Fixed type
4. Movable type
5. Folded type

Flannel/Felt Board
A flannel board is simple and inexpensive to construct. It is easy to store and light to carry. The rigid material (plywood or wooden) covered with flannel cloth/felt sheet/wool/cotton/paper/suede cloth, blotting paper, sponge or any other material with natural adhesion. The items to be displayed (e.g. pictures or drawings, etc.) should have flannel or sand paper pasted on reverse side. It can be used throughout discussion; whenever needed, item can be placed and explained, if the purpose served, items has to be removed. The flannel board is a dynamic medium in that it provides a way of presenting 'mobile' situations and changes can be shown by adding or taking away figures and flash cards. The pictures, which are selected, should be attractive and sufficiently large enough to be clearly seen by all the group members. Do not have too much detail on them.

Three-Dimensional Materials/Aids
Three-dimensional representations of real things, they reduce large object to a size convenient for observation and produce interior view of objects which are normally covered or are otherwise invisible. Non-essentials are removed, so that fundamentals can be more readily observed.

1. Model
Models are substitutes for real things. Models are concrete objects to explain clearly the structure or functions of real things.It is a life size miniature or over size or original size whether workable or not, whether it differs from or not from original size of an object to be studied, which is very useful in teaching. Sometimes they are smaller versions of the real objects. Some models can be commercially bought for teaching purposes and some can

teacher-made. Low cost models made up of clay, pulp, plaster of paris, cotton, cardboard, thermacole, cloth, wood, etc. variety of models can be prepared. Models enable students to have a correct concept of the object, e.g. to teach Anatomy and Basic Concepts in Nursing, Community Health Nursing, etc. teachers can use models to explain the structure in detail. If the teacher places the model in the class, make sure that all the students are given enough time to examine the model.

Essential Qualities
Accuracy, Simplicity in Nature, Utility/ Have Value (Useful), Solidity, Ingenuity

Functions
1. It simplifies reality
2. Concretizes abstract concepts
3. Enables us to reduce or enlarge objects to an observable size
4. It provides the correct concept of an real object, etc.
5. A working model explains the various processes of objects and machines.
6. Promotes creative interest among learners.
7. Models are good for–demonstrating, making an impact, explaining a process, etc.

Types
Scale model: Correct idea of an object can be displayed, e.g. a dam or project.
Simplified model: Gives an idea of an external form of an object, e.g. animal, birds.
Working model: To demonstrate in a simple way of an operation or process, ensure that the model will work, make sure that it is big enough for the students to see, e.g. fetal circulation.
Cross-section model: Inside of an object is visible. Immense value was mainly observed in teaching sciences, e.g. cross-section of blood vessel.

2. Exhibit

It is an arrangement of communication media designed to inform the observer about a specific subject or topic. Educational exhibit offers in an interesting and unique manner of combining multiple media into a small area. It provides an opportunity for learner for own creative participation and developmental thinking. Some times to summarize the work of a unit or course that has been accomplished over a period of days, e.g. after completing first year B.Sc. nursing students will be motivated by nurse educator to arrange an exhibition related to Physiology, Microbiology, for educating general public or school children. The educators will plan competitions and arrange exhibits in a specific subject and motivate the students to participate and give prizes for the winners as a sort of recognition for the sincere efforts made by them. Exhibitions will be arranged in big gatherings like conferences, workshops like books exhibitions will be organised by publishing agencies or in conferences to encourage the students.

3. Specimen

Part of real objects taken from the natural setting. It is simple that shows quality or structure, In Anatomy, Physiology, Nursing Labs the spot specimens will be arranged, e.g. section of lung, thermometer, hot water bag, etc.

4. Mock-up

It emphasizes the functional relationship between the device reality and its workability. Mock-ups of a school TV as a model can be used for narrating stories. To narrate a story, illustrations of the story can be prepared in the series. Certain element of the original reality is emphasized to make it more meaningful for the purpose of instruction, e.g. an artificial kidney to demonstrate dialysis.

5. Moulage

Mould can be made up of plastic material to stimulate some life object, e.g. body which shows evidence of trauma/infection/disease/surgical intervention.

6. Objects/ Realia

Objects are genuine, actual-sized things. Children enjoy bringing objects to school to show to their classmates, brought from its natural setting into the class-room to supply the type of sensory experience that will make instruction more meaningful, vivid and impressive. They make a direct appeal to the senses, e.g. splints, forceps and thermometers.

Uses
- Connects your students to the world outside the classroom
- Makes language learning more relevant and meaningful
- Prepares your students for post-classroom experience
- Motivates students to investigate and use outside the classroom

General principles to be keep in mind when using realia in the classroom
- Tell your students that it is "real"
- Choose realia that is relevant and interesting
- Provide the relevant cultural background beforehand
- Make connections to realia in your students' own culture
- For audio-visual materials, make sure the recording is clear; that you preview the material beforehand; that you have the proper equipment and know how to use it.

7. Diorama

It is a three-dimensional scene in depth incorporating a group of modelled objects and figures in a natural setting. The diorama scene is setup on a small stage with a group of modelled objects kept on the foreground, which is blended into a painted realistic background.

Leaflet

Single sheet of paper folded to make a full page of printed matter on single side.

Pamphlets

Paper can be folded into two or three or five, the matter will be printed either single side or both sides.

Handout/Handbill

Material specially prepared by the teacher, organized the material from different sources, which are not easily accessible, thay are not substitutes for lectures/discussions, the material should be used as supplements to the material being taught. The briefing of a session in a single sheet. Use simple, clear language with short sentences. If needed sketches, graphs can be drawn and labeled. Give titles and sub-titles, underline or bold the key words. Suitable colors can be used. Hand outs may be given well in advance to orient interested group about the purpose, aims and objectives of the presentation or after completion of presentation to leave a record of lesson and for follow-up as an additional reading material, key points within the hand outs should be brought to participants' attention and discussed during class. Improve teaching skills, as it possess readymade material you are going to teach.

The following considerations would be pertinent if you want to ensure that your handouts and materials are purposeful, well-planned and designed:
- Provide a list/lists of books and journals with priority markings for first-line compulsory reading, strongly recommended reading and for reference. These notations and brief comments will guide students through the reading lists. Long comprehensive reading/reference lists without directions will simply overwhelm average students
- Construct handouts that contain outline summaries, worksheets with listing of key issues in diagrammatic/ pictorial forms and so on, consisting of information and key points that are crucial to students' understanding of the subject matter. Such handouts allow students time to see and hear your presentation, and not have to desperately try taking down all the information and details before you move on to the next stage of your teaching plan
- Design handouts in an interactive format by allowing writing spaces between statements or at the margins for students to write notes. For emphasis or direction, ask students to underline a phrase, circle a word or fill blank spaces with key words, etc. as you teach
- Lay your contents in an attractive and uncluttered fashion. Your lettering must be easy to read and not be too decorative or illegible

- Ensure that students know the purpose of your handouts. Start each handout with a title and a statement of objective or introduction
- Use letters or numbers for easy reference and filling. Color code your handouts to indicate that they are of a different subject matter or section.Time your distribution to match the appropriate stage of your presentation. The choice in doing it before, during and after the presentation would depend on your planned objectives, and the desired effect you hope to achieve in using handouts and materials
- Producing and distributing handouts and materials can be time-consuming and expensive, especially when you try to fully cover the course.

Drawbacks
- To be distracted, inattentive and not write their own notes
- To spot examination questions
- Not to attend classes
- Not to read beyond the content as outlined and highlighted

Flash cards
- Small compact cards, which flashed before the class to bring an idea
- 10" × 12" or 22" × 28" in size
- Used for small groups 15 to 30
- Provides variety and activity for group
- The messages has to be brief, Prepare a picture for each idea, which will give visual impact to the idea like simple line drawing or photographs or cartoons by using suitable colors and the contents of each flash card will be written in few lines at the back of each flashcard
- Adapted to local condition
- Ten to twelve cards for one topic can be used
- It needs drill or preview
- It can be used either individually or in combination with other charts

To teach well with flashcards, the teacher should follow certain points.

A series or set of cards can be prepared on a single topic, put in sequential order, before starting the explanation.
- The story on each card must be familiar
- Must use simple words and local terminology
- Hold the cards at chest level where people can see clearly, hold against body and not in air, face different parts of the group, to show cards to all
- Glance down at card, as you are ready to explain and make sure to give correct information
- Use pointer. Don't cover the matter with hand
- Be enthusiastic and enjoy while explaining the matter
- Important point should be written backside, if the trainer forgets any relevant matter, by seeing content in back, easily the teacher will catch the point

Posters
It is good substitute for first hand experience. It varies from a simple printed card to a complicated and artistic design. It should be always a part of campaign, it will serve first to inspire the people and lastly it will serve as a remainder to the group.

Rules to Prepare Poster
- To do a special job
- To promote one point
- To support local demonstration and local exhibits
- Planned for the specified people
- It should stop the people and make them to look
- Tell the message in a single glance
- Use bold letters (20" × 30")

- Use simple, few words which conveys one idea
- Use pleasing colors
- Must be timely
- It contains:
  - First division-announces the purposes of the project.
  - Second division-set out conditions.
  - Third division-recommends actions.
- It should be placed, where people pass or gather together
- Posters can be developed with the help of an artist.

Uses
- To make an instant appeal
- To convey single idea or few ideas
- To understood at a glance
- Comprehensive at a distance and sufficiently clear
- Suitable for patient education, presenting scientific facts, showing safety measures and many other facets relating to health
- Can serve as useful illustrations to aid in the explanation of concepts and principles.

Graphic Materials
It is a combination of graphic and pictorial material designed for the orderly and logical visualization of relationships between key facts and ideas, e.g. comparisons, relative amounts, developments, processes, classification or organization. It includes: graphs, charts, maps and diagrams.

Diagram/Drawing
It is a simplified drawing designed to show inter-relationship primarily by means of lines and symbols, e.g. Stick figures, science figures, geometry diagrams, facial expressions. Drawings can be drawn by hand to convey a variety of ideas, concepts and situations. It can be better used for summary and review.

Standard of a Good Diagram
- Technically correct
- Well-labelled and explained
- Neatly drawn in proper proportions
- It can be moved and seen from all angles

Charts
Charts are versatile and useful visual aids that have been used by teachers for a long time. Visual symbols used for summarizing, comparing, contrasting or performing other services in explaining subject matter. Diagnostic representation of the facts and ideas can be done. A chart is a combination of pictorial, graphic, numerical or vertical material, which presents a clear visual summary. Teacher has to prepare charts by incorporating his own ideas and lines of approach of the specific topic are more useful. Charts usually refer to displays on large sheets of paper or cloth that are designed to be shown to a class or group in the course of lesson. The material on charts are usually larger and easier to read, e.g. Charts are valuable in nursing education, e.g. We can chart a graph showing rise and fall of a patients' temperature. These are highly symbolic representations require skill in interpretation. Symbols should be explained and taught so that the learner comes to see the symbol but he understands the fact or condition for which the symbol stands for.

Purposes
- To show relationships by means of facts and figures
- To present the material symbolically
- To show continuity in process
- To present abstract ideas in visual form
- We can depict the developmental changes or structures

- For creating problems and to stimulate thinking
- Relatively cheap.

How to use Charts effectively
- Involve the students in the preparation of charts. Hand writing skills are necessary
- Every detail depicted in the chart should be visible to all the learners in the class
- It should display the information only about one specific area in the subject
- It should not contain too many details
- It should represent neat and tidy in appearance
- Teacher should make sure that there is provision for hanging the chart at a vantage point
- Use the pointer to point out specific factors in the chart
- Charts should be carefully stored and preserved for use in future.

Types of Charts
1. Wall-Charts
   Displays that are pinned to a wall or bulletin board and are mainly intended for casual study outside the context of a formal lesson. The material on wall-charts clearly distinguishable or legible at a distance, can be studied at close quarters. They contain more complicated and detailed information.
2. Narrative Chart
   Arrangement of facts and ideas for expressing the events in the process or development of a significant issue to its point of resolution or we can show an improvement over a period of years.
3. Cause and Effect Chart
   Arrangement of facts and ideas for expressing the relationship between two systems or between rights and responsibilities or between a complex of conditions and change or conflict, e.g. Showing the relationship between cause and effect in the form of stick diagram or picture form.
4. Chain Chart
   Arrangement of facts and ideas for expressing transitions or cycles, e.g. Life Cycle of an individual
5. Evolution Chart
   Facts and ideas for expressing changes in specific items from beginning data and its projections into the future, e.g. Genesis of specific individual within a specific family system.
6. Strip Tease Chart
   It enables the speaker to present the information step by step. It has great suspense value, which aids in holding attention and building interest. It helps the audience to remember key ideas and maintains interest to the very end of the presentation. It increases the interest and imagination of the audience.
   - The information on the chart is covered with thin paper strips to which it has been applied either by wax, tape or sticky substance or pins, tags can also be used
   - As the speaker wishes to visually reinforce a point with words or symbols, he/she removes the appropriate strip or paper. It aids considerable interest to the presentation by removing the paper
   - It increases learning and aids recall.
7. Pull Chart
   It consists of written messages which are hidden by strips of thick paper. The messages can be shown to the viewer, one after another by pulling out the concealing strips.
8. Flow Chart
   Diagrams used to show organizational elements or administrative or functional relationships. Boxes connected with lines show levels of lines of authority.
   In this chart lines, rectangles, circles or other graphic representations will be used and are connected by lines showing the directional flow, e.g. Organizational Chart of the institution.
9. Bar Chart
   Learners' abilities to recognise concepts such as "more", "greater than", "higher", "taller", "smaller", etc., can easily be developed through graphs. Two types of graphs help us in developing such concepts—Bar graph and Pie graph.

A bar graph is a figure where bars are drawn on a graph paper. The bars can be drawn either vertically or horizontally.

10. **Tabulation Chart**

    The numerical data are presented in a tabular form, used for comparisons or for listing advantages and disadvantages of an organization. It presents information in ordinary sequences, e.g. Comparison tables

11. **Time Chart or Table Chart**

    To show the schedule of an activity or of an individual, e.g. tour chart, timetable of a class. It provides a chronological frame work within which events and developments may be recorded. They develop time sense among the learners, help them to comprehend and visualize the pageant of time and its relationships.

12. **Genealogy Chart**

    To represent historical facets or growth and development of the family. Taking an analogy from the tree, the origin is shown in a single line, rectangle, circle or other representation of the trunk and the various changes or developments are shown, e.g. Family Tree.

13. **Job Chart**

    Job responsibilities of specific categories will be listed out and circulated among its members.

14. **Tree Chart**

    To show the development or growth or the types in the form of a tree, e.g. complications or types of a specific disease.

15. **Flip Chart**

    These consist of a number of large sheets of paper, fixed to a support bar, easel or a display board by clamming or pinning them along their top edges so that they can be flipped backwards or forwards as required. A set of charts related to specific topic have been tagged together and hang on a supporting stand. The individual charts will carry a series of related materials or messages in sequence. The salient points of specific topic will be presented. Hand writing skills are necessary. Used with nonerasable colored pens.

    Advantages:

    Simple to use, inexpensive, portable, suitable for multi-colored display, need no electricity, effectively help to focus your learners' attention, useful for background information, can reveal successive bits of story and can record ideas from discussions and keep for future reference. They contain far more complicated and detailed information with illustrations. To build up sequency and to retain them for further reference. Teacher can prepare before the presentation and keep ready for discussion. A great memory jogger, as it is easy for the teacher to steer the class back to the topic after interruption.

    For example, When the teacher has to present a topic or teach about a disease in medical-surgical nursing a series of charts, e.g. flip chart can be used. She/He can prepare like:

    - Title
    - Definition
    - Prevalence and incidence
    - Causes and risk factors
    - Clinical Manifestations
    - Diagnostic features
    - Management
    - Rehabilitation
    - Prevention

    All charts will be pinned and when the teacher presents the specific sub heading she/he can open that specific chart and explain to group of students.

16. **Overlay Chart**

    It consists of illustrated sheets which can be placed one over the other conveniently and in succession. The drawing or illustration on each sheet forms a part of the whole picture. It enables the viewers to see not only the different parts but also to see them against total perspective when one is placed over the other. When the final overlay is placed, the ultimate product is exposed to view.

17. Pie Chart

A circle will be drawn and the divisions will be made into different sections each section will be coded differently and code key will be given at right corner of the chart as a legend. The circumference is divided into suitable sections. It is relevant for showing the component parts of the total, e.g. A pie graph shows approximate relative weightage given to different subjects in the curriculum.

Maps

Graphic representation of the earth's surface or portions of it are termed as maps. These are flat representations of the earth's surface, which convey the information by means of lines, symbols, words and colors.

Identification of Various Aspects of Maps
- Understanding and interpreting the key of index, lines (e.g. communications, rivers, contours, meridians, and parallels), colors, tints, shadows and symbols
- The top of every map is not north, but the direction of northern pole is north.

Types
1. Relief maps
2. Historical maps
3. Distribution maps, e.g. Vegetation, population, economic, etc.
4. Geographical maps.

Globe

Three-dimensional representation of the earth in a spherical manner. We can see the physical unity of the world, the relation of one part to all rest and the direction of one part of the world relative to another. The examples of graphs were shown after their description.

Graphs

It depicts numerical or quantitative relationship or statistical data are presented in the form of visual symbols. Exact specifications depict specifically quantitative data for analysis, comparison and interpretation.

a. Pie Graph

Pie diagram or circle diagram—The data are presented through the sections or portions of a circle. In determining the circumference of a circle we have to take into consideration a quantity known as, 'Pie'.

It is drawn by first drawing a circle of a suitable radius and then dividing the angle of 360 degree at its centre in proportion to the figures given under:

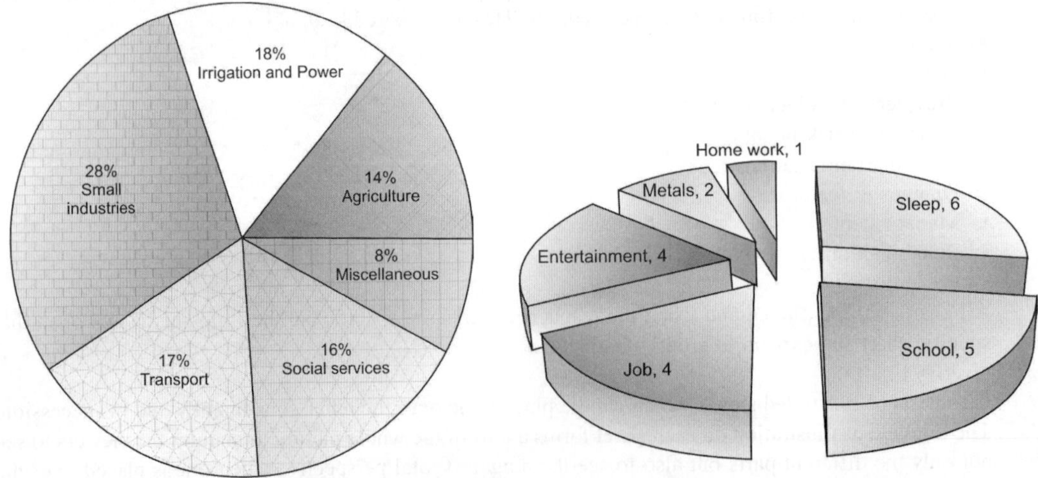

Fig. 7.2: Pie graph   **Fig. 7.3: Segmented pie diagram**

Method of Construction
- The surface area of a circle is to cover 360 degree
- The total frequencies or value is equated to 360 degree and then the angles corresponding to component parts are calculated
- After determining their angle, the required sectors in the circle are drawn
  The numerical data may be converted into the angles of the circle as below

b. Bar Graph

A graphic presentation, which extends the scale horizontally along the length of bars. Each bar must be of the same width, height of the bar over a period represents the corresponding time of the variable. Graphs are available in two forms, i.e. vertical and horizontal.

Types: Simple bar, Double bar, Compound bar, etc.
For example: Simple Bar Graph
- All bars have the same thickness
- Distance between two consecutive bars is the same. The bars can touch each other
- The height of each bar represents the frequency number of students
- The thickness has no significance

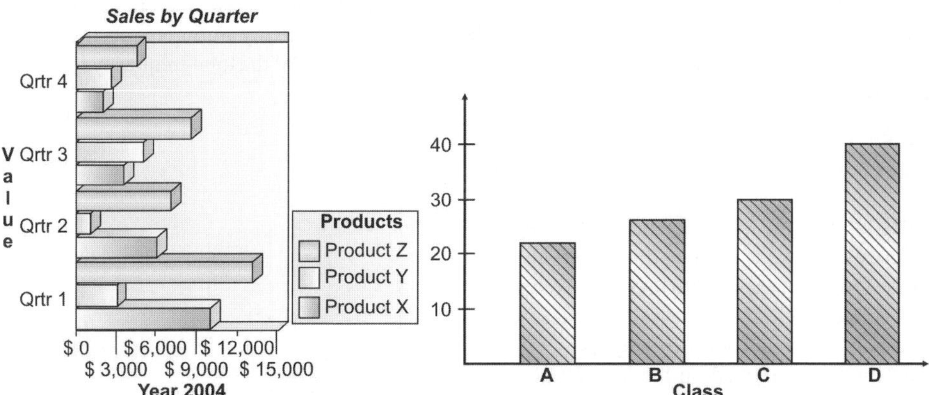

Fig. 7.4: Horizontal bar graph

Fig. 7.5: Vertical bar graph

Double Bar Graph
Double bar or divided bar graph is preferred when we want to compare two sets of related data.
For example:

Class	IX - A	IX - B	IX - C	IX - D
Girls	10	26	18	16
Boys	12	20	12	24
Total	22	46	30	40

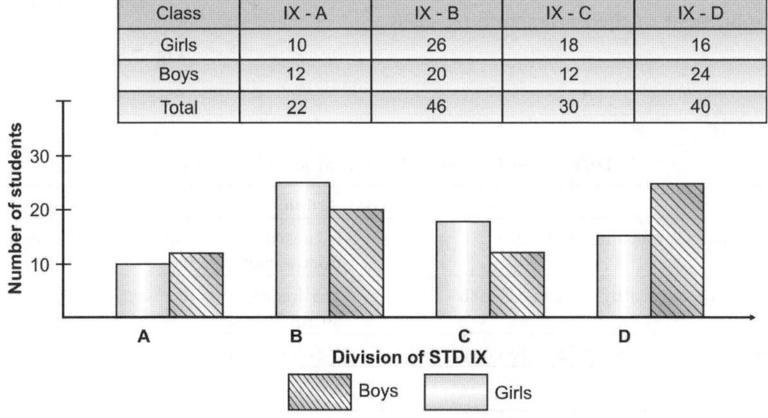

Fig. 7.6: Double bar graph

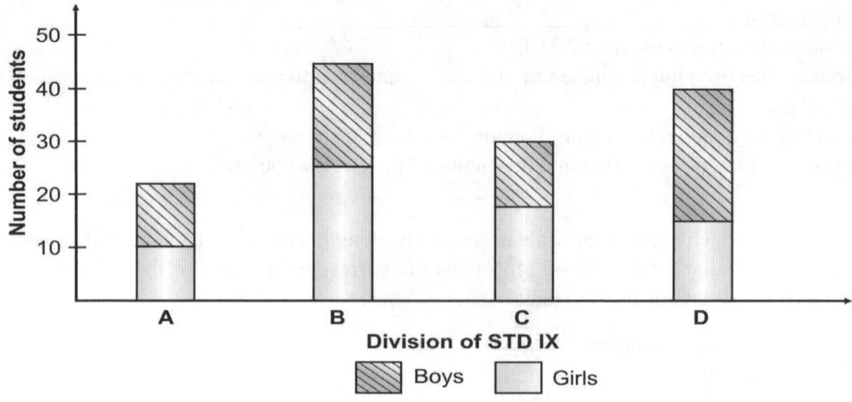

Fig. 7.7: Divided bar graph

Histogram

A two-dimensional frequency density diagram is called a histogram. A histogram is a diagram which represents the class interval and frequency in the form of a rectangle. There will be as many adjoining rectangles as there are class intervals. It represents on acurate picture of the relative proportion of the total frequency from interval to interval (Fig. 7.8).

Steps to be followed in drawing histogram
1. Mark class intervals on X-axis and frequencies on Y-axis.
2. The scales for both the axes need not be the same.
3. Class intervals must be exclusive. If the intervals are in inclusive form, convert them to the exclusive form.
4. Draw rectangles with class intervals as bases and the corresponding frequencies as heights.

The class limits are marked on the horizontal axis and the frequency is marked on the vertical axis. Thus a rectangle is constructed on each class interval.

If the intervals are equal, then the height of each rectangle is proportional to the corresponding class frequency.

If the intervals are unequal, then the area of each rectangle is proportional to the corresponding class frequency.

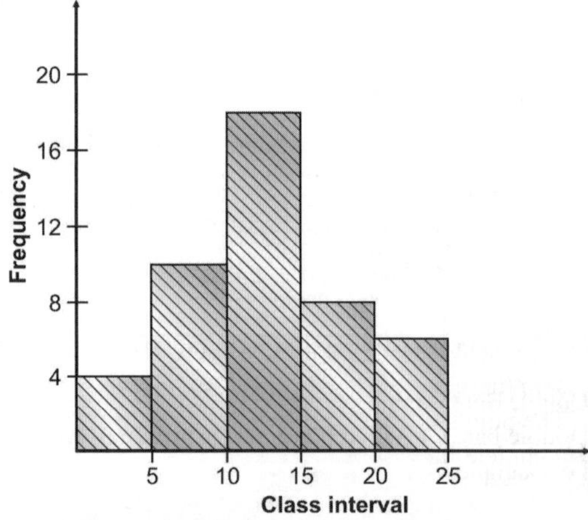

Fig. 7.8: Histogram

Difference between Histogram and Bar grarph

Histogram	Bar graph
1. It consists of rectangles touching each other.	1. It consists of rectangles, normally separated from eachother with equal space
2. The frequency is represented by the area of each rectangle	2. The frequency is represented by height. The width has no significance
3. It is two dimensional (width and height are considered)	3. It is one dimensional (only height is considered)
	4. It is used a visual aid to represent data.

c. The Line Graph (Curve Graph)

To show the trends and relationships, e.g. single line shows the relation and the variation in quantity (Fig. 7.9).

Quantitative data are plotted or when the data is continuous. The concepts are represented with the help of lines drawn either horizontally or vertically. The plotted points are connected to one another, instead of the base, thus producing the curve.

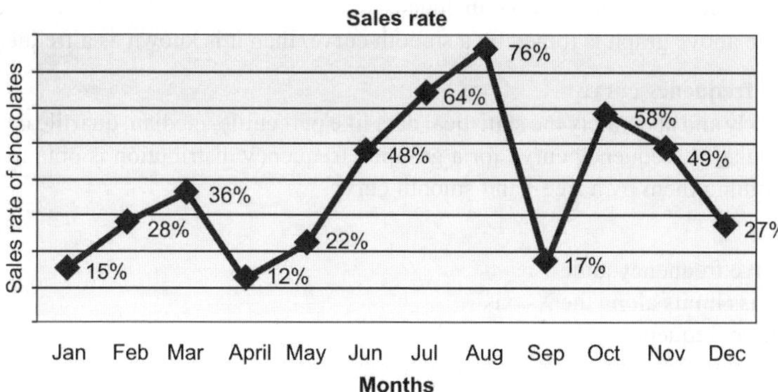

Fig. 7.9: Line graph

d. Pictorial Graph

It is an outstanding method of graphic representation. Pictures are used for the expression of ideas, they are more attractive and easily understood. Vivid pictures will be used to create rapid association with the graphic message, each visual symbol may be used to indicate quantity.

e. Frequency Polygon

A line graph for the graphical presentation of the frequency distribution. A frequency polygon can be constructed for a grouped frequency distribution, with equal-interval, in two different ways:

Method I:
- Represent the class-marks along the x-axis
- Represent the frequencies along y-axis
- Join these points, in order, by straight lines
- The points at each end is joined to the immediate higher (or lower) class mark at zero frequency so as to complete the polygon

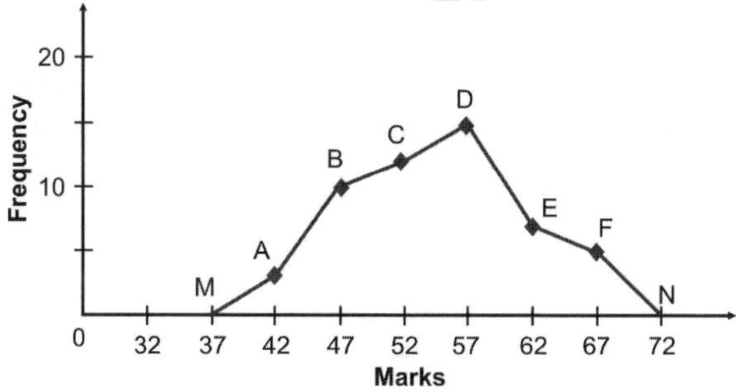

Fig. 7.10: Frequency polygon

Method II:
- Represent a histogram of the given data
- Join the mid points of the tops of the adjacent rectangles by straight lines
- The mid points at each end are joined to the immediate higher (or lower) at zero frequency so as to complete the polygon (Fig. 7.10)
  The two classes, one at each end, are to be included
  For example: If the above graph is joined by a smooth curve, then it is known as a frequency curve

f. Ogive/cumulative frequency curve

To determine quickly and accurately the statistical data like percentile, median, quartile deviation ogive can be used. The cumulative frequency curve for a grouped frequency distribution is obtained by plotting the points and then joining them by a free-hand smooth curve.

Method:
- Form the cumulative frequency table
- Mark the upper class limits along the X-axis
- Mark the cumulative frequencies along the Y-axis
- Plot the points and join them by a free-hand smooth curve.

g. Cumulative frequency graph

A line graph drawn by plotting actual upper limits of the class interval on the X-axis and the respective cumulative frequencies on Y-axis (Fig. 7.11).

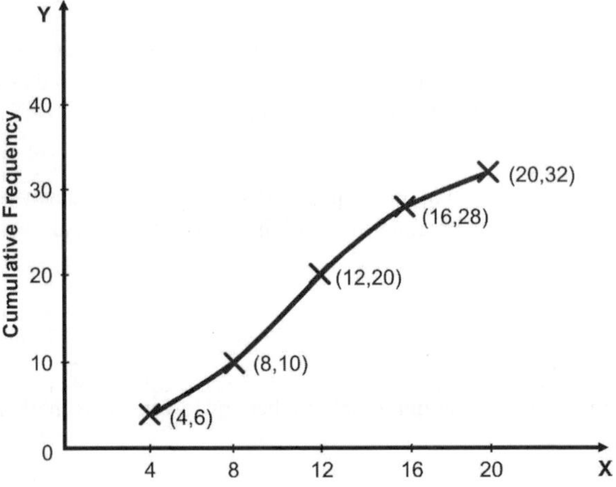

Fig. 7.11: Cumulative frequency graphs

Cartoon

It is a metaphorical presentation of reality. It makes learning more interesting and effective as it creates a strong appeal to the emotions. The cartoon is an interpretative illustration, which uses symbols to portray an opinion, a scene or a situation.

It makes use of
- Personalized humor
- Fantasy
- Incongruity
- Satire
- Exaggeration

The logic of cartoon lies in implication. The quality of the drawing should be high primarily for visual effectiveness, secondly for appreciation. It is simple, clear which tells the story without too much explanation.

The symbols used should be familiar and represent a concept or idea to which the students can react intellectually. The teacher should use the symbols, which the students can understand easily, give time to the students for interpreting the symbols, then the teacher may ask them, to give the meaning and apply to the subject being studied. The teacher should evaluate the point of view being presented. Because of their uniqueness and simplicity, they can be used in appraising, interpreting and emphasizing, e.g. Cartoons can be drawn related to Psychology-mental mechanisms and in Fundamentals of nursing-wrong and correct views of nursing procedures.

Newspapers

The newspaper furnishes many examples which can be used to introduce lessons. Health messages can be published in local languages which can reach to the public easily. The information will be available at low cost, easy to read and understand in simple language. The people may learn to read and interpret the contents along with pictures wherever it is necessary (use adequate and sufficient suitable pictures) to enhance easy grasping.

Puppets

One of the old and popular arts in Indian villages has been puppetry. Puppets can serve as an effective aid to learning. They can be made to illustrate lessons. Events of tales in an interesting and vivid manner, if they are accompanied by effective narratives. It is necessary to have a great deal of action in puppetry as well as plenty of music dancing. Learners or in community, people are very much interested in puppets and puppet shows. Through puppetry you can see puppets doing all sorts of activities-singing, dancing, riding on horse back, fighting, playing a tabla or a sarangi, etc. In writing or selecting a puppet play, the age, background and tastes of the students should be taken into consideration. A short puppet play is always preferable.

Types
- Hand-puppets: which fit in the hand like a glove and are operated from below by fingers. Hand puppets are usually worn on the hand and the hand moments makes the puppet move
- Rod puppets: which are operated from below the stage by a combination of rods and strings
- Marionettes or string puppets: figures with movable limbs operated through strings
- Stick puppets: are fixed on sticks. Many types of fruits/vegetables can be displayed through them
- Finger puppets: are worn on the fingers and are used in describing certain events, e.g. one finger puppet can represent the king and the other the queen. There could be a discussion or a dialogue between these two.

Sketchings

Nature has provided us sand, material, soil and mud which can be very effective, inexpensive and are readily available which will be used to prepare some models or illustrations and to present different ideas.

Publications

To communicate information and findings of research study in an accurate, brevity and clarity form, the articles can be published.

Field trips or school journeys

It brings the learners into direct contact with a real life situation. It is the most concrete and most real of visual technique. Objects and materials can thus be studied first hand in their natural environment.

Value
- They furnish first-hand information to supplement and enrich classroom instruction
- They correlate and blend school life with the outside world, providing direct touch with persons and with community situations
- They create situations which help to develop observation and keenness
- They offer an opportunity to apply that which has been taught
- To verify what has been learned
- They provide actual material for study

- Arouse interest and vitalize instruction, thereby providing motivation
- Effective means of supplementing the subject of the curriculum
- Necessitate planning, cooperation, security of transportation and permission to take the trips and other details of organization
- They give training in shouldering and discharging responsibilities to both learners and teachers.

Museum

It is made up of materials used in classroom teaching cases are collected, classified and exhibited by students with or without the help of a teacher. The activities of museum may be an extra-curricular function of the class or they may be incorporated into a scientific experimental method of teaching.

Objectives
- Permits visual instruction and experimentation with actual museum specimens
- Stimulates enthusiasm for study and research among both teachers and students
- Stimulates interest, cooperation and participation
- To instruct the students in proper scientific methods of laboratory, research and museum conservation and exhibition techniques.

Pictures

Among the various aids in teaching and learning, pictures are important instructional devices at all grade levels. In the class room pictures can make a unique contribution to learning. Pictures are a vital asset to the nurse educator, there are many sources from which highly useful pictures may be obtained. Every teacher should be alert to enrich instruction with these materials.

The study of pictures belongs to the field of observational learning which is a more fundamental and natural process than reading and listening. The training of learners in the habit of purposeful observation which calls for the mental processes of association, reasoning, recapitulation and also the art of interpretation. It provides an environment of 'reality' learner's point of view is the main criterion in the selection of pictures. Pictures have to be integrated with particular lessons. It should be relevant to the topic and it should be colored, accurate and suitable size, watched by all students easily too many pictures should not be displayed in one lesson, after showing the picture, it should be removed from the view of students, sufficient time should be allowed. Select a few key pictures which you feel will best develop understanding. Pictures can be used by individual students for picture reading exercises. Pictures can be collected or selected by students in order to write compositions. We should see that the pictures are suitable, artistic, clear in detail, realistic and effective in color and size. Teacher may encourage students to collect a few pictures on varied themes and present to the group of learners during their class room presentation, e.g. growth and development milestone. Operation procedures; Nursing procedures; with the help of pictures the student teacher can present the topic in a clear way.

Advantages
- Stimulating reading and writing
- Dramatizing a point
- Providing an atmosphere for learning
- Inviting participation
- Creating centres of interest
- Introducing a topic of study
- Reviewing and summarizing the lesson
- Testing and learning
- Developing critical judgment
- Broadening of knowledge
- To speed up understanding
- To create enthusiasm and enjoyment
- Helps the learners to comprehend the subject, situations, conditions, and happenings in out side real life experience

Suggestions to ensure that you have 'good' pictures available when you need to use them
- Build a collection of pictures in varied colors
- Organise your collection by storing and labelling them appropriately. Large pictures should be stored separately from small pictures
- Mount pictures that you are going to use regularly or if the mounting helps them to be shown more effectively
- Make copies, enlarge or minimize the pictures as needed with the help of Photostat Machines.

Factors to be considered when selecting a picture for a particular lesson:
- Appeal: the picture should capture the interest and imagination of all students in the group
- Relevance: the picture should be appropriate for the purpose of the lesson—It must contribute directly to the aim of the lesson. Do not use a picture just because it is attractive or that students find it fascinating
- Recognition: The significant features of the picture should be within students' knowledge and cultural understanding
- Size: If a picture is shown to the whole class, it must be large enough to be seen clearly by all. For pair and group work, the picture can of course be smaller
- Clarity: Avoid crowded pictures—They can confuse and distract the students. The relevant details must be clearly seen. Choose pictures with strong outlines and contrast in tone and color to avoid ambiguity

Cone of Experience

Edgar Dale, the chief exponent of audio-visual aids in teaching is the originator of the, 'Cone of Experience', presented as a diagram in his book Audio-Visuals Methods in Teaching (1964).

Edgar Dale has shown all the learning experiences that can be utilized for classroom teaching in a pictorial device-pinnacle form-that he called the 'Cone of Experience'. If we go up the pinnacle from its base, we find that every aid has been arranged in the order of increasing abstractness or decreasing directness. In simple language, it may be stated that the 'Cone' classifies the audio-visual aids according to their effectiveness in communication-aid at the base of the Cone as 'most effective' and the effectiveness gradually decreases as we go up the Cone, with the pinnacle of the Cone showing the least effective aids.

At the base of the 'Cone', the direct, purposeful experiences are represented. At the pinnacle of the 'Cone', the verbal symbols are represented.

The experiences included in the cone are:
1. Direct, purposeful experience: "An ounce of experience is better than a Tonne of theory as it has vital and verifiable significance". These are mentioned at the base of the cone.
2. Contrived experience: It is a working model which is an editing of reality and differs from the original size and in complexity. If the real object is differ in size, confused or concealed, imitation is preferred for better and easier understanding.
3. Dramatic participation: Real events are presented through the play, pageant, (community drama based on local history), pantomime (actors make movements but will not speak), Tablean (picture line scene in which the characteristics stand still, silently) and the puppets.

USE OF CONCEPT MAPPING IN NURSING EDUCATION

Introduction

"A picture is worth a thousand words".

Concept mapping is a way of representing the organization of knowledge. It is a visual graphic, a web diagram for exploring knowledge and gathering and sharing information. "Concept maps are two dimensional representations of cognitive structures showing the hierarchies and the inter connections of concepts involved in a discipline or sub discipline". It consists of nodes or cells that contain a concept or question and links. The links are denoted by the direction with an arrow or symbol. Labeled links explain the relationship between the nodes, where as the arrow marks describes the direction of the relationship.

Historical overview

The technique of concept mapping was first used by Jospeh D Novak and his team at Cornell University. The concept maps have their origin in the learning movement called constructivism.

Evidence-based Practice

Taylor and Wros describe student's use of a software program to create a visual depiction of a Nursing Care Plan.

All and Haycke narrates Nursing students unique usage of concept mapping in Nursing Theory.

Mac Neil's article describes the benefits of concept mapping in Course Evaluation.

Steps in Preparing Concept Map

- Select: Write down major terms, concepts, key words about a topic
- Rank: Identify the most general, intermediate and specific concepts and rank them as most abstract to most specific
- Cluster: Group the concepts by drawing circles
    - On top most general concepts
    - In the middle intermediate concepts
    - On bottom specific concepts
- Arrange: place concepts into a diagrammatic representation by drawing lines between related concepts
- Link and Label: Use lines and prepositions to link and label the concepts
- Self assessment: Revise the concept map based on the appraisal
- Peer assessment: Get feedback from a peer group
- Finalize: Finalize concept map based on self and peer review and by critical analysis.

Tips used in preparation of concept maps

The following approaches are used to develop nodes and links [Concept]

- Top down approach
- Working from general to specific
- Free association approach
- Brainstorming nodes to developing links and relationships
- Different shapes for nodes to identify different types of information
- Different colored nodes to identify prior and new information
- Cloud node to identify a question
- Question node to gather information

Options for developing concept maps

- Developed by faculty or student
- Open or closed structure
- Computer based concept maps

Types of concept maps

1. Spider Concept Map: The center theme or unifying factor is placed in the center of the map. The subthemes radiate outwardly to the center
2. The Hierarchy Concept Map: The information is presented in a descending order, distinguishing factors determine the placement of the information
3. The Flow Chart Concept Map: It organizes information in a linear format
4. Systems Concept Map: It is similar to flow chart with addition of "inputs" and "outputs"
5. Picture Landscape Concept Map: The information is presented in a landscape format
6. Multidimensional/three-dimensional Concept Map: These describe the flow or state of information or resources which are too complicated for a simple two-dimensional map

7. Mandala Concept: Information is presented within a format of interlocking geometric shapes. A "telescoping" factor creates compelling visual effects which focus the attention and thought processes of the viewer
8. Problem Solution Map: In this students will have a problem statement, definition, causes, and effects, leading to a possible solution. It can be more structured or less structured
9. Process Development Map: There is a beginning and an end with multiple steps and alternatives. Students are asked to create a process for accomplishing a task
10. Persuasive Argument: Students present a persuasive argument. This can be converted to the word processing document
11. Characteristics: Free form of thinking, ask students to think characteristics of something. Can be used for descriptive type of work
12. Research Topic: It is more descriptive asks students to think how, where, why, when research questions
13. Narrative Story Type: It has setting, characters, problem and solution. It is more traditional type

Advantages of concept mapping for Nursing Students
- Demonstrate cognitive synthesis skills with minimum of writing
- Categorize various ideas
- Clarify thoughts
- Define new concept vocabulary
- Illustrate the relationship between ideas/concepts
- Aid in creativity by stimulating generation of new ideas
- Enhance meta cognitive learning abilities to learn and think about knowledge
- Access prior knowledge
- Share knowledge and information generated
- Design structures or processes such as written documents, constructions, web sites, web search, multimedia presentations
- Develop problem solving abilities.

Advantages of concept mapping for Nursing Faculty
- Gain an insight how students' understand the existing knowledge
- Broaden the faculty's understanding on how students' develop the relationship between the facts
- Introduce the topic
- Help in formative assessment/evaluation

Limitations of concept mapping
- If several concepts are included, it will be difficult for the beginning students to understand and comprehend the whole meaning and inter-relationship between the facts
- As key words and phrases are used it may be more challenging to interpret the student's main intent
- A special soft ware is required to create, hence purchase price and training costs should be considered
- Consumes more time in understanding and preparing
- Becomes a nightmare for those who does not have skills in comprehensing the knowledge
- Needs a clear grading rubric, otherwise it becomes subjective
- Faculty need to establish the validity and reliability of their assessment tools

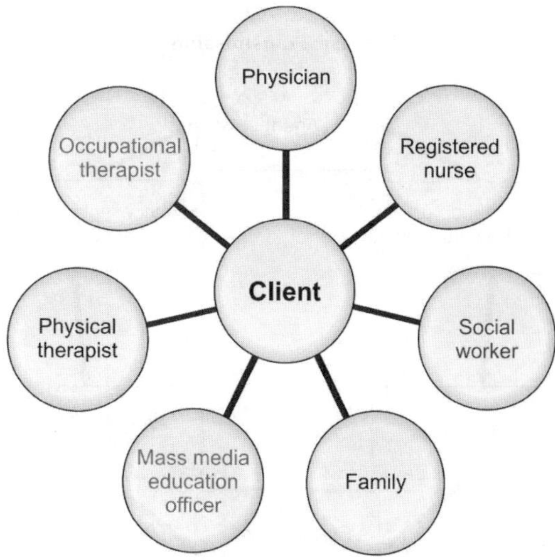

Fig. 7.12: Spider concept map

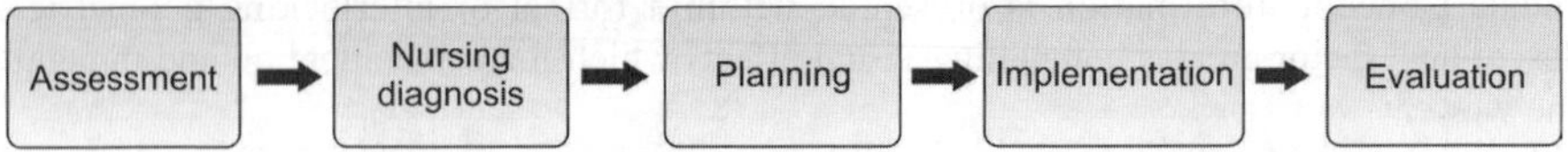

Fig. 7.13: Steps in Nursing Process

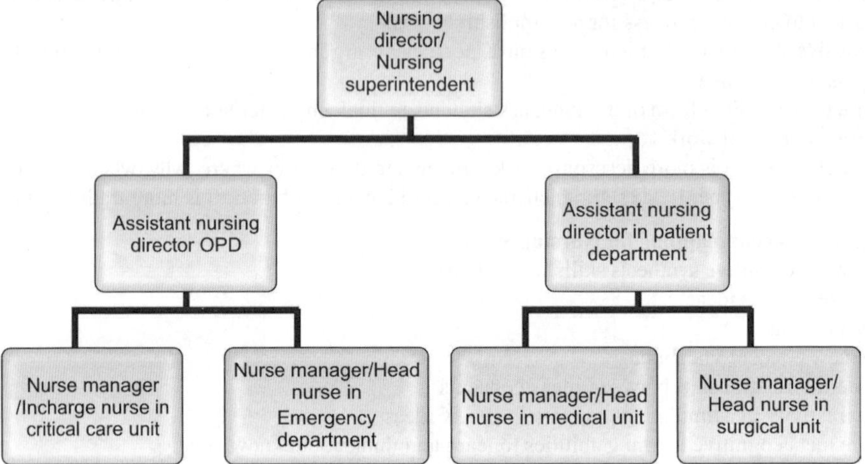

Fig. 7.14: Hierarchy Model – Organization Chart

Health Education—Epidemiological Traid

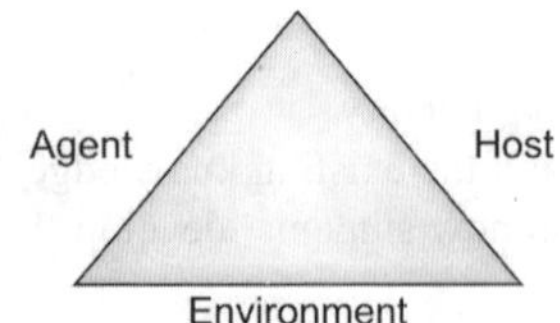

Fig. 7.15: Dimensional Map

Disease Transmission

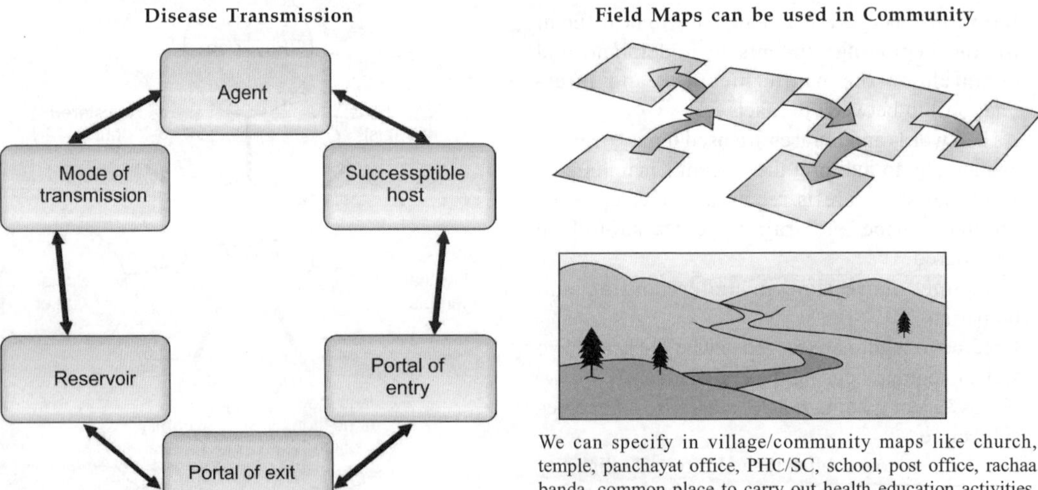

Fig. 7.16: Systems concept map

Field Maps can be used in Community

We can specify in village/community maps like church, temple, panchayat office, PHC/SC, school, post office, rachaa banda, common place to carry out health education activities, setc. pond/lake, north, south, east, west

Fig. 7.17: Landscape concept map

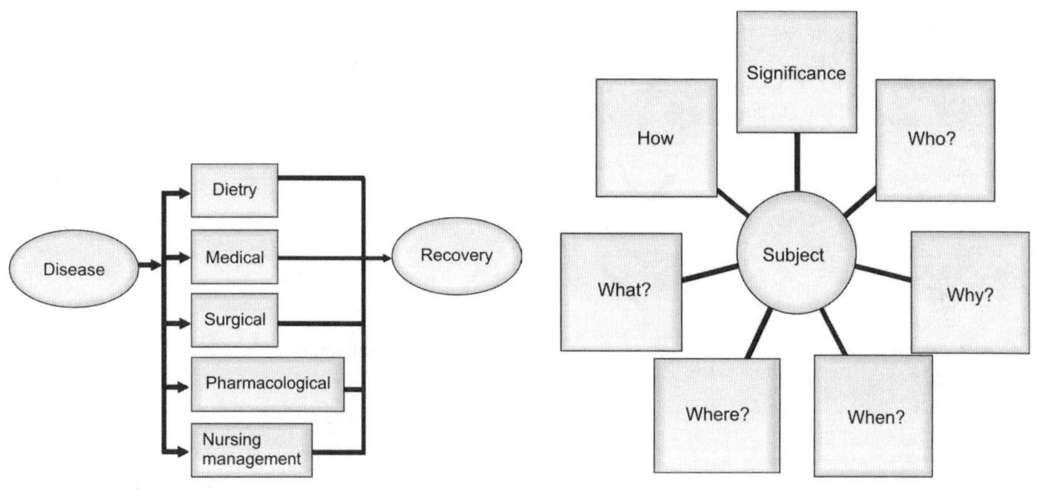

Fig. 7.18: Problem solution map

Fig. 7.19: Research topic

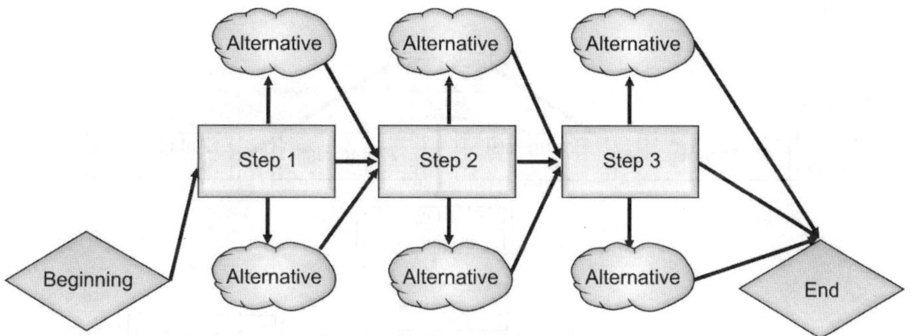

Fig. 7.20: Process development map

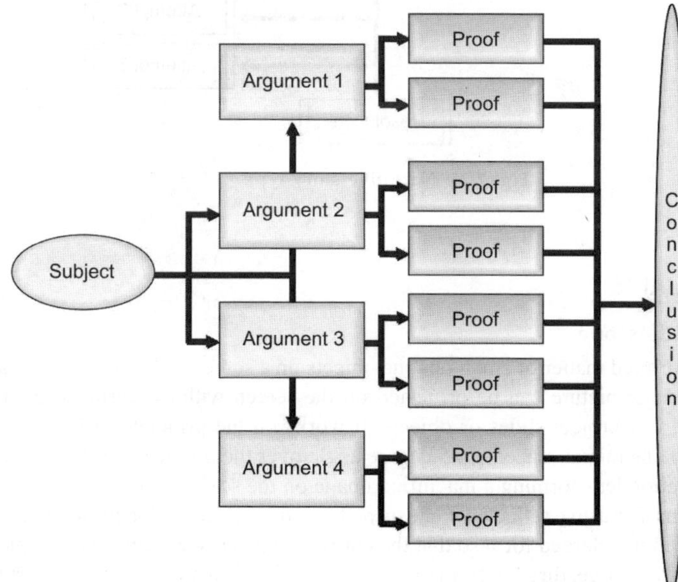

Fig. 7.21: Persuasive argument concept map

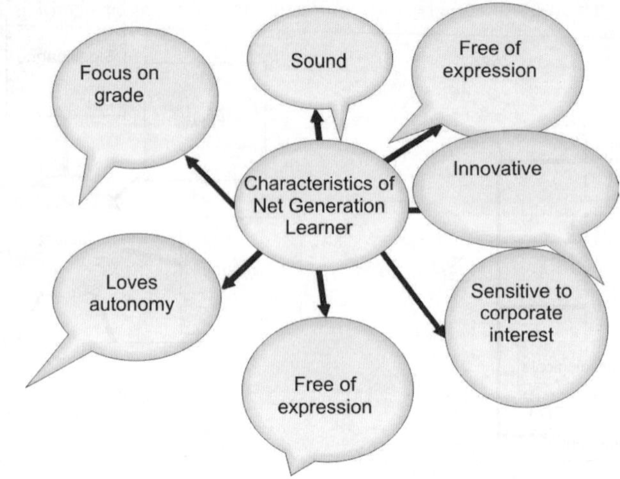

Fig. 7.22: Characteristics concept map

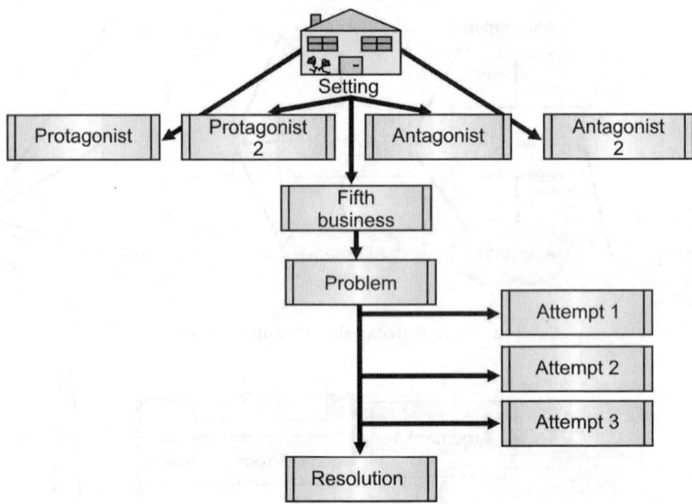

Fig. 7.23: Narrative story type

PROJECTED VISUAL AIDS

Opaque Projector/Epidiascope

It can project images or printed matter or small opaque objects on a screen or it can project images of a 4 × 4 inches slide. Any diagram or picture can be projected on the screen without tearing it off from the book. Through epidiascope we can project slides or objects. It works on the principle of horizontal straight line projection with a lamp, plane mirror placed at 45 degree angle over the projects or reflects the light so that it passes through the projection lens forming a magnified image on the screen.

It is very useful means for using reflected light to pick-up the image or for projection of flat pictures, diagrams, maps to a screen in enlarged form so that the entire group can see them. The opaque projector will project and simultaneously enlarge, directly from the originals, printed matter, all kinds of written or pictorial

matter in any sequence derived by the teacher. It requires a dark room, as projector is large and not readily movable therefore their usefulness is limited.
— on large screen for normal instruction
— an approach to reading

Advantages
- Stimulate attention
- Arouse interest
- Clarify information
- Help students to retain knowledge for a longer period of time
- To introduce subject or topics
- Present specific information
- Test knowledge and ability
- Review instructional problems
- Facilitate cooperative students-teacher participation in problem-solving

Filmstrip

'Filmstrip is a continuous strip of film consisting of individual frames or pictures arranged in sequence, usually with explanatory titles'. Each strip contains from 25 to 75. It is a fixed sequence of related stills on a roll of 35 mm film or eight mm film. Filmstrip can show a process in logical consistency, continuity or the varied aspects of a situation which make up complete presentation. In-still photography, can be used to show the steps in bathing and feeding a patient, in teaching a patient to crutch walking, massage therapeutic techniques and other procedures. It is especially useful in supplementing the motion picture, since it allows time for detailed study.

Advantages
- It is an economical visual material.
- It is easy to make and convenient to handle and carry.
- Takes up little space and can be easily stored.
- Provides a logical sequence to the teaching procedure and the individual picture on the strip can be kept before the students for a length of time.
- Filmstrip can be projected on the screen or wall or paper screen as the convenience and the teaching situation demands.

Instruction to be followed while using Filmstrips
- Preview filmstrips before using them and select carefully to meet the needs of the topic to be taught
- Show again any part of the filmstrip needing more specific study
- Use filmstrip to stimulate emotions, build attitudes and to point out problems
- It should be introduced appropriately and its relationship to the topic of study brought out. After showing the filmstrip, a follow-up discussion and summary is necessary. Learner should develop an interest in the critical viewing and discussion of films seen. Teachers and learners should learn to operate a film projector
- Use a pointer to direct attention, to specific details on the screen.

Slide Projector

The best type to use in the classroom is one which holds a slide tray or carousel and has a long remote control extension cable to allow the teacher free movement and to talk from the front of the class.

A slide is a small piece of transparent material on which a single pictorial image or scene or graphic image has been photographed or reproduced otherwise. Molded slides range in size from 2×2 or 4.5×4 inches. Slides can be made from photographs and pictures by the teachers and learners taking photographs and snapshots when they go on fieldtrips for historical, geographical, literary or scientific excursions. The arrangement of slides in proper sequence, according to the topic discussed, is an important aspect of teaching with them. A teacher needs to use imaginatively and creatively to make the best use of them.

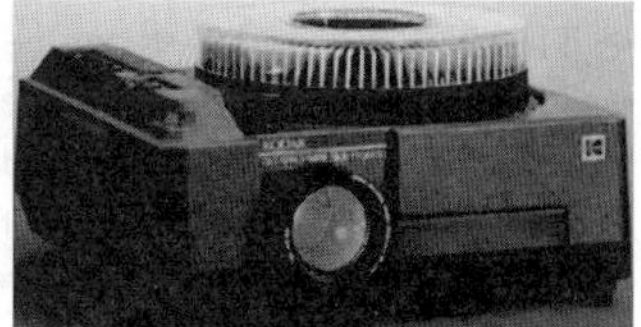

slide projector

Slide must be–Appropriate–Simplicity is the essence, discard inessentials, specially prepared for lectures, graphic presentation is better than tables in presenting facts or data., Legible–Font size 24 to 32 (regular), Title 36 to 42 (bold), Distance between lines 1.5-2, 50 -70 charaters including space and punctuations, don't vary starting point for each line., in a line Accurate–Confirm what you quote, check for graphical data accuracy, Comprehensible–Avoid complicated figures, use brief phrases, one slide per minute, use abbreviations with care and well executed.

Advantages
- There is a change of pace and activity when the slide projector is used and which arouse the interest among the students. The practical preparations of setting up the projector and blacking out the room cause an excitement that something different is going to happen.
- The slides are easy to obtain and produce. Slides can be teacher-made or can be bought commercially.
- They can be arranged and re-arranged into different sets for different uses.
- They create an impact and transport the students beyond the confines of the classroom.
- They can be shown at any speed. The teacher can, for example, hold a picture on the screen for some time to examine it in detail or to facilitate discussion among the students
- Help in retention of the material taught in the minds of the learners
- To convey the information
- To demonstrate teaching skills
- Assist lesson development
- Test student understanding
- Review instruction
- Facilitate student-teacher participation
- Affect attitudes to the individual study or group viewing
- Used for small and large group audience
- Can be used in Class rooms, Workshops, Conferences
- Combined with narration
- Introduces topic, illustration and evidence
  Glass Slide–can be a vivid means of depicting cell structures, tissue layers, body mechanics, etc. 2 × 2 inch film slide.

Over Head Projector

It projects transparencies with screen images suitable for use in a lighted room. The teacher faces the class as he uses OHP and the class views the projections. The teacher can write or draw diagrams on the transparency while he teaches, these are projected simultaneously on the screen by the OHP, thus it is used as aid and tool in teaching-learning situation. The use of transparencies requires the support of an OHP and a Projector screen.

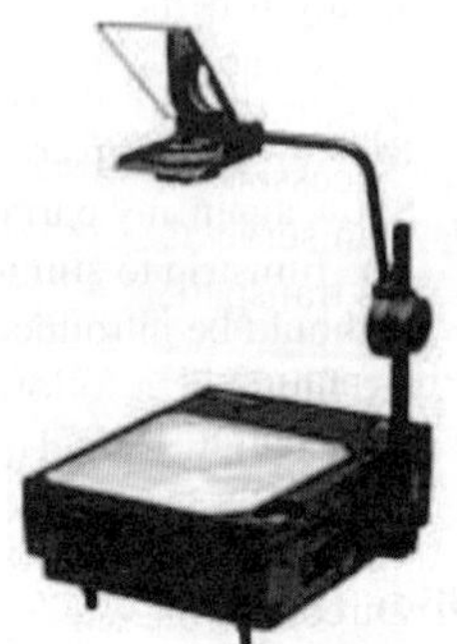

Overhead Projector

Advantages
- It is vivid and interest-catching—Gives a bright image on the screen
- No need to blackout the room—Image is clear even in a bright room
- Teacher can face students while discussing information on the transparency
- Teacher can prepare transparencies ahead of time or write on them during presentation
- The OHP is mobile—It can be moved from room to room or from one part of the room to another part
- There are few technical problems if carefully used
- Image can be projected to high up to enable all to see the image clearly
- Relatively easy to use, very supportive for the beginning teacher to present the topic to the class
- Since the teacher prepares transparency in advance, during the class, he/she can focus much time for explanation of topic, saves time

- Complex diagrams can be taken photocopy on transparency, so even if the teacher doesn't have drawing skills, it does not bother much
- The transparencies are easily carried around and stored
- Teacher and their collegues can build up a collection of transparencies for general use
- Can be used in different ways to convey information, teach skills or affect attitudes
- Useful for instructing large groups
- Projector located in front of room and near speaker for easy access
- Can be used to focus audience's attention
- Effective in a fully-lighted room, audience can follow handouts or take notes
- Ability to modify transparencies during presentations
- Less expensive
- Sequence of material can be modified during presentation
- Short time for preparation of transparencies, different colors used for writing the topic
- It permits the teacher to stand in front of the class while using the projector, thus enabling her/him to point out features appearing on the screen by pointing to the materials at the projector itself and at the same time and observe the students' reactions to the discussion
- It is flexible tool for teaching because a wide variety of materials can be used for many different teaching purposes
- Materials projected can be changed easily and quickly, shapes can be presented and compared, colors may be included and exposure can be controlled
- To develop concepts and sequences in a subject matter area, each component part can be presented, as the teacher senses the student, readiness for the next step
- To make marginal notes on the transparencies for the use of the teacher that can be carried without exposing them to the class, when projected
- To test students' performances, while other classmates observe
- To show relationships by means of transparent overlays in contrasting color
- As a recording device for presenting minutes of a group discussion visually
- To give the illusion of motion in the transparency, e.g. Blood circulation through the use of a special device attached to the OHP termed as " technimation".

Disadvantages
- Bulky, difficulty to carry and shift or transport
- Use on and off switch to focus attention—On to focus attention on visual, Off to focus attention to speaker
- Totally dependent on Electricity
- Accessories like Screen, a stand or table to place OHP, an extension board, sockets, etc. are required
- Can serve as a distraction
- As transparencies can be reused, so same old transparencies will be used for long time.

Presentation techniques for OHP
- Concentration on message being covered
- High light the headings by using different color marker pens
- Use codes and explain them in legend
- Direct attention to the point being covered, avoid distraction
- While preparing transparencies—Avoid overcrowding, limit only six to seven lines, six to seven words per line, six mm smallest letter size, for titles five words per line, three cm margin from each side
- Never use faded pens or markers as they affect clarity of text
- Write only key points and the ideas, don't overcrowd the transparency
- Remember teacher is the focal point of the presentation use the aid is only to support the talk, not to deliver it.

How to use the OHP effectively?
- Keep the OHP clean especially the glass surface and the lens
- Don't jerk the OHP and move it when the lamp is on or when it is still hot
- Face the audience, not the screen when using the OHP

- Avoid blocking the students' view of the screen
- Focus the OHP in advance
- Get your transparencies in the right order–putting paper in between them helps
- Check that the transparencies are place right way up and all text is visible on screen
- Point to the transparency with a pen or use a pointer to highlight information you want your students to pay attention:
    - Cover words or sections of the transparency that you are not referring to
    - Leave the transparency long enough on the OHP for your students to jot down important points or review the information thoroughly
    - Prepare transparencies of complicated diagrams ahead of time, using different color pens to highlight important information
    - Use several overlays, rather than one "crowded" display, to progressively develop a diagram or concept.

Transparencies

Single image, i.e. seen by means of a light passing through a visual project, is usually given to those materials which are projected in the overhead projector.

Stereograph

The still picture gives an illusion of space, the observer receives the impression of reality. Hence, it is known as three-dimensional photographs. The stereofilm is a double photograph made by the stereoscopic cameras, the two photographs being taken from a slightly different angle. The two pictures are enlarged and merged into one view when seen through the lenses of the stereoscope.

Advantages

Present realistic view, stimulates interest among students.

Microfilm

Microfilm and microfiche are used widely for storage and retrieval of information. Microfilm contains photographed reading material on 35 mm film, each frame being the reduced photo of a printed page. Thus, printed matter of a book can be stored in a small loop of 35 mm film. When the microfilm is passed through a microfilm reader, an enlarged image approximately of the size of the printed page is formed on a ground glass (rear-view) screen and the observer can read the matter by moving the film through the microfilm reader images of different pages can be obtained and read.

Micro Projector

It consists of a projection lens, a plane mirror at 45° angle to the vertical plane and a vertical ground glass screen.

Document Cameras

Document cameras are located in many of the general purpose and technology enhanced classrooms on campus. With a document camera, you can display documents, books, graphics, e.g. pictures, charts and maps, and three-dimensional objects and project them so even students in the back of the class can see.

In most cases, the same rules that apply to the use of the chalkboard also apply to overhead projectors. Overheads, however, have several advantages — Transparencies can be prepared in advance of the class, and it is easier to prepare graphics and pictures for the overhead than for the chalkboard.

Tips for Using the Document Camera
- The camera is best turned off when you are not directly referring to information on it. Many instructors use a piece of blank paper to cover part of a document so that only the point being developed is revealed. When preparing documents for display on the camera, use fonts such as Arial, Helvetica or Tahoma in a 24 pt. or larger font size. Margins should be set at 1½ inches to avoid information being cut off the sides. When writing on displayed documents, use a medium to wide stroke marker and print clearly
- Avoid using white paper as it produces a glare when projected. Blue paper or other similar pastel is a better choice. Likewise, three-dimensional objects are projected more clearly when placed on a darker background rather than on white paper or directly on the camera platform. Practice with different backgrounds to see which works best for you

- Glossy paper in magazines and books may not project well because of glare. Practice with the camera settings before class to reduce glare or if possible consider copying the image onto different paper
- Avoid the rapid paper flip. Consider placing your stack of papers on the cameral platform and sliding a sheet off when you are finished rather than taking off and repositioning a new sheet every time you change documents. Leave the document on long enough so the students have time to take notes but not pass the point where you are finished talking about it.

AUDIO-DEVICES

Radio

Radio is the most significant medium for education in its' broadcast sense, as a supplement to classroom teaching the benefits are unlimited. By utilizing the rich educational and cultural offerings of the radio, children and adults in the community, however remote, have access to the best of the worlds' store of knowledge and art. The most commonly used modes in educational broadcast radio are: 1. Radio talks by individual speakers (experts in the field) on specific theme, talks are supplemental for learners for their class room learning, as the speakers will use the common language, simple terms, with adequate examples. 2. Panel discussions about a specific theme where 3 to 4 speakers will be speaking about the same topic in different angles, interview–Eminent persons in various fields can be interviewed for motivating the learners to emulate them, their values, their work and their success. 3. Radio drama—Very useful for inculcating values as well as for creating interest in literature, it enables the listeners to concentrate on the content and substance. 4. Documentaries—is a creative of presenting a real story, event or issue. Truth and reality are the essence of documentary. 5. Phone in programs—Interactive, participating, interesting are the three key factors in phone in programs.This enables the listeners to ask questions and to get the answers. Listening to a radio program needs prior training in listening skills. One type of radio program is called education. Radio broadcasts—Which provide scope for participation of teachers and students.

They also supplement school activities. You along with your students may listen to the program and take notes on them. As a follow-up activity, discuss the program, the main events, the content, the dialogue, the characters, etc. with the students to evaluate and consolidate their learning. The second category of radio programs are those where a general discussion on social issues, health and diseases, about the universe etc. is held. Those programs which you consider useful for your students may be recorded and used to supplement your presentation inside the classroom.

Characteristics of audio experiences through radio and recordings are
1. Immediacy: Radio can describe events as they happen.
2. Emotional impact: Through the combined effect of voice, environmental sound and music, the student's interest can be captured and their imagination stirred.
3. Authenticity: It is possible, (through audio media) for experts to visit any classroom at any time. Students' knowledge of a subject can be enriched by listening to an expert, discuss the topic understudy on the radio. In this way, radio can bring the outside world into the classroom.
4. Conquest of time and space: Through simulated programs, audio-media actually can overcome, the barriers of time and space.
5. One-way communication: No possibility of students' feedback.
6. Audition: Cannot be auditioned, to determine their educational value.

Uses

- Bringing the school in contact with the world around
- Enrichment of school curricular program
- Furnishing up–to–date information
- Developing critical thinking
- Developing leisure time interest and appreciation
- Providing opportunities for students participation
- Promoting National and International integrity as it has no boundaries

- To develop increased skills in listening participation and evaluating what is heard
- To set the stage for student discussions by presenting opinions of outside experts from remote sources
- To provide interest and varied sources of new knowledge and to contribute to the development of appreciation and attitudes
- It keeps the nurse well-informed on all sources of information relating to health preservation and education, so that not only she/he will be well-informed herself/himself but also he/she can help in the health education of her/his patients
- Radio, can help the nurse with background and understanding, for listening attentively
- To acquire information about the cultural background of many different ethnic groups
- To understand the patient better, their likes and dislikes, their idiosyncrasies
- The religion, social factor which the nurse must take into consideration in her/his work, through radio, the student can learn about the teachings of the major faiths, as well as personally receive inspirational values from religious programs. She/he can be able to assist patients in meeting the religious needs
- To call attention to social problems, which frequently involve health
- To build attitude, appreciation and understandings of the great medical and nursing personalities, their struggle in bettering man's health and lengthening his lifespan
- They acquaint the student with the social effects of scientific discoveries
- To keep well-informed in literature, history and current events, to develop a complete well-rounded personality increased understanding and appreciation of them
- Bringing the school into virtual contact with the world around timely. Presenting and interpreting events, while they are either happening and thus keeping students well- informed about what is taking place all over the world
- It is one of the mass-media that can be used to inform the public of the objectives and the needs of Nursing and Nursing Education
- Public shall be informed, permitted and encouraged to participate in maintaining and raising health standards
- Enrichment of the school program
- Developing critical thinking, leisure time, interest and appreciation
- Broadcasts are effective means of presenting music, drama and discussions for study and appreciation
- These are actually team-teaching demonstrations
- Nurse educators can give lectures on health topics like Nutrition, Health Promotion, Prevention of Communicable diseases through radio program and they can counsel the community by answering their health issues through radio.

Principles and the Procedure for the effective utilization of Radio

1. Preparation of instructor
   - Objectives has to be clearly stated. It will help the educator to select specific content to be prepared
   - To evaluate the effectiveness of media in a particular teaching-learning situation
   - Teacher also have noted down a few points for a further discussion on the topic
   - Gathering advance information
   - Motivation.
2. Develop student readiness
   - Everybody has his/her own copy and pencil to take notes
   - Learners know in general what to note down
   - Reception involves proper listening, can be facilitated by providing suitable physical conditions in the classroom
   - Preliminary comments, questions, defining key word, reference readings.
3. Listening to the program
   - Learners will be able to grasp the program by listening to it once
   - Encourage the students to develop good listening habits
   - Concentrate on the program, thinking about what is said and what it really means
   - Listen with an open mind and with willingness to hear another point of view
   - Listen quietly and with courtesy to others in the room

- Consciously relate what is heard to problems and questions that were set up in the audition period and take notes on the radio program
- Note-taking develops the ability to determine salient points from broadcast, to state facts, issues, arguments clearly
- It teaches the student to look for speech out-lines, dramatic organization and conflicting issues.

4. Discussion and application

After the program, a group discussion should follow to clarify her/his thinking and enrich critical thinking.

5. Follow-up

A proper follow-up of students understanding of the information, to remove fallacies and misunderstandings.

Problems and Limitations

- No concentrated attention
- One-way communication
- Educational value is based on sense of hearing alone
- Adjustment
- No pre-hearing and re-usability
- Administrative problems
- Broadcasting timing does not suit all educational institutions
- Students may be uninterested and inattentive in gaining learning experiences.

Educational Recordings

Teacher should listen to the records from various sources and select those most useful for the subject and the topics they are going to teach. The voices and speeches of many professional leaders can be heard on records and discs; classroom teaching can be enriched and made interesting and meaningful by their appropriate use. Recordings should be handled carefully.

Record players—are a means of audio play-back, 7, 10, 12 and 16 inches records are in common size. The use of recorded pieces in education has great value in language learning. The needed selection for a particular learning situation can be easily identified by the specific microgroove ring it occupies on the record.

Types

- Phonograph records or disc recording
- Wire recording
- Tape recording.

Advantages

- Recordings can be stopped at will
- To discuss passages
- To answer questions
- To clarify certain points
- It eliminates the time-adjustment problems of radio
- Recordings can be made to play at desire and teaching need
- Recording can be heard and evaluated (to see how far they are suitable to fulfill the objectives for which they are meant)
- Recording offer a wide range of helpful material
- The school can have its own recording
- Recordings are to the ear—Reconstruct direct reality as faithfully as possible, both enable us to overcome of time and space so that we can receive the original experience whenever we chose.

Recordings can be used

- For introducing a lesson
- For illustrating some facts or skills
- For enriching classroom activity
- For summing up a topic.

Gramophone Record

A gramophone record, commonly known as a phonograph record, vinyl record (when made of polyvinyl chloride), or simply record, is an analog sound storage medium consisting of a flat disc with an inscribed, modulated spiral groove. The groove usually starts near the periphery and ends near the center of the disc. Phonograph records are generally described by their size ("12-inch", "10-inch", "7-inch", etc.), the rotational speed at which they are played ("33 rpm", "45 rpm", "78 rpm", etc.), their time capacity ("Long playing"), their reproductive accuracy or "fidelity", or the number of channels of audio provided.

In 1877, Thomas Edison developed the phonautograph into a machine, the phonograph, that was capable of replaying the recordings made. The recordings were made on tinfoil and were initially intended to be used as a voice recording medium.

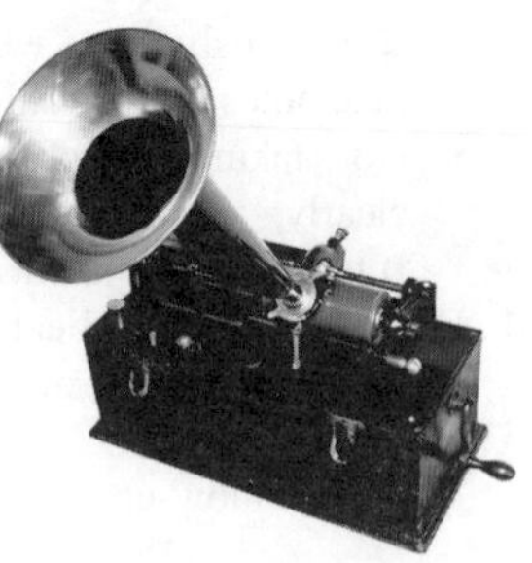

Edison cylinder phonograph 1899

Uses

* To mend speech defects in one's own language
* To teach good pronunciation in a foreign language
* For co-curricular activities in the school, e.g. song, dancing, back-ground music.
* To inculcate a love of good music, to listen to songs, to hear spiritual speech, famous speech, to learn languages and good pronunciation skills.

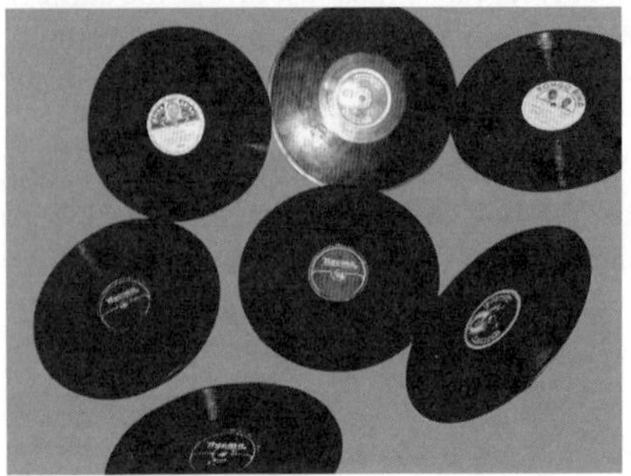

Example of congolese 78 rpm records

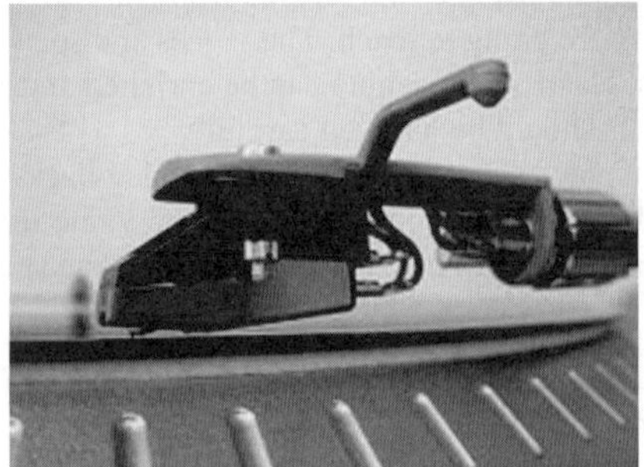

A modern 12 inch vinyl album being played. Note the stylus's contact with the surface.

The normal commercial disc is engraved with two sound-bearing concentric spiral grooves, one on each side, running from the outside edge towards the centre. The last part of the spiral meets an earlier part to form a circle. The sound is encoded by fine variations in the edges of the groove that cause a stylus (needle) placed in it to vibrate at acoustic frequencies when the disc is rotated at the correct speed. Generally, the outer and inner parts of the groove bear no intended sound.

Tape Recorder

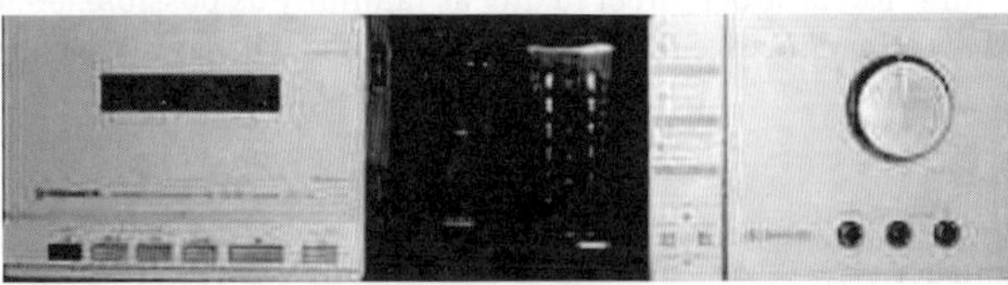

Tape recorder

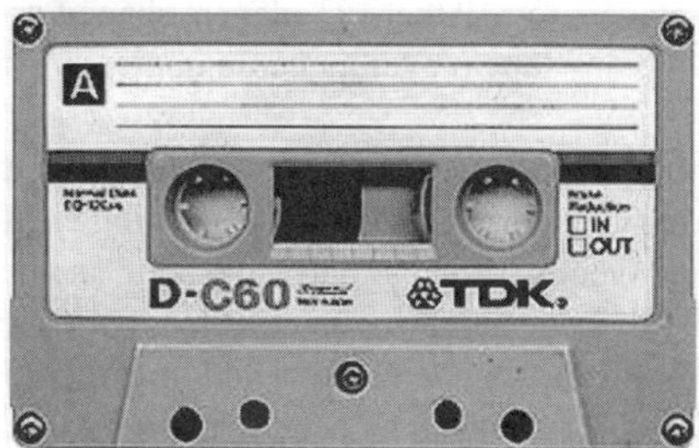

A TDK D-C60 cassette, a common speech-quality tape with a 60-minute playing time, in a housing similar to that of the original Compact Cassette specification

Media type	*Magnetic tape*
Capacity	Usually up to 30 or 45 minutes of audio per side. Some cassettes have 60 minutes of audio per side. mostly used for short messages and answering machines. There was also a C180, 3 hour tape, but due to the extremely thin tape (often causing tape entanglements) it was only used for long time recording. Later the material was copied to normal tapes for durability.)

The Compact Cassette, often referred to as audio cassette, cassette tape, cassette, or simply tape, is a magnetic tape sound recording format. Compact Cassettes consist of two miniature spools, between which a magnetically coated plastic tape is passed and wound. These spools and their attendant parts are held inside a protective plastic shell. Two stereo pairs of tracks (four total) or two monaural audio tracks are available on the tape; one stereo pair or one monophonic track is played or recorded when the tape is moving in one direction and the second pair when moving in the other direction. This reversal is achieved either by manually flipping the cassette or by having the machine itself change the direction of tape movement.

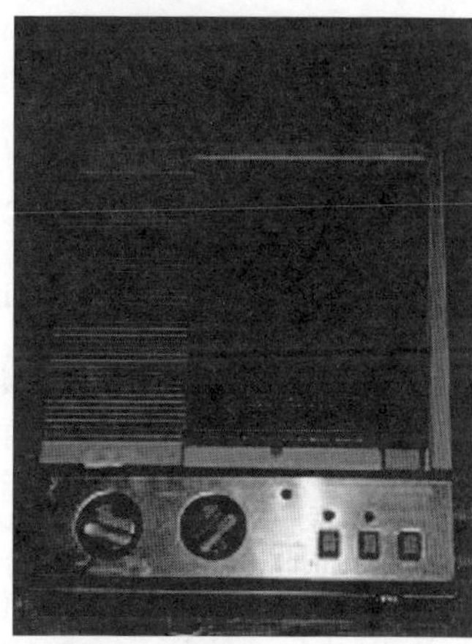

A dual compact cassette tape based answering machine

Audio-The Compact Cassette was originally intended for use in dictation machines. In this capacity, some later-model cassette-based dictation machines could also run the tape at half speed ($\frac{15}{16}$ in/s) as playback quality was not critical. The Compact Cassette soon became a popular medium for distributing prerecorded music.

Most home computers of the late 1970s and early 1980s could use cassettes for data storage as a cheaper alternative to floppy disks, though users often had to manually stop and start a cassette recorder.

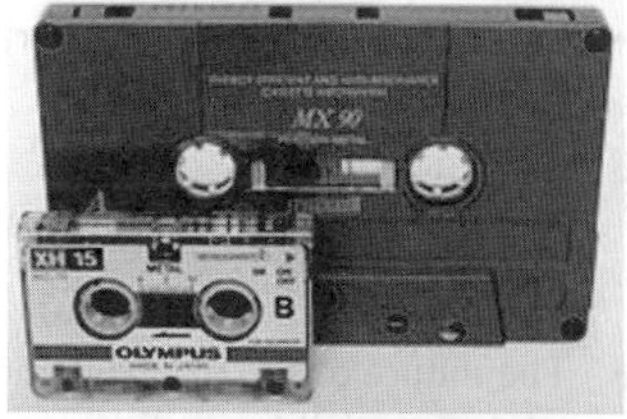

The microcassette has in many cases supplanted the full-sized audio cassette in situations where voice-level fidelity is all that is required, such as in dictation machines and answering machines. Even these, in turn, are starting to give way to digital recorders of various descriptions. Since the rise of cheap CD-R discs, and flash memory-based digital audio players, the phenomenon of "home taping" has effectively switched to recording to Compact Disc or downloading from commercial or music sharing websites.

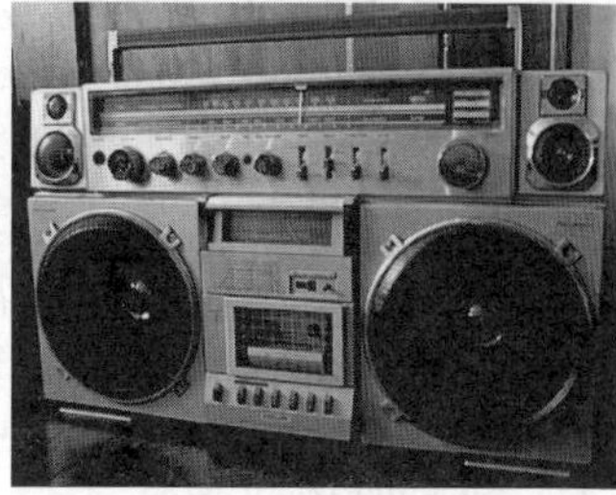

As the Compact Disc grew in popularity, cassette-shaped audio adapters were developed to provide an economical and clear way to obtain CD functionality in vehicles equipped with cassette decks. A portable CD player would have its analog line-out connected to the adapter, which in turn fed the signal to the head of the cassette deck. These adapters continue to function with MP3 players as well and are generally more reliable than the FM transmitters that must be used to adapt CD players to MP3s. MP3 players shaped as audio cassettes have also become available, which can be inserted into any tape player and communicate with the head as if they were normal cassettes.

The audio-cassette tape recorder is commonly available in schools. In fact, most teachers and students own one of their own. Thus, taped audio materials can be easily incorporated into the teaching and learning context of the classroom. However, to obtain maximum effectiveness of such materials, their use must be carefully planned and organised. Tape recordings are not easily damaged and can be replayed many more times. If any scratches or damages, repair can be made on the spot. It enables one to listen and hear recordings previously made. Provides for the learner to hear their own voice and events which occur in their own school. Language learning is facilitated by the use of tapes. The class can tape their own singing or discussion programs and listen into them in order to improve them later on. The teacher and learners should operate and record on the tape-recorder with facility.

Advantages
- The tape recorder is simple to operate and it is portable
- It provides a change from hearing the teacher's voice
- It is an ideal substitute for a live presentation
- It exposes your students to the different ways the English language is spoken, including the way English is spoken by native speakers
- The audio tape can be played repeatedly without changing the intonation and content of the speech
- You can stop the tape or re-play earlier sections at your discretion. The tape can also be edited or erased and reused
- It provides a change of pace and activity and this could arouse the interest of your students
- To record
  - Radio programs for classroom use
  - To develop Learners' listening skills, discussions, debates, round table talks
  - Speeches at celebrations, ceremonies, political rallies
  - Interviews with workers, businessmen, community leaders
  - Extracts, from disc records, with comments
  - Plays classroom dramatizations, puppet shows
  - Student participation in assemblies
  - Corrective work in speech
- Can serve to document or summarize topic
- To record interviews, case studies or role playing situations
- Can be used to record descriptions or instructions for procedures for the listener to review, practice or respond to verbally.
  - To listen music, songs
  - To learn languages and good pronunciation skills.

Producing own audio materials
- The nature of the material and the purpose for which it is to be used
- Highest possible quality
- Try to optimize the recording environment by making sure that:
  - It is free from extraneous noise
  - It has the appropriate acoustic properties
  - Use appropriate equipment and materials such as:
    An external microphone (not one built into the tape recorder) of sufficient quality to do justice to the rest of the equipment the best tape recorder available, assuming it is suitable for the job in hand a good quality tape of suitable grade and of sufficient length to give the required playing time at the tape speed you intend using, e.g. preparing a casette by recording the heart sounds pattern in Patients' with Cardio Vascular Disorders.

AUDIO-VISUAL AIDS

Motion Pictures

Communicating through sound and sight simultaneously, the motion pictures blends pictures, words, objects, motion and even color to make impact on the children's minds.

The viewer sees motion that can be recreated. The time factor can be controlled in any series of events, objects can be enlarged or reduced; processes hitherto a mystery may now be visualized. By the use of straight photography and special effects, motion pictures may transport the viewer into another world. Thus, this medium can bring to the student a realistic portrayed of the trials.

Education Value

1. Enriches the learning process and leads to greater all round achievement
2. Directly modifies beliefs in desirable directions and causes students seek additional information about subject studied
3. Helps in the improvement of educational achievement by different subjects
4. Compels attention
5. Makes the experience almost first hand
6. It is an edited version of reality
7. Control the time factor in any operation or series of events
8. Provide an easily reproduced record of an event or an operation
9. Offers common denominator of experience
10. Influence and even change attitudes
11. Assist the learners to understand abstract concepts, encourage thinking and thus leading them to further reflect on human relationships
12. Brings variety to instructional materials
13. Offers a satisfying experience.

Uses

- Teach factual materials effectively over a wide range of subject matter, ages, abilities and conditions of use
- Effective in teaching perceptual-motor skills
- Films can be made more effective as learning tools through the use of various teaching techniques
- Films can modify motivations, interests, attitudes and opinions if they are designed to stimulate or reinforce existing beliefs of the audience
- Films are greatly influenced in their effectiveness by audience-learner characteristics.

Purposes for which films may be used

1. To provide a background of sensory experience
2. To provide concrete experiences which serve as a basis for thinking, reasoning and problem solving
3. To provide an easily accessible fund of knowledge which stimulates interest and motivates the students to further study and learning activities
4. To present a large amount of information in a short period of time
5. To increase the amount of initial learning and permanency of learning
6. To develop attitudes, appreciation and better social relationships
7. To promote unitary learning
8. To review
9. To introduce a unit by presenting a whole range of problems to students to attack
10. To demonstrate a process
11. To emphasise and bring out the underlying principles of nursing procedures
12. To supplement laboratory instructions
13. Unexcelled for presenting actions, for showing changes, for portraying attitudes and relationships
14. Its' special devices–Slow motion, time lapse, microscopic photography to make it a facile teaching instrument, it can take the student to a favored seat in famous clinics or to a hospital room in which a rare disease is being treated
15. Replaces the first hand experience.

Educational Television

Television is the electronic means by which sound and light energy are transmitted from one place to another. Technically, it is an electromechanical system of converting the energy contained in sound and light patterns into electrical and electromagnetic energy when it is then reconverted back into sound and light. Television is the electronic blackboard of the future, which is brought to life. It offers vitality and newness, which attracts attention, creates interest and stimulates a desire to learn. Television is a multi dimensional and general medium of communication. It is an instrument of encoding, transforming, transmitting or projecting or re-transforming and then presenting the encoded patterns of meaningful information. These processes are performed so that the information input has correspondence with the information output.

Two kinds of licensed television stations: Commercial Television and Educational television.

Educational Television/Enrichment Television

Designed towards enriching learning, but is not directed towards any particular course of study nor is it presented in any particular learning sequence, e.g. demonstration of nursing procedures and house safety precautions.

Instructional Television

Broadcasts designed to aid instruction i.e., it is planned in relation to educational objectives and is presented in an orderly and sequential arrangement of learning experiences.

1. **Total television**
   - The student is on his own
   - Only direction that he receives is through instructions given in the telecast, the syllabi, the books, etc.
   - The student must be highly motivated and sufficiently mature to direct his own study efforts.
2. **Major resource teaching**
   Teaching takes over the main burden of the formal course presentation, but the student's learning is directed and facilitated by a classroom teacher.

   This may be done through:
   - Class assignments
   - Small group discussions
   - Use of audio-visual materials, e.g. filmstrip recordings demonstrations
3. **Observational television**
   Broadcasts over a closed circuit system. It provides a closer view of important phenomena, e.g. a telecast of a nursing procedure can give every student in a large nursing class a front row seat from which she/he can see clearly every step of the procedure.

Functional Characteristics of Television

1. Image multiplication: The simultaneous display of some information at two or more physically separated locations
2. Image magnification
3. Image association
4. Image transportation.

Educational Value of Instructional TV

1. The voice of the broadcaster as well as his figure; his movements, the illustrations used by him, the demonstrations presented by him, etc. are transmitted simultaneously.
2. Educational TV combines sight and sound together and thus makes the experience real, concrete and immediate.
3. TV offers uniformity of communication even the back bench feels the pleasure of front row seat.
4. TV is a versatile educational vehicle. Any telecast may use a battery of audio-visual aid materials like models, charts, exhibits, blackboards, etc.
5. It stimulates and reinforce ideas, beliefs and tendencies already possessed by the onlooker.
6. It offers opportunities of seeing and listening to the scenes and events, e.g. inaugurations, etc.

7. It enables the viewers to profit from leisure and recreational activities by participating vicariously in sports, or play, etc.
8. It makes better use of faculty time, by sharing the lecture portions of their classes, many teachers will be able to spend more time in discussion with individual students, in preparation of better lectures, and in independent research or study and self-improvement. Some teachers are better at learning, some at small group sessions. TV is helping teachers to specialize, so that each does what he can do best.
9. It can teach large number of student at one time and is particularly adaptable for demonstrations of close ups.
10. It provides resources often unavailable to classrooms. TV can bring immediate events with great realism into the class-room without changing the events themselves. TV can bring resource persons from the local, state or national community to many classes simultaneously in many different schools.
11. Skills, knowledge and time are required to prepare effective televised instruction.
    - A thorough knowledge of the subject
    - Pleasing personality
    - Ability to work cooperatively as a member of a team
    - Ability to take directions and suggestions as well as give them
    - Time and resources at their disposal for preparation, rehearsal and telecasting.
12. It provides excellent learning opportunities for both pre-service and in service education of teachers. Good TV teaching is providing inspiration and good example to many new and inexperienced teachers.

Limitations

1. One way communication.
2. Listening to and viewing a particular TV program in school hours would very often require the teacher to rearrange the school schedule.
3. Classes cannot be made to work identical timings.
4. Financial problem, not all schools can afford a TV set.

Videotapes played through TV

Prerecorded videotapes can be played through TV in the classroom. Video films on educational topics shown through TV in the classroom. The arrangement is compact and require little space and time for manipulation, e.g. Demonstration of Nursing Procedures, Panel Discussions, Nutrition Lab Procedures.

Video Cassettes

Control of the equipment and the learning process is placed in the hands of the learner through control over the mechanics of the machine i.e., stopping, starting, timing, reviewing and previewing and consequently the capacity to order the sequence of events, controls the rate of learning and facilitates practices sequences. A wide range of motor, intellectual, cognitive, interpersonal skills as well as affective aspects will be promoted. These are useful in distance education programs to update skills and techniques of workers in the field.

Video Recorder

The videocassette recorder (or VCR, more commonly known in the UK and Ireland as the video recorder or video machine), is a type of video tape recorder that uses removable videotape cassettes containing magnetic tape to record audio and video from a television broadcast so it can be played back later.

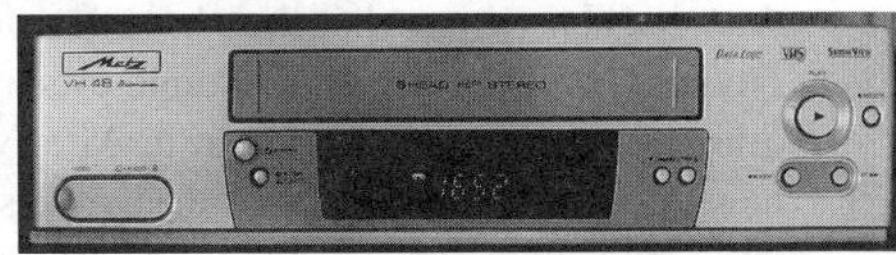
Videocassette recorder

Most VCRs have their own tuner (for direct TV reception) and a programmable timer (for unattended recording of a certain channel at a particular time). These began as simple mechanical counter-based features similar to those available on contemporary audio equipment.

Visual of using the Video
The video recorder and tapes are now common teaching aids available in many schools.

Uses of Video
- Generate interest and stimulate students' imagination
- Provide a common experience for all your students
- Offer a different approach to a topic
- Connect their students to far away places or to experiences unavailable in the classroom
- Demonstrate abstract ideas
- Stimulate the development of critical thinking skills
- Promote critical viewing skills and media awareness.

Suggestions to ensure an effective lesson using the video and to encourage students to become active viewers.

Before Viewing
- Check the room's lighting, seating, picture and sound quality to be sure that everyone can see and hear the video when it is played
- Preview the video to see if its content is appropriate for lesson's objectives
- Review related print material, especially the teacher's guide that may accompany the video
- Decide whether you will need to use the entire tape or only relevant segments that illustrate your lesson's objectives
- Remember that there is no rule that we must use the whole tape; in some cases, a few minutes of video can be effective.

Tips to selecting a video program
- Select programs that model language and provide settings and events that are familiar to your students' real-life experiences
- Select video that provides background images for student reading
- Prepare the classroom environment and video equipment by
  - Making sure that you are familiar with the features on television and video recorder, especially the record and memory functions. Teacher has to delegate the job of operating the video recorder to responsible students
  - Using low light to increase the dramatic effect and brighter light to help eliminate distractions in order to enhance the learning experience
  - The teacher has to plan to position in such a way that it maximise "facilitator" role. If teacher stand close to the TV monitor, he/she find it easier to point to the screen and explain unfamiliar information or he/she may prefer to move freely among students and control the video image by using the remote control
  - Planning to have students sit together on the floor during viewing in order to elicit discussion or personal response and to encourage group empathy
  - Carry out previewing activities with students by stimulating their pre-existing knowledge, e.g. Brainstorm the class a list of words related to the video topic. Ask students to write down what they are sure and know about the video topic and what they think they know. After viewing the video, let students revise their lists based on what they have learned.
  - Divide students into small groups to summarize what they already know about the topic and identify questions they may have about it. After viewing the video, these groups can answer questions, discuss new information and formulate new questions.
  - Give students a focused viewing assignment. This makes viewing more meaningful as it encourages active viewing and evaluation of content. For example; A task for viewing, something they are responsible for gathering, such as, interesting facts or personal responses.
  - Ask them to look for specific information or answer to a question.

During Viewing
- Use video as the jumping-off point for active learning. Teacher can add a short segment of video at the beginning, middle or end of a lesson in order to stimulate co-operative learning, writing and hands-on activities

- Use a short segment at a time and find segments that support your specific objectives
- Control the pace and amount of information your students receive in any given viewing
- Classify, analyse and discuss each segment thoroughly
- Increase your students' observation and listening skills through repeated viewing or showing similar segments from different sources, e.g. Consider showing a given segment in its entirely; then show it again in smaller increments, drawing your students' attention to specific topics
- Show different videos to reinforce learning and experience various presentations of related content. Evaluate the different information gained and presentation methods of each
- Use the "pause" button often:
  - Let your students ask for a pause so you can give immediate feedback based on their interests and comments.
  - Stop to hypothesize and predict answers whenever a question is asked.
  - Clarify new points as it is used in context.
  - Take time to identify and clarify what your students are watching.
  - Encourage your students to be aware of production values and techniques.
  - Ask them to watch for elements of the production such as camera angles, shot choices and music.
  - Ask them to consider what effects these techniques have on the delivery of the content, how the director manipulate the viewers' reactions.

  Try viewing without the sound:
  - Give your own video commentary and eliminate any narration that may be inappropriate for your students
  - Ask your students to narrate in order to identify their prior knowledge or assess what they have learned
  - Encourage your students to share their own questions as they view without sound. Then, view the video with sound to discover whether their questions have been answered.

  Try "viewing" without the picture:
  - Turn down the brightness control and have your students concentrate on the sound. What roles do the music, visuals and narration play?
  - After listening to a video, have your students create their own visual images and compare them with the video images.

After Viewing

Brainstorming:
- Present a key vocabulary word or concept from the video and ask your students to form small groups to generate related concepts.
- Select a group representative to record the ideas and present a summary of the responses to the entire class. Allow your students to question their classmates about particular ideas they have generated.
- After each group has reported, summarize the ideas of the entire class and provide additional information or clarification as needed.

Comparing and Contrasting:
- Divide your students into groups to compare and contrast ideas by making Similarities/Differences charts
- Have the groups present their charts.
- Supply additional information, if necessary.

To encourage "media literacy" among your students, pose the following questions for discussion:
- What is the message?
- Who is the target audience?
- How was the video made?
- Why was it made in that way?
- What is the context in which it was created?
- How might this impact you, your community, the bigger society?

LCD Projectors (Liquid Crystal Display Projectors)

The University has invested heavily in modernizing classrooms and lecture halls to take advantage of instructional technology, including LCD projectors. LCD's used with a computer project an image onto a screen or blank

A line array speaker system and subwoofer cabinets at a live music concert
- The "main" system (also known as "Front of House", commonly abbreviated FOH), which provides the amplified sound for the audience, will typically use a number of powerful amplifiers driving a range of large, heavy-duty loudspeakers including low-frequency speaker cabinets called subwoofers, full-range speaker cabinets, and high-range horns. A large auditorium may use amplifiers to provide 3000 to 5000 watts of power to the "main" speakers in auditorium; an outdoor concert may use 10,000 or more watts
- The "monitor" system reproduces the sounds of the performance and directs them towards the onstage performers (typically using wedge-shaped monitor speaker cabinets), to help them to hear the instruments and vocals. In British English, the monitor system is referred to as the "foldback". The monitor system in a large auditorium may provide 500 to 1000 watts of power to several foldback speakers; at an outdoor concert, there may be several thousand watts of power going to the monitor system.

At a concert in which live sound reproduction is being used, sound engineers and technicians control the mixing boards for the "main" and "monitor" systems, adjusting the tone, levels, and overall volume of the performance.

Acoustic feedback

All PA systems have a potential for audio feedback, which occurs when sound from the speakers returns to the microphone and is then re-amplified and sent through the speakers again. Sound engineers take several steps to prevent feedback, including ensuring that directional microphones are not pointed towards speakers, keeping the onstage volume levels down, and lowering gain levels at frequencies where the feedback is occurring, using a graphic equalizer, a parametric equalizer or a notch filter.

Large-scale PA systems are used to amplify sound for concerts or theater productions. Often called sound reinforcement or SR systems, these versions are much more complex than the simple ones found in schools and offices. SR systems frequently use a dual broadcast system, projecting the sound from the stage into the audience, and also into backstage monitors that keep any off-stage personnel informed of what is happening on stage. These systems may have dozens of microphones feeding into them, and may need several technicians to operate correctly.

How to Set Up a PA System

Basic instructions on setting up the type of personal address system
- Place the speakers on the stands at a height of approx 5' to 6' high and 6' minimum apart
- Plug the speaker leads into the connectors provided at the back or side of the speakers and amplifier. Some connectors plug straight in, others require inserting then turning (usually clockwise) to 'lock' them in place. If you are using a mixing desk the outputs are sometimes located at the back of the unit or on the top right hand section above the volume meters
- If using a minidisc, CD, audio cassette or other player for your backing tracks or interval music, plug the phono leads into the back of the player and the jack or phono plugs into one of the equivalent sockets (located at the front of the amplifier or top of the mixer)
- Plug the microphone lead into another socket of your amplifier and connect the other end to the microphone. Cannon to Cannon leads are preferred for microphones and Jack to Jack leads for Instruments, Effects, Tone Generators and Sequencers
- If you have a monitor you will usually find the slave or monitor outputs marked clearly at the front or rear of the amplifier, use a speaker lead to connect the amplifier to the monitors input socket. (Most Slave and Powered Monitors have an input and output socket so you can link the sound out to more than one monitor if required). Powered monitors are also connected to the mains using a normal power lead
- Check that all volume levels and power switches are OFF and all leads are connected correctly before switching on the mains power. (At the end of the gig turn off everything including the mains power before disconnecting plugs and leads)
- Use your extension power leads and plug the amplifier and player in-switch on should be up and running.

DO
- Keep your LEADS neat and tidy-use tape on trailing leads to avoid trips and wires being pulled out of the sockets
- LOOSLY wind the speaker leads around the stands or use tape to keep them neat and prevent accidents

- ALWAYS use an extension lead or plug with a safety cut off feature. Extension leads should always be fully extended and checked for breaks or kinks in the wire before use
- Clean your leads regularly with a soft (slightly) damp cloth and check for wear and tear
- Perform regular maintenance checks on all equipment, cables, leads, plugs and accessories
- Carry spare fuses/batteries/strings/plugs/screwdriver/pen/paper and a torch!

DON'T
- Have glasses full of liquid on stage or placed on speakers/amps or equipment-Drink from a screw top or resealable bottle (less likely to tip and ruin your electrical equipment and cause electrocution or severe equipment damage!)
- Plug anything but Speaker Leads into the Speaker Outputs!
- Use leads or plugs that are split or broken
- Cover the aeration vents on any equipment
- Block emergency exits with equipment
- Have loose trailing leads that people can trip over!

Types of Players

The following list gives a few 'player' options to help you choose which is best for your act:
- Midi Controlled Devices using floppy disks i.e, computer with sound card, tone generator or sequencer
  - PRO'S—Midifiles can be easily configured to your requirements. Changing the pitch, speed, volume, velocity and adding, muting or re-allocating instrument sounds are all options you can access with a good music software package.
  - CON'S—Data on floppy disks can become corrupted and you need some musical and technical knowledge to use them effectively.
- CD Players, now available with record and rewrite facilities, uses......CD'S!
  - PRO'S—No technical knowledge required, easy to use, transport and set up, good sound quality.
  - CON'S—Have a tendency to jump, sensitive to temperature changes and transporting.
- Minidisk Recordable Players are a more compact and manipulable version of the CD Player and use small minidiscs. You can record, move, combine or delete tracks as required.
  - PRO'S—Easy to use, temperature and transport tolerant, great if you want to change your set list regularly.
  - CON'S—Will sound distorted if over recorded and must be cleaned regularly. Currently no commercial instrumental backings available so must record from your own midifiles or cd's although some companies do provide backings on minidisc.
- Tape Machines are a well recognized piece of equipment which you probably already own!
  - PRO'S—Tons of commercial tapes available from high street stores. Cheap option if you are on a tight budget. Durable, transport and temperature tolerant.
  - CON'S—Tapes can stretch or break and playback quality is poorer than the other options. Songs must be recorded in the order you require, no flexibility in jumping to a track further in the set.

Equipment Repairs

Switch off and unplug everything before attempting any repairs.

Amplifiers, Mixers and Monitors

Sometimes its the simple things that go wrong and the most basic solution is the answer. If an amplifier ceases to work take a look at the fuses.

There are usually two on a powered amp/mixer-one inside the plug (check and replace this first), and the other inside the amplifier. It is not usually necessary to open up the amp to replace the fuse on newer models which is normally placed at the rear of the amplifier and marked 'fuse'. Open this, check and replace if required. Always replace the fuse with the same type and ampage as the manufactures recommendation.

Speakers

Nasty crackles or no sound from one or both of the speakers can be caused by loose or incorrect connections.

Check to ensure that all leads are plugged in firmly into the correct connectors which should also be tightened if loose.

Split and broken leads can also cause crackles so try using different leads.

Microphones

If you have a microphone that 'pops', 'crackles' or just won't work then it's worth taking a look at the inside to see what the problem is.

Check the base of the microphone for bent or loose pins repair/replacement by a qualified repairer advised. A temporary repair for microphones whose plugs are loose is to wrap a piece of electrical tape around the lead and base of the microphone. This prevents the lead from dropping out or moving around.

Unless the microphone is a one piece unit you should be able to unscrew the top. Inside there is a diaphram with wires leading to it-check these are securely in place. If a wire has come loose from its connection re-attach or solder it back in place.

If you are unsure of where to connect the wires and have a spare microphone of exactly the same make and model then open it up to check where the wires should be before attempting to repair-if in doubt take it to a qualified repairer.

Leads

These are often the main culprits for drop out or crackles and should be checked regularly for splits and breaks in the wires. Invariably the problem is easily fixed by tightening the plugs connections but some repairs or replacements may be necessary.

Cannon Leads

Undo the screw at the side of the cannon plug, carefully remove the center from the casing to it's limit (tugging and pulling may disconnect the wires) and check that the wires inside are firmly soldered. A wire that has become detached should be re-soldered into place.

Jack and Phono Leads

Unscrew the casing and lower gently, check that the wires are firmly in place and re-solder if necessary. Do not tug or pull the wires or their connections inside the plugs as you may inadvertantly disconnect them! It should also be noted that some leads are solid units which are unable to be opened or unscrewed.

Plugs

Every singer should learn how to change the fuse on a three pin mains plug!

Many power leads and plugs supplied with musical equipment are sealed units, some of which may provide access to the fuse without the necessity of opening the unit. In some cases the fuse is covered by a sliding or flip top often red in color. This allows the user to replace the fuse without disturbing the inner components. If the fuse is not accessible the plug unit should be replaced with a new unit purchased from the instrument/equipment retailer or manufacturer.

Some amplifiers and PA systems are connected to the mains with 'kettle leads'. The mains plug can often be unscrewed at the back and opened to reveal the fuse within a small holder plus two or three wires secured by adjustable screws. Check and replace the fuse with one of the same ampare if required.

Dead Fuse Detection

In most cases an inoperative fuse can be detected by it's darkened or burnt appearance. Clear glass fuses allow you to view the thin wire contained within the fuse, if this is broken or discolored either inside or on the outer casing then the fuse should be replaced.

Important to remember

1. Always replace the fuse with same amp rating as the manufacturers recommendation. Equipment plug ratings can usually be found in the instruction manual or specifications supplied when purchasing. Plug amp rating is usually written on the base of the plug.
2. Seek advice and supervision from an experienced person until you are confident and competent at performing minor maintenance and repairs. Children should NEVER attempt any repairs or maintenance unless instructed by a qualified adult.

3. Always read the equipment manufactures instructions FIRST and NEVER open electrical equipment without switching off and unplugging everything unless you are a qualified or experienced electrician!
4. Opening equipment can affect the guarantee or warrantee conditions and should be undertaken with extreme caution.

Survival Kit

Anyone who possesses or has regular use of a sound system should have a survival kit on hand. This includes:
- Tape—electrical, duct, masking
- Several of every kind of adapter imaginable
- A set of Allen keys (useful for guitar repairs and various other things)
- Markers for the console
- Soldering Iron and solder
- Nine volt batteries
- Voltmeter for testing cables, batteries, AC lines
- Set of very small screwdrivers, wire cutters, wire strippers, sharp razor knife
- Small flashlight
- Ear plugs
- Spare cables and speaker wire
- Headphones to do line checks during set changes.

Computer

Advancing technology has opened many doors in education. It has been a long time since TVs and VCRs began being used in teaching. After something has been taught conventionally, teaching the topic visually adds a new level of understanding for the student. The next step in this direction would add interactivity to teaching. Not only would the student be able to see what is involved, but he or she would be able to learn from hands on experience. Using computers can be a very effective way of accomplishing this. Computers can also be used to design and access supplemental references. These can be effectively used before a lab to increase familiarity with certain lab procedures. Changes in health care delivery and styles of learning in medical education have forced a need to use and critically evaluate a variety of new teaching tools, including the computer. Computers have begun to show up in classrooms recently, as they have become cheaper, more powerful and easier to use. There have been many software titles written as well for the purpose of education and for use in the classroom. In Nursing Education, Computer Applications in Nursing was added as a subsidiary subject in Nursing Curriculum by INC and the affiliated universities, whereby the Nursing students got an opportunity to Practice Computers and save the files related to Patient care and documentation of Nursing care rendered by them.

Potential Roles for the Computer
- In medical education, computers are useful as there is such a need for learning and presenting large amounts of data, getting and comparing accurate study and test results and effectively monitoring patients
- In Nursing Education-An educator, use the computer to show Nursing students PowerPoint presentations that simplify the large amounts of text often needed in Medical and Nursing Sciences. Stick to the basics in the visual presentations. Educator also may use computers to present video data of Nursing and Medical policies or procedures or for slide shows of diseases or traumas and their treatments
- Simulations–As Nursing and Medicine involves hands-on work, Professional students need to practice procedures before they do the procedure for real on a patient. Use computer programs that simulate procedures to meet this need. The use of virtual reality in simulated procedures is a new application of computers in medical education. Procedures can be standardised and trainees able to test and practice their skills. The most valuable clinical experience a student can gain is by talking to and examining real patients. At present the use of computers in this area is minimal and prohibitively expensive
- Informational Storage-Computers can store massive amounts of data. Use a computer to store data this makes it much easier to find the medical information you need when discussing the patient and reduces the physical amount of papers and texts you need to carry with you

- Testing and Self Evaluation-Use computers to take tests on Nursing subjects or to quiz yourself on Common examinations like Practice tests in TOFEL, ILETS. The advantage of this is that you can get immediate feedback and do not need to depend on your instructor to review information or to find out how well you have learned. If you use this method, keep your tests or reviews short and use them often rather than having huge long tests and reviews
- The multimedia, decision-making and immediate feedback facilities can all be used to build realistic case studies in which students can explores, solve problems, analyze data and make decisions without any detrimental effects to either the patients or the students themselves. This type of resource in increasingly in use in teaching institutions
- Library resources-The modern library places an increasing amount of its material in electronic format and increasing numbers of journals are available either on CD-ROM or over the Internet. This represents a considerable saving in storage space and manpower. Many students who wish to persue their studies using library facilities can now do some in electronic fashion and CD-ROM will prove a useful educational resource
- Teachers and teaching forums-The lecture is the standard format for the delivery of information. A good lecturer will provide a relatively small amount of fact, stimulate the audience, ensure that they remember something of what was said and are motivated to go away and learn more
- The computer can be a tool used to provide material traditionally delivered in lecture format-either as text on the screen replacing lecture note handouts or slide presentations duplicating what was previously the lecture. There are many websites which illustrate this change from traditional to electronic delivery of lecture material. There is little evidence that passive text on the computer screen in any better than the same material delivered in lecture form. However, providing this information in electronic forms makes it easier to update and correct. It also has the potential to save significant administrative time and money, freeing up resources, which might be used to better effect elsewhere
- Apart from the lecture, the mainstay of medical education has been the tutorial. A good tutorial should be a dynamic activity, capable of fostering active learning. It is possible to construct programs that are designed to provide students with an experience similar to tutorials. Students may develop a greater understanding of data analysis with computer-based materials, but there is no clear-cut advantage of one resource over the other software which will allow students to learn as well in this environment as in the small group tutorials
- Another educational concept is distance education which has entered a new are with the advent of the internet and multimedia teaching. For those with minimal facilities and without access to current information the electronic environment may be a blessing, but while students may be able to work at their own pace and in their own time, they lose the dynamics of group interactions with students, teachers and patients. Working in isolation may appeal to many students, but in a profession where communication skills are of paramount importance, there is much to be gained by focussing as much learning as possible in a team or group.

Critical Evaluation of the Computers as an educational tool
- Users and critics of computer-based education need to be convinced about the value of the medium. In many cases, this means showing that the computer can be at least as effective as the resource it is intended to replace or supplement
- In any evaluation of the computer as a teaching and learning tool, two issues must be addressed. What is the value of the medium and what is the value of the content? It is too easy to be seduced by the medium and the content ignored. Short-term retention of fact is not a particularly useful educational activity and assessment of analytical processes, problem-solving abilities and cognitive skills would have more validity.

Computer Basics Equipment (Hardware)

COMPUTER	A machine that processes information and performs computations.
Tower or Desktop	The "box" or case that holds the parts that make up a computer: CPU, hard disk drive, floppy drive, memory chips, power supply, interface cards, etc.
CPU	Central Processing Unit, or "brains" of the computer.
Monitor	An output display device (looks similar to a TV) in a computer system. You see information on the monitor's screen.
Screen	The viewing area on a monitor or the information or image displayed.
Disk Drive	A device that reads data from (input) or records data onto a disk for storage (output).
Floppy	Floppy Drive
Hard Drive	The main device that a computer uses to store information. Most computers come with a hard drive, called drive C, located inside the computer case.
CD-ROM	ROM means Read-Only-Memory-you can only "read" information, not save. A CD can store a large amount of data including documents, photographs, software, and music (about 20 songs).

CD Drive

Compact Disk

CD-RA CD-Recordable drive can put data onto a disk in just one session, and then is "closed"-one "burn" only-you can't add to it after you create it.
CD-RWA CD-ReWritable drive can be written onto more than once-similar to a floppy or hard disk.

DVD-ROM	Digital Video Disk-Read-Only—Memory Used to store full-length **CD's, CD-R's, CD-RW's, and DVD's** all look the same. You must read the label to determine what type of media it is. Both CD's and DVD's are optical storage media. Optical technology uses a laser or light beam to process information.

USB Flash Drive	These can hold documents, picures, and music. Some flash drives are also MP3 players.
Mouse	A hand-held input device you roll on your desk to point to and select items on your screen. When you move the mouse, the mouse pointer on the screen moves in the same direction.
Mouse pointer	The little symbol on your screen that you move with your mouse. You use the mouse pointer to point to and select items on your screen. The mouse pointer changes shape, depending on its location on your screen and the action you are performing.
	Left Mouse Button-usually use this button. Right Mouse Button-occasionally use this button for "special" actions.
	Scroll Wheel-the mouse wheel may work differently from program to program and it may not work in some programs. In most word processing programs, you can rotate the wheel to move up or down the page, equivalent to using the PAGE UP or PAGE DOWN keys on your keyboard or to clicking the scroll bar. Due to various problems it is best if you do not use the scroll wheel in the computer lab.
Click	Press and quickly release the button on a mouse.
Double Click	Press and quickly release the mouse button twice.
Drag	Move objects or data around on the screen through the use of a mouse. Keep the left mouse button pressed while you move the mouse.
Speakers	Output device that produces sound and music when connected to the computer. Speakers come in different shapes and may even be in the monitor's case.
Headphones	Output device for listening that is held over the ears by a band worn on the head.

Microphone	Input device in which sound energy is changed into electrical energy for the sending or recording sound (your voice).
Scanner	Input device that reads copy as an image and digitally records the image.
Digital Camera	Records and stores images as a digital file, operates similarly to a "normal" camera, but no "film" is needed.
Projector	Output device for displaying onto a large surface (projection screen) what appears on the computer monitor.
Printer	A device that produces a paper copy of the information on your screen. The printer on the left is an INK JET PRINTER, and the other is a LASER PRINTER.
Hub	Hubs are devices that have many ports into which network cables are plugged. A hub takes the signal from each computer and sends it to all of the other computers through the network. Hubs come in different sizes and colors. The hub must be plugged in and turned on for the network to work-be sure you see green lights.
Keyboard	Input device-choose letters, symbols, and actions by pressing keys.
Key	Any of the buttons on a keyboard that the user presses to input data (information) or to type commands.
Escape	Usually pressed while you are working in a software application to stop the current activity, back out of a menu (or screen), or return to a previous screen.
Enter	Used to move the cursor to the beginning of a new line. It may also be called the return key. In some applications, pressing Enter tells the computer to stop waiting for more input and begin processing. Notice the arrow symbol on the Enter key; it is sometimes used in instructions and means to press the enter key.
Backspace	Moves the cursor one space to the left, erasing any character that is in its path

Spacebar (split spacebar)	Moves the cursor one space to the right, leaving a small blank white area (space) on the screen. If the spacebar is "split", the left "spacebar" acts like the backspace key-it erases the character to the left of the cursor.
Shift	Does nothing by itself, but when pressed and held down with another key it makes either a capital letter or the upper character on a key. Pressing Shift with a letter key when the CAPS LOCK key is "on" makes a lower case letter.
caps lock	Makes all letters uppercase without having to use the shift key-it is best to only use this when you are going to make many letters uppercase-don't use for just a few capital letters
Tab	Marked with two arrows, one pointing left, the other, right. If pressed by itself, it moves the cursor to the next tab on the right. When pressed with the Shift key, it moves the cursor to the previous tab stop on the left.
Alt	Does nothing by itself. When pressed with another key, it performs a special function. For example, pressing Alt-F4 may quit a currently running program.
Ctrl	Does nothing by itself. When pressed with another key, it performs a special function. For example, pressing Ctrl-S may "save" a document.
Num Lock	Typically "on" at start up. When "on", it changes the keys on the numeric keyboard from cursor control arrows to numbers arranged in a typical ten-key calculator keypad.
Delete	On "Windows" computers (P) it erases the character to the right of the cursor. It performs a "forward erase".
End	The key you press to move the cursor to the end of the current line. Many programs also use keyboard shortcuts such as Ctrl+End to move the cursor to the end of a document.
Insert	Changes between insert mode and overstrike mode in word processing programs. In insert mode, all characters typed are placed at the cursor position (or to the right of the insertion point). As you type, anything to the right of the cursor moves to the right to make room for the new typing. If insert mode is turned off, typing then overwrites (erases) the old characters instead of putting the new ones before the old ones. This is often called overwrite mode. Most PC keyboards have an Ins or Insert key that lets you switch back and forth between insert and overwrite modes. Many word processing programs display OVR in a status bar at the bottom when overwrite mode is on.
Home	The key you press to move the cursor to the beginning of the current line. Many programs also use keyboard shortcuts such as Ctrl+Home to move the cursor to the beginning of a document.
PgDn	The function of this key is usually software specific. Typically, it scrolls a document backward one screen or one page.
PgUp	The function of this key is usually software specific. Typically it scrolls a document forward one screen or one page.

Arrows/navigation keys	Four keys that move the cursor in the direction the arrow points.
Function Keys (F1, F2, ...)	Special keys that perform a number of important tasks. Their exact functions are software dependent. F1 usually is reserved for Help, while F10 frequently exits or quits the program.
Print Screen	It directs the computer to copy whatever is displayed on the screen to the clipboard for pasting later. It doesn't really "print" in Windows.
Scroll Lock	Its function is often software specific. In spreadsheets, it usually locks the cursor on its current screen line and scrolls text (rather than the cursor) up or down whenever an up or down cursor control arrow is pressed.
Pause	Not usually used with Windows. Pressing this key under DOS temporarily stops a screen display or freezes rapidly scrolling information.
Windows Key	The WINDOWS key acts as another special function key. If you press the Window key by itself, the Start Menu will open. Windows +E will launch Windows Explorer.

Desktop Computer System

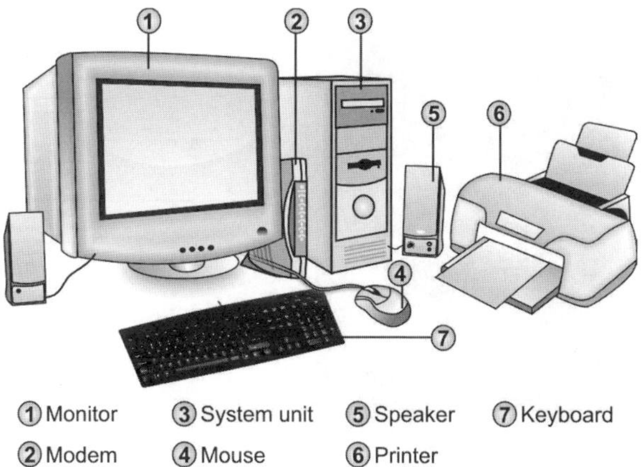

Storage

Computer has one or more disk drives—devices that store information on a metal or plastic disk. The disk preserves the information even when your computer is turned off.

Hard Disk Drive

Computer's hard disk drive stores information on a hard disk, a rigid platter or stack of platters with a magnetic surface. Because hard disks can hold massive amounts of information, they usually serve as computer's primary means of storage, holding almost all programs and files. The hard disk drive is normally located inside the system unit.

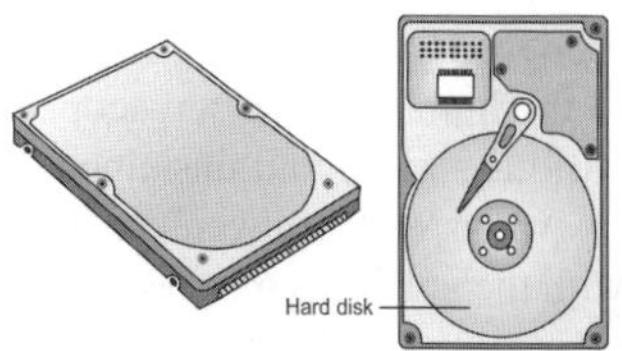

Hard disk drive

CD and DVD Drives

Nearly all computers today come equipped with a CD or DVD drive, usually located on the front of the system unit. CD drives use lasers to read (retrieve) data from a CD and many CD drives can also write (record) data onto CDs. If you have a recordable disk drive, one can store copies of their files on blank CDs. Use a CD drive to play music CDs on computer.

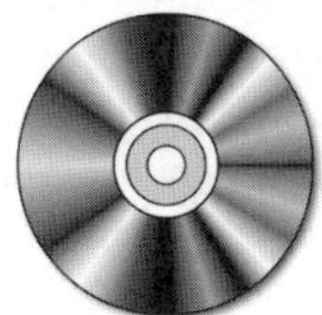

CD

DVD drives can do everything that CD drives can, plus read DVDs. With DVD drive, one can watch movies on your computer. Many DVD drives can record data onto blank DVDs.

A recordable CD or DVD drive, periodically back up (copy) your important files to CDs or DVDs. That way, if your hard disk ever fails, you won't lose your data.

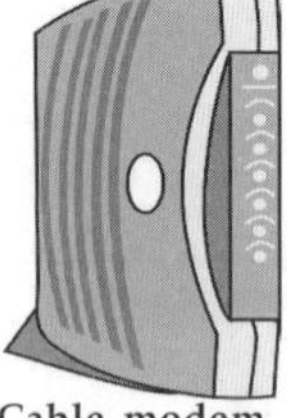

Modem

To connect your computer to the Internet, you need a modem. A modem is a device that sends and receives computer information over a telephone line or high-speed cable. Modems are sometimes built into the system unit, but higher-speed modems are usually separate components.

Cable modem

THE MICROSCOPE

Reliable microscopy is a mainstay of primary health care. For effective diagnosis to occur, the entire health care team must function effectively. The microscopist must perform the examination and report the results to the doctor promptly and accurately for effective identification of the condition, treatment and betterment of the patient.

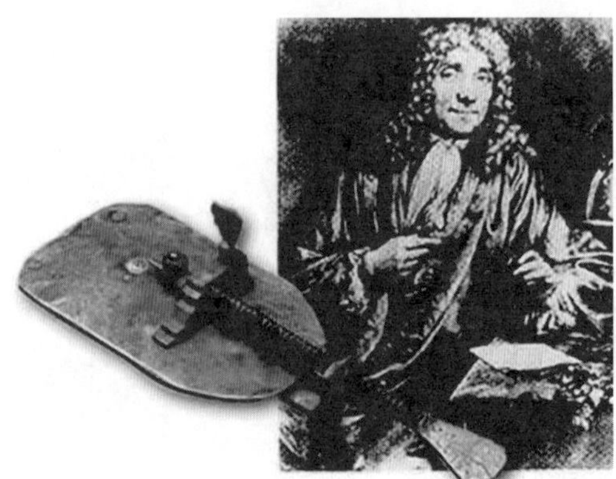

Anton Von Leeuwenhoek

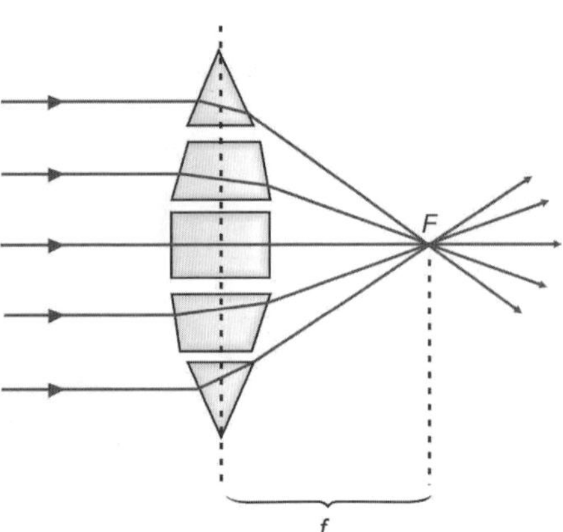

Lense bending light

Introduction

The microscope is a valuable instrument. There are many small objects or details of objects which cannot be seen by the unaided human eye. The microscope magnifies the image of such objects thus making them visible to the human eye. Microscopes are used to observe the shape of bacteria, fungi, parasites and host cells in various stained and unstained preparations; along with the tissue specimens obtained in the pathology lab.

Anton Von Leeuwenhoek (1632-1723) was the first person to accurately identify the microscopic structures with the aid of his microscope. He is also called as The Father of Classical Microbiology.

Lenses and bending of light

To understand how a light microscope operates, one must know something about the way in which lenses bend and focus light to form images. When a ray of light passes from one medium to another, it bends (refracted). The refractive index is a measure of how greatly a substance slows the velocity of light, and the direction and magnitude of bending is determined by the refractive indexes of the two media forming the interface. When the light source is distant so that parallel rays of light strike the lens, a convex lens will focus these rays at a specific point, the focal point 'F' and the distance between the center of the lens and the focal point is called the focal length 'f'. The shorter is the focal length, higher the magnification. Our eyes cannot focus on objects nearer than about 25 cm or 10 inches.

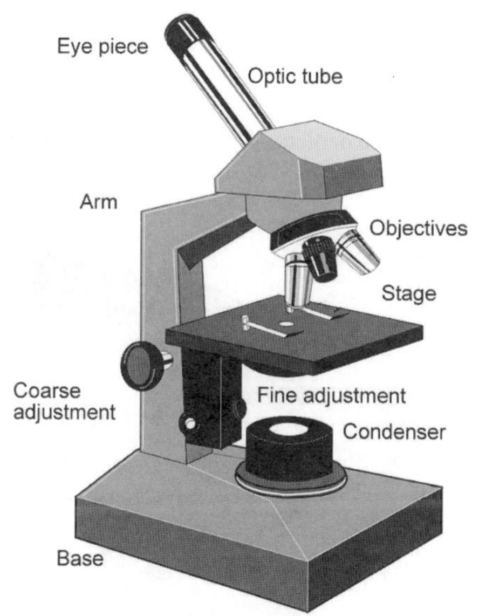

Simple Microscope

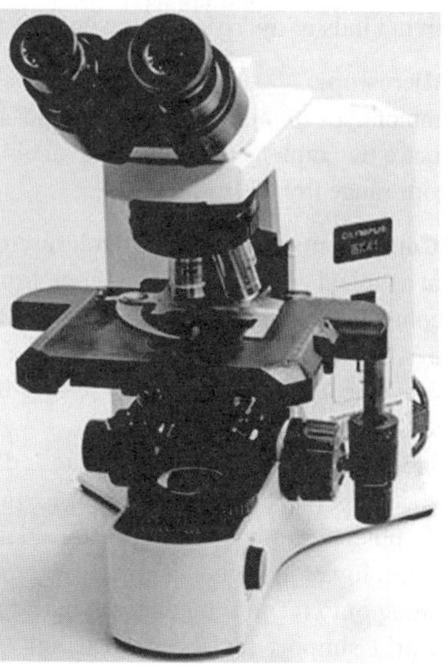

Compound Microscope

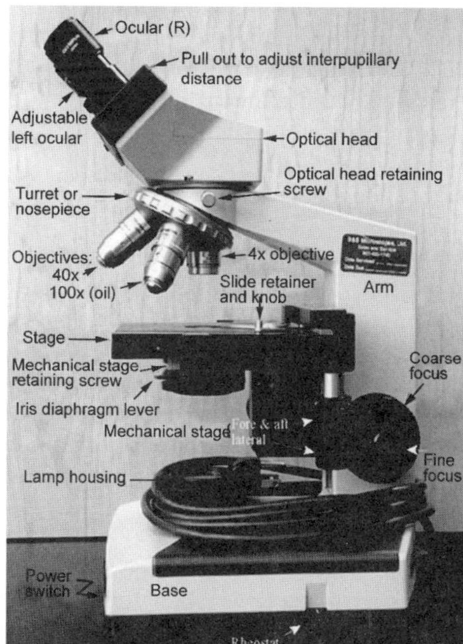

Compound Light Microscope

Types of Microscopes

Microscopes used in clinical practice are light microscopes and they use a beam of light to view specimens. A compound light microscope is the most common microscope used in microbiology. It consists of two lens systems (combination of lenses) to magnify the image. Each lens has a different magnifying power. A compound light microscope with a single eye-piece is called monocular; one with two eye-pieces is said to be binocular.

Several different kinds of microscope can be found in use in biomedical laboratories:

Compound Microscope

The most common type of microscope. It contains two or more hence the term "compound" and utilizes visible light to produce a two dimensional image of an object viewed through the oculars. Typical magnifications of a light microscope range from 50x to 1000x.

Mechanical Components of a compound microscope

If one looks at a typical compound microscope from the top down, the basic mechanical components are:

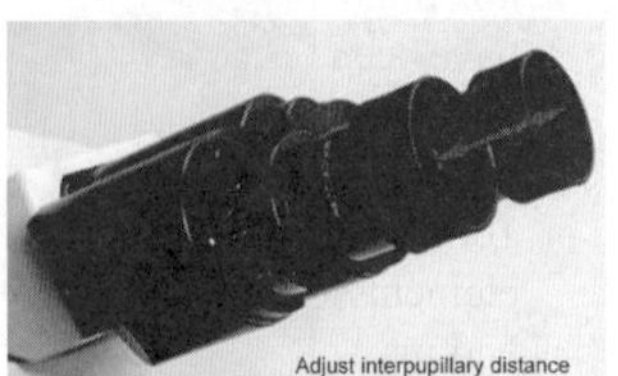

1. Binocular head—Sits on top of the stand and is equipped with two oculars (eyepieces); adjustable for setting individual inter-pupillary distance.
2. Nosepiece—The nose-piece is attached under the arm of the microscope tube. The nose-piece houses the objectives and rotates them. The objectives are arranged in sequential order of their magnifying power, from lower to higher. This helps to prevent the immersion oil from getting onto the intermediate objectives.
3. Arm—Solid support for the optical and mechanical parts of the microscope.
4. Stage—Platform on which the specimen is placed; may be equipped with a specimen holder and mechanical stage for moving specimen around on stage.

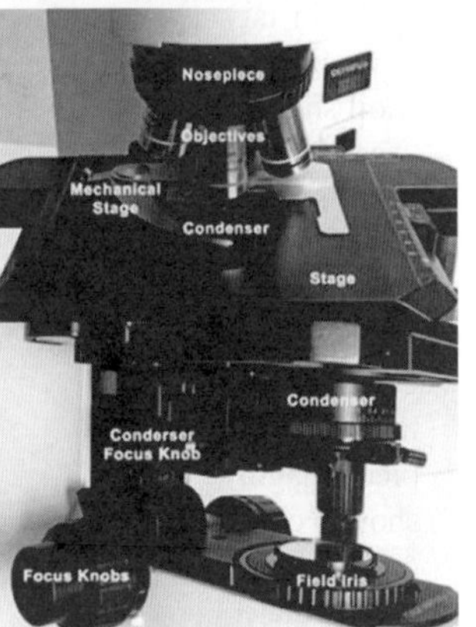

5. Condenser Carrier and Focusing Knob—Holds the condenser and allows it to be moved up and down for critical alignment of the light path.
6. Focus Knobs (coarse and fine)—mechanical means of focusing the microscope.
7. Base—Supports the microscope.
8. Field Iris—Located in the base, it limits the area of the specimen that is illuminated.
9. Illuminator—Contains light source and consists of mirror centering knob, bulb centering knob, and collector lens focus knob for critical alignment of light source; modern compound microscopes contain pre-set lamps which do not need centering and/or alignment.

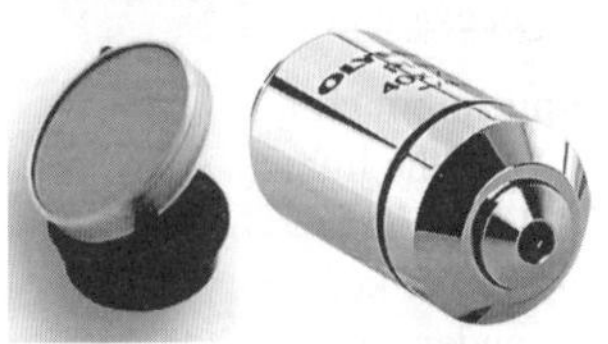

10. Two-Sided Mirror—Is the simplest illuminator. The two-sided mirror provides necessary illumination through reflection of natural or artificial light. It has two surfaces, one plain for artificial light and other concave for natural light. It is supported on two sides by a fork fixed on a mount in a way that permits free rotation.

Optical Components of a Compound Microscope

There are three main optical pieces in the compound light microscope, which are essential for a sharp and clear image. These are:

1. Oculars (eyepieces)—lenses which provide secondary magnification of the specimen image and project the image into the viewer's eye; available in various strengths (10x/20x); available in "high-eye point" configuration for eye glass wearers; adjustable to viewers eyes.
2. Objectives—lenses which magnify (10x, 40x, 100x) the specimen and resolve critical elements of the specimen.
   a. Objectives are of two general types:
   i. Dry—Never allow oil or other fluid to get on the optical surface.
   ii. Oil—Must be used with immersion oil for maximum resolution; the oil actually becomes part of the optical path. Any synthetic non-drying oil with a refractive index of 1.5 and/or as recommended by the manufacturer should be used.

b. Objectives have various magnification "power"

i. 10x (low power)—Used primarily for slide scanning and to locate specimen elements or areas for more detailed examination. When scanning a slide, begin at one edge of the specimen and scan using a back-and-forth or up-and-down motion.

ii. 40x (high dry)—Used to examine smaller elements that have been located with 10x objective. This magnification is useful for identifying cells, yeast and parasites. Immersion oil is not used with this objective.

iii. 100x (oil)—Used for critical viewing of specimen elements at maximum magnification. Focus is critical and may not be possible if the specimen is too thick. Immersion oil is always required with this objective to obtain clear specimen views, gather light from the specimen and to optimize the optical path. Cedar wood oil should not be used as it leaves a sticky residue on the objective. If cedar wood oil is used, particular care then needs to be taken to ensure that the objective is thoroughly and promptly cleaned with xylene after each session of use. Petrol can be used in place of xylene for cleaning if xylene is not available.

Magnification	Numerical apperture
10x	0.25
40x	0.65
100x	1.25

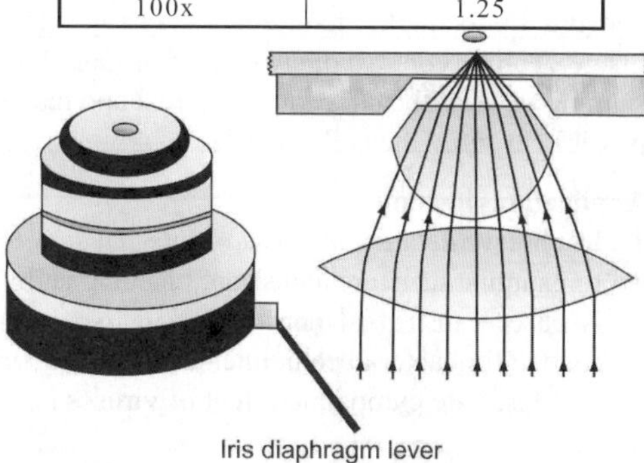

The numerical aperture (NA) is the measure of light-gathering power of a lens. The NA corresponding to the various magnifying powers of the objective is:

A high NA indicates a high resolving power and thus useful magnification

3. Condenser—The condenser illuminates the object by converging a parallel beam of light on it from a built-in or natural source. The objective forms a magnified inverted (upside down) image of the object. The eyepiece magnifies the image formed by the objective. This image is formed below the plane of the slide. In short, a condenser focuses light onto the specimen; alignment is critical to the resolution of the microscope; condenser iris determines specimen contrast and depth of field.

To calculate image magnification, multiply the ocular magnification by the objective magnification:

For example: 10x (ocular) X 40x (objective) = 400x magnification

Some important things to note while using a microscope

- With the light intensity knob, decrease the light while using the low magnification objective
- When placing a specimen slide on the stage, make sure the slide is not placed upside down
- Always keep the condenser up, adjusting the light intensity by using the illuminator regulator. Open the condenser iris diaphragm to 70%–80% to adjust the contrast so that the field is evenly lighted
- Only the 100x objective can be used for viewing under immersion oil. All other lenses are to be used without immersion oil; keep them dry and avoid applying oil or any liquid to these lenses
- When using oil immersion, increase the light by turning the intensity knob until a bright but comfortable illumination is achieved
- If immersion oil was used, wipe it from the objective with lens paper or muslin cloth at the end of each session of use. In general, avoid wiping the objective except when it seems to be dirty. Do not use bad quality facial tissue or coarse cloth to clean the lens as the coarse fibers can scratch the surface of the lens
- Do not clean lenses frequently. This may cause scratching and chipping of lenses
- Cover the microscope with polythene or a plastic cover when not in use and take necessary precautions against dust and fungus.

Other Microscopes

Stereo/Dissecting Microscope

A stereo microscope uses light from two different paths to produce a three dimensional view of the specimen. Stereo microscopes have high depth perception but low resolution and magnification. These microscopes are best used for dissecting and viewing large specimen, i.e. whole insects.

Phase Contrast Microscope

Phase contrast microscopy is an optical microscopy illumination technique in which small phase shifts in the light passing through a transparent specimen is converted into amplitude or contrast changes in the image. A phase contrast microscope does not require staining to view the slide. This microscope made it possible to study the cell cycle.

Applications include

- To observe detailed analysis of internal structure
- To examine structure and shape of living cells
- To observe microbial motility
- To look for bacterial components like endospores
- To appreciate cytopathic effect of viruses

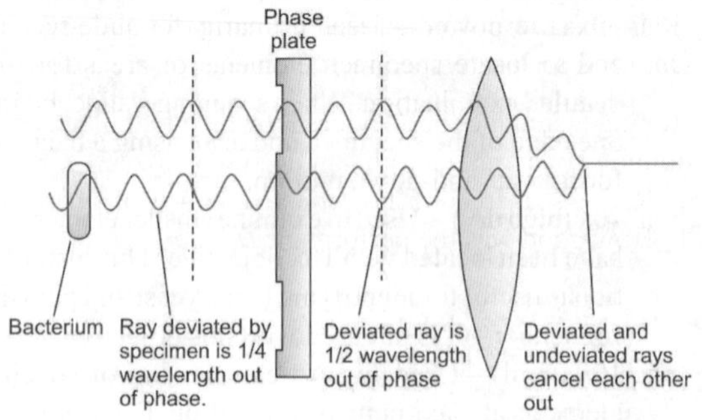

Fluorescence Microscope

It is one of the most important tools in diagnostic medicine. It is based on the principle that fluorescent objects can emit light on their own. If the specimen cannot emit light by themselves, fluorochromes stains such as acridine orange stain, Auramin-Rhodamine stain, etc. are tagged to them. But some bacteria like *Cyclospora* and *Pseudomonas species* can emit light on their own.

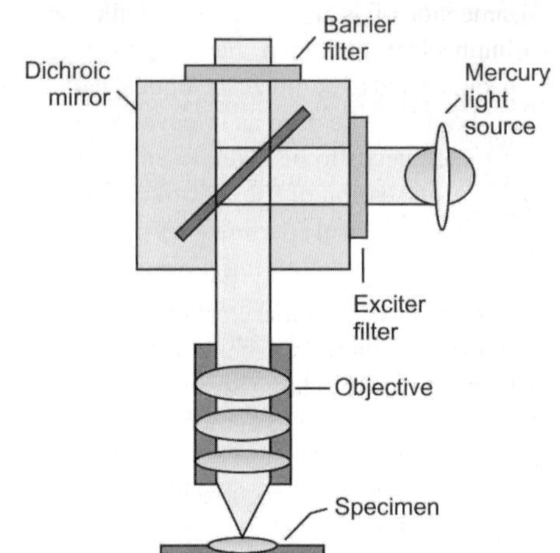

Transmission Electron Microscope (TEM)

The TEM utilizes magnets to focus a beam of electrons and pass it through an object placed within the beam path to produce a two dimensional image. Samples for observation must be completely dry and no more than one cell thick, but may be viewed at magnifications of up to 200,000x.

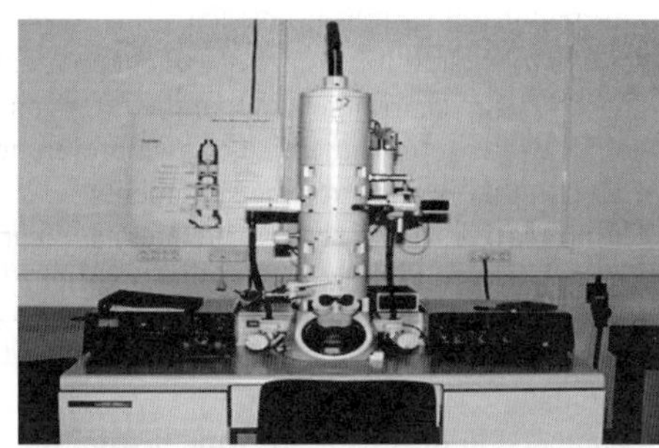

Scanning Electron Microscope (SEM)

It focuses an electron beam onto an object, but in this case, the focused beam knocks electrons from the objects surface which are then collected and reconstructed to provide an image of the objects surface. Samples must also be completely dry as with TEM. Possible magnifications range from 15x to 200,000x.

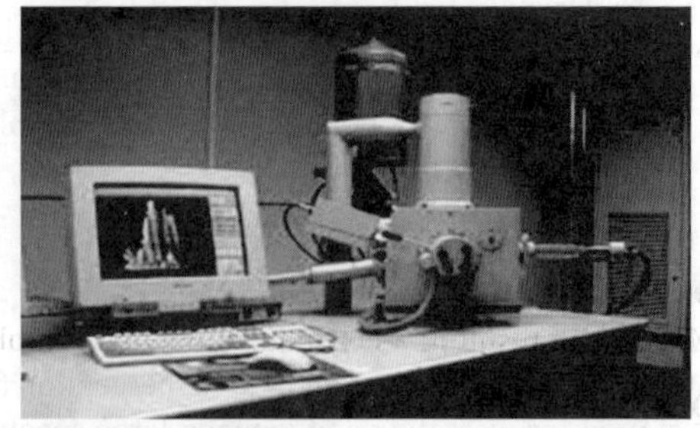

Confocal Microscope (CM)

It utilizes one or more laser beams and "scanning mirrors" to take the surface of the specimen with a point light of specific wavelength. Reflected or fluoresced light from the scan is then detected by the "scanning mirrors", transmitted to a photo-multiplier tube (PMT) through a pinhole (or in some cases, a slit), and the output from the PMT is built into an image and displayed by a computer. Laser scanning confocal microscopy has the ability to produce three dimensional images of specimens that

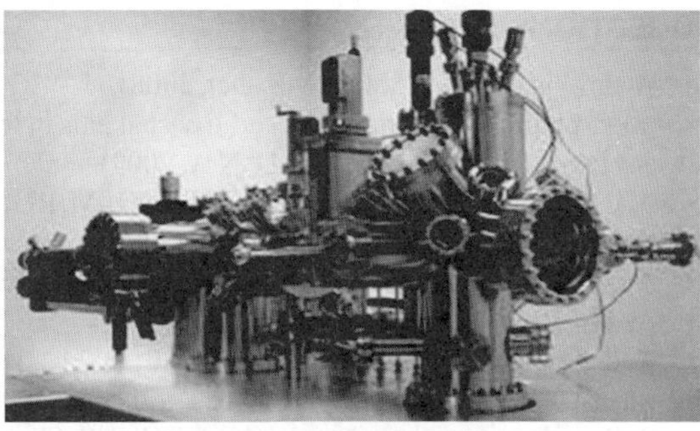

have a thickness ranging up to 50 micrometers or more. The compound microscope consists of mechanical and optical components which are both essential to the function and use of the microscope. Mechanical components provide a rigid and stable platform onto which are mounted the optical components in precise alignment to allow high magnification viewing of specimens.

Uses of Microscope in Nursing Education and in Medicine

- Microscope has played a pivotal role in Science and Medicine
- In health care, a microscope is used in a laboratory to determine the amount or number of analytes (measured substances) present in a specimen, such as blood, urine, sputum or stool, etc.
- To detect disease or to quantify the risk of future disease
- To establish or exclude a diagnosis
- Individual cells can be examined for abnormalities and tissues can be studied for the presence of a disease
- Cell biologists use microscopes to better understanding the cells and the individual compartments within a cell
- The diversity of organisms in samples can be diagnosed with the help of microscopes, to gain a better understanding of the characteristics of microbes
- Many medical tests require the use of a compound microscope for evaluation. These include:
  - Biopsy: Tissue examined for cancer or any other abnormalities.
  - Blood cells: Identification of abnormal red and white blood cells, immature cells.
  - Bone marrow aspiration: Examination of marrow from hip bone or breastbone under a microscope for abnormalities of blood cell precursors and bone marrow tissue.
  - Chorionic villus sampling: Examination of chromosomes of fetal cells under the microscope to determine if an abnormal number are present or if there is structural damage.
  - Papanicolaou (Pap) test: Microscopic examination of cells scraped from the cervix to detect cancer.
  - Microbiological exam: Microscopic examination of specimens (some normally sterile) for the presence of bacteria, parasites, yeast, and fungi. Most often this involves use of the gram stain or acid-fast stain.
  - Cytological exam of body fluids: Examination of urine, cerebrospinal fluid, pleural, pericardial, and synovial fluid for blood cells, malignant cells, crystals, bacteria, and other cells.
  - Seminal fluid exam: Determination of sperm concentration, viability, and morphology (appearance).
- To assess the severity of a disease
- To direct the selection of interventions
- To monitor the progress of a disorder
- To monitor the effectiveness of a treatment
- To diagnose the cause of crime investigations in Forensics
- Microscopes also can be used as an aid in surgical procedures
- Microscopes can help a student to appreciate how different components work together to create a functioning system
- Microscope helps to improve an understanding of life and also in depth of understanding of medical conditions
- Microscope has become a discipline.

QUESTIONS

- Audio-visual aids (15M, NIMS, Oct, 2008).
  (a) Explain the importance of audio-visual aids in teaching nursing (b) Describe the principles in the use of any two aids (7+8 = 15 M, MGU, Nov, 2009).
- Audio-visual aids and their use in teaching (10M, RGUHS, Oct, 2009 and 15M, NIMS, Oct, 2009) Explain with suitable examples (10M, NIMS, Oct, 2008).
- Audio-visual aids in nursing education (10M, RGUHS, April, 2007 and Oct, 2006).
- Audio aids (5M, NTRUHS, June, 2010).
- Audio-visual aids (5M, RGUHS, Aug, 2010).
- Black board / chalk board (5M, Baba Farid UHS, 2009; 2M, RGUHS, Sept, 2009).
- Bulletin board and its principles (5M, RGUHS, Sept, 2009 and Aug, 2010).
- Chalk board (2M, RGUHS, Aug, 2009 and Feb, 2010).
- Define audio-visual aids and write the advantages of using audio-visual aids in Nursing Education (5 M), List the various types of audio-visual aids, discuss how black board is a simple and effective visual aid used for teaching (6 M, NIMS, Dec, 2009)
- Define audio-visual aids, State different types of audio-visual aids, explain in detail about black board as a simple and effective Audio-visual aids used in Nursing Education (15M, NIMS, Sept, 2010) .
- Differentiate between Chalk board - Bulletin board (5M, MGU, Dec, 2008).
- Educational Communication Media (5M, NTRUHS, July, 2008).
- Effective use of OHP (5M, Baba Farid UHS, 2008).
- Elicit the role of teacher in using teaching aids effectively (10M, RGUHS, May, 2010).
- Enumerate criteria for selection of audio-visual aids (10M, Rajasthan UHS, March, 2010 & 6M, Feb, 2008).
- Explain method of Selection of Media for Public Educational Programmes in a rural area (10 M, Baba Farid UHS, Faridkot, Punjab, 2008).
- Explain OSCE & OSPE (10M, Baba Farid UHS, 2008).
- Flash cards (2M, RGUHS, Aug, 2010 and 5 M, MGRUHS, Aug, 2007).
- Importance of black board (5M, RGUHS, Aug, 2010).
- List the purposes of audio-visual aids in Nursing Education and elaborate the need for computer in Nursing Education . (15M, NTRUHS, June, 2008 & 10M, Rajasthan UHS, March, 2010 & Feb 2008).
- List the types of audio-visual aids (5M), Discuss about Three Dimensional Aids help in Nursing Educational System (9M, Baba Farid UHS, 2009).
- Mention the Three Dimensional Aids (2M, MGRUHS, Feb, 2010).
- Over Head Projector (5M, MGRUHS, Nov, 2010, 7.5M, Baba Farid UHS, 2010).
- Poster (2M, RGUHS, Sept, 2009).
- Principles of audio-visual aids (5M, NTRUHS, June, 2009).
- Principles of using Bulletin Board (2M, RGUHS, Feb, 2010).
- Projected Teaching Aids (4M, NTRUHS, June, 2009; 5M, RGUHS, Feb, 2010; 2M, RGUHS, Sept, 2009).
- Puppets (2M, RGUHS, Feb, 2010).
- Slide Projector (5M, MGRUHS, Feb, 2009).
- Tape recorder (2M, RGUHS, Aug, 2010).
- Three dimensional aids (5M, RGUHS, Aug, 2010 & Aug, 2009; 5M, NIMS, May, 2008) .
- Three principles in the use of audio-visual aids (3M, MGU. Oct, 2007).
- Three purposes of audio-visual aids in teaching (5M, MGU, Dec, 2008 & 5M, MGU, Dec, 2006) .
- Uses of flannel board (2M, RGUHS, Feb, 2010).
- What are the types of Chalk Boards? (2M, MGRUHS, Feb, 2009).
- What do you mean by educational media? Explain in detail about audio-visual aids (15M, NTRUHS, Nov, 2010).
- Write the classification of films (2 M, MGRUHS, Aug, 2008).

8

Evaluation

INTRODUCTION

The realization of educational goals and objectives in the educative process are based on the accuracy of the judgments and inferences made by decision-makers at every stage. To arrive at a good decision, the test, measurements and evaluation are being used in all educational situations. Thus, evaluation has become a part and parcel of every system of education to determine the achievement of educational goals by the students in a given period.

CONCEPTS

Test: It will be used in the narrowest and restricted means.

"It is a device or procedure for confronting a subject with a standard set of questions or tasks to which the student is to respond independently and the results of which can be treated as a quantitative comparison of the performance of different students".

The test results in a measure (numerical value) of characteristics of the students that yields only a verbal description.

MEASUREMENT

"Any device, e.g. rating scale, observation, etc. which allows the students to obtain information in a quantitative form."

"It is an act or process that involves the assignment of a numerical index to whatever is being assessed".

"The process of obtaining numerical description of the degree to which an individual possesses a particular characteristic."

"The extent or quantity of something, it has an intimate relationship with human beings, e.g. height, weight, age, intelligence and abilities."

Some of the measurements are physical in nature, tools used are meter, litre, grams, etc. measurement are simple, direct and very accurate.

Types of Measurements
- Direct measurement
- Indirect measurement
- Relative measurement.

Evaluation
- "An act or process that allows one to make a valuable judgment about the desirability or value of a measure"
- It includes both qualitative and quantitative means, e.g. Quantitative—description of learners' achievement; qualitative—description of learner's ability, value judgments about achievements and abilities
- It implies a systematic, continuous process based upon certain criteria process and emphasizes the broader personality changes

- It provides a basis for value judgments that permit better educational decision-making and revise if necessary
- It begins with a clear and meaningful definition of its objectives
- Evaluation of the performance of learners, the effectiveness of teachers and techniques has been attained the quality of program and courses, it can be done in relation to educational objectives
- Evaluation is a broader term than measurement, "it is not only concerned with the determination of results but also involves judgment of the desirability of those results. It includes techniques of testing or measurement, which can be utilized. It is a cooperative process or the activity in which the principal, the teacher, learners and parents will participate"—*Lesler D Crow*
- "Evaluation is essential and never ending process, vicious cycle of formulating goals, measuring progress towards them and determining the new goals which emerge as a result of new warnings"—*Chara M*
- "A process by which, changes in behavior of learners are studied and guided towards goals sought by a school"
- "A process of making judgments to be used as a basis for planning. It consists of establishing goals, collecting evidence concerning growth towards goals, making judgments about the evidence and revising procedures and goals in the light of judgments. It is for improving the product, the process and even the goals in themselves"—*Wiles*
- "The process of determining to what extent the educational objectives are being realized"—*Ralph Tyler*
- "The process of determining: The extent to which an objective and goal is being attained or accomplished and the effectiveness of the learning experiences provided in the classroom."— *NCERT*
- "An act or process that allows one to make a judgment about the desirability or value of a measure"
- "A foundation stone for future planning. It implies the use of relative and flexible standards"
- "A continuous process of collecting, recording, assembling and interpreting the information"
- It includes both measurement (quantitative) and appraisal (qualitative).

Educational Evaluation

- It emphasises for the development of more adequate techniques of assessing a learner's growth and development
- It caters to the child's psychological needs, interests, aptitudes and appreciation
- Puts more stress on learning than teaching.

Meaning

- 'To evaluate' means 'to ascertain the value or amount of appraise carefully'
- It is the judging of the worth or value of something that represents the satisfaction of a human need, e.g. An object/event/activity/process/product
- It denotes more than estimation of the results of activities that have already been completed, it also includes the judging of actions that will take place in the future
- It signifies estimating the probable worth of activities involved in the teaching—learning relationship, judging the worth of methods or devices used in pursuit of those activities and estimating at various stages the outcomes resulting from the activities
- 'Measure' means 'the act or process of ascertaining the extent, dimensions, quantity, etc. of something, especially by comparison with a standard'
- Measurement connotes appraisal in terms of some fixed and absolute standard
- Evaluation includes measurement, but adds to the concept of factors that are in tangible and not subject to quantitative determination. The intangible factors refer to human factors, i.e appraisal of the student as a whole, whereas in measurement our appraisal is confined to those elements or factors which can be reduced to a quantitative basis. Thus evaluation is more comprehensive than measurement
- In education, we will measure the changes that have occurred in the students as a result of teaching and experience and judging the desirability and adequacy of those changes (performed by evaluation)
- The manner in which an individual organizes his behavior patterns is an important aspect to be appraised. Information gathered as a result of measurement or evaluation of activities must be interpreted as a part of the whole

- It helps the student to understand himself/herself better and he/she will consider that life is worthwhile
- The nature of measurement and appraisal techniques used, influences the type of learning that goes in the classroom
- A wide range of evaluation activities covering various objectives of a course will lead to varied learning and teaching experiences within a course
- The development of any evaluation program is the responsibility of the professors, school administrators, and the student's maximum value can be derived from the participation of all concerned
- Evaluation process is concerned with provision of learning experience, increasing the capabilities to perform certain functions
- Thus, evaluation should provide data for improvement of teaching as well as an insight for enhancement of learning on the part of the learner
- Evaluation requires bold initiation and creative thinking on the part of the teachers as well as the planners
- Evaluation can guide teaching, when it furnishes diagnosis of specific strength and weakness in the learner's achievements or capacities. This knowledge will help the teacher to attain maximum accomplishment
- Evaluation may again motivate learner's learning experiences. What the learner will study and seek to learn is determined largely by what he expects the measure of his learning to be
- Evaluation is an act or a dynamic process that allows one to make a judgment about the desirability or value of a measure
- The teacher has to stimulate the learner's growth in understanding, application of what has been understood attitudes, appreciation, interests, powers of thinking and personal social adaptability.

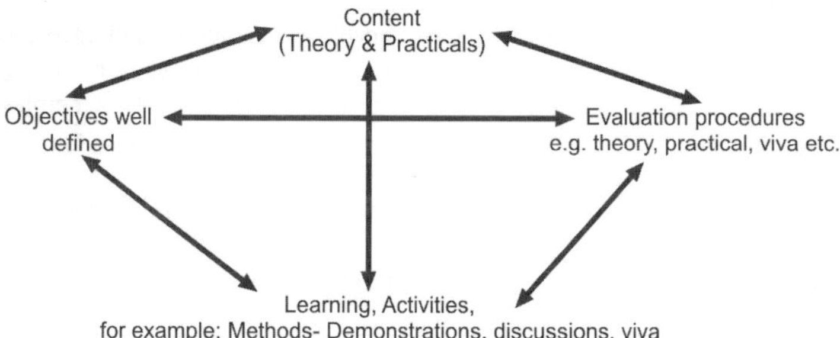

Fig. 8.1: Aspects of educational evaluation

Scope of Evaluation

- Value judgment
- Ascertaining the extent to which the educational objectives have been attained
- Effectiveness of appraisal or methods of instruction
- Identifies learner's strengths and weaknesses, difficulties, issues and problems, needs and demands
- Provides baseline for guidance and counseling
- Placement and promotions in jobs
- Development of attitudes, interests, capabilities, creativity, originality, knowledge and skills, etc.
- Development of tools and techniques
- Development of curriculum for its revision
- Interpretation of results and identify the strengths and Weaknesses of Curriculum implementation
- Helpful for curriculum planners and administers to improve the curriculum pattern.

The Philosophy of Evaluation

Each individual should receive
1. Education that most fully allows him to develop his potential.
2. Placed that he/she contributes to the society and receives personal satisfaction in doing so.
3. Fullest development of the individual requires recognition of his/her essential individuality along with some rational appraisal by himself/herself and others.

4. The judgments required in assessing an individual's potential are complex in their composition, difficult to make and filled with error, which can be reduced but never eliminated. Hence any evaluation can never be considered as final.
5. Composite assessment by a group of individuals is likely to be in error than assessment made by a single person.
6. A conscientious group of individuals has to put efforts to develop more reliable and valid appraisal methods lead to the clarification of the criteria for judgment and reduce the error and resulting wrongs.
7. Every form of appraisal will have critics, which is a spur to change and improvement.

Measurement	Evaluation
• Refers to quantity describing in terms of pupil's attainment in a subject • For example, how much an individual's performance has taken place, i.e. score in one subject • It describes a situation, e.g. 50 out of 100 marks in nursing education • It is only a tool to be used in evaluation	• It is measured in terms of quality and value judgment, e.g. Good, bad, Normal, etc • For example, how good an individual's performance has taken place • Evaluation judges its work and values it as average • Evaluation includes measurement and signifies a wider process of judging students' progress

The Psychology of Evaluation

- Evaluation techniques should consist of and what we know to be the best and most effective psychological principle
- Student will be ready to have the evaluation of his/her abilities when he understands and accepts the values and objectives involved
- Learner tend to carry on, those activities which have success associated with their results, i.e. law of effect. The type of evaluation device used to determine to a great extent, the type of learning activity in which students will engage in the classroom, e.g. If a test requires students to apply principles, interpret the data or solve problems, the students will study with the idea of becoming best fitted to do well on the types of test items
- Individuals learn better when they are 'constantly' appraised in a meaningful manner as to how well they are doing
- Motivation of the student is important. A person's top performance on a test is directly related to his/her motivation
- Learning is most efficient when there is activity on the part of the learner.

Characteristics of a Good Evaluation Instrument

- It should show how far the educational objectives have been achieved
- It has to measure the knowledge and overall personality development of the individual learner
- It is a continuous process, therefore it should have formative, summative and terminal evaluation (quarterly, midterm, semifinal and final test or examination)
- Evaluation technique should be reliable and valid
- To identify how far changes have taken place among the students in the teaching learning process
  1. **Validity:**
     The accuracy with which a test measures whatever it is intended/supposed to measure, the efficiency with which a test measures what it attempts to measure, the accuracy with which a test reliably measures what is relevant, e.g. a test may be valid for specific purpose but not for general. The validity of a test must determinate with reference to the particular use for which the test is being considered. The validity pertains to the results of a test or tool and not to the instrument itself. An evaluation procedure is valid to the extent that it provides an assessment of the degree to which learners have achieved specific objectives, content matter and learning experiences. Validity is the most important consideration on the selection and use of testing procedure.
     - It is an inclusive term.
     - It is a matter of degree i.e., high, moderate, low. It does not exist on an all or none basis.
     - Specific.

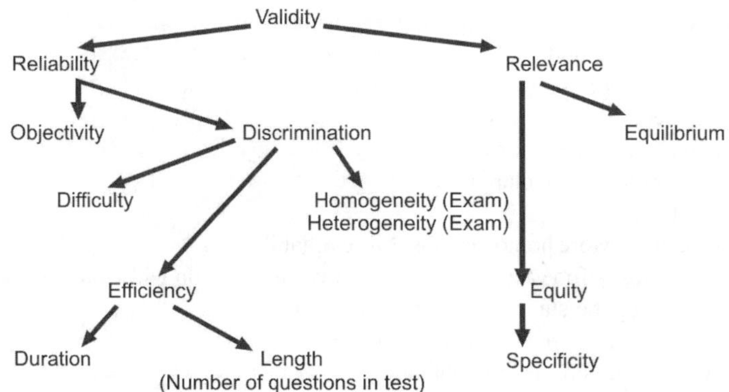

Fig 8.2: Relationships between characteristics of measurement

Factors Affecting Validity
- Unclear direction results to low validity
- If reading vocabulary is poor, the students fail to reply to the test item, even if they know the answer
- Difficult sentences are difficult to understand, unnecessarily confused, which will affect the validity of the test
- Use of inappropriate items will lead to disorganization of matter leads to lower validity
- Medium of expression—English, as the medium of instruction and response for non-english medium students creates more serious problem, affects the validity of a test
- Difficulty level of items: too easy or too difficult test items would not discriminate among learners; thereby the validity of a test will be lowered
- Influence of extraneous factors, e.g. style of expression, legibility, mechanics of grammar, handwriting, length of the answer and method of organizing the matter
- Inappropriate time limits—if no time limit is given the results will be invalidated
- Inadequate weightage to sub—topics or objectives forms a question of validity of a test
- Quiz items—To assess students' ability to understand a test item, guess and respond quiz items will be formulated. This would lower the validity of the test item.

Types of validity
- Content validity: All major aspects of the content area must be adequately covered by the test items and in correct positions. A good judgment may ensure content validity.
- Predictive validity: The extent to which a test can predict the future performance of the students. The tests which are used for classification and selection purposes.
- Concurrent validity: The relationship between scores on measuring tool and criteria available at the same time in the present situation. To diagnose the existing status of the individual rather than predicting about his future outcome.
- Constructive validity: It refers to the extent to which a test reflects and seems to measure a hypothesized trait.
- Face validity: When one looks at the test, he thinks of the extent to which the test seems logically related to what is being tested. This explains the face validity. The common sense approach gives, 'face validity.'

2. Reliability

The degree of accuracy, consistency with which an exam test measures what it seeks to measure a given variable. 'The degree of consistency among tests scores.'
- A test score is called reliable, when we have reasons for believing it to be stable and trustworthy.

Methods of Estimating Reliability
Reliability is expressed by a coefficient of correlation is called as 'the reliability coefficient.'
Approaches
- Test re-test method
- Alternate or parallel forms method

- Split-half method
- Rational equivalence method.

Factors Influencing Reliability
- Data collecting method
- Interval between testing occasions
- Test length (higher the length, more reliable)
- Speed of the method
- Group homogeneity—More homogeneous, More reliability
- Difficulty of the items—Too easy or too difficult tests for a group will tend to be less reliable because the differences among the students in such tests are narrow
- Objectivity of scoring is more reliable than subjective scoring
- Ambiguous wording of items is less reliable
- Inconsistency in test administration, e.g. Deviations in timing, procedure, instruction; Fluctuation in interest and attention of learners; Skills in emotional attitude, make a test less reliable
- Optional questions: If optional questions are given, the same student may not attempt the same items on a second administration; thereby the reliability of the test is reduced.

Relation between Validity and Reliability
- Validity is truthfulness, while reliability is trust worthiness. These both are the two aspects of efficiency
- A test cannot be valid unless it is reliable
- A test has single reliability coefficient estimated by statistical procedures whereas no single validity index for a test
- Validity includes reliability.

3. **Objectivity**

A test is objective when the scorer's personal judgment does not affect the scoring. It eliminates fixed opinion or judgment of the person who scores it. The extent to which independent and competent examiners agree on what constitutes a good answer for each of the elements of a measuring instrument.
- The objectivity is a prerequisite of reliability and validity
- The objectivity of a test can be increased by:
- Using more objective type items, e.g. Multiple choice, short answers, true or false
- Preparing scoring key
- Two independent examiners (equally competent teachers) evaluating the test and using the average score of the two as final score, e.g. Practical examinations.

4. **Practicability (usability)**

The overall simplicity of use of a test for both constructor and for learner. It is an important criterion used for assessing the value of a test. Practicability depends upon various factors like ease of administrability, scoring, interpretation and economy. This includes the case of administering the test with little possibilities for error in giving directions, timing, ease and economy of scoring without sacrificing accuracy and the ease of interpretation.

5. **Relevance:** The degree to which the criteria established for selecting the item so that they conform to the aims of the measuring instrument.

6. **Equilibrium/Equity:** Achievement of the correct proportion among questions allotted to each of the objectives and teaching content.

7. **Specificity:** The items in a test should be specific to the objectives.

8. **Discrimination:** The basic function of all educational measurement is to place individuals in a defined scale in accordance with differences in their achievements tents. such a function implies a high discriminating power on the part of a test. The quality of a test directly affects its validity. The discriminating power of a test item refers to the degree to which it discriminates between good and bad students in a given group or a variable. This suggests that learners with superior ability should answer the item correctly more often than learners who do not have such ability.

9. **Efficiency:** It ensures the greater possible number of independent answers per unit of time.

10. **Time:** The required time to answer items should be provided to avoid hurry, guessing, taking risks or chances etc.,
11. **Length:** The number of items in the test should depend upon the objectives and content of the topic.
12. **Test usefulness:** Grading or ranking of the student can be possible with items in the test.
13. **Precise and Clear:** Items should be precise and clear so that students can answer well and score marks.
14. **Comprehensiveness:** The total content and objectives has to be kept in mind while preparing items for the test.
15. **Adequacy:** A measuring instrument should be adequate, i.e. balanced and fair. The test should include items, measuring both the objectives and the content. A blueprint will be very useful.
16. **Ease of administrability:** Provision should be made for the preparation, distribution and collection of test materials.
    - Instruction should be simple, clear and concise
    - Practice exercises will be illustrated
    - Illustrations should be clear cut and easily tied up with the appropriate test items.
17. **Ease of scoring:** Simple scoring is good. Algebraic manipulations should not be used to get the scores.
18. **Ease of interpretation:** The raw scores of a test should be easily converted into meaningful derived scores.
19. **Economy:** It should be computed in terms of the validity of the tests per unit of cost. economy refers to the cost as well as the time required for administering and scoring a test.
20. **Comparability:** A test possesses comparability when scores resulting from its use can be interpreted in terms of a common base that has a natural or accepted meaning. comparability of results used for standardized tests are:
    - Availability of:
      - Equivalent (parallel) forms of test
      - Adequate norms.
21. **Utility:** It serves a definite need in the situation in which it is used.

Principles of Evaluation

The principles or guidelines will serve as self-checking devices for the teacher.
- The value of evidence is gained through careful appraisal of teaching-learning process
- Evaluation is a continuous process, the teacher should make a plan of evaluation to cover the entire course
- The objectives should be stated in terms of behavior and content, in which the behavior is to operate
- It determines to what extent the objectives of the course are being met
- Identifying and defining the educational objectives for maximum benefit
- Methods of evaluation should be selected on the basis of purpose to be served for and type of behavior to be measured
- Comprehensive evaluation requires variety of evaluation techniques
- Proper use of evaluation technique requires awareness about limitations as well as their strengths
- The worth or value of teaching method/learning method or the materials of instruction is known until their effect being measured
- Adequacy of experience should be made in terms of excellence of performance and quality of experience
- Records for practice should reflect the objectives of practice and give evidence to the extent of achievement of these objectives.

Purposes of Evaluation

Evaluation occupies an important component in the educational process. It occurs in every aspect of teaching-learning relationship. The teacher must use some form of evaluation when he/she is selecting a course of action.
- Essential for sound educational decision-making
- Attains educational goals and to ascertain the extent to which these goals have been realized

- For an adequate teaching learning situation, evaluation techniques are essential
- Clarifies the aims of education
- Helps in the improvement of the curriculum
- Assists in developing a scientific approach to educational problems
- Appraises the status and changes in learner's behavior
- Discloses learner's needs, possibilities, strengths, weaknesses and to suggest remedial measures for solution of the problem
- Aids learner teacher planning
- Expands the concept of worthwhile goals beyond pure achievement
- Familiarizes the teacher with the nature of Students' learning, development and progress
- Relates measurement to the goals of the instructional program
- It facilitates the selection and improvement of measuring instruments
- It appraises the teacher's/supervisor's competence
- It serves as a method of improvement
- It serves as a guiding principle for the selection of supervisory techniques
- To determine the level of knowledge and understanding of the students in her/his classes at various times
- To determine the level of student's clinical performance at various stages
- To become aware of specific difficulties of individual students
- To encourage students' learning by measuring their achievement and informing them of their success
- To help the students to acquire the possible attitudes, efficient skills and self-direction in their study
- Evaluation provides opportunity to practice critical thinking, the application of principles and making judgments, etc.
- To estimate the effectiveness of teaching learning techniques, instructional media to reach the goals
- To gather the information needed for administration purpose, e.g. formation of standards for selection of students for different courses, promotion, placement of students for advanced studies, meeting graduation requirement
- It serves as a means of improving school and community relation
- Grading of students with the intention of grouping and promoting them
- To determine how far the objectives of teaching in a particular subject are being realized or to see whether the teacher's method and the experiences, which he organizes for children, are fulfilling his expectation and appraisal of learner's attainment is always necessary
- For both formative and summative purposes
- It provides feedback to the staff to enable revisions and refinements to be made to the content and presentation of a course
- It may also be used to assist in the annual review of staff performance.

Functions of Evaluation in an Educational Program

- To provide a basis for the modification of the curriculum, syllabi or courses
- It forms a basis for the introduction of experiences to meet the needs of students
- To motivate learner towards better attainment, growth and development
- To pinpoint areas where remedial measures are needed
- To make provision for guiding the growth of individual learners
- To diagnose the weaknesses and strengths of the program
- To improve instructional activities and educational program
- To test the efficiency of teachers in providing learning experience and effectiveness of instruction and classroom activities
- To achieve educational goals
- It helps to know the rate of progress in different areas of learning
- To bring out the capabilities of a student, e.g. Attitudes, habits, skills, etc.
- To know the rate of progress in different areas of learning

Evaluation and Teacher

- It provides him with knowledge concerning the students' entire behavior
- In setting, refining and clarifying realistic objectives for each student
- In determining, evaluating, refining his instructional techniques or learning activities to improve classroom procedures
- To test the efficiency of teachers in providing learning experiences
- To find out how far educational objectives have been achieved
- To know the efficiency of instructional methods used in the teaching-learning situation
- To diagnose the strengths, weaknesses of students and to classify the gifted, bright and slow learners.
- To provide guidance and counseling services in order to plan remedial measures
- To inform student's progress to parents
- Motivates the teacher to evaluate critically her/his teaching practices and plan cooperatively to work together for the improvement of the curriculum.

Evaluation and Administrator

- To find out whether the school has achieved educational objectives or not
- To bring about various activities in the school
- It is the basis for modification of curriculum
- To introduce appropriate learning experiences.

Evaluation and Students

- Communicating the teacher's objectives. If the students clearly know what the teacher expects from them; they will try to fulfil/realize the objectives directly or indirectly
- Increasing motivation. It motivates the students to learn better and perform effectively; thus, evaluation facilities learning
- Encourages developing good study habits, abilities and skills
- Evaluation summarizes and reports student's progress
- Evaluation provides feedback where the students' strengths and weaknesses will be identified and it serves the purpose of guidance.

Types of Evaluation

Evaluation of education must begin with a clear and meaningful definition of objectives. The teacher's responsibility is to convince the student that his/her education is directed towards wider aims. Evaluation is continuous ongoing process.

R.D. Tennyson in his book, 'Educational Technology' described four basic interactive phases.

Phase-I: Feasibility evaluation.

Phase-II: Formative evaluation or diagnostic evaluation.

Phase-III: Summative evaluation or certifying evaluation.

Phase-IV: Maintenance evaluation.

1. Feasibility evaluation:

This activity occurs concurrently with the instructional development problem analysis phase, teachers and other potential developers should first identify the instructional problems and then provided recommendations concerning the need for developing instructional materials. Documentation of procedures, Sources of data used in the needs assessment should be specified. Educational policies and educational organizations which will help for standardizing the policies, rules and regulations of educational institutions have to be identified.

2. Formative evaluation:

- It provides the student with information on his/her progress or gains
- It must be continuous, it starts with commencement of the program until the time he completes it
- Informs the student about the extent of learning is needed to reach the educational objectives

- Enables learning activities to be adjusted in accordance with progress made or lack of it
- The anonymity of the students has to be maintained by using code of choice
- Is controlled in its use by the student (results should not appear in any official record)
- Useful in guiding the student and prompting him to ask for help
- It is carried out frequently whenever the student or teacher feels it as necessary
- Provides the teacher with qualitative and quantitative data for modification of his/her teaching.

3. Certifying evaluation or summative evaluation

'We do not care how hard the student tried, we do not care how close he got ……….. until he can perform he must not be certified as being able to perform'—*RF Mager.*
- Certifying evaluation is designed to develop competent personnel from practicing
- To place the students in order of merit
- Justifies the decisions as to whether they should move upto the next class or be awarded a degree or diploma
- Carried out less frequently at the end of a unit or period of instruction.

4. Maintenance evaluation

For placing the qualified people in jobs or to select suitable candidates for filling up of the vacancies or promotions. To maintain the level upto the mark or the standards. The maintenance evaluation will be carried out.

5. Evaluation of teaching—Informal evaluation

Self-appraisal

A conscientious teacher would wish to continually appraise his/her performance. This may be done by checking periodically with such questions as:
- Am I achieving the desired goals?
  You may find it useful to use the *Teaching Goals Inventory*
- Do I convey clearly the aims, objectives and demands of the course?
- Do I establish rapport with my students?
- Am I helping my students to learn what they should?
- What other methods/techniques/materials might I use to enhance learning?
- What were the most, and the least, successful features of a particular session?
- An *item bank* providing a much fuller list is provided to facilitate the drawing up of a personalized checklist. It can also be used in designing your own questionnaire to obtain feedback from students.

Student Feedback

This may be obtained by administering a questionnaire, preferably one designed by teacher, herself/himself. Dialogue with students can be highly effective. The discussion should have some structure, be fairly specific and the agenda should include input by students.

Peer Observation and Feedback

Arrangements can be made with a colleague to observe your classroom performance. Feedback may be solicited on the design of the course, course content, planning, presentation and the reaction of the students. If the arrangement is reciprocal, mutual trust and confidence can be developed between colleagues.

Other Sources of Informal Feedback

Some indication may be obtained by
- Noting class attendance, which could indicate the usefulness of sessions to students
- Assessing the atmosphere in the class (e.g. attentiveness of students, noise level, student posture and activity)
- Observing the performance of students in class work, projects and so on.

Evaluation of Teaching: Formal Evaluation:

Performance Appraisal

This is done for appointments, reappointments, promotions and tenure. It includes appraisal of scholarship, teaching and service.

Appraisal of teaching/teacher is based on information from various sources:
- Student feedback
- Peer review of modules taught (e.g. classroom teaching, curriculum design, teaching materials and assessment)
- Teaching portfolio
- Others (e.g. interview with candidate, interview with students, letters from students, alumni and colleagues, candidate's reports on theses supervised, interviews with supervises)
- Teacher appraisal will be done only for promotions and tenure. Peer review of modules will be done every three years as it is required for reappointment and teaching awards.

Student Feedback
- A *common questionnaire* is used across all faculties, though some faculties have appended some additional, discipline specific items. The evaluation is administered at the end of each module and students submit their feedback online. The results are also made available online—Individuals have access to their own results— and are available within a week after all the examination results in the respective faculties have been released. To encourage frank responses, anonymity of the respondents is maintained and the feedback obtained is made available to staff only after the final examinations.

Peer Review
- There will be a comprehensive review which covers the entire spectrum of a teacher's contribution to student learning, including classroom teaching (lectures/tutorial/seminars), curriculum design, printed and electronic teaching materials and assessment tasks (questions/problems for continuous assessment and final examination). Such reviews are necessary for critical administrative decisions (e.g. reappointment, promotion, tenure, teaching awards)
- Copies of peer review reports will be given to the teachers under review as soon as the reports are completed. These reports should be included in the teaching portfolios submitted for tenure, promotion, reappointment and teaching excellence awards
- If a teacher feels that a particular peer review report is unfair or prejudiced, he/she may defend himself/ herself in writing on the negative points raised by the report. The teacher's defense will be an integral part of the teacher appraisal exercise
- As far as possible, at least two reviewers should be assigned to each teacher for a given peer review exercise. Reviewers should be assigned to a teacher on a rotating basis across years
- Wherever possible, the reviewer should have sufficient familiarity with the subject matter of the modules being reviewed
- The reviewer and the candidate being reviewed should not be in competition for the same position.

6. Student Evaluation
Aims
- Conventional role of examinations is to determine the success or failure on the part of the student
- To provide feedback for the student
- To inform upto what level the student is receiving instruction and the extension of his/her achievements
- To make him/her aware of the questions whether he/she has understood or not
- To modify the style of teaching to ensure that what he/she wishes to communicate to the student is correctly understood
- The reputation of the school will be represented by the percentage of the results the institution got
- Selection of students in courses
- Motivates the student to learn
- For modification of learning activities
- Certify whether he/she has succeeded or failed in the due course
- Maintains school public relations
- Protects the society by certifying competency.

Steps

1. The criteria or acceptable level of performance of the educational objectives. The objectives should be stated clearly in measurable terms before any course or program was planned.
2. Defining changes in behavior expected as educational outcomes:
   - The faculty should specify the behaviors that will be used as the basis for assigning grades
   - To determine the student's ability to apply their knowledge to different situation
   - To determine whether the student has an adequate base of knowledge and skills to pass onto the next state of his/her learning
   - The teacher will plan to evaluate systematically the educational objectives, the teaching-learning procedures, the progress of students and the outcomes in each of her/his classes
   - Teacher will involve the students in the total evaluation process in a profitable manner.
3. Describe the situations that give opportunity for the expression of desired behaviors
   When the learning situations has provided, in which the students would be expected to display the desired behavior, so that evidence can be obtained regarding the extent of change in the students' behavior pattern.
4. Development and use of appropriate measuring instruments.
   Standardized impersonal tests should be given to students so that comparisons can be made for individual students. The effects of inconsistencies in problem presentations and teacher bias will be reduced.
5. Interpretation of measurement data by deciding on ways of recording and summarizing the behavior on the basis of evidence collected.
   - Scoring, rating and describing the learning situations
   - Project assignments
   - Case analysis
   - Term papers
   - Rating scales
   - Checking validity, reliability and difficulty of the measures used.
6. Establishing conditions that permit the student to give her/his best performance.
7. Assigning scores to permit achievement of the purposes of evaluation.
8. Determine the students' progress and learning outcomes for assessing effectiveness of the program.
9. Formulation of judgments and taking of appropriate action.

ACHIEVEMENT TEST

Introduction

Achievement test is an important tool in school evaluation and has a great significance in measuring instructional progress and progress of the students in the subject area. Achievement means one's learning attainments, accomplishments, proficiencies, etc. It is directly related to learner's growth and development in educational situations where learning and teaching are intended to and so on.

Definition

'Any test that measures the attainments or accomplishments of an individual after a period of training or learning'—*NM Downie.*
'The type of ability test that describes what a person has learned to do'—*Throndike and Hagen.*
'A systematic procedure for determining the amount a student has learned through instruction'—*Groulund.*

Functions

- It provides basis for promotion to the next grade
- To find out where each student stands in various academic areas
- It helps determination about the placement of the student in a particular section
- To motivate the students before a new assignment has taken up
- To know how effectively the student is performing in the theory as well as the clinical areas
- To expose learner's difficulties which the teacher can help them to solve.

Characteristics of a Good Achievement Test
- It can be tried out and selected on the basis of its difficulty level and discriminating power
- Directly related to educational objectives.
- It should possess description of measure behavior in realistic and practical terms
- Contains a sufficient number of test items for each measured behavior; concerned with important and useful matter; comprehensive brief, precise and clear
- It should be divided into different knowledge and skills according to behaviors to be measured
- Standardized the items and made instruction clear so that different users can utilize it
- Rules and norms have to be developed so that various age groups can use at various levels
- It provides equivalent and comparable forms of the test
- A test manual has to be prepared, which can be act as a guide for administering and scoring.

Steps of Achievement of Test Construction
Step I
- Stating the objectives in terms of achievements be verified
- Spelling out the actions that are necessary for the attainment of objectives
- Spelling out the criteria by which the attainment of objectives to be assessed
- Spelling out the personnel whose judgments are involved in each component of the plan

— Shipman M (1979) School evaluation.

Step II
1. *Determining the purpose of testing:*
   Test may be divided into categories like:
   - Pre-testing: Readiness and placement
   - Testing during placement
     - Formative test
     - Diagnostic test
     - End testing—summative test.
2. *Developing the test specifications:*
   - A list of instructional objectives
   - An outline of the course content
   - A two-way chart.
3. *Selecting appropriate type of questions:*
   A balanced selection of:
   - Essay type
   - Short-answer type
   - Objective type questions.
4. *Preparing relevant test items*
   - Matching the test items with the learning outcome
   - Selecting most representative items
   - Preparing test items
   - Avoiding all possible barriers in test items which prevent examinees from responding
   - Avoid providing any clues to answer which may help examinee to answer correctly even if they lack the necessary achievement.
5. *Assembling the test:*
   After preparing relevant test items, the test constructor has to follow the process.
   - Writing each item on a separate card
   - Reviewing the test items
   - Arranging the test items according to well-defined criteria
   - Providing proper instructions to the examinees.
6. *Administering the test:*
   Suggestions to administer the test
   - Long announcements before or during the test should not be made

- Instructions should be given in writing
- The test administration should not respond to the individual problems of the examinees.

7. *Scoring the test should be done objectively.*
8. *Appraising the test or item analysis.*

Item Analysis/Appraising the Test

The procedure used to judge the quality of an item is called, 'Item analysis.'

To ascertain whether the questions/items do their job effectively. A detailed test and item analysis has to be done before a meaningful and scientific inference about the test can be made in terms of its validity, reliability, objectivity and usability.

A systematic analysis aims at finding the performance of a group.

- The central tendency of marks obtained by them, e.g. Normal/average; positive or negative skewness high or low value
- The variability characterized by standard deviation (SD) indicates the nature of spread of marks, the greater the spread and the greater will be the value of standard deviation
- Coefficient of reliability for the test indicating the degree of consistency with which the test has measured the students' abilities. A high value of this means that the test is reliable and it produces virtually repeatable, scores for the students
- Item analysis is useful in making meaningful interpretations and value judgments about students' performance
- A teacher or paper setter comes to know whether the items had the right level of difficulty and whether there was discrimination between more able and less able students
- Item analysis defines and maintains standard of performance, ensures comparability of standards
- To understand the behavior of items
- To become better item writers, scientific, professional and competent teachers.

Steps

- For each item, count the number of students in each group who answered the item correctly. For alternate response type of items, count the number of students in each group who choose each alternative
- Award of score to each student.

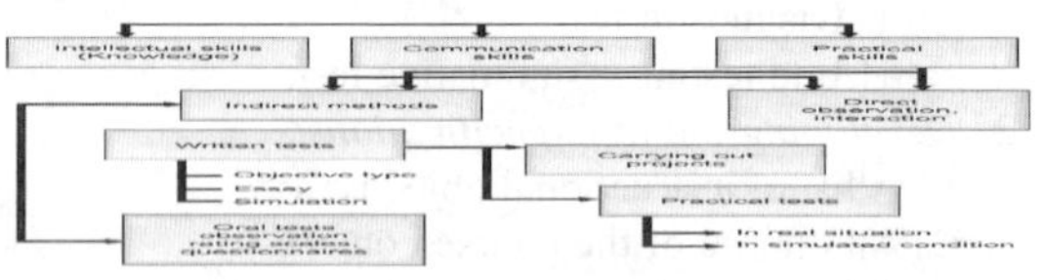

A practical, simple and rapid method is to perforate on your answer sheet the boxes corresponding to the correct answer; placing the perforated sheet on the student's answer sheet the raw score can be found almost automatically.

Ranking in order of merit and identifying high and low groups.

- Arrange the answer sheets from the highest score to the lowest score
- Make two groups, i.e. highest scores in one group; lowest scores in other group or top and bottom halves

Calculation of difficulty index of a question

For each item, compute the percentage of students who get the item correct is called 'item difficulty index.'

1. $D = R/N \times 100$.

   R: Number of learners who answered the item correctly.

   N: Total number of learners who tried them.

   The higher the difficulty index, the easier is the item.

   Difficulty level/facility level of a test; it is an index of how easy or difficult the test is from the point of view of the teachers. The index is a ratio of the average score of a sample of subjects on the test to the maximum possible score on the test. It is usually expressed in percentage.

2. Difficulty level =

$$\frac{\text{Average on the test}}{\text{Maximum possible score}} \times 100$$

3. Difficulty index $= \dfrac{H + L}{N} \times 100$

   H: Number of correct answers to the high group
   L: Number of correct answers to the low group
   N: Total number of students in both groups
4. Find out the facility value of objective tests first
   Facility value $=$

   $$\dfrac{\text{Number of students answering questions correctly.}}{\text{Number of students who have taken the test.}} \times 100$$

   If the facility value is 70 and above, those are easy questions; if it is below 70 the questions are difficult ones.

Estimating Discrimination Index (DI)

The discriminating power (validity index) of an item refers to the degree to which a given item discriminates among students who differ sharply in the functions measured by the test as a whole.

Formula - 1

$$DI = \dfrac{RU - RL}{\frac{1}{2}N.}$$

RU   = Number of correct responses form the upper group.
RL   = Number of correct responses from lower group.
N   = Total number of pupils who tried them.

High discriminate value questions are needed for selection purposes.

Formula - 2

$$DI = \dfrac{\text{No. of HAQ} - \text{LAQ}}{\text{No. of HAG}}$$

No. of HAQ: Number of students in high ability group answering the questions correctly.
No. of LAQ: Number of students in low ability group answering questions correctly.
No. of HAG: Number of students in high ability group.

Using Item Analysis Results

- It helps to judge the worth or quality of a test
- Aids in subsequent test revisions
- Lead to increase skill in test construction
- Provides diagnostic value and help in planning future learning activities
- Provides a basis for discussing test results
- For making decisions about the promotion of students to the next higher grade
- To bring about improvement in teaching methods and techniques
- For making decisions about the promotion of students to the next higher grade
- To bring about improvement in teaching methods and techniques.

Test Construction

Planning the Test

a. Unit plan has to be developed, i.e. teachers' careful analysis of the content and his plan for promoting learner's learning.
   Promotes objective based teaching.
   Brings the relationship between the content objectives, methodology, economizes the time plan.
b. Preparing weightage tables
   To enhance content validity—objective has to be prepared in terms of knowledge, understanding and application oriented, number and usability of concepts.
   By difficulty index face validity can be enhanced.
   Objectivity, reliability, practicability of items has to be maintained.
   Weightage to form of question, i.e. construct validity has to be given, e.g. Essay type questions, short answer questions, objective type questions, etc.

Blue Print

It is a three dimensional chart which has a provision for giving weightage for objectives content and the form of questions. It depicts the true nature and purpose of the test. It describes feasibility of items, guides to select correct questions, helps the students to advance plan for development of study/learning experiences.

Preparing the Test

The teacher has to prepare the test in accordance with the blue print. Arranging the test items in ascending order of difficulty. Prepare instructions for students in writing principles of valuations, fix norms for grading.

Administering the Test

It plays a vital role in enhancing the reliability of the test scores. Test should be administered in a congenial environment strictly as per the instructions planned and assure uniformity of conclusions to all the people tested.

Scoring the Test

The principles of valuation should be followed in scoring the test. It enhances the objectivity and reliability of the test.

Evaluating the Test

Learning activities are "The methods, techniques which the class teacher employs to help pupils to learn the content and realize the objectives." The means of determining the extent to which learning activities have been effective are termed as, 'evaluation procedures or testing.'

The test scores must be evaluated in relation to the objectives and learning experiences planned so that these components may be modified. To evaluate the individual performance and progress his/her score must be compared with peer group scores and his previous scores. It helps to uplift the total pedagogic program.

The Process of Evaluation

a. Identifying and defining general objectives
- Determine what to evaluate—set down educational objectives
- What kind of abilities and skills should be developed when a learner studies.

b. Identifying and defining specific objectives

Learning is a modification of behavior in a desirable direction. The teacher is more concerned with a student's learning. Changes in behavior are an indication of learning. These changes, arising out of classroom instruction are known as the 'learning outcomes.' What type of learning outcome is expected from a student after he/she has undergone the teaching-learning process is the responsibility of the teacher, hence the teacher has to identify and define the objectives in terms of behavior changes, i.e. learning outcomes.

The specific objectives will provide direction to teaching-learning process. It is useful in planning and organizing the learning activities and in planning and organizing evaluation procedures.

The specific objectives determine two things:
1. The various types of learning situations to be provided by the class teacher to group of learners.
2. The method to be employed to evaluate both the objectives and the learning experiences.

c. Selecting teaching points

Through teaching points objectives can be realized. After setting up of educational objectives, the content has to be decided.

d. Planning suitable learning activities

The teacher has to coordinate objectives, teaching points and learning activities. The learning activities have to realize the objectives and help him to determine the evaluation procedures to be used in future.

e. Evaluating

The teacher observes and measures the changes in the behavior of learners through testing. While testing, the teacher has to keep in mind the objectives, learning activities and learning outcomes. Select appropriate evaluative device and administer.

f. Using the results as feedback

The results will act as feedback, the teacher observes the results and plans appropriate modality/learning activity to consider, reorganize and to achieve the objectives. He/she will retrace his/her steps to find out the drawbacks in the objectives or in the learning activities he/she has provided for his/her students. This is known as "feedback". Whatever results the teacher gets after testing learners should be utilized for the betterment of the students.

Evaluation Tools

Evaluation of the student is a continuous ongoing process. It is necessary to consider the major objectives or purposes of any course in order to set up the testing program. In planning and preparing any examination, the teacher must make adequate provision for considering all the important outcomes of his/her instruction. There are different ways, which have devised for measuring the learning abilities of students.

Methods of Evaluation

The methods of evaluation used in nursing education related to the assessment of:
1. Knowledge
2. Attitude
3. Skills.

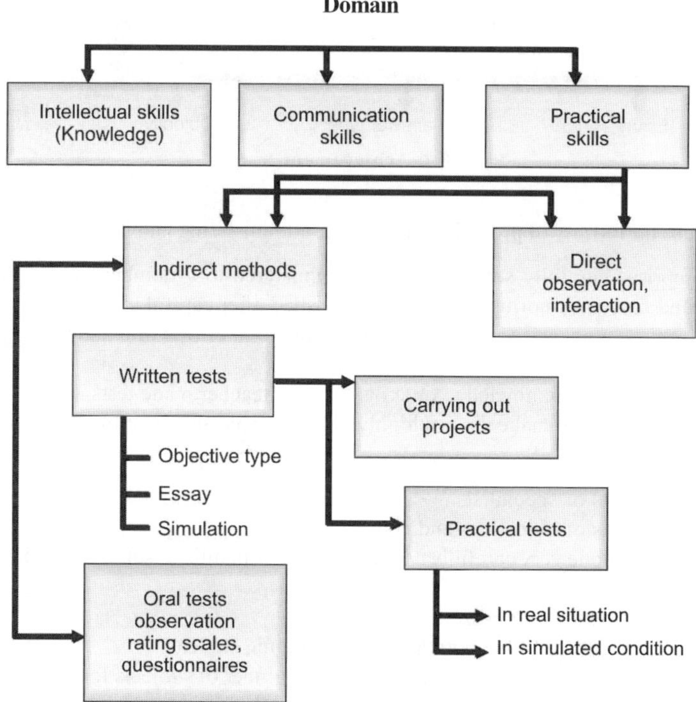

Fig. 8.3: Methods of evaluation

Evaluation methodology according to domains to be evaluated

The methods use for assessment of knowledge are:
a. Subjective type: Essay type (Descriptive-Narrative type, comparison, amplification, precise-writing, short-notes.)
b. Objective type: Multiple choice type, matching type, true - false, fill in the blanks, sentence completions, etc.
c. Problem-solving type, situational, analysis.

Methods of assessing attitude

Interview, Assignments, Cumulative records, Assessing documentation, Anecdotal records, Observation during performance, Attitude scales, Critical incident technique and Discussion, etc.

Tools to assess Skills

Performance appraisal, Rating scale, Observation checklist, Anecdotal record; Cumulative record; Critical incident technique.

Cognitive Tests

To assess the intellectual levels of students, cognitive tests will be performed, e.g. Written examinations—Theory, Practical Examinations, Viva or Orals.

Educational test or Achievement Tests

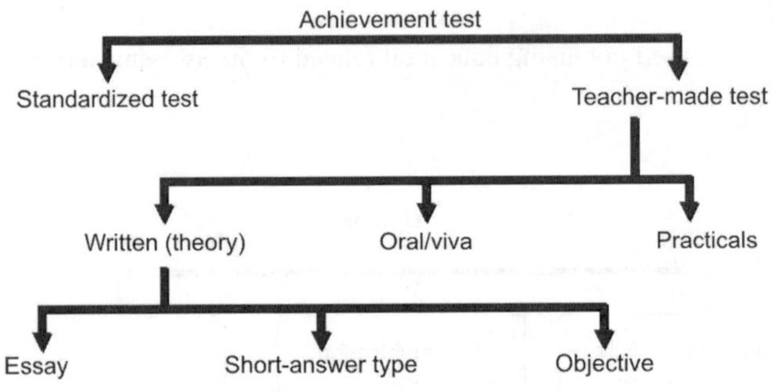

Fig. 8.4: Achievement tests

Standardized Tests

'Standardization means uniformity of procedure in scoring, administering and interpreting the results.'

'The tests which comprises carefully selected items, administered to a number of sample or group under standard conditions and for which norms have been established after careful evaluation.'

- It is produced by some test agency and is the product of the joint efforts of a number of persons including test experts
- It deals with larger segments of knowledge or skills than the teacher made tests
- Every possible effort is made to make the test highly valid, reliable and discriminating.

Characteristics

- Constructed by test experts or specialists
- Covers broad or wide areas of objectives and content
- Selection of items will be done very carefully and the validity, reliability, usefulness of the test is ascertained in a systematic way
- Procedure of administration is standardized
- Test has clear directions and it will be motivating, encouraging students
- Before finalization, test is tried out and administered on a number of subjects for the expressed purpose of refining its items
- Scoring key is provided
- Test manual provides norms for the test.

Teacher-made Test

These are very useful in evaluating the student's progress report to parents and administrators.

Uses

- To know the ability and achievements of students
- Helps the teacher to assess the strengths and weaknesses of student
- Motivates the students
- Provides continuous evaluation and feedback to the teacher
- Helps to achieve particular objectives
- Helps the teacher to adopt better instructional methods.

Limitations
- Tests are often ambiguous and unclear
- They are either too short or too lengthy
- Tests do not cover the entire content
- Tests are usually hurriedly conducted
- Supervision is not proper
- Lot of scope for copying
- Conducted as rituals only
- Answer books not marked with care.

Qualitative Techniques

a. Observational techniques: For example, Charts, Checklists, Rating Scales, Anecdotal Records.
b. Sociometric techniques: For example, Peer Appraisal, Nominating technique (Sociogram, Social distance scales)
c. Self-report techniques: For example, Interview, Inventories or Questionnaires, Attitude scales.
d. Projective techniques: For example, Sentence Completion, Doll play, Perception of inkblots, Interpretation of pictures.

Essay type examinations or Essay Test

'An essay test presents one or more questions or other tasks that require extended written responses from the persons being tested' —*Robert LE and David AF.*

'It is a test containing questions requiring the student to respond in writing. It emphasize recall rather than recognition of the correct alternative'—*Gilert Sax.*

'It requires the student to structure a long written response up to several paragraphs'—*William W and Stephen GJ.*

In essay type question, the student prepares her/his own answers. It evaluates the knowledge areas alone. Handwriting, spelling, neatness, organization, ways of expressing ideas may be considered in scoring the items.

The element of subjectivity can be reduced by careful preparation of the questions for the selected content areas to be tested in advance.

Features
- No single answer can be considered throughout and correct
- The examinee is permitted freedom of response
- The answers vary in their degree of equality or corrections.

Types
Based on the amount of freedom given to a student to organize his ideas and write his answer. The essay questions are divided into two types.
1. Extended response
2. Restricted response

Extended Response
- No restriction is placed on the student as to the points he/she will discuss and the type of organisation he/she will use
- Most important, pertinent and relevant material whatever he/she wishes can be used. This type of question permits a student to demonstrate his ability to
- Recall and evaluate factual knowledge
- Organize his ideas in a logical, coherent fashion.

Restricted Responses
Student will have less scope, limited nature in the form because he/she is told specifically the context in which his/her answer has to be made.

Principles for Preparing Essay Type Test
- Do not give too many lengthy questions
- Avoid phrases, e.g. 'Discuss briefly'
- Questions should be well-structured with specific purpose or topic at a time
- Words should be simple, clear, unambiguous and carefully selected
- Do not allow too many choices
- According to the level of students' difficulty and complexity items has to be selected.

Scoring Problem
- For every question, set out the elements which according to you, should appear in the answer by point scoring system
- Score the answers of all students for one question, before going on to the scoring of another question
- When two or more teachers correct the same test, they should agree on the scoring procedure before the test and correct the answer scripts
- The time allowed and the marks allotted will act as a guide to the students to answer the questions.

Advantages
- Tests the ability to communicate in writing, depth of knowledge and understanding
- The student can have free to communicate her/his ability for independent thinking
- The student can demonstrate her/his ability to organize ideas and express them effectively in a logical and coherent fashion
- It requires short-time for the teacher to prepare the test and administer
- It can be successfully employed for all the school subjects.

The Abilities like
- Organises ideas express them effectively
- Criticizes or justifies the statement
- Interpretation of ideas, thoughts etc., will be more clearly put into writing and freedom for the student to write, whatever he/she wants to respond
- The mental processes like logical thinking, critical reasoning, systematic presentation can be best developed
- Induces good study habits like making outlines, summaries, organizing the arguments for and against, etc.
- The students can show their initiative, originality of their thought and imagination, as they are permitted freedom of response
- The responses of the students need not be completely right or wrong
- Eliminates guessing.

Disadvantages
- Lack objectivity
- Provide little useful feedback
- Takes long-time to score
- Limited content sampling
- Subjectivity of scoring
  Essay type possesses relatively low validity and reliability because of the factors like contaminated by extraneous factors like spelling, good hand writing, colored writing, neatness, grammar and length of the answer.
- Biased judgment by previous impressions
- Good verbal ability even in the absence of relevant points
- Mood of examiners
- First impression
- Improper comparison of answer, of different students (Bright and dull)
- Ambiguous wording of questions may be misinterpreted results in guessing and bluffing on the part of the students
- Laborious process both for corrector and for the student
- Only competent teachers can assess it
- Scoring costs.

Short Open Answer Type Tests (Restricted Response Tests)

The student responds by selection of one or more of several given alternatives by giving or filling in a word or phrase. It does not call for an extensive written response. Questions should be drafted in such a way that, the answer calls for a predetermined and precise concept. The answer is expected in short and can be expressed in different forms. Ideally, only one answer is acceptable.

Principles for Preparing Short type Item
- Use action oriented precise verbs
- Each item should deal with important content area
- Question can be as long as possible, but answer should be short
- Use precise, simple and accurate language in relation to the subject matter area
- Provide the necessary space for answers below each question asked.

Advantages
- Easy to score, reliability of the score is improved, quick response

Disadvantages
- Difficulty in construction of reliable items.

Objective Type Tests

To seek more objective measurement of teaching-learning results. A set of standardized stimuli that elicit samples of behavior. These tests can be used to measure rating modern, application of principles and different abilities as well as actual knowledge depending on the way they are prepared. It refers to "any written test that requires the examinee to select the correct answer from among one or more of several alternatives or supply a word or two and that demands on objective judgment when it is scored."

When questions are framed with reference to the objectives of instruction, the test becomes objective centered test. If it is objectively scored, it is called as objective type test item.

The system of scoring is objective and it will not vary from examiner to examiner.

Forms of Objective Type tests

1. Teacher Made Tests
a. Recall type—Simple recall; Sentence completion items.
b. Recognition type—Multiple choice type; Matching; Alternative response (True or false).
c. Others—Rearrangement; Analogy; Identification; Context—dependent type (Pictorial form, Interpretative).

Merits of Objective Type
- Easy for scoring
- Objectivity in scoring
- It will not vary from time to time or from examiner to examiner
- More extensive and representative sampling can be obtained
- It reduces the role of luck or cramming of expected questions
- Greater reliability and better content validity
- Economy of time; takes less time saves a lot of time for scoring
- It eliminates extraneous factors, e.g. Speed of writing, fluency of expression, neatness, literacy style etc.
- It measures the higher mental processes of understanding, application, analysis, prediction and interpretation.

Disadvantages
- Takes a lot of time and effort in preparing the test
- Provides little or no opportunity for measurement of students' ability to organize and to express thoughts.

Limitations
- Ability to organize matter, Ability to provide matter logically coherent fashion cannot be evaluated
- Guessing is possible
- The construction of items is difficult, requires special abilities and is time consuming
- Printing cost is high.

2. Multiple Choice Items

These are the most flexible and most effective of objective type test items and consists of two parts.
- The stem—which presents the problem, presented in the form of an incomplete statement or a question
- The options or responses—the list of possible/correct answers/possible distractors.

Directions for preparation of multiple-choice items
- Have enough content in the stem with less distracters
- Avoid lengthy stem
- Use positive statement in the stem. If negative statement has to be used then underline it or write in capital letters, so that it will not be overlooked
- Stem consists of complete statement, not just a single word
- Place all common elements in the stem to add up simplicity and compactness to the item
- The stem of one should not suggest the answer to another
- Eliminate all unrelated details from an item
- Use plausible or logical distractors
- Avoid the use of clues that may suggest correct answer
- Be sure that the distractors and the correct response possess homogeneity, i.e. they should be fairly similar in content or in the total number of words
- Be cautious of the use of 'none of the above' as a distractor or as a correct answer
- If it is impossible to obtain more than three plausible responses, do not waste time trying to invent some others
- When dealing with items that have numerical answers, arrange them in order in a sequential manner
- Arrange the place for the correct answer, in such a way that, for the test as a whole, no letter corresponding to a given answer appears more frequently than some other letter.

Advantages
- Ensure objectivity, reliability and validity
- Provides constructive criticism
- The range and variety of facts can be sampled in a given time
- Provide precise and unambiguous measurement of the higher intellectual processes
- Provide detailed feedback for both students and teachers
- Easy and rapid to score.

Disadvantages
- Takes a longtime to construct items in order to avoid arbitrary and ambiguous questions
- Careful preparation is required to avoid questions testing only recall
- Provide cues that do not exist in practice
- Expensive, when the group is small to respond.

Variations of the Multiple-Choice Format

One correct answer

Simplest type. The student is required to select the one correct answer listed among several plausible, but incorrect options.

Best answer

The student is told to select the best answer.

Analogy type

The student is required to deduce the relationship that exists between the first two parts of the item and then apply it to the third and fourth parts. Usually the third part is given and the missing fourth part is selected from the list of options on the basis of the relationship existing between the first two parts.

For example: Lack of iron content: Anemia, Lack of iodine content: …………
a) Cretinism, b) Myxoedema, c) Goitre.

Reserve type/Negative variety of multiple choice item
All but one of the responses is correct. The student is asked to select the incorrect response. This method is not recommended, unless it is a must.

Limitations of multiple-choice items
- Difficult to construct
- Requires more skill and more time to prepare
- Teachers cannot always think of plausible distractors
- Tendency for teachers to write multiple choice items demanding only factual recall
- Requires more time for students to respond to
- Not well-adapted for measuring the ability to organize and present ideas
- Require more space per item.

3. The Alternate-response Items
It is essentially a two-response item in which only one of the answers is presented and the student judges the truth or falsity of the statement.
Types: True/false; Yes/no; Right/wrong; Cluster variety; Correction variety.

True/False items
Question or declarative statements followed by yes/no or true/false.
- The student is asked to tick mark the correct response
- Easy to prepare, takes comparatively much less time when compared to matching type or multiple choice.

Directions for preparation of true or false items:
- Give single idea clear and direct in the statement
- Avoid ambiguous statements
- Avoid using clues like: Usually; No; Sometimes; Should; None; Always; Nothing; May, etc.
- Avoid 'trick' and 'catch' items
- Have equal number of 'true' and 'false' items
- Determine the order of 'true' 'false' by chance.

Right/wrong Variety
Some pairs of words will be given, if two words have opposite meanings, write an 'R' in the blank, and if not, write 'W'.

Cluster Variety
One incomplete statement with several suggested answers to be judged as true or false. It permits the item - writer to ask many questions using a single stem and thereby conserving space and reading time.

The Context - dependent Items
Items are based on an external source that may be pictorial or verbal. If the teacher interested in learning whether his/her students can read and interpret a graph or a table. The learner has to use it as his frame of reference to answer items based on this external material.

a. Objective test item based on pictorial materials
The pictorial form is a medium used to present the material to the examinee.
- Useful to young children or those having reading difficulties
- To count, to measure and to discriminate pictorial material is an excellent medium
- For measuring some of the more complex skills, e.g. Reading graphs or table or using an index pictorial material is ideally suited
- When picture is equal to use many hundreds of words, then using pictorial form is best.

b. Interpretative test
It consists of
- Introductory statement

- Pictorial material
- Series of questions that measure in part the students' ability to interpret the material etc.

Uses
1. The structuring of the problem assists both examiner and examinee.
2. Measurement of understanding, interpretation and evaluation can be done.
3. Complex material can be measured with a series of different items based upon a single introductory passage, graph or chart.
4. Minimizes the influence of irrelevant factual material.
5. Can demonstrate thinking and problem-solving skills.

Limitations
- If they are based on a paragraph, they make a heavy demand on a student's reading skills
- Difficult to prepare
- More time required for administration
- Selecting appropriate interpretative material is somewhat difficult.

Advantages of Alternate Response Items
- Good for young children with poor reading habits
- They can cover a large portion of the subject matter in a relatively short space and short period of time
- Provide high reliability per unit of testing time
- Can be scored quickly, reliably and objectively
- Suitable to test beliefs, misconceptions, superstitions
- Adaptable to most content areas
- More easily constructed than other objective type items
- Directions are easily understood
- Time-saver
- Conveniently used to measure the ability
- To identify the correctness of statements
- To distinguish fact from opinion
- To recognise the cause and effect relationship
- It carefully constructed, they can measure the higher mental processes of understanding comprehension, application and interpretation.

Limitations
- Undue influence by good or poor understanding or luck in guessing
- More susceptible to ambiguity, misinterpretation, therefore low reliability
- Lend them most easily to cheating
- Tend to be less discriminating.

4. Matching Type Item
These items form a special form, prepared in two columns. One set is called the 'response column' and the other is called 'stimulus column' the items have to be matched. The examinee is required to make some sort of association between each premise response. He pairs the corresponding elements and records his answers.

Directions for preparation of Matching Type Items
- The matching items should be of same kind in nature
- The number of choices should be more than the required answer, e.g. 7 choices for 5 answers; 14 choices for 10 answers
- Number of items should be short
- Keep the stimuli and response columns on the same page
- Give some heading to both the column like 'A' or 'B'
- Items in one of the two columns may be listed in some logical order, but the item in the other must have a random sequence, so that item position does not give a clue to that which it matches

- Clear cut directions should be given regarding columns to be matched, how the response is to be written, e.g. in words, letters or numbers
- An answer choice may be used more than once.

Advantages
- It should be used only when the teacher is constructing multiple-choice items and discovers that there are several such items having the same alternatives
- Used if the teacher is interested in testing the knowledge of terms, definitions, dates, events and other matters involving simple relationships, etc.
- Used to determine whether a learner can discriminate among nouns, verbs, adjectives, adverbs, etc.
- They require little reading time, many questions can be asked in a limited period of testing time
- Provides an opportunity to have a large sampling of the content, which ultimately increases the reliability of the test
- Amenable to machine scoring or even with hand-scoring, they can be scored more easily than the essay or short-answer test
- Can be constructed easily and quickly
- Space can be saved
- Less opportunity for guessing because all the responses are plausible distractors for each premise.

Limitations
- If sufficient care is not taken in their preparation, they may encourage serial memorization rather than association
- It is sometimes difficult to get clusters of questions that are sufficiently alike so that a common set of responses can be used
- Items are likely to include irrelevant clues to the correct answer
- They cannot be successfully used to measure understanding or the ability to discriminate due to the difficulty of finding homogeneous responses that are answers to a certain premise and that are, for other premises; distractors requiring careful thought before rejection.

5. Problem-situation Test

It describes the situations followed by possible solutions or conclusions and a series of plausible reasons supporting these solutions are given. The student by applying various principles and basic concepts is expected to select the best solutions to the problem, gives reasons to substantiate her/his choice of a solution. The problem is so constructed, the solution and the supporting reasons can be indicated by the student quickly and easily with minimum amount of writing.

Advantages
- Used to represent those patterns of behavior that constitute nursing competence
- Specification of acceptable level of competence
- Less time consuming for the student to answer
- Useful to determine ability to apply principles to new or relate situations.

Disadvantages
- Time consuming to prepare
- Requires greater skills to prepare valid, reliable problem situations
- Require more space than other objective type.

6. Oral Examinations

An examination consisting of a dialogue where the examiner asks questions and the candidate will reply.
- Short open answers based on educational objectives
- MCQ
- A series of questions not necessarily interrelated questions.

This type exam suffers from a scarcity of examiners who are really capable of making the best use of it in practice.

Aims
1. To assess student's ability to communicate orally with another person.
2. To use simulation methods, e.g. Role-play, Telephone conversation.
3. To improve student's memory, vocabulary skills, understanding and comprehension of subject.

Advantages
- Provides direct personal contact with the candidates
- Provides opportunity to take mitigating circumstances into account
- Provides flexibility in moving from candidates' strong points to weak points
- The candidate has to formulate his own replies without cues
- Possibility to question the student, how he arrived at an answer
- Opportunity for simultaneous assessment by two or more examiners.

Disadvantages
- Lacks standardization, objectivity and reproducibility of results
- Permits favouritism and possible abuse of the personal contact
- Suffer from undue influence of irrelevant factors
- Shortage of trained examiners to administer the examination
- Costly in terms of professional time and limited time to get in depth of/value of the information.

7. Practical Examination

To develop appropriate professional skills over a period of time with consistent practice. Transportation facilities should be provided to take the students to the place of examination.

Purposes
The practical examination should be conducted in actual fields, i.e. hospital, clinic and health centers associated with parent school of nursing. To assess
- The ability of student to give care in a practical situation
- The attitude of the student towards client
- Able to meet the needs of the client and work along with others
- Expertise in practicing nursing techniques
- Ability to give the best nursing care possible according to the facilities available in the field
- Ability to give need based health education
- Documentation Skills (recording and reporting)

Physical Arrangements for conduct of examination
- College faculty has to meet hospital Superintendent and ward in-charges or medical officers, subcenters in community facility and obtain Written permission to conduct the examination in the hospital. Faculty along with the cooperation of clinical staff will select and arrange the center for examination
- Examination centers should be selected in advance based on learners' requirement depending upon the specialities offered
- The varieties of nursing care situations, adequacy of facilities of equipment and supplies, place for examiners and other factors should be kept in mind while selecting the place of examination
- To implement nursing procedures required equipment has to be kept ready
- The examiners both internal and external has to be assisted by junior faculty in conduction of practical examination.

Procedure
- Examiner has to arrive one day prior to the examination, to visit the clinical area selected, held discussions with the Administrator and coexaminer along with other school faculty and the clinical staff to assess nursing care situations available
- Examiners must prepare a written plan of the assignments, areas they plan to give to the students
- General plan for examining and grading the students should be discussed among the examiners
- They will allow the students to do systematized care based on nursing process

- Each examiner will examine 10 to 15 students per day
- Evaluate the performance of the student in a practical situation and the procedure of carrying out the assignments
- The teacher has to give assignments in writing by lottery method
- The examiners has to provide conducive environment for the students to perform care in nursing situations
- Examiner has to allot case, prior to that she/he has to prepare list of clients along with diagnosis in single chits, allotting the clients by lottery method; 30 to 45 minutes will be given for each student to collect the history of client and to assess and diagnose the problems of the client and intervene specific nursing activities to meet their needs by applying the principles of nursing process
- Examiner should test the student's knowledge of the principles underlying the nursing care carried out for the patient
- All aspects of total client care should be considered for total evaluation
- Examiners make sure that the students should have their register number, admission cards, hall tickets, and necessary files, cumulative record with them
- Examiners will observe the care given by the students and educational activities carried out by them; depending upon convenience either bedside viva or separate viva will be conducted.

Advantages
- Provides the opportunity to test all the senses in a realistic situation
- Possibility of performance evaluation in clinical situation
- Tests for investigate abilities, apply ready-made recipes
- Attitudes of the students can be observed and tested including the responsiveness to a complex situation.
- Rapport will be established
- Provide opportunity to observe and test attitudes and responsiveness to a complex situation
- Provide opportunity to test the ability to communicate under pressure and to arrange the data in a final form.

Disadvantages
- Lacks standardized conditions in bedside examinations/providing care/doing a procedure with patients of varying degrees of cooperativeness
- Lacks objectivity and suffers from irrelevant factors
- Limited feasibility for large groups
- Difficulties in arranging for examiners to observe candidates demonstrating the skills to be tested
- Emergencies in the wards may act as hindrances
- Takes longer time to complete the examination for the entire group
- Unavailability of required cases with specific diagnosis
- In community many of houses will be locked after 8 am, as elders in family go for work, some times it is very difficult to identify the needs of family by collecting history as health professionals are unable to meet the elders in home, if practical exam is conducted after 10 am in community
- Non cooperation of community some times.

Assessment Techniques of Affective and Psychomotor Domain
Scaling Techniques
In social research, scaling techniques are used to measure the attitude and behavior. One can make judgment about some characteristic of an individual and place him/her on a scale which is measuring for that characteristic.

Definition
"A scale is a continuum from the highest to the lowest points and has intermediate points in between these two extremes. The scale points are related that the first point indicates a higher position than the second, the second point is higher than the third point and so on."

The scaling technique consists of questionnaires where the score of individual's responses gives him/her a particular place on the scale.

Factors Influenced Scaling Phenomenon
The factors are logically interrelated and should be capable of continued measurement.

1. Reliability of the Scale

The methods used to test the reliability of the scale.

a. *Test Retest method:* The same scale can be applied twice to the same population to achieve the same objectives and if the two results are similar. The scale is regarded as reliable. The test can be done on two similar groups also.

b. *Multiple form:* The same population is subjected to 2 or more types of scales will be administered, in case the results are more or less similar, the scales may be regarded as reliable.

c. *Split-half method:* The scale may be divided into two equal parts. Each part is taken as a complete scale and measurement is made separately. The correlation between the two scores is obtained. If the degree of correlation is high, the scale may be regarded as reliable.

2. Validity of Scale

a. *Logical validity:* The scale must conform to common sense, reasoning, and therefore is partly subjective.

b. *Known groups:* The scale is applied to the known category of people, the result obtained is compared with the known facts. If they are similar, the scale is considered to be valid.

c. *Opinion of jury:* The opinion of many jurists who will not have bias will be considered, if several jurists are of same opinion then it will be valid.

d. *Independent methods:* Independent criteria will be used to measure a thing and if the results are similar, the scale is said to be valid.

Uses

- To utilize simultaneously a number of observations on a respondent
- Meaningful responses are logically arranged in the analysis of attitude and behavior.

Difficulties in Scaling

- To assess directly the validity, it is not possible
- Since human behavior is flexible, heterogeneous, unpredictable and variable, a scale can be applied to a particular group only and often there is a dichotomy between the expressed attitude and overt action
- Social phenomena are complex and qualitative in nature
- No universal recognized measuring rod
- The intangibility of social phenomena is an obstacle to scale construction
- The social phenomena cannot be experimented in a controlled way.
  Thus, the scale cannot measure all the causative variables involved.

Types

Nominal Scale

Simple method: It consists of 2 or more named categories into objects, individuals, responses are classified. It is possible to distinguish 2 or more categories relating to the specified attribute, e.g. classification of individuals according to religion.

Ordinal Scale

The order of position will be measured. The numbers are assigned to indicate only the relative position. The ranks will be given to the individual along the specified continuum. It does not measure the distance between the positions, e.g. 'X' is regarded as more beautiful than 'Y'; 'X' is greater than 'Y'; but he cannot say by how much.

Interval (Cardinal) Scale

It has equal units of measurement. Thus, it is possible to interpret not only the order of scale scores, but also the distance between them.

Ratio Scale

One can compare both differences in score and the relative magnitude of score. It incorporates the properties of an interval scale together with a fixed origin or zero point, e.g. time, length and weight.

Rating Scales (Directed Observation)

Rating is the assessment of a persoadann by another person.

Definition

'Rating is a term applied to expression of opinion or judgment regarding some situation, object or character. Opinions are usually expressed on a scale of values'—*Barr and others.*

'Rating techniques are devices by which judgments may be qualified. A rating scale is "a device by which the opinion concerning a trait can be systematized.'

Rating scale records how much or how well it happened. Quantitative and qualitative terms will be used, e.g.

1. How good was the performance?

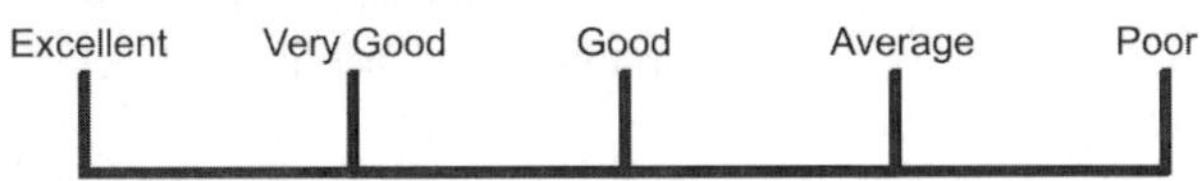

2. How many times you will discuss with your friend to take decisions?

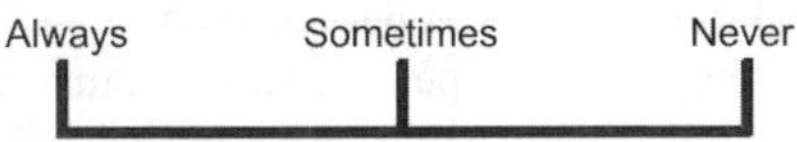

Assuming numerical positions to individuals so that variations in degree may be ascertained. In preparing rating scale, the rater places the individual at a particular point along a continuum, a numerical value is attached to the point. 'It is a characteristic that can occur in varying degrees; the instrument is so designed as to facilitate appraisal of a number of traits or characteristics by reference to a common qualitative scale of values.'

Types

1. **Descriptive rating scale:** Provide for each trait a list of descriptive phrases from which the rater selects the one most applicable item being rated, selected usually by means of a check mark.
2. **Numerical rating scale:** (Specific rating scale/Specific category scale/itemized rating scale).
   The rater assigns a code number and approximate number to each trait of the person being rated or to the descriptive phases. Arranged in order of the degree, level, intensity or frequency with which they indicate possession or lack of occurrence of each trait. The number of specifications depends on the nature of research problem.
3. **Graphic rating scale:** Descriptive phrases closely correspond to the numerical points on the scale printed horizontally at various points from the lowest to the highest. The rater indicates the performer's standing in respect to each trait by placing a check mark at an appropriate point along the line. Here, the degree of each characteristic is arranged so that the rater can make as fine distinctions as he/she wishes to make. This will help the rater to indicate his/her own preference. It ensures fineness of scoring. By this scale, one can avoid vague, unlikely and extreme statements.
4. **Comparative rating scale:** The rater has clear knowledge of the activities of the given groups or individuals. The positions on the rating scale are explicitly defined in terms of a given population or group or in terms of people with known characteristics. The rater may be asked to specify the comparative ability of a teacher with reference to the teaching in a college.

Uses

To evaluate skills, product outcomes, activities, interests, attitudes and personal characteristics.

Advantages

- Easy to administer and to score
- Can be used for a large group of students
- Wide range of application
- Clarity of feedback to students.

Disadvantage

Misuse can result in a consequent decrease in objectivity.

Qualities

Clarity, Variety, Simple, Relevance, Objectivity, Useful, Precision and Uniqueness.

Principles for Preparing Rating Scales

- It directly relates to learning objectives
- Needs to be confined to performance areas that can be observed
- Clearly define the specific trait or mode of behavior
- The trait or behavior should be readily observable, it should be observed in number of situations
- Allow some space in the rating scale card for the rater to give supplementary remarks
- 3 to 7 rating positions may need to be provided
- There should be provision to omit items, the teacher feels unqualified to judge
- Pooled ratings from more than one observer's participation in instrument development will make the scale more objective, clear, valid and reliable
- All raters should be oriented to the specific scale as well as the process of rating in general
- The rater should be unbiased and trained
- Consider evaluation setting, feedback and student participation
- All raters should be aware that rating scales are open to errors resulting to subjective judgments required of the observers. Errors may be due to leniency, contrast error and halo effect etc.
- Have expert and well-informed raters
- Change the ends of the scale, so that the 'good' is not always at the top or always at the bottom
- Assure the rater that his/her anonymity will be maintained.

Limitations for Rating Scales

- It is difficult or dangerous to fix up rating about many aspects of an individual
- Halo effect in the judgment may take place
- Chances like the rater may over estimate the qualities of a known person and underestimate those of unknown persons
- The rater does not want to make extreme judgment, chances of subjective evaluation; thus the scales may become unscientific and unreliable.

Rank Order Scale

- It is a method of comparative and relative rating
- The rater is required to rank the individuals in relation to one has to another from highest to lowest
- Self-rating also can be done, useful in measuring the attitudes like intensity, importance, liking and so on.

1. Paired Comparison

Two stimuli are presented before the judges, out of which the better one has to be selected. The continuum is properly defined. It is rough and simple method, e.g. Jobs suitable for ladies can be determined. The scale value also can be assessed by the number of preferences of all persons for a particular trait is added and is divided by the number of people who are giving the preferences. The scale values explained numerically.

2. Horowitz Method

Individual preferences and attitudes can be measured, e.g. it is applied a ranking scale for testing racial prejudices. Pictures of blue, green and red colors will be taken and given to the students and were asked to indicate their preferences.

Attitude Scales

- These are used for measuring the social attitudes
- Questionnaire is prepared, by the items in the questionnaire are the attitudes of an individual towards a matter thing and object or system and score will be allotted for each item
- We will ask the individual to express his/her response towards an object or system, on the basis of his/her responses, he/she is assigned a score which indicates the position
- Some relevant and indirect statements will also be used to reveal the attitude
- The scale also specifies the crucial shades of opinions.

Types

1. Point Scale

Method—1
- Select the words which will give the opinion
- The respondent is to cross out every word, i.e. more annoying than pleasing to him/her
- The attitude of a respondent is known by calculating the numbers of words crossed or not crossed. The words selected should be suggestive of an attitude and the opposite words should also be given at the same time
- One point is given to each agreement or disagreement whichever has to be chosen

Difficulties in this method
- The words may not be dichotomous in nature
- The neutral or confused opinions cannot be represented
- Adequate number of words expressing the same attitude may not be found.

Method—2
Two sets of words indicating both favorable and unfavorable opinions are given. The unfavorable items may be crossed and favorable items may be left unscored.

2. Differential Scale (LL Thurstone scale)
These scales are used to measure the social phenomenon. The researcher will collect varied number of statements related to attitudes. Judges will determine the positions on the scale. The position is determined by the method of equal appearing intervals. Judges will work independently to classify these statements into 11 groups.
1st group—Unfavurable statements to the specified issue (score—11)
2nd group—The next unfavorable statements and so on.
11th group—Favorable statements (score—1)
6th group—The point at which the attitude is neutral.

The scale value of a statement is computed as the 'mean' or 'median' position to which it is assigned by the judges.
- Avoid ambiguous, vague and irrelevant statements
- The evaluated statements that spread out evenly from one extreme to the other.

At the same time of administration of the scale questionnaire, the respondents are asked to check the statements with which they agree. The scale values are not shown in the questionnaire and the statements are arranged randomly. The mean or median of the scale values of the items are checked by respondent indicates his/her position in the scale. A series of statements whose positions have been determined neutrally by the judges. The scattered responses of an individual imply that the respondent has no definite and organized attitude towards the phenomenon.

3. Summated (Likert) Scale
To measure the social attitude Likert type scale is used. It uses only the definitely favorable and unfavorable statements. It excludes intermediate opinions. It consists of a series of statements to which the respondent is to react. The respondent indicates the degree of agreement or disagreement. Each response is given a numerical score and the total score of a respondent is found out by summing up his different scores for different purposes. This total score indicates his position on the continuum.

The Likert scale uses several degrees of agreement or disagreement, e.g. strongly approve, approve, undecided, disapprove, strongly disapprove. These five points will constitute the scale. Each point of the scale carries a score. "Strongly approve" is given the highest score (5 or +2) and " Strongly disapprove" is given the least score (1 or −2). Other points will have the scores accordingly (i.e., 5,4,3,2 and 1).

For example: Statement 1: Prohibition of alcohol should be made compulsory.

1	2	3	4	5
Strongly Approve	Approve	Undecided	Disapprove	Strongly Disapprove
(5 or +2)	(4 or +1)	(3 or 0)	(2 or −1)	(1 or −2)

The Method of Construction of a Likert Type Scale
- The researcher gathers a large number of statements which clearly indicate favorable or unfavorable attitude towards the issue in question
- The questionnaires consisting of the above five points with respect to a statement are administered to the respondents who indicate their responses
- The responses will imply various scores. The scores are consistently arranged either from the highest to the lowest, or from the lowest to the highest
- By adding up the different scores of an individual, the total score is calculated (i.e., summation of different scores for different statements)
- The researcher should identify the items, which have a high discriminatory power. The responses are interpreted to determine which of the statements discriminate very clearly between high scores and low scores on the total scale. It has to be ensured that the questionnaire is consistent. To achieve this, the items with low discriminatory power or those having no significant correlation with the total score are eliminated.

Advantages of Likert Scale over the Thurstone Scale
a. The method of construction of Likert type scale is less cumbersome.
b. It supplies more precise and definite response towards an issue. The intermediate vague points are absent in this scale.
c. The Likert scale permits the revelation of several (five) degrees of agreement or disagreement; but Thurstone scale is based on only two alternative responses i.e., acceptance or rejection. Thus, Likert scale is more informative and reliable than the Thurstone scale.
d. In a Likert type scale, any item or statement empirically consistent with the statement may be included. In Thurstone scale, only the strictly related items are included. Thus, Likert type scale has a broader area of reference and has also a method of checking internal consistency which is conspicuous by its absence in Thurstone scale.

Defects in Likert Type Scale
1. The judgment on the basis of total score, which is estimated by calculating the mean or median, is not scientific. The total score values may be the same in many cases, but the attitudes may be different towards an issue.
2. The scores on the Likert type scale may be helpful for making an ordering of the people, but such an ordering will not have any scientific and objective basis.
3. There is no objective basis for expressing different degrees of agreement or disagreement. However, despite some limitations, it remains an important ordinal scale.

Cumulative scale/Bogardus social distance scale
In the cumulative scale, a respondent is given a number of questions, to express agreement or disagreement over an issue. The items are arranged in such a way that a respondent who responds favorably to item number 2 also replies favorably to item number 1 and one who relies favorably to item number 3 also replies favorably to items 1 and 2 and so on. Therefore, the individuals who answer favorably have higher total score than those who answer unfavorably. The score of an individual is computed by counting the number of items he/she answers favorably. His/her scores indicate for him a particular position on the scale. The intervals between the positions may not be equal. The items may be arranged from favorableness to unfavorableness in a systematic manner or may be randomly selected.

The purpose of social distance scale is to measure the attitude towards a particular racial group or groups.

The social distance can also be calculated mathematically. In order to do this, weights are attached to different categories of relationships. Thus, if there are only five categories, the weights such as 1, 2, 3, 4 and 5 can be assigned to the first five categories respectively. The following procedure is generally adopted for the measurement of social distance:
1. Place the weights and percentage response for each category in rows.
2. Multiply the percentage response by its weight.
3. Add up the product, and this will be the social distance.

In the Bogardus type scale, the score does not indicate the exact extent or degree of preference of a group over the other. One important difficulty in this type of scale is that one may not be fully acquainted with a group and hence it is not possible for him/her to state the attitude. The influence of an individual member or members may not be eliminated from the mind while making preferences.

5. Scalogram (Guttman) Method

According to Guttman, a 'universe of content' can be considered to be unidimensional only if it yields a perfect, or nearly perfect cumulative scale. The Scalogram technique is based on 'reproducibility criterion' i.e., it is possible to reproduce the responses of the respondent about each item from the score item. This is a major test of the Guttman scale.

The Scalogram analysis is a simple method of testing the 'scalability' of the statements. The views of judges are not necessary in this case. A diagram in which individual responses are laid out is called a Scalogram. In the Guttman technique, the perfect scale implies that a person who answers a given question favorably will have a higher total score than a person who answers it unfavorably. The Guttman scale is analytically complex, apart from the fact that there is no guarantee that the various items will scale, and even if they do, the universe of content may remain narrow in coverage.

Guttman model is deterministic in nature. It assumes that a person who responds positively/negatively to one item must respond positively/negatively to a series of others. The model can be made probabilistic rather than deterministic. This attempt has been made by 'Latent Structure Analysis,' as developed by Lazarsfeld.

Guttman has developed another technique. According to this, the respondent not only gives his/her view (agreement or disagreement) but he also mentions the intensity (degree) which is classified into five categories. For each respondent, we thus get two scores (content score and intensity score) which can be plotted against each other on a graph. The result often gives U-shaped curve. The more extreme views have highest intensity. The content score at the lowest point of the curve may be regarded as the dividing line between favorable and unfavorable responses. The lowest point suggesting favorable response is not affected by the form and the wording of the individual items. Hence, this method is objective.

6. The Q-sort Scaling Technique

The method is widely applied in the study of personality. The individual can make a study of changes in his/her own image, or in his/her ideal person and so on. The data yielded by the Q-sort can be summarized into a single score, as in a summated scale, to yield a scale on 'adjustment.' The adjustment score of the control group can be compared with the therapists' ratings of the success of therapy, and the extent of agreement can be known. The technique can also be applied to the study of various types of socio economic attitudes.

7. Semantic Differential Attitude Scale

Osgood, Suci and Tannen-baum developed Semantic Differential Attitude Scale. Its main objective is to examine the meaning of certain concepts. The semantic differential makes the measurement and comparison of various objects or concepts possible. In order to form an attitude scale, what is required is to decide the description of the issue to be evaluated and to choose suitable adjective pairs for it. A respondent's total score is the measure of his/her attitude. In a semantical differential, there is only one issue to evaluate.

Check List

A checklist consists of a listing of steps, activities or behavior which the observer records when an incident occurs. While preparing a checklist teacher must keep in mind what kinds of behavior are important to record and what kinds of objectives are to be evaluated. A checklist enables the observer to note only whether or not a trait or characteristic is present.

Suggestions to follow while using checklist:
- Checklist should relate directly to learning objectives
- Checklist needs to be confined to performance areas that can be assessed sufficiently by examining positive and negative criteria and when sufficient opportunity for observation exists
- Use checklist only when you are interested in ascertaining whether a particular trait or characteristic is present or absent

- Clearly specify the traits or characteristics to be observed
- Have a separate checklist for each candidate. Individual observations can be recorded on a master checklist
- The observer must be trained how to observe, what to observe and how to record the observed behavior
- Multiple observations provide a more accurate assessment of performance than a single observation
- Students should be evaluated in the natural setting or one as closely as possible to the real situation
- A completed checklist should be given to each student for review followed by an individual session with the student, to discuss the strength and weaknesses of the performance and formulate a plan to improve the performance.

Peer Appraisal Method
- It is a very good supplement in the evaluation program
- In evaluating characteristics like: Popularity, Leadership ability, Concern for others.
  Fellow students are often better judges than teachers.

Principles
- The traits to be rated should be within the student's experiential background
- Complete anonymity and confidentiality must be maintained.

Technique
Each learner is given a list of descriptions and asked to name the pupil who best fit each description. One may include one's own name if one believes the description suits. The teacher can readily see which pupils are mentioned most frequently, seldom or not at all for each characteristic.

Anecdotal Record
'It is a brief description of an observed behavior that appears significant for evaluation purposes.'

'A factual record of an observation of a single specific, significant incident in the behavior of a student.'

'A verbal snapshot of an incident'.

'A simple statement of an incident deemed by the observer to be significant with respect to a given pupil.'

'The spot description of some incident, episode or occurrence i.e., observed and recorded as being of possible significance.'

'An objective description by the teacher of a significant occurrence or an episode in life of the learner.'

'It is the written description of a specific incident for which a teacher has observed.'

Meaning
- Informal device used by the teacher to record behavior of students as observed by him/her from time to time
- It provides a lasting record of behavior which may be useful later in contributing to a judgment about a student
- It gives useful information concerning an individual. The observer should be objective and has to mention various kinds of social relationships in which the individual takes part, e.g. Parent-child, Pupil-teacher, social interaction, etc.
- Teachers will note down the important happenings pertaining to a learner for future reference
- The teacher describes the events he/she observed carefully and writes his/her comments, takes the signature of student, he/she will also sign and keep it into the file and will be considered for evaluating the particular student.

Characteristics (content)
- A factual description of an event, how it occurred; what happened; when it occurred and under what circumstances the behavior occurred will be described by the observer i.e., objective description of learner's behavior recorded from time to time, along with observer's comments, the treatment (The interpretation and recommended action should be noted separately from the description)
- Each anecdotal record should contain a record of a single incident
- The incident recorded should be one, i.e. considered to be significant to the pupil's growth and development.

Purposes
- To furnish the multiplicity of evidence needed for good cumulative record
- To substitute for vague generalizations about student specific exact description of behavior
- To stimulate teachers to look for information i.e., pertinent in helping each student realize good self-adjustment
- To understand individual's basic personality pattern and his/her reactions in different situations
- The teacher is able to understand his/her learner in a realistic manner
- It provides an opportunity for healthy pupil-teacher relationship
- It can be maintained in the areas of behavior that cannot be evaluated by other systematic methods
- Helps the students to improve their behavior, as it is a direct feedback of an entire observed incident, the student can analyse his/her behavior better
- Useful in supplementing and validity observations made by other means
- Can be used by students for self-appraisal and peer assessment

Advantages
- Supplements and validates of other structured instruments
- Provision of insight into total behavioral incidents
- Use of formative feedback
- Economical and easy to develop

Disadvantages
- If carelessly recorded, the purpose will not be fulfilled
- Subjectivity
- Lack of standardization
- Difficulty in scoring
- Time consuming
- Limited application

How to use Anecdotal Record effectively
- Specify the behavior to be assessed in advance
- Limit observations to those categories or qualities
- Record enough of the situations to decrease subjectivity
- Avoid too much dependency on memory by recording it time to time. It will increase its objectivity, validity and reliability
- A single specific incident has to be recorded (positive and negative aspects) and consider both in making inferences
- Relates anecdotal records directly to the clinical objectives.

Items in Anecdotal Record
To relate the incident correctly for drawing inferences the following items to be incorporated:
- Name of student, Class and School, date of observation
- Setting background of the incident
- Signature of the observer
- Interpretation of the behavior
- Recommendations concerning the behavior.

Identified unacceptable behavior and number of times noticed	Brief description of indent how and what happened and its consequences
Signature of student and date	Signature of Instructor and date

Critical Incident Record
To evaluate performance, the evaluator records specific critical incidents of effective and ineffective behavior, two sides or aspects of a performance record i.e., effective and ineffective performance. The incident presents only the facts of the performance.

- Effective behavior (positive behavior): Contributing to patient care service
  - Completion of an assignment or achieving of an objective
  - Maintenance of quality in nursing care of patients.

  For example: anticipated needs of the clients.
- Ineffective behavior (negative behavior)

  Which interfere with good nursing cares or leads to poor nursing care. For example Failed to organise nursing care for maximum patient benefit.

  Critical incidents are outstanding happenings, which indicate the presence or absence of the quality or characteristic or behavior pattern to be analysed.

'An incident will be considered critical, when it occurs in a situation, where the purpose or intent of the act seems fairly clear to the observer.'

'An analysis of incidents helps in breaking down broad statements of objectives into specific components needed for evaluation.'

The description of incident should be explained in detail, what a student did or said that made a teacher to believe he really understood something or failed to understand it.

Criteria for Using Critical Incidents

- Observer has to observe actual behavior and must be reported
- All the relevant factors in the incident must be given
- Definite judgment about the behavior, i.e. considered to be critical

How to record the Critical Incidents

- Total period of observation has to be written in the form
- Number of incidents, effective and ineffective behavior has to be recorded
- Space for signature of the evaluator and the person who is being evaluated should be provided

Sociometry and Sociogram

To study the interaction of children, *JL Moreno* developed the sociometric technique by using Sociogram.

- It enables the teacher to get a comprehensive picture of the structure of social relationship in the entire class by means of certain instruments and methods of interpreting and applying the results obtained
- It is a special method of obtaining the information through oral questions, written responses and analyzing the records in studying the group
- It is a technique whereby each member is asked to state the kind of relationships, which he/she holds towards other members. These responses have been recorded graphically and represented in Sociogram
- The sociometric status, the individual relationship with other members in a group perception of other members, etc. will be revealed in Sociometry
- It is a method used to determine the degree to which individuals are accepted or rejected in a group and group structure, sub-divisions of the group/based on sex. Age, caste, family, profession, cultural affinity, etc. group positions (popular stars, leaders, isolates, rejects, etc.) and so on
- This technique is simple in use and speedy in administration
- The curricular and co-curricular activities formation of groups, choosing companions, partners for specific activities or occasions can be drawn in Sociometry.

Sample Questions

- With whom would you like to sit and to be friendly?
- With whom would you like to work?
- Whom would you like last to work on a committee?

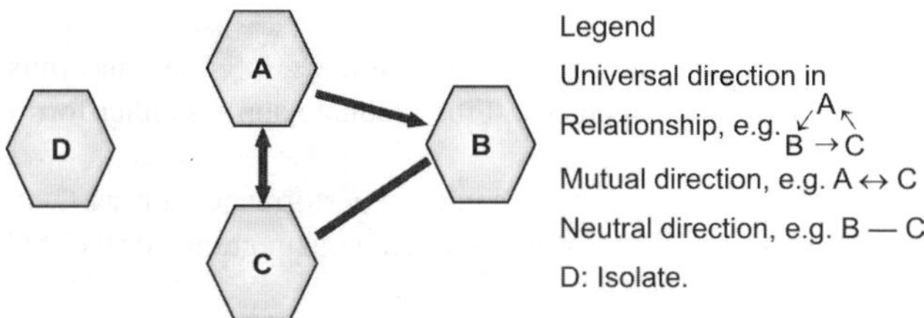

Fig. 8.5: Sociogram

For example: the student is asked to nominate the persons with whom he would like to work, sit, study, or play. It provides data relevant to the existing social relationships in the class.

With this technique, we are interested in who made the nomination as well as who has nominated. The relationships between group members will be shown.

Instruction

Take a paper, write your name and mention other three persons in order of preference, with whom you would like to study. The results are tabulated in a matrix and a graphic picture of the data matrix (Sociogram) is prepared. From the Sociogram, we can identify the students, who are most popular (stars), those who receive no choices (isolates) and those who receive only a single choice (neglectees).

Cumulative Record

It is an account of the learner's history in the educational institution. It begins as soon as the learner enters the school and continues till he/she leaves the school. It contains the total duration of the course his/her activities during the program like varied learning experiences, subjects being taught, different assignments, evaluation and judgments held from time to time, cumulative record gives information regarding all aspects of the life of the child, i.e. his/her physical, mental, psychological and social. It seeks to give comprehensive picture and total personality of the student. The significant information about the student and his/her activities will be gathered from various techniques like tests, inventories, questionnaires, observation, interview, case study, case conferences, etc. will be assembled in summary form on a cumulative record.

Definition

"It is a record of information concerned appraisal of an individual learner in all academic years, maintained by teacher incharge for a specific group of students in a card and kept in administrators' room in college or school.

Form

1. Card sheet contained in an envelope
2. Printed folders
3. Booklet

Contents

- Personal data
- Milestones of growth and development
- Health information
- Psychological report
- Vocational plans
- Personality characteristics
- General overall remarks
    - Over all performance in theory and practicals, grade obtained
    - Leisure time activities
    - Extracurricular activities participated like NCC, NSS
    - Any Awards, Medals obtained
    - Cocurricular activities.

Purposes

- Helpful to the principal, at the end of the course of each trainee, to issue transcripts
- To write credential reports for foreign agencies, if the graduate applies either for futher education and for employments in abroad
- To send the regular reports to parents about the student's performance during the training program
- To recommend the professional organizations to issue scholarship grants for the student during the training program.

Question Bank

A question bank is a planned library of test items designed to fulfil certain predetermined purposes. Question bank has to be prepared with utmost care so as to cover the entire prescribed text. Question bank should be exhaustive and cover entire content with different types of questions. Question bank contains questions which are pretested for their validity and practicability.

The questions may be arranged is as follows:

- Objective/behavior aspect/(abilities in cognitive, conative and affective domains)
- Content/subject area aspect
- Form of the question aspect like essay type, short answer type and objective type
- Weightage aspect.

Purposes

- To improve the teaching-learning process
- Through instructional efforts the learners' growth and development will be obtained
- To improve evaluative process
- A pool of test items can be used for formative and summative valuation of the learners
- It is a pool of readymade quality questions is made available to teachers and examiners so that they may select appropriate questions to assess predetermined objectives.

The paper setters and examiners find it difficult to prepare the questions for the tests, they will try to select the items from the question bank. It is the teacher's responsibility to prepare a large number of questions (of various forms) on different topics of the total subject which she/he is entrusted to teach. Therefore, the teacher should prepare a pool of quality questions, which are reliable and valid.

Teacher Evaluation

Teaching is an interactive process between a teacher and the taught. This technique is used in basic and inservice and continuing education programs.

I. Classroom Interaction Analysis Technique

It is used to:

- Improve classroom teaching
- Provides insight into the nature of classroom communication
- Modify teacher's behavior
- Evaluate the teaching competency of a teacher
- Minimizes the difficulties in teaching
- Evaluate behavioral modification for both the teacher and the taught.

Definition

'Any system for coding spontaneous verbal communication arranging the data into a useful display and then analyzing the results in order to study patterns of teaching and learning.'—*Chauhan* (1979).

Teacher Behavior

It plays an important role in achieving the desired behavioral modifications among students.
Teacher's behavior is classified as:

- Verbal behavior, e.g. explanation, teaching, questioning, demonstrations, illustrations, etc.
- Non-verbal behavior, e.g. movements, using audio-visual aids, etc.

Two types of observational system is used in analyzing the behavior
1. *Sign system:* A list of observable behavior has to be made. The observer note down the teacher's behavior and put the check, which he has observed.
2. *Category system:* The observer observes the teacher's behavior in a stipulated time in a systematic way. The teacher's behaviors are divided into varied categories.

II. Flander's Interaction Analysis Category System
In 1960 Heada Flander, Minnesota university invented, interaction analysis. He has classified teacher-interaction into three categories.
1. Teacher's behavior
    a. *Direct influence*: Lectures, questioning, directing and criticizing
    b. *Indirect influence*: Accepts feelings, praising or encourages
2. *Student talk:* Initiation, response
3. *Silence or confusion*: The observer has to learn the code numbers and sit in a convenient place and per every 3 seconds one observation has to be made, for every minute 20 to 25 observations has to be recorded in a matrix table. The observer has to sit in a convenient place and records the code numbers. The data is analysed by the observer depending on the numbers in the matrix table, the percentage of teacher talk, student talk and silence is calculated. Based on the percentages decisions to be made. For example: If the percentage of teachers talk is more, teacher is very active

Precautions
- Trained observers in the process to be appointed as observers
- It relates to observation only
- To improve validity two trained observers should be appointed
- The observer should record the code numbers in the vertical order

Advantages
- It provides an opportunity to evaluate classroom interaction
- Determines the validity, reliability and objectivity
- One can observe what is happening in the classroom and evaluate the desired behavioral modification both in the teacher and the taught
- Possibility to encourage good teaching and learning strategies
- Scope to alter the teaching and learning methods
- Estimate the teachers' efficiency

III. Verbal Interaction Category System
In 1967 Edumund Anidon and Elizabeth Hunter developed this technique. The interaction between teacher and the taught is a main concept.

Concepts
1. To stimulate taught by teaching activities.
2. To maintain discipline.
3. To develop teaching-learning activities.

Categories
- To give information
- Introduce the topic through motivation
- Give instructions
- Encourages the subject matter by questioning
- Initiates and accepts students responses
- Responds for students' stimulus
- It initiates the teacher to follow innovation of new and modern techniques
- It develops enquiry spirit among student teachers
- It provides objective recapitulation
- To develop teaching strategies

IV. The Reciprocal Category System
- Activities are related to classroom
- It helps to use teaching strategies
- It helps to prepare teaching principles.

Observation System
- Observer notes the category numbers
- Calculation of percentages
- Explanation of data.

Uses
- It provides equal value for both the teacher and the taught
- It helps to formulate teaching strategies
- It encourages the observational procedures
- It helps to start classroom activities
- To develop reinforcement and principles of learning
- It helps to evaluate teachers' activities
- It helps the researcher in the field of education.

Defects
1. No scope to develop skills
2. No scope to determine unfavorable behavior
3. It helps only the interaction.

Converting Measures of Outcomes into Grades
Evaluation of the results of teaching would be complete without a consideration of the real significance of test scores and other measures of outcomes, once they have been obtained. Test score is a numerical value or credits, that a student acquires on a given test or examination, i.e. students' achievement in that subject, his/her status in terms of knowledge, ability, skill or accomplishment in it. Marks are an outcome or evaluation of students' work in terms of the whole group. Students' marks represent educational progress in school and generally are based on an estimation of outcomes.

Before valuation the teacher has to determine or she/he has to keep certain points in her/his mind:
- How many points are satisfactory?
- How many points should be required for passing or failing?
- How many points should be required for different marks in a relative grading system?
- Satisfactory standards, i.e. quality of attainment
- The traits of students (perseverance, study, attitude, regularity, sincerity, etc.) in their grades as these qualities are of value in directing the formation of good habits and the personality development
- The assignments, records maintenance
- Achievements and traits are rated together.

Grading by Percentage Plan
Students' achievement is graded on a percentage basis. A fixed passing mark is set up, e.g. 50% is pass mark, 50% to 59% is second class, 60% to 74.5% is first class, above 75% is distinction. Below 50% is fail. This plan is applied to tests, examinations used to measure the results of learning.

The Relative Grading System
It is based on relative values, marks are determined according to order of merit. The distribution of marks is either by normal curve or percentage.

Principles basic to Good Marking System
To make a system of marks valid, reliable, definite, objectives, comprehensive and practicability certain principles has to be followed by the teachers.
- A marking system should be based on a definite purpose

Criteria for evaluating student-teacher

Name of the student-teacher:　　　　　　　　**Date:**　　　　　　**Time:**
Lesson:　　　　　　　　　　　　　　　　　　　　**Name of the Evaluator:**
Level of students:

	0	1	2	3	4

I. Plan of Teaching
1. Central objective-clear, adequate and appropriate.
2. Contributory objective—clear, adequate and appropriate.
3. Introduction—Relevant and motivating.
4. Subject matter—Well selected sequentially organised.
5. According to time limit and level of students and complete.
6. Scientific principles—adequate and relevant.
7. Problem solving approach used.
8. Summary—Clear and includes all points.
9. Well selected books and journals for students and teacher.
10. Questions for students—different types based on objectives.
11. Arrangement on classroom and equipment—neat and orderly.

II. Audio-visual Aids
1. Good selection and appropriate.
2. Observed principles in preparation.
3. Observed principles in use is visible/audible.
4. Audiovisual aids other than chalk board and overhead projector.

III. Presentation
1. Student participation/maintains inter-personal relationship.
2. Development of subject and make the subject interesting.
3. Subject matter—Complete, valid and accurate.
4. Mastery of content.
5. Objectives made clear.
6. Evaluation of previous knowledge.
7. Eliciting and stimulating recall.
8. Assignments clear, creative and appropriate.
9. Sequencing information.

IV. Personality and Communication
1. Voice and speech clear, easy to follow, audible and expressing. Modulated and carries conviction, clear and free of distractions.
2. Language—Correct use of terms grammar and spelling, simple and clear, is easy to follow.
3. Non-verbal communication—Pleasant, humorous and observation.
4. Dress and posture—Appropriate, good and grooming maintains, good posture.

V. Principles of Teaching and Learning
1. Simple to complex, Concrete to abstract.
2. Known to unknown.
3. Others.

VI. Methods of Teaching
1. Lecture makes it effective by examination and illustration.
2. Uses opportunities for demonstration.
3. Observes principles in the methods used.
4. Other methods used.

Total Marks

Remarks:

Date:　　　　　　　　　　　　　　　　　　Signature of the Evaluator and
　　　　　　　　　　　　　　　　　　　　　Professor signature and HOD

- Measurement is always a means to an end and never an end in itself
- Course objectives
- Organization and management of the course
- Teaching techniques and procedures
- Assignments
- Examination and other evaluation of students' performance
- The teacher herself/himself, his/her qualifications, Educational background and personal characteristics, e.g. voice, mannerisms, approachability, etc.

Valuation
- Write/frame the questions first
- Put the questions in order (objective type/short answer question/essay type)
- Write the answers next day
- Prepare the key for objective questions
- Score sheet proforma has to be used.

Sl no	Name of the student	Objective type	Short answers	Essay type	Total marks obtained.

- Under conducive environment, test has to be administered
- Collect the answer scripts and valuate the same question for all the candidates, again start the next question
- After validating, marks have to be entered in the score sheet and internal assignment register
- Arrange the answer scripts in descending order of merit and give to the students, explaining his/her demerits or weak points for enhancing improvement in the next test.

Internal Assessment
Evaluation is an integral part of the instructional program. It includes quantitative, qualitative assessment and value judgment. It can be done by the examining body either university or board and teaching faculty of the respective institution. These are supplement of external examinations.

Purposes
In the teaching-learning situation
- To have a regular, systematic appraisal
- To observe educational decisions into effective
- To assess the progress of students' internal assessment examinations will be conducted
- To give comprehensive picture of the students' learning, viz. academic achievements, personality traits, achievement of three domains objectives. Thus internal assessment improves the teaching-learning process effective

  Objectives of affective domain (attitudes, interests and appreciation) and psychomotor domain (skills) can be followed through internal assessment. During the annual examination or the external examination, weightage is given to the internal assessment. This internal assessment will work as motivating factors for students to study and provides a basis for feedback.

Procedure
- Internal assessment should be built into the total educational program and used for improvement rather than for certifying the level of achievement of the student—*The Education Commission (1964 to 66)*
- All the items of internal assessment need not follow qualified scoring procedures. The result should be kept separately. It has to be combined with other results to form aggregate scores
- Through internal assessment, teachers can change the attitudes of students favorably towards the day-to-day school program
- Internal assessment should be objective, unbiased.

Components of Internal Assessment System

The school should provide as many activities as possible and detailed records of students' participation should be scrupulously maintained.

The items of activities may be as follows:

Weightage to Items of Internal Assessment

Due weightage should be given to the different items mentioned. Below is given a sample. It is subject to change, depending upon the curriculam as per subject-wise and school/college and objectives philosophy, etc.

a. Subject-wise Assessment

The suggested weightage is given below

Unit tests	25
Two term tests	25
Performance tests	10
Home work and class work	10
Term papers (two per subject)	10
Assignments (ten in each subject)	20
	100

The final maximum score in a subject should be 100. A student must obtain a minimum score of 50 in order to gain promotion to the next higher standard.

b. Assessment of Co-curricular Activities

Library work	20
Sports and games (at least 2 activities)	20
Debates, elocution, drawing, music, etc.)	20
Study circle (any one)	20
Visits (excursion, educational visits, field trips etc.)	20
	100

A student must obtain a minimum score of 50 in order to gain promotion to the next higher standard.

c. Assessment of Personality Traits

Here, the assessment in terms of scores is not possible. Various grades may be assigned to different traits as suggested below:

Traits	Very much	Not at all
Cooperation		
Initiativeness		
Honesty		
Leadership		
Followership		
Perseverance		
Confidence		
(More traits may be added)		

With the help of this scheme, percentage scores or grades may be determined and reported separately. The minimum expected score or grade for promotion to the next higher standard should be made known to the learners.

Validity of Internal Assessment

Though internal assessment is a powerful tool in the hands of a teacher, there is a likelihood of its misuse. It becomes invalid if the teacher is biased, has prejudice against a pupil, shows favoritism or antagonism towards

Items and tools of internal assessment

Sl no	Item of assessment	Tools for assessment written tests	Number of tests in a year
1	Practical tests	Written tests	Unit tests depend on the number of units
	a. Unit tests	a) Standardised unit tests	Two term tests
	b. Term tests	b) Teacher-made tests	Two term tests
2	Oral tests (mostly for languages)	Interview technique	Two (one in a term)
3	Laboratory work—Practical tests (for science)	Practical tests Observational techniques	Two (once in a term)
4	Library work—Reading and preparing notes	Observational techniques— Interest inventories	Two (once in a term) and casual inspection
5	Term papers	Written assignments	Two (once in a term) per subject
6	Study habits		
	a. Home work	Written assignments	Continuous in day-to-day teaching At least ten assignments in each subject
	b. Regular assignments	Written assignments	
7	Participation in sports/games	Observation Cumulative record card	At least two sports activities
8	Co-curricular activities: Debates, Elocution, Drawing, Music, Mimicry, Dramatics, School magazine, and Exhibition	Interest inventories Rating scales	At least two activities
9	Study circles (Clubs): Language, Science, Mathematics, Social studies	Interest inventories Rating scales Check lists	At least in one study circle
10	Personality tests: Cooperation, Initiative, Honesty, Leadership, Followership	Observational techniques Rating scales Questionnaires, inventories, Standard tests	During the whole year
11	Visits Educational visits, Hikes and excursions, Picnics and field trips	Interest inventories Questionnaires Check lists	Once per term Twice per term Once per term

a pupil. The tool of internal assessment is a very good tool if the assessment is made objectively and is free from bias.

Advantages
1. No undue weightage is given to the final or annual or external examination. This is logical, psychological and scientific.
2. Proper study habits are likely to be developed. For example:
   a.   Students will be engaged in study throughout the year
   b.   They will be more regular, alert, sincere in their studies, e.g. in doing class work, homework, assignments.
   c.   Undue emphasis on eleventh-hour preparation, in most of the cases cramming will be reduced to the minimum.
3. Students will pay attention to all the activities organized by the school and they will try to participate in these activities.
4. Internal assessment helps us to minimize anxiety and nervous breakdown on the part of students, which otherwise are possible at the time of the final examination.
5. It gives us a comprehensive picture of a learner's progress.
6. It helps as to diagnose the weaknesses and strength of learners. On the basis of this, remedial teaching is possible.
7. It can be used as a good device for motivating students.

8. It brings about a change in the attitude, interests and appreciation of students and teachers towards school programs.

9. It gives an ample opportunity to the teacher to assess his/her own students. It is completely in accordance with the principle: "The teacher who teaches is the best to assess student's performance".

10. If internal assessment has to a considerably high weightage in the promotion of a student to the next higher standard, not only teachers but also students and even parents should feel more responsible for the entire syllabus during the whole year.

Disadvantages

- A teacher may misuse it
- It can cause a great harm in the hands of an inexperienced, insincere, inefficient and dishonest teacher
- It will lose its validity if favouritism, personal prejudices and subjectivity, if assessment are subjective.

Objective Structured Clinical Examination (OSCE)

Introduction

An OSCE is a modern type of examination often used in Health Sciences (like Medicine, Chiropractic, Physical therapy, Radiography, Nursing, Pharmacy and Dentistry) to test clinical skill performance and competence in skills such as *communication, clinical examination*, medical procedures/prescription, exercise prescription, joint mobilization/manipulation techniques and interpretation of results.

The term 'OSCE' is an acronym that stands for 'Objective Structured Clinical Examination'.

Definitions

- "An exam whereby 'students demonstrate their competence under a variety of simulated conditions". – Watson, 2002
- "Examinations in which the student is required to perform specific skills and behaviors in a simulated clinical or patient care environment".

Purposes

An examination of students' clinical skills OSCEs:

- Used in both formative and summative assessment in health professional education
- Identify objective performance criteria for the skill being examined
- Structure the performance criteria in a checklist to facilitate identification of desired clinical skills
- Use a set structure to encourage parity between students
- Use 'Stations' designed to assess a specific skill or component of health professional clinical practice
- A requirement for accreditation in many health professional programs
- Encourage a collaborative approach between HEI and practice in the creation of health professionals who are 'fit for purpose'
- Adaptable across professions and clinical skills in all academic levels
- Have potential for peer feedback and assessment
- Promote development of functioning knowledge
- Have scope for application outside the health arena: Objective Structured Professional Examination (OSPE)
- Identifying the performance criteria for advanced practice skills or 'expertise' can be challenging
- Experts as examiners must be liberated to assess using global judgement alongside set performance criteria
- Knowledge associated with specific advanced practice skills can be assessed within a viva subsection of the OSCE checklist
- Important to differentiate between academic levels in OSCE, not just in the advanced skills performance required but in the higher challenge for and expectations of these students
- "Teachers, Examiners and Students" feedback on the Masters Level OSCE is very positive.

Conventionally, students move between multiple OSCE 'stations,' each one focussing on a different skill, so students demonstrate the breadth of skills required for clinical practice expected at their stage of learning and development. During an OSCE, the examiner will assess learners' performance with regard to four distinct elements which includes "Knowledge and understanding underpinning the skill (K); Motor or technical aspects of the skill (M); The affective aspects (A), i.e., the professional attitude associated with the performance; and structure (S), i.e. how you approach the skill in terms of being systematic, logical and organized." A simple acronym that can help to remember these components is KMAS (Knowledge, Motor skill, Attitude, Structure).

An OSCE usually comprises a circuit of short (usual is 5 to 10 minutes although some use upto 15 minute) stations, in which each candidate is examined on a one-to-one basis with one or two impartial examiner(s) and either real or simulated patients (actors). Each station has a different examiner, as opposed to the traditional method of clinical examinations where a candidate would be assigned to an examiner for the entire examination. Candidates rotate through the stations, completing all the stations on their circuit. In this way, all candidates take the same stations. It is considered to be an improvement over traditional examination methods because the stations can be standardized, enabling fairer peer comparison and complex procedures can be assessed without endangering patients health.

Objective (O)

'O' in the word OSCE stands for "objective and objectivity" is a defining feature of this type of assessment.

All candidates are assessed using exactly the same stations (although if real patients are used their signs may vary slightly) with the same marking scheme. In an OSCE candidates get marks for each step on the mark scheme that they perform correctly which therefore makes the assessment of clinical skills more objective rather than subjective, where one or two examiners decide whether or not the candidate fails based on their subjective assessment of their skills. By the nature of their role, assessors have the responsibility of making professional judgments about the performance of students whom they are assessing.

The assessor is required to make decisions based on two key judgments:

1. The extent to which a student has met the learning outcomes and standards of the particular course or subject that is being examined.
2. Whether the student has demonstrated the level of competency that is expected and consequently, whether the student is able to practice safely in the clinical setting.

The OSCE is designed to achieve transparency by minimizing potential bias.

Clinical practice and what you have seen while working in the practice environment, you will recognize that most practitioners have a preferred way of doing something. For example some nurses might like to set up a sterile field in preparation for a wound dressing in a particular way, while still making sure that the key principles of asepsis are maintained. Likewise, you may have seen a colleague make a hospital bed in a slightly different way to how you or other nurses like to make it. For example: They may like to position the pillows facing away from the door while another colleague may be concerned about folding the bedspread in a specific way. Regardless of this, it is almost certain that the key principles underlying both techniques used for bed making are the same.

However, if an examiner had a specific way of assessing student performance in accordance with her/his own particular likes, dislikes or habits, this could cause difficulties in terms of equity and consistency, especially if there were more than one examiner assessing the same skill. Problems would arise if students were not assessed objectively on their competence but instead on how well their performance complied with the examiner's likes and dislikes. You can see that if this were to happen, the assessment process would not be fair. In fact, it could be considered biased towards the examiner. Therefore, it is very important that the clinical exam is free from any prejudice or bias. In other words, it needs to be objective.

Structured

The letter 'S' stands for structure. To achieve objectivity in the assessment of competency, a clinical skill or procedure is typically broken down into component parts in a very structured way.

Stations in OSCEs have a very specific task where simulated patients are used detailed scripts are provided to ensure that the information that they give is the same to all candidates, including the emotions that the patient should use during the consultation. Instructions are carefully written to ensure that the candidate is given a very specific task to complete. The OSCE is carefully structured to include parts from all elements of the curriculum as well as a wide range of skills.

When planning for the OSCE, a team of course lecturers will spend time considering in detail each of the skills that will be examined. Each skill will be broken down into its component parts, and marking criteria, in the form of a checklist, will be developed. Essentially, this is a list of the key components of the skill that the student should perform in order to demonstrate that he is competent, safe and thorough.

During the examination the assessor will use the checklist to mark each student's performance. This is typically done by observing if each part of the skill has been performed and whether it has been demonstrated correctly and safely. By using such a structured approach, any examiner's bias is substantially minimized as they can only mark a student's performance in accordance with whether the student has or has not met each criterion set out on the marking sheet. The allocation of marks between different stations will be agreed upon by the examiners in advance of the OSCE and the student's final score will usually be based on the overall number of correct responses on the marking criteria checklist.

Another way in which OSCEs can be considered to be a structured form of assessment is the way in which they are organized. OSCEs consist of different types of assessment tasks we will consider the most typical OSCEs, which consist of a circuit or series of short activities, each of which must be performed at a different 'station.' These activities are timed and students are assessed at each station by one examiner using the predetermined, objective marking sheet. In this way, each student is assessed in both a structured and standardised way, thereby eliminating the risk of inequality and inconsistency.

Clinical (C)

A clinical examination: The OSCE is designed to applied clinical and theoretical knowledge. Where theoretical knowledge is required (E.g. answering questions from the examiner at the end of the station) then the questions are standardized and the candidate is only asked questions that are on the mark sheet (if they are asked any others then there will be no marks for them).

You may know from experience that a typical clinical environment is often busy with multidisciplinary team members working to meet the needs of the numerous patients or clients for whom they are caring. Sometimes when performing a clinical skill in the practice setting, it is not unusual to be interrupted or distracted by what else is happening. But clinical skills are fundamental to nursing practice and specific skills are often needed for patients who are very ill, experiencing pain or who are emotionally distressed. Therefore, in many cases it would be inappropriate or even unethical for an examination to be conducted in the clinical setting or for a skill to be demonstrated several times by many different students using a real patient. Likewise, it would be unrealistic to expect a patient to recount his history repeatedly for the purpose of an OSCE. To overcome these issues, simulation is commonly used for OSCEs in order to create an environment similar to that of the clinical setting. A variety of approaches can be used.

For example: A simple model of the skin can be used to enable the student to demonstrate how to give an intramuscular injection

To set the scene at the beginning of each station, the student will be given a short scenario to read. This will provide the information necessary to establish the context in which the specific set of skills is to be performed and will identify the skills being examined.

Examination (E)

An examination is the process of testing competence or knowledge. As such, in an OSCE, clinical competency is assessed by breaking it down into its various components. In this way students are required to demonstrate not only *what they know* but also that they *know how* to perform a clinical skill. Therefore, they must also *show how* to perform it competently by demonstrating the necessary *actions* required for the execution of the skill in a safe, appropriate and competent manner.

Preparation

Preparing for OSCEs is very different from preparing for an examination on theory. In an OSCE, clinical skills are tested rather than pure theoretical knowledge. It is essential to learn correct clinical methods and then practice repeatedly until one perfects the methods. Marks are awarded for each step in the method; hence, it is essential to dissect the method into its individual steps, learn the steps, and then learn to perform the steps in a sequence. Most universities have clinical skills labs where students have the opportunity to practice clinical skills. It is often very helpful to practice in small groups with colleagues, setting a typical OSCE scenario and timing it with one person role playing a patient, one person doing the task and (if possible) one person either observing and commenting on technique or even role playing the examiner using a sample mark sheet. In doing this, the candidate is able to get a feel of running to time and working under pressure.

From acquiring knowledge to applying knowledge

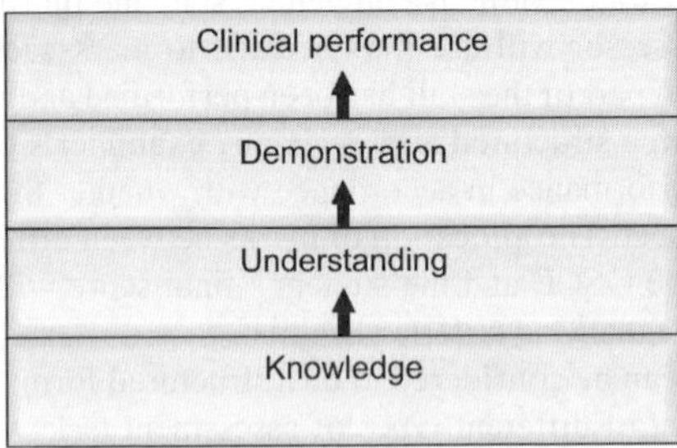

Miller (1990) recommends that, in order to demonstrate competency, 'knows', 'knows how', 'shows how' and 'does' are necessary. This means that, in terms of demonstrating clinical competency, knowledge (knows), competence (knows how), demonstration (shows how) and clinical performance (does) are all important.

Knowing, Showing, Doing, e.g. Pain Assessment

As part of an OSCE, you were required to undertake a pain assessment on a simulated patient/client, the examiner would assess you on the following clinical competences.

Knowledge

This is at the bottom of the triangle, indicating that it is the most basic and broadest component in the framework. It relates to having the appropriate knowledge that underpins practice. Pain is a very complex phenomenon. Because of this, adequate knowledge and understanding of the potential physiological, psychological and emotional elements of pain is required in order to effectively undertake a pain assessment. Knowledge and understanding of the different types of pain and how these may relate to an individual is also important.

Understanding

This is a higher component in the framework because it depends on *knowing how* to do something and *understanding why* it should be done in a certain way. In the given example, this would involve demonstrating knowledge and understanding of how pain assessment can be effectively undertaken, including the use of appropriate communication skills. Knowledge of different pain assessment tools and how to use them is important. Likewise, knowing how to interpret data obtained from a pain assessment is also essential.

Demonstration

This is a further step up in the framework because it depends on demonstrating or *showing how* to do something. It requires familiarity with the process of pain assessment and with demonstrating how to perform the assessment in a systematic and structured way.

Clinical performance

The performance or the 'doing' part is the most important and sometimes, most challenging part. It requires integrating all three previous points and performing the skill in a professionally competent way. In this example, it includes communicating with the patient, assessing pain using an appropriate method, documenting it and interpreting the findings.

If we reconsider the key requirements of an OSCE one has to recall that they need to be objective and structured. To meet these requirements the OSCE is conducted in a simulated environment and all students are assessed in the same way, by examiners using a structured checklist. It is also important that any actors playing the role of a patient behave in a consistent manner. This will help to maximize standardization and consistency of the examination.

For example: If a patient interview scenario was being used to assess communication skills, it would be important that the patient role player communicates the same information to each student. Likewise, if an actor/patient role player's pulse rate was being measured as part of an OSCE station, it is important that this is stable and free from any significant fluctuations that might compromise standardization. In practice, such standardization is not possible, as every patient is different. Furthermore, the environments in which they are cared for are also very different.

The OSCE provides an opportunity for an assessment of competency within a simulated environment. However, the 'doing' part requires this competency to be demonstrated in practice.

Types of OSCE

1. OSCEs comprising a number of short stations within a circuit, these are known as 'short cases' or 'multi-station OSCEs' used for the students in the beginning of the program, e.g. the OSCE may last an hour, during which time students rotate around six stations, demonstrating a simple clinical skill at each station. In this case each station would be 10 minutes' duration.

2. In addition to skills, some OSCEs may also comprise knowledge stations, which a number of skills are assessed referred as 'long cases' or 'single stations' and are most commonly used for assessing competency in skills for final year students. They are typically used to assess competency in the integration of skills. This type of OSCE may be one hour long, but comprise just one station, lasting the whole hour or two stations, each one of 30 minutes duration. As part of a 'long case,' knowledge may be tested while a procedure is undertaken or after the skills component has been completed.

Example 1

A nursing student approaching the end of first year, an OSCE has to be conducted to assess clinical skills in the course that are fundamental to nursing practice. It is likely that the OSCE for this student would focus on the assessment of competence in a range of fundamental skills taught and above all, the student would be required to demonstrate knowledge of key principles such as safety and accuracy. In this type of OSCE the stations would be developed with a focus on discrete skills, such as aseptic technique, hand washing technique, measurement of vital signs, First Aid, etc. rather than on the more complex integration of skills

Example 2

For Final Year students, the clinical component of the course requires to demonstrate competency in skills related to clinical specialities in that academic year. It is likely that the OSCE for this course would focus on assessing competence in the skills learnt, but also be expected to demonstrate the integration of those skills like the ability to effectively answer any questions in the scenario may ask. In other words, the OSCE is designed to assess competency in skills that are fundamental to nursing practice and to do so at different levels of complexity, depending on what stage the student has reached in the program.

The first OSCE is to assess how you perform the basic skills required for a range of different tasks while later OSCEs assess how well you are able to integrate appropriate skills in specific patient scenarios.

Using peer assessment in formative OSCE

- Peer involvement is beneficial to the students by promoting deeper learning as they increase their effort knowing peers will be evaluating their work and by making students rethink their understanding of the skill in order to be able to provide appropriate feedback
- Providing peer feedback prepares students for professional practice where assessment of peers and students is expected
- Peer assessment using formative OSCE provides the student with a clear understanding of the performance criteria required for clinical practice
- Peer involvement in teaching and learning helps by improving the success of student learning and by empowering students to progress through feedback.

RECRUITMENT

Introduction

Recruitment has become the most challenging human resource management (HR) function and it is one of the activities that impact most critically on the performance of an organization. Recruiting strategy must follow certain considerations, viz. 1. Aggressive growth plans, 2. Retention, 3. Recruitment Costs, 4. Time factor,

5. Intellectual Property 6. Impact on quality and safety. A well planned and well managed recruiting effort will result in high quality applicants. Acquiring and retaining the employees is high-quality talent and critical to an organization's success. An organization needs to analyse the benefits and disadvantages of recruiting its personnel through internal or external sources and whether formal or informal systems has to be used.

Successful recruitment begins with proper employment planning and forecasting. In this phase of the staffing process, an organization formulates plans to fill or eliminate future job openings based on an analysis of future needs, the talent available within and outside of the organization and the current and anticipated resources that can be expanded to attract and retain such talent. The success of a recruitment process are the strategies, an organization is prepared to employ, to identify and to select the best candidates for its developing pool of human resources. Organizations seeking recruits for base-level entry positions often require minimum qualifications and experience.

Poor recruitment decisions continue to affect organizational performance, limit goal achievement and also can produce long-term negative effects among them.

Definitions

"The set of activities and processes used to legally obtain a sufficient number of qualified people at the right place and right time, such that the people and the organization can select each other in their own best short and long term interests."

"The Process of searching for and obtaining applicants for jobs, from among whom the right people can be selected."

"It is the process of finding and attracting capable applicants for employment. The Process begins when new recruits are sought and ends when their applications are submitted. The result is a pool of applicants from which new employees are selected."

"The recruitment process provides the organization with a pool of potentially qualified job candidates from which judicious selection can be made to fill vacancies."

Purposes

- Provides a pool of potentially qualified applicants for specific jobs
- Selects the suitable candidates for specific jobs
- Determines the present and future requirements of the organization in conjunction with its personnel planning and job analysis activities
- Enhances the success rate of the selection process
- Limits under qualified or overqualified job applicants
- Retains the employees for long time
- Represents the first contact a company makes with potential employees
- Meet the organizations' legal and social obligations regarding the composition of its workforce
- Increases organizational and individual effectiveness in the short term and long term
- Evaluates the effectiveness of various recruiting techniques and sources for all types of job applicants.

Elements in Recruitment Strategies

- *Specialized recruitment managers:* To develop a suitable strategy for the organization, a recruitment manager must have a overall understanding of the profession as well as a good understanding of his own company's procedures, policies, products and services. Strong personnel-oriented managers should know the right kind of people for the company and be able to develop strategies to attract them, for this position
- *Consolidation of recruitment efforts on a global scale:* To derive maximum benefit for the organization, promoting an organization by making the organization more visible at career fairs and other activities
- *Raising the Company's Profile:* Market the organization by understanding the main things that people want out of a career like opportunity for development, travel opportunities, to be part of a great culture, to work with a great manager and to make money
- Identifying new talent pools and countries where you can recruit massively

- Identifying and developing good headhunters for starters to work further on developing ways to attract them
- *Improving candidate's* selection: Building long-term relationships with universities and educational institutions where they are offering professional courses
  - University and Technical School Relationships: Graduates are raw potential talent that companies can develop in-house due to their ability and proven appetite to learn quickly. They are cost-effective labor at the start, bring a fresh perspective and provide future leadership talent
  - Developing relations can involve attending career fairs, conducting company or technical presentations, providing internships, awarding scholarships, conducting joint studies and regularly making visits to ensure that faculty members know the organization
- *Recruitment Resources:* Ensure that resources will identify the best sources for talent and establish good relationships with agencies in places where talent pools exist but where the company may not have operations. Work on developing relationships with a wide network of top-notch headhunters and keep track of successes with them. This is a good way to tap into the passive talent pool
- *Developing strategic Workforce Planning:* To properly implement a new and more aggressive recruiting strategy, first understand long-term requirements are going to be, many of the positions that we recruit for
- *New Talent Pools:* Both inside and outside of an organization and in new places that have not been tapped into heavily
- *Recruitment Technologies:* Once a candidate has been attracted to the organization, must ensure that he/she can easily apply for a position and that his/her information is professionally managed.

New Realities Call for New Strategies

Old Reality	New Reality
Recruiting is like purchasing	Recruiting is like sales and marketing: the organization is the product
Recruit from traditional sources	Look at diverse pools of talent and be prepared to train and develop
People accept offers	People demand much more
Recruit to fill today's vacant positions	Hunt for talent all the time, every time and plan ahead, much further ahead

Recruitment Process

The process of finding and attracting capable applicants for employment, it will inform qualified individuals about jobs and employment opportunities, create positive image of the organization, so that applicants can make comparisons with their qualifications, interests and generate enthusiasm, interest among the best candidates, such that they will apply for vacant positions. The process begins when new recruits are sought and ends when their applications are submitted. The result is a pool of applicants from which new employees are selected.

The effectiveness of process can play a major role in determining the resources that must be expended on other HR activities and their ultimate success.

Steps/Stages

- Planning
- Strategy Development
- Searching
- Screening
- Evaluation and Control.

Processes in Successful Recruitment

1. *Development of a Policy:* Employment equity policies and programs are about fairness in the workplace, it is achieved when no one is denied employment opportunity and no one benefits for reasons unrelated to ability. Employment equity programs attempt to change the composition of the work force so that employees better reflect the community.

2. *Needs assessment:* To determine the current and future human resource requirements of the organization. If the activity has to be effective, the human resource requirements for each job category and functional division/unit of the organization must be assessed and a priority assigned
3. *Identification:* Human resource pool—Within and outside the organization of the potential and the likely competition for the knowledge and skills resident within it
4. *Job analysis and job evaluation:* To identify the individual aspects of each job and calculate its relative worth
5. Assessment of qualifications, profiles, drawn from job descriptions—Identify responsibilities and required skills, abilities, knowledge and experience
6. Salaries and benefits—Determination of the organization's ability to pay salaries and benefits within a defined period
7. Procedural transparency—Identification and documentation of the actual recruitment process and selection to ensure equity and adherence to equal opportunity and for audit and other purposes of special, important documentation that is in conformity with:
   - Criteria and procedures for the initial screening of applicants, for the selection of interview panels; interview questions; interview scores and panel lists comments
   - Criteria for generating long and short list
   - Results of tests (if any administered)
   - Results of reference checks (if asked).

Recruitment Strategies

Openness and transparency in recruitment and selection practices are crucial.

a. Internal recruitment: Seeks applicants for positions from those who are currently employed, through Promotions and Transfers.

Advantages
- Maintains effective interpersonal relationship
- Encourages competency in employees
- Good Performance is rewarded
- Improves the probability of good selection
- Acts as a training device for developing middle level and top level managers
- Control the internal job posting process
- "*Insiders*" know the organization, its strengths and weaknesses, its culture and most of all, its people.
- Promotions from within build motivation, enhances employee's morale, organisational commitment and job satisfaction. Skilled and ambitious employees are more likely to become involved in developmental activities, as it will lead to promotion
- Internal recruitment is less expensive and quicker than advertising in various media and interviewing "*outsiders*". Time spent in training and socialisation is also reduced
- Organizations have better knowledge about the internal candidates.

Disadvantages
- It perpetuates the old concept of doing things
- It abets raiding
- Candidate's current work may be affected
- Politics play a greater role
- Morale problem for the personnel who were not promoted
- Sometimes it is difficult to find the "right" candidate within and the organization may settle for an employee who possesses a less than ideal mix of competencies or lack of new talents
- If the vacancies are being caused by rapid expansion of the organization there may be an insufficient supply of qualified individuals above the entry level. This may result in people being promoted before they are ready or not being allowed to stay in a position long enough to learn how to do the job well

- In times of rapid growth and during transitions, the organization may promote from within managerial positions. Transition activities and rapid organizational growth often mask managerial deficiencies; it is not until the growth rate slows that the deficiencies become apparent and then, the organization finds it difficult, if not impossible, to undo the damage
- Personnel decisions involving internal candidates are more likely to be affected by the political agenda of the decision makers.

Methods of Internal Recruitment
Before posting a vacancy, management needs to decide whether:
- It tends to retain the job in its present form and with its present title, remuneration and status
- Selected attributes of the job, e.g. skill or experience
- The existing organizational policy on recruitment is still applicable (e.g. whether referrals, by staff members of friends and family are still an acceptable way of filling vacancies)
- Flag imminent vacancies throughout the organization to ensure that the recruitment process is timely
- Ensure that no candidates are lost but, instead, move through the process and are kept informed of their status
- Ensure that good candidates whose applications are pending are kept in touch to maintain their interest in the organization
- Assist in analysing hiring, transfer and exit trends and provide other data that are helpful in planning, evaluating and auditing the recruitment process
- Identify any adverse impacts of the recruitment process on vulnerable groups.

1. **Promotions**
   a. *Job posting:* The purpose of posting vacancies is to bring to the attention of all interested persons (inside or outside of the organization) the jobs that has to be filled. A strategy of placing notices on manual and electronic bulletin boards by publicizing an open job to employees and listing its attributes, such as criteria of knowledge, qualification, skill and experience. Announcing at staff meetings and inviting employees to apply.
   b. *Personnel records*: Helpful as it indicates their educational achievements and skills acquired, effective guide for consideration of promotions.
   c. *Skill banks*: Lists current employees who have specific skills.
2. **Transfers**
   Provides employees a broad based view of the organizations, necessary for future promotions, recruiting the present employees without promotion.
3. **Through office memoranda/notices**
4. **Employee Referrals:** Employees can develop good prospectus for their families and friends by acquainting them with the advantages of a job with the company, they will introduce and encourage them to apply, provides a large pool of potential organizational members. Most employees know from their own experience about the requirements of the job and what sort of persons the company is looking for. Individuals are likely to be similar type, to those who are already working for the company.
5. **Former Employees:** Retired people or the persons who worked with the organization for long time, who knows in and out of the organization and willing to help the institution may come back again to work for higher emoluments or recommend someone who will be beneficial for the organizational growth.
6. **Previous Applicants:** Those who have previously applied for jobs can be contacted by mail, a quick, inexpensive way to fill an unexpected opening, e.g. Professional openings can be filled by applicants to previous jobs.

Informal recruiting methods
Informal recruiting methods are commonly used for hiring clerical and other base-level recruits who are more likely than other groups to have submitted unsolicited applications.
- Rehiring former employees

- Choosing from among those "walk-in" applicants whose unsolicited resumes had been retained on file. Direct applications can provide a pool of potential employees to meet future needs
- The use of referrals also constitutes an informal hiring method
- Former students who participated in internship programs may also be easily and cheaply accessed.

External Recruitment

Searching the labor market more widely for candidates with no previous connection to the organization

1. Walk-ins—Direct applications can also provide a pool of potential employees to meet future needs. From employees' view point, walkins are preferable as they are free from the hassles associated with other methods of recruitment.
2. Write-ins—Are those who send written enquiries. These jobseekers are asked to complete application forms for further processing.
3. Talk-ins—Job aspirants are required to meet the recruiter, on an appropriate for detailed talks, no application is required to be submitted to the recruiter.
4. Consultants—The agencies in the profession are retained by organizations for recruiting and selecting managerial and executive personnel. Consultants will have nation-wide contacts and lend professionalism to the hiring process. They also keep prospective employer and the employee anonymous, but the cost can be a deterrent factor. Most of them charges some percentage of the first year salaries of the individuals placed.
5. Contract—are used to recruit casual workers.
6. Employment agencies and executive search firms to "head hunt" to recruit skilled workers.
7. Using Mass Media Resources—Radio and Television are used to reach skilled workers. Government agencies certain times will use them to announce recruitments, Private agencies may feel that advertising by mass media is expensive.
8. Acquisitions and Mergers—Staffing Organizations is a result of the merger or acquisition process. When organizations combine into one, they have to handle a large pool of employees, some of whom may no longer be necessary in the new organization, consequently the new organization has, in effect, a pool of qualified job applicants, although they are current employees.
9. Competitors – Rival forms can be a source of recruitment, Popularly called 'Poaching' or 'Raiding' , this method involves identifying the right people in rival companies, offering them better terms and luring them away.
10. Professional Associations—Vacancies will be posted in Professional journals, and can be placed in workshops, conferences organized by them.
11. On-line via the Internet/e-Recruiting

    Networking, therefore, continues to be a viable mechanism for recruiting, especially at the senior management level. Online applications/recruiting on the internet—Using the Internet is faster and cheaper than many traditional methods of recruiting. Jobs can be posted on Internet sites for a modest amount (less than in the print media), remain there for periods of thirty or sixty days or more at no additional cost and are available twenty-four hours a day. Candidates can view detailed information about the job and the organization and then respond electronically. Most homes and workplaces are now using computerised equipment for communication; the Internet is rapidly becoming the method of choice for accessing and sharing information. First-time job seekers are now more likely to search websites for job postings than to peruse newspapers, magazines and journals. The prevalence of e-advertising has made it easier. The Internet speeds up the hiring process in three basic stages:

    - Faster applicant response—Jobs posted on the Internet and requiring responses via the same medium receive responses on the same day
    - Faster processing of resumes—An applicant sending a resume electronically can immediately have the application processed, receive an acknowledgement, be screened electronically, and have details of the application and resume dispatched to several managers at the same time
    - Online recruiting provides access to passive job seekers, that is, individuals who already have a job but would apply for what appears a better one that is advertised on the Internet. These job seekers may

be of a better quality since they are not desperate for a job change as are the active job seekers who may be frustrated, disgruntled workers looking for a new position. Organizations that are likely to advertise online usually have a website that allows potential candidates to learn about the organization before deciding whether to apply, thus lowering the incidence time-wasting through the submission of unsuitable applications

- Take advantage of the fact that Internet job advertisements have no space limitations so recruiters can use longer job descriptions to fully describe the organization, job requirements and working conditions offered
- The website can be used as a tool to encourage potential job seekers to build an interest in joining the organization
- Job websites offer unlimited space which can be used, by management
  The site can then be used, not only to post vacancies, but also to publicize the organization, that will allow candidates to become more familiar with the company, know what skills the company is looking for and get to know about its culture. Most importantly, the system will provide a proper path to secure quick responses to job openings
- Online recruiting facilitates the decentralization of the hiring function by making it possible for other groups in the organization to take responsibility for part of the function
  Drawbacks in Internet recruiting:
- Some applicants still place great value on face-to-face interactions in the hiring process. Such applicants are likely to ignore jobs posted, impersonally, online
- Companies are overwhelmed by the volume of resumes posted on the Internet. This can, in fact, lengthen the short-listing process. If the screening process is not well done, the quantity of applications/résumés logged-on may be more of a hindrance to the process that an aid to selection
- Job seekers who demand confidentiality in the recruitment process may be reluctant to use the Internet as a job search mechanism. For effectiveness in the use of the strategy of e-Recruiting, companies are advised to use specialised Job Sites that cater to specific organizations, thoroughly assess the service level provided by Job Sites to ensure that they maintain the level they claim to provide
- Use valid Search Engines that will sort candidates effectively, but will not discriminate against any persons or groups
- Encourage employees to e-mail job advertisements to friends.

12. College recruitment—Sending an employer's representatives to college campuses to prescreen applicants and create an applicant pool from that college's graduating class. It is an important source of management trainees, entry-level candidates and professional and technical employees. To get the best out of this hiring strategy, the organization and its career opportunities must be made to stand out. The organization that will succeed, then, is one can show how the work it offers meets students' needs for skill enhancement, rewarding opportunities, personal satisfaction, flexibility and compensation.

College recruitment offers an opportunity for recruiters to select the potential employees with the personal, technical and professional competencies which they require in their organization. The personal competencies identified may include: a positive work ethic, strong interpersonal skills, leadership capacity and an ability to function well in a work team.

Advantages

- The cost (which is higher than word-of-mouth recruiting but lower than advertising in the media or using an employment agency)
- Convenience (since many candidates can be interviewed in a short time in the same location with space and administrative support provided by the college itself)
- Career planning workshops are used mainly as information giving tools which the school leaver can use to make informed career choices

Disadvantages

- Unfortunately, suitable candidates become available only at certain times of the year, which may not always suit the needs of the hiring organization

- College recruiting is the lack of experience and the inflated expectations of new graduates
- The cost of hiring graduates for entry-level positions that may not require a college degree
- College recruitment is relatively expensive and time consuming for the recruiting company. The process involves screening the candidate that is, determining whether he/she is worthy of further consideration and opportunities for internships.

13. Job fairs and career fairs—to bring those interested in finding a job into those companies who are searching for applicants. Job fairs are open floor at which employers can exhibit the best their companies have to offer so that job seekers can make informed choices. They are considered one of the most effective ways for job seekers to land jobs. At the job fair, employers have a large pool of candidates on which to draw, while job seekers have the opportunity to shop around for dozens – sometimes hundreds of employers, all in one place. Not-withstanding the fact that the atmosphere at the fair is more relaxed than at an interview, employers are still on the look out for qualified, potential employees who have interest, dedication and initiative.

    At least one representative of the company present to provide information. The fairs usually have a common theme or are specific to a certain field or area of interest. Interested individuals browse through the information provided by each organization and then decide if any, they would like to apply to. They have the opportunity to talk with a current employee of specific companies to learn more about the employment experience.

14. Advertisements—Want Ads – Ads may be placed in common medium like Professional journals and news papers describing the job, its benefits, employer and address, qualification, experience required, areas of interest of advertisers expected salary, procedure how to apply and specific requirements.

    Blind Ads – Large organizations with national reputation will be filling the lower level positions by blind ads, It can assist recruiters in finding qualified applicants.

15. Public Service—Entry may follow the procedures like: Application on prescribed forms; Selection on the basis of seniority of application, age limits for entry into certain defined grades/classes, The use of written examinations and/or competitive interviews as the basis for/selection.

Evaluation of external recruitment

Advantages
- The organization will have the benefit of new skills, new talents and new experiences
- The management will be able to fulfill reservation requirements in favour of the disadvantaged sections of the society
- Scope for resentment, heartburn and jealousy of present employees can be avoided by recruiting from outside.

Disadvantages
- Better motivation and increased morale associated with promoting own employees are lost to the organization
- Expensive
- If Recruitment and selection processes are not properly carried out, chances of right candidates being rejected and wrong applicants being selected
- Chances of creeping in false positive and false negative errors
- Adjustment of new employees to the organizational culture takes longer time.

Application forms for seeking employment

Whatever be the type of recruitment, the job seekers must submit application forms seeking employment, certain times application blanks will be provided by the organizations or the applicants are expected to prepare their own application forms and submit on or before the expiry of the stipulated date.

Purposes
- Reason for applying i.e., applicant's desire or ambitions will be known
- Profiles of applicants
- Basic personnel records for applicants who later become employees.

Screening of Applications

It is an integral part of recruiting process, the selection process will begin after the applications have been scrutinized and short listed. Applications received in response to advertisements are screened and only eligible applicants are called for and an interview is conducted by a selection committee. Effective screening can save time and money. Care must be exercised, in screening, clear job specifications will be judged on the basis of their knowledge, skills, abilities and interests required to do the job. The techniques used to screen applicants vary depending on the candidate sources and recruiting methods used. For example: Walk-ins: Interviews and application blanks., for Campus recruiters and agency representatives use interviews and resumes., Reference checks are also useful in screening.

Evaluation of Recruitment Process

Objective of searching for and obtaining applications from job seekers in terms of sufficient numbers and quality. The evaluation include:

- Return rate of applications sent out
- Number of suitable candidates for selection
- Retention and performance of the candidates selected
- Cost of the recruitment process
- Time lapsed data
- Comments on image projected.

Evaluation of Recruitment Methods

- Number of initial enquiries received which resulted in completed application forms
- Number of candidates:
  At various stages of the recruitment and selection process, especially those shortlisted.
  Recruited are retained in the organization after six months.-

Evaluation and Control

- Salaries for recruiters
- Management and Professional time spent on preparing job description, job specifications, advertisements, agency liaison etc.
- Cost of advertisements or other recruitment methods i.e. agency fees
- Cost of producing supporting literature
- Recruitment Overheads and administrative expenses
- Costs of overtime suitable candidates for the selection process, statistical information on the cost of advertisements, time taken for the process and the suitability of the candidates for consideration in the selection process should be gathered and evaluated.

Philosophies of Recruiting

The traditional philosophy of recruiting has been to get as many people to apply for a job as possible. A persuasive agreement can be made that matching the needs of the organization to the needs of the applicants will enhance the effectiveness of the recruitment process. The result will be a workforce which is likely to stay with the organization longer and performs at a higher level of effectiveness.

Approaches

1. Realistic Job Preview

   It provides complete job related information (both positive and negative) to the applicants. The information provided will help jobseekers to evaluate the compatibility among the jobs and their personal ends before hiring decisions are made. It will result self selection process. Job applicants can decide whether to attend the interviews and tests for final selection or withdraw themselves in the initial stage. RJPs are more beneficial for organizations hiring at the entry level, when there are innumerable applicants per position and under conditions of relatively low employment.

2. Job Compatibility Questionnaire

   To determine whether an applicant's preferences for work match the characteristics of the job. It is designed to collect information on all aspects of a job which have a bearing on employee performance, absenteeism, turn over and job satisfaction. It measures job factors which are related to performance, absenteeism, turn over and job satisfaction. It consists of 400 items cover the following factors: task requirements, Physical environment, Characteristics of job seeker, peer interaction, leadership skills, compensation preferences, task variety, job autonomy, physical demands and work schedule. The JCQ is administered to job seekers who are very familiar with either a specific position to be filled, they have to indicate the extent to which each item is descriptive of the job or position in the study.

Performance Appraisal/Employee appraisal/Performance review/Career Development Discussion

'Evaluation' aims at 'objective' measurement, while 'appraisal' includes both 'objective and subjective' assessment of how well an employee has performed during the period under review. Thus performance appraisal aims at ' assessment, feedback and development'. The process of performance appraisal will concentrate on the job of an employee, the environment of the organization and the employee. These three factors are inter-related and interdependent. The appraisal system has to be individualized, subjective, qualitative and oriented towards problem solving. It is based on clearly specified and measurable standards and indicators of performance. Since what is being appraised is performance and not the personality; personality traits which are not relevant to job performance should be excluded from the appraisal framework.

Definitions

"The evaluation of work done (quantity, quality and the manner it is carried out) during a specified period against the background of the total work situation."

" A method by which the job performance of an employee is evaluated (generally in terms of quality, quantity, cost and time) typically by the corresponding manager or supervisor"

"A part of guiding and managing career development."

"The process of obtaining, analyzing and recording the information about the relative worth of an employee to the organization."

"Analysis of an employee's recent successes and failures, personal strengths, weaknesses and suitability for promotion or further training."

"The judgement of an employee's performance in a job based on considerations other than productivity alone."

"A structured formal interaction between a subordinate and supervisor, that usually takes the form of a periodic interview (annual or semi-annual), in which the work performance of the subordinate is examined and discussed, with a view to identifying weaknesses and strengths as well as opportunities for improvement and skills development."

"The process of examining and evaluating the performance of an individual."

Concept

Performance appraisal is a management tool, which is helpful in motivating and effectively utilizing human resources. Assessment of human potential is difficult, no matter how well designed and appropriate the performance planning and appraisal system is. It should be correlated with the organizational mission, philosophies and value system; It covers assessment of performance as well as potential for development; take care of organizational as well as individual needs and help in creating a clean environment by linking rewards with achievements, generating information for the growth of the employee as well as of the organization and suggesting appropriate person task matching and career plans.

Feedback is an important component of performance appraisal. While positive feedback is easily accepted, negative feedback often meets with resistance unless it is objective, based on a credible source and given in a skilful manner.

Aims

The organization's main resources are its employees and their interest cannot be neglected. Performance appraisal aim at the mutual goals of the employees and the organization. This is essential because employees can develop only when the organization's interests are fulfilled. Goals can stimulate employee effort, focus attention, increase persistence and encourage employees to find new and better ways to work, to identify and correct existing problems and to encourage better future performance. Thus the performance of the whole organization will be enhanced. Mutual goals simultaneously provide for growth and development of the organization as well as of the human resources. They increase harmony and enhance effectiveness of human resources in the organization. Information needed by the organization for administrative purposes providing information about human resources and their development measuring the efficiency with which human resources are being used and improved; providing compensation packages to employees and maintaining organizational control.

- Increases mutuality between employees and their supervisors so that every employee feels happy to work with their supervisor and thereby contributes their maximum to the organization
- To align responsibility and accountability at every organizational level by establishing and uphold the principle of accountability
- To provide data for management decisions concerning merit, salary, increments, incentives, rewards, promotion, transfer, demotion or discharge from service
- Document criteria used to allocate organizational rewards
- To evaluate employees objectively and the need to encourage and develop them can be balanced
- Form a basis for personnel decisions: salary increase, promotions, disciplinary actions and bonuses etc.
- Provide the opportunity for organizational diagnosis and development
- Facilitate communication between employee and administration
- Validate selection techniques and human resource policies to meet government equal employment opportunity requirements
- To improve performance through counseling, coaching and development
- To weed out low performers
- To Identify employee training needs and development needs
- Recognize the need for training more pressing and relevant by linking it clearly to performance outcomes and future career aspirations
- Provides a regular and efficient training needs audit for the entire organization
- Give employees/students feedback on performance
- To consider the employee's suitability for different types of assignments/work allotments/Distribution of work/Delegation of Authority
- To have on hand information required for purposes like letters of recommendation, domestic enquiry, avoidance of arbitrary on the spot decisions and reemployment
- To create a desirable culture and traditions in the department (as per organizational policy or council norms)
- To meet the University and Council requirements for manpower planning and organizational development like employee's strengths they can build on and what specific weaknesses they need to overcome
- Provides employees with recognition for their work efforts. The power of social recognition as an incentive has been long noted
- To monitor the effectiveness of changes in recruitment strategies
- To assess whether the general quality of the workforce is improving, staying steady or declining
- Based on employee's capabilities, strengths organizations will be assign specific role and function
- Assist each employee to understand more about their role and become clear about their functions by providing an opportunity to each employee for self-reflection and individual goal-setting, so that individually planned and monitored development takes place
- To be instrumental in helping employees for better understanding their strengths and weaknesses with respect to their role and functions in the organization
- Act as a mechanism for increasing communication between employees and their supervisors. In this way, each employee gets to know the expectations of their superior and each superior also gets to know the difficulties of their subordinates and can try to solve them. Together, they can thus better accomplish their tasks
- Provide an opportunity to each employee for self-reflection and individual goal-setting, so that individually planned and monitored development takes place

- Help employees internalize the culture, norms and values of the organization, thus developing an identity and commitment throughout the organization
- Prepare employees for higher responsibilities in the future by continuously reinforcing the development of the behavior and qualities required for higher-level positions in the organization
- Be instrumental in creating a positive and healthy climate in the organization that drives employees to give their best while enjoying in doing so.

Difficulties in Conducting Performance Appraisal

- Lack of support from the top levels of management
- Organization and culture
- Appraisers may fear the possibility of repercussions—Both for themselves and the appraise
- Consistently poor appraisal results will indicate a need for counselling, transfer or termination. The exact remedy will depend on the circumstances.

Important considerations in designing a performance appraisal system

- Ensure that the performance appraisal system is in alignment with evolving organizational goals
- Goal—The job description and the performance goals should be structured, mutually decided and accepted by both management and employees
- Reliable and consistent—Appraisal should include both objective and subjective ratings to produce reliable and consistent measurement of performance
- Practical and simple format—The appraisal format should be practical, simple and aim at fulfilling its basic functions. Long and complicated formats are time consuming, difficult to understand and do not elicit much useful information
- Regular and routine—While an appraisal system is expected to be formal in a structured manner, informal contacts and interactions can also be used for providing feedback to employees
- Participatory and open—An effective appraisal system should necessarily involve the employee's participation, usually through an appraisal interview with the supervisor, for feedback and future planning. During this interview, past performance should be discussed frankly and future goals established. A strategy for accomplishing these goals as well as for improving future performance should be evolved jointly by the supervisor and the employee being appraised. Such participation imparts a feeling of involvement and creates a sense of belonging
- Rewards—Both positive and negative—should be part of the performance appraisal system. Otherwise, the process lacks impact
- Relevance and responsiveness—Planning and appraisal of performance and consequent rewards or punishments should be oriented towards the objectives of the program in which the employee has been assigned a role, e.g. if the objectives of a program are directed towards a particular client group, then the appraisal system has to be designed with that orientation
- Commitment—Responsibility for the appraisal system should be located at a senior level in the organization so as to ensure commitment and involvement throughout the management hierarchy
- Organizing logistics—Data can be gathered by or in: Written surveys, Intranet or internet, Individual discussions and Group meetings
- The process can be coordinated by—Employee, Manager, Human Resources and an outside professional (External Examiner)
- Follow up for the organization—Use aggregated ratings for gap analysis and needs assessment, Track performance appraisal statistics to measure the success of the management development system, Train new hires and periodically retrain reviewers about how to evaluate reviewees and give useful feedback.
- Giving feedback—Follow up for the individual can include: A written development plan with goals, timelines and responsibilities, progress reports, additional meetings with manager, training to build on strengths and address needs, "Stretch" assignments or rotations, coaching and mentoring .
  - Unless feedback is timely, it loses its utility and may have only limited influence on performance. Performance can be appraised after each project is completed, after a milestone is reached, quarterly, Semi-annually or annually

- Feedback must be impersonal, Open and noticeable, if it is to have the desired effect. Personal feedback is usually rejected with contempt and eventually demotivates the employee. The staff member being appraised must be made aware of the information used in the appraisal process. An open appraisal process creates credibility
- Feedback meetings can include: Discussion of strengths and development needs, compensation ,team challenges and opportunities, development and career planning, goal setting for upcoming performance cycle, upward feedback
- Feedback reports can be (or not be): Filtered or summarized by manager , for an employee's file, shared with others, reviewed and approved by others and inclusive of tables or graphics
- Feedback reports can include: Attributed ratings and comments, Anonymous ratings and comments, statistics and comparisons—Weighted or unweighted ratings by competency or by reviewer and competencies necessary for advancement
- Feedback is most useful when it is: Honest, specific and actionable, based on more than one incident or example or based on more than one person's view, framed positively and constructively, behaviorally based rather than personality based and Summarized and integrated into key themes
- Feedback is least useful when it is: Inaccurate or untrue, biased due to favoritism or politics, insensitive, unduly critical and not specific or actionable, constituted by orders or ultimatums.

Performance improvement

Employee's objectives

- For self improvement and for achieving individual and organizational goals
- Employee gets a feedback of his or her performance which motivates him or her to perform better. It tells a subordinate how he or she is doing. It brings about awareness of the strengths and weaknesses and suggests needed changes in attitudes, skill or knowledge of the job
- To recognize that problems left unchecked could ultimately cause more harm to an employee's career than early detection and correction
- Frequent mini-appraisals and feedback sessions will help to ensure that employees receive the ongoing guidance, support and encouragement they need
- To review the priorities and values that it has instilled in its supervisory ranks
- Need to understand that the ingroup/outgroup bias, e.g. for instance reduces the morale and motivation of their subordinates
- Employee develops role clarity with regard to the job, especially when told what is expected of him or her (Job Responsibilities)
- Employee is able to clarify his or her career plan in the organization.

Appraiser's objectives

- Superior gets feedback on how well the institutional objectives have been communicated to the subordinates, facilities provided for their effective performance and ability to motivate them to perform; Manager can identify whether institutional objectives achieved or not. If not, the improvements need to be identified
- Review of the work situation with the employee and identification of the resource requirements and helps the appraiser in defining his or her own and department's contribution to institutional objectives.

Process of Performance appraisal System

Performance appraisal involves an evaluation of actual against desired performance. It also helps in reviewing various factors which influence performance. Managers should plan performance development strategies in a structured manner for each employee. In doing so, they should keep the goals of the organization in mind and aim at optimal utilization of all available resources, including finance. Performance appraisal is a multistage process in which communication plays an important role.

Craig, Beatty and Baird (1986) suggested an eight-stage performance appraisal process:
  i. Establishing standards and measures
  - To identify and establish standards and measures which would differentiate successful and unsuccessful performances. These measures should be under the control of the employees being

appraised. The methods for assessing performance should be decided next. Basically, management wants to know the behavior and personal characteristics of each employee and assess their performance and achievement in the job

- There are various methods available for assessing results, behavior and personal characteristics of an employee. These methods can be used according to the particular circumstances and requirements.

ii. Communicating job expectations

Communication is at the core of an appraisal system. Communicating to employees the measures and standards which will be used in the appraisal process. Such communication has to clarify expectations and create a feeling of involvement.

Communication can be either upward or downward. Downward communication is from upper management levels to lower levels, and passes on a judgement of how the employees are doing and how they might do even better. As the information flows downward, it becomes more individualized and detailed. Upward communication is from lower to higher levels. Through this process, employees communicate their needs, aspirations and goals. As information flows upward, it has to become brief and precise because of the channels through which it has to pass.

iii. Planning

The manager plans for the realization of performance expectations, arranging for the resources to be available which are required for attaining the goal set. This is an enabling role.

iv. Monitoring performance

Performance appraisal is a continuous process, involving ongoing feedback. Even though performance is appraised annually, it has to be managed each day, all year long. Monitoring is a key part of the performance appraisal process. It should involve providing assistance as necessary and removing obstacles rather than interfering. The best way to effectively monitor is to walk around, thus creating continuous contacts, providing first-hand information and identifying problems, which can then be solved promptly.

v. Appraising

This stage involves documenting performance through observing, recalling, evaluating, written communication, judgment and analysis of data. This is like putting together an appraisal record.

vi. Feedback

After the formal appraisal stage, a feedback session is desirable. This session should involve verbal communication, listening, problem solving, negotiating, compromising, conflict resolution and reaching consensus.

vii. Decision making

On the basis of appraisal and feedback results, various decisions can be made about giving rewards (e.g. promotion, incentives etc.) and punishments (e.g. demotion). The outcome of an appraisal system should also be used for career development.

viii. Development of performance or professional development

By providing opportunities for upgrading skills and professional interactions. This can be done by supporting participation in professional conferences or by providing opportunities for further study. Such opportunities can also act as incentives or rewards to employees.

Approaches in performance appraisal

- Performance appraisal is a multistage process involving several activities, which can be administered using a variety of approaches. Some of these approaches are based on Einstein and LeMere-Labonte, 1989; and Monga, 1983
- Intuitive approach—A supervisor or manager judges the employee, based on their perception of the employee's behavior
- Self-appraisal approach—Employees evaluate their own performance using a common format
- Group approach—The employee is evaluated by a group of persons
- Trait approach—This is the conventional approach. The manager or supervisor evaluates the employee on the basis of observable dimensions of personality, such as integrity, honesty, dependability, punctuality etc
- Appraisal based on achieved results—appraisal is based on concrete, measurable, work achievements judged against fixed targets or goals set mutually by the subject and the assessor

- Behaviorial method—It focuses on observed behavior and observable critical incidents
- Teacher Evaluation/Appraisal by teacher—Appraisal of performance on the job/clinical skills is most frequently carried out by the superior/teacher
- Essay appraisal method—The assessor writes a brief essay providing an assessment of the strengths, weaknesses and potential of the subject. In order to do so objectively, it is necessary that the assessor knows the subject well and should have interacted with them. Since the length and contents of the essay vary between assessors, essay ratings are difficult to compare
- Peer appraisal—It is possible to have peers to rate him/her, usually done in educational institutions., but very seldom done in a hospital situation. In organizations which primarily render service, the beneficiaries of the service may be primary appraisers
- Self appraisal—Appraisal of one's own job performance is advocated, because, each individual knows himself/herself best and he/she is aware of his/her strengths and weaknesses and of his/her efforts to achieve his/her personal and organization's goals.

Self appraisal is an important factor in participative management and in the achievement of individual and organizational goals. However, self appraisals are not widely used, the reasonsare Individuals do not wish to reveal their weaknesses and short comings on the job, more so as this information may be used against them when administrative decisions are taken.

In general, self appraisals are 'inflated' as most employees or students have an unrealistically favorable perception of their own performance.

Formats for appraisal

A common approach to assessing performance is to use a numerical or scalar rating system whereby managers are asked to score an individual against a number of objectives/attributes.

A performance appraisal system could be designed based on intuition, self-analysis, personality traits, behaviorial methods and result-based techniques. Different approaches and techniques could be blended, depending on the goals of performance appraisal in the organization and the type of review. For example, management by objectives, goal-setting and work standard methods are effective for objective coaching, counseling and motivational purposes. Critical incident appraisal is best suited when supervisor's personal assessment and criticism are essential. A carefully developed and validated forced-choice rating can provide valuable analysis of the individual when considering possible promotion to supervisory positions. Combined graphic and essay form is simple, effective in identifying training and development needs and facilitates other management decisions.

Techniques of Appraisal System

Several techniques exist for appraisal of employees in an organization. Each has its own combination of strengths and weaknesses. No one technique by itself is able to achieve all the purposes for which management institutes depends on three major factors:

- Utilization criteria why is performance evaluation being done
  The objective may be candidate/employee for selection or training, development, promotion, feedback or for any disciplinary action etc
- Qualitative criteria consideration of organizational constraints—Assumptions of the method, relevance of evaluation criteria, data availability, practicality, potential for equivalence and interpretability
- Quantitative criteria—Psychometric properties of the evaluation—Reliability, discriminability, accuracy, inherent rating errors.
  A technique which is potentially less subjective and more objective than another is preferred. 'Objectivity' is the ability of the format to bring out impartial, reliable and valid information about the individual, many formats are available.

1. Creating metrics/Rating scales

Ratings will be done on the basis of: General or specific standards or expectations, Improvement on past performance, Rankings or comparison to others.

Rating scales differ in terms of definition of ratings, number of possible ratings, Presence or absence of a midpoint.

Types

Forced distribution technique

Forced-choice rating method does not involve discussion with supervisors. Although this technique has several variations, the most common method is to force the assessor to choose the best and worst fit statements from a group of statements. These statements are weighted or scored in advance to assess the employee or candidate. The scores or weights assigned to the individual statements are not revealed to the assessor so that she or he cannot favor any individual. In this way, the assessor bias is largely eliminated and comparable standards of performance evolved for an objective. However, this technique is of little value wherever performance appraisal interviews are conducted.

The main advantage of this technique is that all employees cannot be given average or good ratings, some must be rated better than others. Though it is the best format when a supervisor has to evaluate a large number of subordinates, the scale is not frequently used.

- It is 'too gross' and does not discriminate between individuals in a group
- Problems occur with 'borderline' cases.

The scale does not explain the reasons for a certain performance gradation and the employee does not know what specifically he/she must do to improve his/her performance.

Forced choice rating method (Mixed standard scale)

A scale containing a number of statements. The appraiser is required to indicate those statements which best fit the employee and those which least describe the individual. The appraiser does not know which statements are indicative of high performance and which represent low and undesired behaviors or traits. Each statement carries a weight or score, but these scores are not revealed to the appraiser. After the evaluator completes the ratings, the personnel department arrives at an index of performance of the employee using the scoring key. For example: In Nursing Educational Institutions, Teachers will observe student's clinical performance and indicate student's performance in clinical areas by scale which will aid for clinical assessment and keep as a record in administrators' office, at the end of the academic year, the teaching faculty as a form of encouragement, give special awards like Best Clinical Nurse, Best Outgoing student, etc. which will be boost or motivating force for other students to perform better in future.

Advantages

- Performance evaluation is made more objective
- The scale reduces halo effect and leniency error and improves reliability of ratings
- The scale can be used for self appraisals.

Drawbacks

- The construction of the scale takes a great deal of time and effort
- The rating procedure tends to irritate appraisers who feel that they are not being trusted
- The method is not useful for appraisal interviews.

The ranking methods

Ranking methods however have a significant advantage in that they can be used even by untrained appraisers.

Ranking aims at establishing a rank order of employees/students based on their relative merit. In the method of alternation ranking the names of employees/students are listed in random order. The supervisor is asked to choose the 'most valuable' or 'intelligent' student/ employee, cross his/her name off and note it at the top of a list. He/she next selects the 'least valuable'/ least 'intelligent' employee/student, crosses him/her off and notes the name at the bottom of the list. The supervisor/educators continues this procedure on the remaining list of students/employees till all the rates have been ranked.

Paired comparison ranking entails that each employee is compared with each other employee. This method is much simpler than alternation ranking, requiring the appraiser to judge which of the two workers being compared is superior. The appraiser puts a tick mark on each slip against the individual whom he considers the better of tally marks against each name.

Drawbacks:

- It is too cumbersome to rank individuals when their number is 20 or more

- Comparisons involve an overall subjective judgment
- It is difficult to rank students/employees apart from and between the top and bottom extremes.

Some of the important forms of ranking for performance appraisal are based on Oberg, 1972; and Monga, 1983:

a. Alteration ranking method—The individual with the best performance is chosen as the ideal employee. Other employees are then ranked against this employee in descending order of comparative performance on a scale of best to worst performance. The alteration ranking method usually involves rating by more than one assessor. The ranks assigned by each assessor are then averaged and a relative ranking of each member in the group is determined. While this is a simple method, it is impractical for large groups. In addition, there may be wide variations in ability between ranks for different positions.

b. Paired comparison—The paired comparison method systematizes ranking and enables better comparison among individuals to be rated. Every individual in the group is compared with all others in the group. The evaluations received by each person in the group are counted and turned into percentage scores. The scores provide a fair idea as to how each individual in the group is judged by the assessor.

c. Person-to-person rating scales—The names of the actual individuals known to all the assessors are used as a series of standards. These standards may be defined as lowest, low, middle, high and highest performers. Individual employees in the group are then compared with the individuals used as the standards and rated for a standard where they match the best. The advantage of this rating scale is that the standards are concrete and are in terms of real individuals. The disadvantage is that the standards set by different assessors may not be consistent. Each assessor constructs their own person-to-person scale which makes comparison of different ratings difficult.

d. Checklist method—The assessor is furnished with a checklist of pre-scaled descriptions of behavior, which are then used to evaluate the personnel being rated (Monga, 1983). The scale values of the behavior items are unknown to the assessor, who has to check as many items as she or he believes describe the worker being assessed. A final rating is obtained by averaging the scale values of the items that have been marked.

Graphic rating scale/ Merit Rating scale/ Summated rating Scale

A graphic scale assesses a person on the quality of his or her work (average; above average; outstanding or unsatisfactory). Assessment could also be trait centered and cover observable traits such as: reliability, adaptability, communication skills, etc. Although graphic scales seem simplistic in construction, they have application in a wide variety of job responsibilities and are more consistent and reliable in comparison with essay appraisal. The utility of this technique can be enhanced by using it in conjunction with the essay appraisal technique.

An attempt is made to ascertain the degree of presence in the employee/student of certain characteristics—personality traits, knowledge, abilities, skills, quantity and quality of work. The responses, which can vary from three points on a horizontal scale may be just enumerate numerically (e.g. 5, 4, 3, 2, 1) or the scale points may be defined to indicate the degree of applicability of the criterion as: 'excellent, good, average, poor, very poor or always, often, sometimes, seldom, never'.It is easy and inexpensive to develop and administer; It provides information about the employee on a number of characteristics and the degree of their applicability; A composite score of each individual can be obtained. This enables study of an individual's performance over time as also comparison of the performance of two or more individuals at varying points of time.

Pitfalls

- Composite scores are deceptive. An identical total score may be obtained by two employees having significantly different specific traits
- The graphic rating scale is invariably associated with a great deal of subjectivity because personality traits are generally focused upon
- The graphic rating scale is subject to a number of errors: halo leniency, central tendency, logical, contrast, similar and proximity.

Field review method

Since individual assessors differ in their standards, they inadvertently introduce bias in their ratings. To overcome this assessor related bias, essay and graphic rating techniques can be combined in a systematic review process. In the field review method, 'a member of the HRM staff meets a small group of assessors from the supervisory units to discuss each rating, systematically identifying areas of inter-assessor disagreement.' It can then be a mechanism to help each assessor to perceive the standards uniformly and thus match the other assessors. Although field review assessment is considered valid and reliable, it is very time consuming.

The Behaviorally anchored rating scale

First developed by Smith and Kendall for staff nurses in 1963, It consists of sets of behaviorial statements describing good or bad performance with respect to important qualities. These qualities may refer to inter-personal relationships, planning and organizing abilities, adaptability and reliability. These statements are developed from critical incidents collected both from the assessor and the subject. The BARS assumes the following:

- A person's effectiveness on the job can be best inferred from the behavior on the job rather than on personality traits. Evaluation of behaviors is more objective than judging personality traits
- The employee's performance is complex and results from several dimensions. The amount or degree of each dimension can be effectively recorded through statements rather than by mere numerical gradation
- During the evaluation process, BARS forces appraisers to focus on an employee's actual behavior. The instrument is less subjective and shows higher validity and reliability and less halo effect.

Limitations

- The process of BARS construction is time consuming
- With a situation of high turn over amongst appraisers, the new appraisers no longer feel they have been involved in BARS construction
- BARS developed for one situation cannot be easily used in another situations the job requirements may be different in another situation.

2. The critical incident method

Supervisor describes critical incidents, giving details of both positive and negative behavior of the student or an employee. These are then discussed with the student /employee. The discussion focuses on actual behavior rather than on traits. While this technique is well suited for performance review interviews, it has the drawback that the supervisor has to note down the critical incidents as and when they occur. That may be impractical and may delay feedback to students/employees. It makes little sense to wait six months or a year to discuss a misdeed, a mistake or good display of initiative.

The critical incident approach to performance appraisal requires the appraiser to record factual incidents involving the student/employee which have been critical to the latter's effective or non effective performance. The usual procedure is to have the supervisor record (in a 'little book') actual incidents of positive or negative critical job behaviors concerning the subordinates appraisal form when required. A modification of the above method entails preparation of an extensive checklist of behaviors critical to the professional tasks, the supervisor has to review the same and recollect specific behaviors observed in the employee during the relevant period.

Advantages

- Evaluation of the individual is less subjective as the supervisor/teacher is forced to focus on behaviors specific to the job rather than on vaguely defined traits
- Appraisal interviews and counseling become easier when factual incidents can be cited to the employee
- This technique is effective when objective work standards or quantitative goals are not available.

Drawbacks

- The idea of the 'man with the little hook' hovering in the background and taking notes on conduct is hardly consistent with a mature attitude
- This method requires that supervisors' jot down incidents on a daily or at least a weekly basis. This can become a chore
- Appraisers are often seen to differ in their understanding of what behaviors are critical and hence have to be reported. this is partly overcome by having the behavioral checklist
- Critical or outstanding incidents happen relatively infrequently. This may result in the supervisor not having enough critical incidents to report for a large number of employees
- The technique tends to push the observer recorder towards picking up things to criticize.

3. Work standard approach

In this technique, management establishes the goals openly and sets targets against realistic output standards. These standards are incorporated into the organizational performance appraisal system. Thus each employee has a clear understanding of their duties and knows well what is expected of them. Performance appraisal and interview comments are related to these duties. This makes the appraisal process objective and more accurate. However, it is difficult to compare individual ratings because standards for work may differ from job to job and from employee to employee. This limitation can be overcome by some form of ranking using pooled judgment.

4. Appraisal by objectives

The employees are asked to set or help set their own performance goals. This avoids the feeling among employees that they are being judged by unfairly high standards. This method is currently widely used, but not always in its true spirit. Even though the employees are consulted, in many cases management ends up by imposing its standards and objectives. In some cases employees may not like 'self-direction or authority.' To avoid such problems, the work standard approach is used.

In this appraisal format the employee and his superior review the achievement of the former's objectives which had been previously setup and agreed upon. The focus is on analysis of actual performance rather than on appraisal of traits or behaviors. It concentrates on what an employee does rather than what his superior thinks of him.

Appraisal by objectives involves the following processes:
- The top management should formulate the goals for a definite period
- Departmental heads next translate the organizational objectives into specific departmental objectives and lay down priority in terms of key result areas
- Staff of a department review the key result areas and evolve a results involvement—matrix showing the major contribution, minor contribution or advisory involvement of the person
- Each individual then lists out specific time bound action plans to achieve the key task. The supervisor coordinates this process
- At the end of a specified period (six months to one year) the individual and his superior meet again to review the former's performance in the light of objectives setup earlier.

Appraisal by objectives has much to recommend
- The focus is on analysis of performance and not on a judgment of personality or of behavior
- The subordinate is no longer a 'passive' object being evaluated. He/she is an active agent responsible for his/her own career, growth and development and striving to achieve individual and organizational goals
- The employee develops clarity regarding his/her work and the contribution required from him. He/she is involved in decision making, thus contributing towards increase work motivation
- The method is not favorable if the data generated from appraisals are to be used primarily for administrative and control purposes.

5. The appraisal interview

The appraisal interview is held periodically, between the superior (appraisor) and subordinate (appraisee). The latter is given a feed back on how his/her work performance during the period under review has been perceived by the superior. Depending on the nature of the interview, the discussions may include reactions the subordinate may have to the appraisal, analysis of the factors facilitating or inhibiting his performance, additional resources that may be required by the subordinate for effective performance, setting up of specific performance objectives for the future, discussion of the indvidual's career in the organization, identification of his/her training needs, superior—subordinate interaction, etc. the appraisal interview, though desirable, is not an essential part of the appraisal process.

Appraisal interviews may follow:
- The tell and sell method, where the supervisor informs the subordinate in the best manner possible of his ratings and advices him on how to improve
- The tell and listen method, where the appraiser communicates his evaluation to the employee and allows the subordinate to react to the appraisal

- The problem solving approach, the focus being on 'analysis' rather than on 'appraisal' and what needs to be done to improve performance.

Objectives
- Providing legitimate feedback to the individual on how his/her performance is perceived by his/her superior
- Information communicated through such interviews may be a source of satisfaction and motivation to the employee, especially if feedback is positive
- The employee can, at such a discussion, achieve role clarity with regard his job
- The subordinate, while coming to know of his/her weaknesses, can focus on corrective action. The superior can also plan training programs, continuing education etc.
- The employee obtains greater knowledge of the organization, his/her superior expectations, clarifications of his/her career plan in the organization, etc. however, appraisal interviews are not often held because
  - The discussion of rating with employee often results in traumatic experiences for the subordinate and in superior—Subordinate conflicts which affect the work situation
- Negative ratings can result in demotivation and decreased performance, especially when the individual considers himself/herselfbetter than the superior's assessment of him/her
- Appraisal in often associated with salary decisions, promotions, transfer, dismissals, etc. the employee is, thus, defensive during appraisal discussions when negative appraisals are likely to have an untoward effect on him
- The superior feels inadequate about justifying the rating to his/her subordinate by citing relevant critical incidents
- Many supervisors shown progress interviews as they fear opening a situation which they will not be able to cope with such as if the employee asked for a raise, he questions the manner of running the department, etc.

It is important to ensure that appraisal interviews do not cause ill will. This can be ensured by having the supervisor ask himself/heself at every stage, 'will what I am about to say, help this man'? appraisal interview are effective if the employee participates actively in the discussion, is involved in setting specific performance goals for himself/herself, and if the interview is designed primarily to improve an employee's performance rather than be connected to his/her salary or promotion.

Periodicity of appraisal
Performance appraisal is most often conducted as an annual activity, though for trainees and new recruits, quarterly frequency is usually the norm. Thus employees may be rated at the same time during the year or on the anniversary date of employment of the respective individual.

Most appraisals attempt at gathering information for administrative purposes and also for self improvement and growth of the individual. Simultaneous attainment of both these objectives is not practicable as the moment data are required for control purposes, critical information pertaining to weaknesses of the person is not revealed in the appraisal process. The organization should therefore be clear about what objectives are to be achieved through the appraisal processes.

Focus on traits versus behaviors
Assessment of personality traits in preference to work behaviors is associated with grave implications, in that the ratings are not reliable, they tend to focus on an individual's personality rather than on his/her contribution to the organization, and the interpretation of traits varies markedly with people and therefore tends to be subjective.

Multiple criteria scores versus a composite score
Composite scores are often required when comparing the performance of several individuals for selection, placement, promotion, incentives, etc. however, they have the drawback that the facts of performance are not brought out through composite scores are not useful for feedback and for analysis of the individual's performance.

6. Assessment centers
This technique is used to predict future performance of employees were they to be promoted. The individual whose potential is to be assessed has to work on individual as well as group assignments similar to those they

would be required to handle they were promoted. The judgment of observers is pooled and paired comparison or alteration ranking is sometimes used to arrive at a final assessment. The final assessment helps in making an order-of-merit ranking for each employee. It also involves subjective judgment by observers.

Components of the appraisal format

Key performance areas, self-appraisal, performance analysis, performance ratings and counseling are the important components of a performance appraisal system oriented to development of human resources in an organization. The appraisal format should be designed in consonance with the objectives of the performance appraisal system and generate information on a number of important aspects including

- Identification of key performance areas—The first step in an appraisal process is identifying key performance areas and setting targets for the next appraisal period. This may be done either through periodic discussions or at the beginning of the year, as in research institutions or end of the year as in Academic areas
- Self-appraisal by the subject—At the end of the appraisal period, employees/students appraise their own performance against the key performance areas, targets and pre-identified behavior. Information on these issues is provided in an appraisal format. The students/employees also write their self-evaluation reports and hand them to their supervisors
- Analysis—The supervisor reflects on the performance of the employee and identifies the factors which facilitated or hindered the employee's performance. The manager then calls the employee for a discussion to better understand his or her performance and provide counseling on further improvements. During this discussion, appraisal records (such as notes, observations, comments, etc.) are exchanged. The manager then gives a final rating and recommendations regarding the developmental needs of the individual. These are shown to the subject and his or her comments are recorded on the appraisal form. The appraisal form is then transmitted to the personnel department for the necessary administrative action. The personnel or human resource development department uses these forms for identifying and allocating training, rewards and other activities
- Identification of training needs—The use of a development-oriented performance appraisal system is based on a good understanding of the concept of human resources development. The need for developing employee capabilities, the nature of capabilities to be developed and the conditions under which these capabilities can be developed have to be appreciated. During the discussion between the supervisor and the employee, the development needs of the subject are identified and goals set for the next period
- Identification of qualities—The supervisor may also identify the qualities required for current as well as future tasks and assess the employee's potential and capabilities to perform jobs at higher responsibility levels in the organization.

Attributes considered in evaluating performance

There are many personality traits which could be considered when evaluating performance and methods to facilitate such consideration include scaling methods that differentiate employees on a series of given traits. The important personality traits fall into two categories: personal qualities and demonstrated qualities

Management problems in evaluating performance

Some of the important problems faced by managers in evaluating performance are identification of appraisal criteria, problems in assessment and policy-related problems.

1. Identification of appraisal criteria

Performance of a student or employee has to be measured in toto/the whole, qualitative assessment and quantitative assessment, as an integral part of the an academic program as it is multi dimensional.

2. Assessment problems

It is difficult to observe behavior and interpret it in terms of its causes, effects and desirability. Rating behavior on an appraisal form is quite difficult. The human element plays a significant role in the appraisal process and introduces subjectivity and bias. This can be minimized by: documenting performance from time to time; basing criteria for evaluation on observable behavior; training the supervisors and effectively communicating the expectations which management requires.

Personal and demonstrated personality traits

Personal Qualities	Demonstrated Performance Qualities
Adaptability: Adjustment with new or changing situations or people. *Appearance and bearing:* Having good bearing and appearance. *Decisiveness:* Ability to arrive at conclusions promptly and to decide on a definite course of action. *Dependability:* Ability to consistently accomplish allocated jobs without supervision. *Drive and determination:* Ability to execute job vigorously and resolutely, and induce others to do so. *Ingenuity:* Resourcefulness and ability to creatively devise means to solve unforeseen problems. *Initiative:* Ability to take necessary and appropriate action independently. *Integrity:* Ability to maintain an honest approach in all dealings. *Loyalty:* Ability to faithfully, willingly and loyally support superiors, equals and subordinates. *Maturity:* Understanding and balance commensurate with age and service. *Stamina:* Ability to withstand and perform successfully under protracted physical strain. *Tenacity:* Ability to preserve in face of odds and difficulties. *Verbal expression:* Ability to express oneself clearly and concisely. *Written expression;* Ability to express oneself clearly and concisely in writing.	*Professional knowledge:* Ability to apply professional knowledge to assigned duties so as to achieve a high standard of performance. *Administrative ability:* Having administrative ability to use resources economically and judiciously. *Responsibility for staff development:* Ability to fulfil responsibilities in the development and training of staff. *Foresight:* Ability to display foresight and plan beyond immediate needs. *Delegation:* Ability to delegate responsibilities and exercise required degree of guidance and supervision. *Motivation:* Ability to motivate subordinates effectively to produce desired results. *Morale:* Ability to maintain morale and look after the management of staff. *Control:* Ability to exercise control over subordinates and gain their confidence.

(**Source:** Adapted from an appraisal form of an organization illustrated in Monga, 1983.),

3. Policy related Problems
The results of the appraisal system should be followed up through a set of well designed and enforced policies and translated into positive forms like rewards and negative forms like punishments, demotions or failures. Performance is sometimes difficult to assess. An assessor/Educator/Manager has to balance between employees'/ students' creativity and organizational goals.

CONCLUSION
Despite the numerous problems associated with appraisal, most organizations continue to have the formal and good appraisal program to maintain quality.

A sound appraisal program must satisfy the following basic requirements:
- The system must be consistent with the management style and philosophy, work technology, Organizational policy, goals and socio cultural characteristics of the individuals concerned
- It should be in tune with other personnel program such as the system of rewards, compensation schemes, training programs, etc.
- The technology in use should have the cooperation of the appraisers. It should have the ability to assess, in as objective manner as possible, the performance and effectiveness of an individual as related to his/her job.

QUESTIONS

- Advantages and disadvantages of essay type of questions (5M, RGUHS, Feb, 2010)
- Advantages and disadvantages of Practical Examinations (5M, RGUHS, Aug, 2009)
- Advantages of multiple choice questions (5M, RGUHS, Sept, 2009)
- Anecdotes (4M, NTRUHS, Dec, 2007)
- As a principal College of Nursing explains your responsibilities related to the Clinical Evaluation of the students. (10 M, RGUHS, April 2007)
- Assessment (5M, NTRUHS, Dec, 2007)
- Briefly explain philosophy and aims of education (5M, RGUHS, Sept, 2009)
- Checklist (5M, Rajasthan UHS, Feb, 2008 & March, 2010)
- Criteria for selection of Evaluation Devices(4M, NTRUHS, June, 2009)
- Define Evaluation (2 M), List the Criteria of Evaluation (3 M), Explain the Methods of Evaluation of students in clinical area, write the Merits and Demerits (15 M, MGRUHS, Aug, 2006)
- Define evaluation and explain its importance. Discuss the method of assessment of skills in a nursing students (10M, RGUHS, Aug, 2010)
- Define evaluation, (b) Explain qualities of evaluation tool (c) Prepare a rating scale to assess the clinical performance of I year B.SC Nursing students (2 +4 + 4M, MGU, Dec, 2006)
- Define evaluation. What are the principles of evaluation? Prepare four multiple choice questions on prevention of dengue fever (10M, RGUHS, Feb, 2010)
- Define Evaluation? Write its importance and steps in evaluation (5M, NTRUHS, Dec, 2007)
- Describe OSPE and OSCE with examples (15M, Baba Farid UHS, 2010)
- Describe the purpose of evaluation, Role of teacher in evaluation (5+10M, NTRUHS, Nov. 2010)
- Describe the types of Reliability (5M, MGRUHS, May, 2008)
- Differences between Formative Evaluation -Summative evaluation (5M, MGU, Oct, 2007 and 5M, MGU, Nov, 2006)
- Disadvantages of Multiple Choice Questions (2M, RGUHS, Feb, 2010)
- Discuss different Methods of Evaluation the Nursing students in the class room and Clinical field situations. (15 M, RGUHS, April 2006)
- Essay type Questions (5M, NIMs, Dec, 2009)
- Explain likert attitude scale (5M, MGRUHS, May, 2008)
- Explain the steps in constructing a test(10M,RGUHS, Aug, 2010 & 10M, MGRUHS, May, 2010)
- Explain validity (10M, RGUHS, May, 2008)
- Functions of Evaluation (5 M, MGRUHS, Feb, 2009)
- Give examples of Multiple Choice Questions (9M, Baba Farid UHS, 2008)
- How can attitude be measured and changed (10M, RGUHS, May, 2010)
- Important Steps in Evaluation (10 M, RGUHS, April, 2009)
- Internal assessment (5M, MGU, Dec, 2008)
- List the criteria for Selection of Assessment Techniques and Methods (5M, RGUHS, 2010),
- List the purpose of educational evaluation, Explain the qualities of an evaluation tool, Describe the evaluation tool used to assess the clinical performance of students (3+7+10 = 20 M, MGU, Dec,2008)
- List the tools used in assessing the skill of students. Prepare a check list to assess the student's performance on hand washing (10M, RGUHS, Aug, 2010)
- MCQ (5M, NTRUHS, June & Nov2010)
- Mention two differences between Measurement and Evaluation (10 M, MGRUHS, Aug, 2008)
- Methods of Internal assessment (5M, MGU,Oct,2007)
- Name any four Standardised Tests (10 M, MGRUHS, Aug, 2008)
- Objective Structured Clinical/Practical Examination (5M, NIMS, Sept, 2010)
- Objective Tests (5M, MGRUHS, Nov, 2010 & 5M, MGU, Dec,2006)
- Objective type of questions (5M, MGU, Nov, 2009; 5M, MGU, Dec,2008)
- Principles of educational evaluation (5M, MGU, Oct, 2007)

- Principles of Evaluation (5M, Rajasthan UHS, March, 2010)
- Principles of test construction (5M, MGU,Oct,2007)
- Purposes of Evaluation (5 M, MGRUHS, Aug, 2008 & Nov, 2010)
- Qualities of Evaluation Tool(5M, MGRUHS, Nov, 2010)
- Rating Scale (5 M, MGRUHS, Aug, 2008)
- Scope of Evaluation (5M, Rajasthan UHS, Feb, 2008)
- Steps in Evaluation (4M, NTRUHS, June, 2009 and 5M, RGUHS, 2009)
- Teacher's Evaluation (5M, NTRUHS, Dec, 2007)
- Technique of questioning (2M, RGUHS, Feb, 2010)
- Three advantages of essay tests (3M, MGU, Dec, 2006)
- Three principles of objective type test (3M, MGU, Oct, 2007)
- Three types of standardized tests (3M, MGU, Dec, 2006)
- Tools of Evaluation (5 M, MGRUHS, Feb, 2009)
- Validity (2M, RGUHS, Aug, 2010)
- What are the different tools and methods used in Clinical Evaluation and write in detail on any one of the method (15M, NIMS, Oct, 2008)
- What are the major considerations in the Evaluation of a Text Book (2M, MGRUHS, Feb, 2009)
- What are the prerequisites to successful Questioning (2M, MGRUHS, Feb, 2009)
- What do you understand by the term "Evaluation"? (2M, MGU, Dec, 2006)
- What do you understand by the term Evaluation? Discuss different methods of evaluation the Nursing students in the class room and clinical field situations. (10M,RGUHS, Oct, 2006)
- What is item analysis (2M, MGRUHS, May, 2008)
- What is a Check List? (2M), Differentiate between Rating Scale & Check list (3M), Write a sample Check list for Ryles Tube Feeding Procedure (10M, MGRUHS, Aug, 2007)
- What is Item Difficulty , Item Analysis (2M + 5M, MGRUHS, May, 2008 & 10M May, 2010)
- Write in detail about method of evaluation in Nursing Education (15M, RGUHS, May 2010)
- Write in detail about Performance appraisal(10M,RGUHS, M.Sc.(N), Aug, 2010, 5M,NTRUHS, June 2009 & Nov, 2010)
- Write the meaning of Evaluation and measurement, Describe the characteristics of a good evaluation tool that may be used in the clinical area, prepare a tool to evaluate baby bath procedure(15M, NIMS, Sept,2010)

Communication

INTRODUCTION

Communication is the exchange of ideas, facts, feelings, thoughts, opinions and information which is vital in facilitating human interaction through (written or spoken) words, symbols or actions. Communication is essential for progress of any individual and it is the back bone in establishing good interpersonal human relationships. To adapt, to change or to develop the abilities, an individual incorporates the spirit and artful skills of communication into every step of his plan of activities.

DEFINITIONS

"Anything that conveys meaning, that carries a message from one person to another; from student to teacher, from student to student, from teacher to student, from administrator to teacher and so on"–Field of Education

"Imparting, conveying or the exchange of ideas, knowledge, meanings, etc. among individuals through the medium of a sign of some kind", e.g. Symbol.

"A process by which two or more people exchange ideas, facts, feelings or impressions in ways that each gains a 'common understanding' of meaning, intent and use of a message"–*Paul Leagens*.

"Communication is a two way process of sharing and transmitting ideas, information and messages between two or more individuals".

Meaning

"A dynamic process, emergent, containing unprecedented elements, a contingent sequence of events, interactional, interpersonal, intrapersonal, subjective narratization of thoughts, within an environment of ever changing situations, conditions, creating shared meaning, succeeding in its stated aims, goals or objectives, shared codes, through a verbal or nonverbal system that appear to be symbolic, with a wide vocabulary and semantic sensitivity, intentionally sent, transmitted with previous knowledge of idea, desire and hope for outcome of the sender or source and with the potential for feedback from another with the capability of returning by word or deed the intent of the communicator".

Effective communication requires knowledge of the symbols, the cues, stimuli to which other persons will react.

It consists of 6 small messages
1. What do you mean to say?
2. What do you actually say?
3. What the other person hears?
4. What the person thinks he hears?
5. What the other person says?
6. What do you think the other person says?

Ways of communication
1. Oral or written
2. Sign/Signal or Symbol
3. Action
4. Object

Purposes/Goals
- Communicator formulates behavioral objectives like information on awareness, action, continuation and updating
- Promotes clear thinking
- Brings change in desired direction
- Helps in achieving predetermined objectives
- Specific and meaningful information will be transferred
- People communicate in consistent ways
- Regulates the behavior
- Creates a positive environment
- Facilitates verbalization of feelings
- Identifies the teaching topic, objectives/goals, issues to be attacked in dealing with a specific session, methods, formulates teaching learning activities, adapts techniques of evaluating receivers' level of understanding
- The concept or the content of the message has to be communicated clearly by using simple terms
- Utilizes multiple techniques/methods (verbal, mechanical and Non verbal means) to convey message
- Understands and verifies the extent of comprehension capacity of decoder/receiver
- Acceptance of message which has to be communicated
- Obtains feedback from the learners about the effectiveness of the session
- Promotes mental development of the learner/audience
- Increases the knowledge, brings change in the existing patterns of behavior and attitude among learners
- Acquires new skills
- Sharing of information and ideas
- Influencing people for behavioral change in attitudes and beliefs
- Persuasion and negotiation of predefined issues
- Motivates for efficiency in knowledge and skills
- Provides instructions
- Reaching decisions and coming to conclusions
- Builds human relationship
- Entertainment.

The Communication Process

It begins with the sender who encodes an idea, which can be sent in oral/written/visual/in some or other form to the receiver. The receiver decodes the message and gains an understanding of what the sender wants to communicate, this in turn may result some change or an action in their behavior.

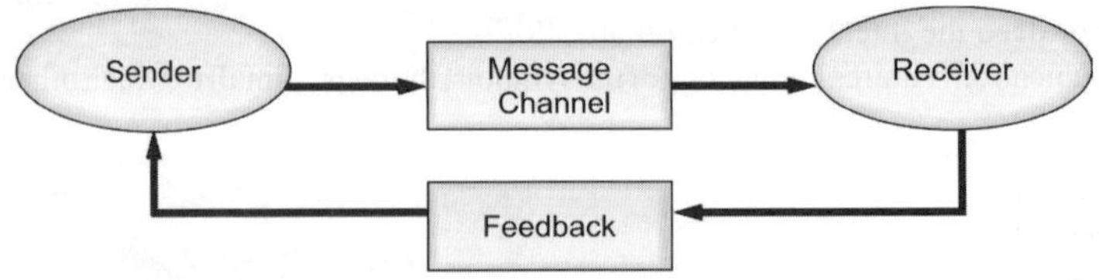

Fig. 9.1: Communication process

Elements:

Communication is an interactive process of 5 elements which ensures
- Who?
- Says What?
- What Channel?
- To whom?
- With what effect?

The transmission model of communication has five main parts according to Karen Reynolds
- Information source–where the message is produced
- Transmitter–where the message is encoded
- Channel–where the signal is carried
- Receiver–where the message is decoded
- Destination–where the message ends up

Components
- Source/Sender/Encoder/Communicator
- Message/Content/Medium
- Channel/a transmitter/Medium
- Receiver/Decoder /Audience
- Feedback/Effect/Impact

1. The Source/Encoder/Teacher/Sender

The teacher who wishes to affect the behavior of a student or a group serves as the source for communication by originating or perceiving an idea or purposes, which they want to communicate in order to produce a particular response. This purpose must be encoded (transformed) into the form of a message which can be transmitted. The teacher may directly encode their message through perceiving, thinking, reasoning, judging, speaking, writing, drawing, gesturing, demonstrating etc., into iconic or digital signs designed to attain the desired response from the student.

On the other hand, the teacher may use a mediated source to convey the desired message or to assist them in conveying their own message to the student. In this case, the message has been originated and encoded by a source.

Varied factors within the teacher (source) will influence the effectiveness of the communication.

a. Communication skills

Factors which will influence the skills of communicator
- The words they have at their command
- The way they put them together—It affects; how they think about
- Think thrice before communicating, e.g. speak or act
- Effective/"active" listening in which the provider gives small verbal or nonverbal feedback that indicates to the client that (s) he/she is being heard and understood
- Rephrasing what the client has said to make sure it is correctly understood
- Asking open-ended questions, asking the client to answer questions with more than one word answers
- Making eye contact
- Providing complete attention, not being curt or showing a condescending attitude toward the client

b. The verbal skills constitute the primary communication skills in man are
- Speaking and writing (encoding skills)
- Listening and reading (decoding skills)
- Intellectual skills (perceiving, memorizing, reasoning, judging and abstracting)

Words are digital (abstract) signs used to convey meaning, the clarity, the preciseness of language, it facilitates in effectiveness of the communication of the message. It will affect what she/he thinks about and how she/he thinks about it, her/his ability to speak and to write clearly will influence her/his effectiveness as a communicator.

The information and the understanding that the teacher possesses related to which she/he wishes to communicate effectively with her/his students.

Teacher needs to know the symbols, the cues, the stimuli to which students will react, so he/she can select appropriate media and signs which will help to communicate the messages he/she has selected to attain the desired responses of her students.

c. Attitude

It is the tendency or predisposition to act in a particular direction to a thing, person or an event.

The character of sender/Resource/Encoder

Attitude towards

- Themselves
- Subject
- Others
- The receiver/the decoder/the learner
- Teaching

For example, if the teacher lacks self-confidence, does not respect their students or is bored with the subject, blocks the communicative process

Conversely, if she/he has self-confidence, respects her/his students, shows interest and enthusiasm for subject, the communicative process will be facilitated.

d. Knowledge

The extent or mastery over the subject matter will affect the confidence levels in delivering lecture/content/message will be communicated with maximum effectiveness

e. Socio-cultural System

The source/encoder communicates as a free agent without being influenced by his/her position in the serial set-up–the position one holds influences the communication. Therefore we need to take into account the personal factors in the source, communication skills, attitudes, knowledge of the subject and the kind of social system in which he/she is operating influences the quality of communication. Greater familiarity of the source, greater will be the communication. The people in different social class communicate differently, word choices people makes, the purposes they have for communicating, the choice of receivers, the channels they use etc., also influences the effectiveness of communication. Perception of the sources position in a social and cultural context will affect general communication behavior. The social system, the roles fulfilled in that system, the functions performed, all influences communication behavior. Self expectations of the teacher and the expectations of others, (students/learners, parents, school administrators) in the teaching-learning setting have definite influence in the communication process.

2. Message

The message is some desired behavior in physical form, it is the translation of the ideas, the purposes and the intentions of the teacher (source) into a code, i.e. a systematic set of iconic and digital signs. A sign is a strong determiner of behavior. Message is what is transmitted in the communication process and message content is related to the behavior that needs to be changed or encouraged. Messages should be transmitted in the local language, in appropriate tone and at the appropriate time. It always has to be pretested.

a. Natural sign: A part of the larger thing or event or condition signified by it. For example: Blood on surgical dressing is a sign of hemorrhage.
b. Non-natural signs: Which symbolize something is designated.
c. Iconic sign: A sign is like the thing it signifies.
d. Digital sign: Independent of their physical parameters for their meaning. For example: pattern, size or stimulus intensity.

The more the sign it represents, the more dependency for its meaning on its physical parameters and the greater in its iconicity. For example: A picture of a patient in a body cast is more like an actual plaster cast than live drawing of a patient in a cast and thus possesses more iconicity.'

Teacher communicates to her/his students not only the intended message but also certain aspects of personality and feelings of which she/he is unaware some times. The 'selective inattention' on the part of a speaker creates what has been frequently called the 'arc of distortion' between a speaker and the listener. The speaker (source) always communicates at least two things–the intended, as well as the unintended, if these two messages are inconsistent, the listener (receiver) may wonder which of them should determine her/his response. The 'arc of distortion' is further complicated by the listener's 'selective inattention'. One way of reducing the 'arc of distortion' on the part of both listener and speaker is to have the receivers' 'feedback' to the sender what she/he thinks she/he was saying.

Characteristics of an Effective Message
- Useful and comprehensive
- Precise and clear
- Correct and complete
- Relevant and interesting
- Has to motivate and lead to behavior change
- Message has to reach the person through all five senses
- Message should be as per the existing social norms and felt needs of community and should not contradict prevalent beliefs and practices
- Message has to improve the knowledge and skills of audience
- Message should be specific and scientific
- Message should seek attention, persuasive and convincing
- Different messages are required for different target groups
- Too many messages should not be given at the same time
- We need to make our messaging more effective by following certain essential principles, such as:
    - Keep the messages simple
    - Humanize them by stressing how they affect people's lives
    - Stress the positive, not just the negative
    - Communicate the science in understandable terms

Components
a. Message code: Any group of symbols that can be structured in a way that is meaningful to same person, e.g. Language.
b. Message content: The material in the message i.e., selected by the source to express with purpose or meaningful objectives based on felt needs and demand needs
   In a book, the message content includes the assertions that one makes, the information i.e., presented, the inferences drawn and the judgments proposed contents like codes has both elements and structure. It has to be presented in clear, specific, accurate, timely with adequate, interesting, understandable, fitting the audience in a correct order in a sequential and logical manner
c. Message treatment: The source encoder has choices available to him and in coding you can choose one or another set of elements from within the code. In this, sender demonstrates his/her style of communicating. We can define treatment of a message as the decisions which the communication source makes in selecting, arranging both codes and content.
   The form of the message will be influenced by the purpose and the intent of the source and by the type of channel selected to transmit the message.

3. Channel

In order to encode the purpose of the source into a message, some type of channel, e.g. media is needed between encoder and decoder. Channel is "A means of carrying information or a message from the communicator to the target audience", e.g. In face-to-face communication, the encoding function is performed and channeled directly by the intellectual, the sensory and the motor skills of the source, e.g. vocal mechanism for oral communication; muscle system for the writing words or the drawing of pictures, posture and gestures, facial expressions for non-verbal communication. These messages are transmitted from the source via some channel, e.g. sound waves carry the spoken word. When the teacher transmits the desired message by other means than through her/his own vocal mechanism, the various media eg: Audio-visual aids are used. We need a vehicle carrier. So in communicating the source has to choose a channel. The media buyers chose the best message vehicle. The media selection is determined by what is available? What are the source preferences and how much has to be spent on it? Which channels are received by the most of the people? Which channel has the most effect? Which channels are adaptable to the objectives and content of the message? The proper selection and use of channel results in successful communication. A combination of variety of methods of channels may be required to accomplish educational purpose, helps the learners/receivers to understand their situations and choose actions that improves their abilities.

Classification
- Mass Communication Channel
  Means of communicating messages to a large group of people or masses
- Group Communication Channel
  Means of communicating messages to a small group of people simultaneously and not to an individual
- Interpersonal Communication Channel
  Means of communicating messages to an individual face to face

Points to remember while selecting a Channel
- Availability
- Purpose and suitability
- Type of audience
- Type of messages
- Preference of audience
- Communication skills of communicator
- Cost effectiveness.

Media
Media is an agency through which communication takes place
Media of communication are:
    Electronic Media—Print Media
    Folk and Traditional Media—Alternate Media (Nukkad Natak, Street Play, etc.)

Points to remember while selecting a Media:
Educational level of target audience.
Media habits of target audience.
- Electronic media can have a better reach among a particular section of society and can be used for creating awareness and reinforcement of messages
- Print Media has limited use in areas with low literacy levels
- Folk and traditional media is more popular in rural and tribal areas
- Media-mix approach or use of various media forms at the same time is more effective.

4. Receiver/decoder/learner
The person at the other end of communication process is the receiver,may be a single person or group of persons. If the receiver does not have the skills of communication he will not be able to receive and decode the message that the source encoder has encoded. Sender must tune to the frequency of receiver, i.e. to his intellectual capacity. Importance of communication is to improve others in all (sources) spheres. The learner (student) for whom the message is intended is considered as the receiver in the communication process in the teaching-learning situation. The student (receiver) has to decode the message, i.e. must listen, read, think, interpret, reason and judge the message. The teacher who wishes to communicate effectively with their students, either directly or with the help of audio-visual aids will need to know her/his students abilities and their level of understanding the knowledge.

Types of Receiver/the Audience/Decoder
a. Controlled/Homogeneous Group
   A group of persons held together with a common interest. Effective communication takes place since the group possess common interest/felt need to acquire new information and getting benefit out of it, e.g. a batch of students in a specific educational training programme
b. Uncontrolled Group/Free Audience
   A group of individuals gathered together, who has curiosity to acquire or more inquisitive to learn and enrich their knowledge, interested to lead qualitative life by practicing adequate health practices. These people will pose a challenge to the ability of an Educator, e.g. a group of young adults attending for an Health Education session in a selective communication

Types of communication

Comparison between One-way and Two-way Communication

1. One Way Communication (Didactic Method)	2. Two Way Communication (Socratic Method)
Appears neat and efficient to an outside observer, less or no feedback from audience	Audience will understand very easily
Accuracy is less	More Accurate than One Way communication
Orderly, systemic	Receivers are more sure of themselves and make correct judgments of how right or wrong they are
Sender is more psychologically comfortable	Sender finds himself psychologically under attacked, as receivers pick up his/her mistakes
Knowledge is imposed	Much more trial and error method

3. Interpersonal Communication

It is a process in which the communicator and the communicatee engage in a face-to-face interaction, e.g. interviews, group meetings. It is the process of sending and receiving information between two or more people. It differs from other forms of communication in that there are few participants involved, the interactions are in close physical proximity to each other and feedback is immediate. The campaigner should introduce himself/ herself to local authorities, local leaders and community and brief them about the programme. This will make the work easier and help the programme managers to get adequate support from everybody. Group meetings, focus group discussion, different indoor games like ludo, jig-saw puzzle, building blocks, as well as outdoor games, jingles, slogans, pada yatra, adopting influence of the community and religious leaders, senior citizens/elderly person etc. are part of interpersonal communication. The campaigner should take a round of the village, go from door to door to know the people, talk to them, try to find their day to day problems and gain their confidence. Some of the institutions that could be effectively involved for creating awareness are school teachers and children, Anganwadis workers, scout and guides, NSS, NCC, religious and charitable organization and community based organizations.

a. Dyadic communication—It allows for more specific tailoring of the message and more personal communication than do many of other media, e.g. Telephone interview

b. Public speaking, e.g. organizing health awareness campaign, Spiritual retreats

c. Small group communication, e.g. clinical discussions

It is considered important for insuring comprehension of a communication, in identifying barriers to communication and in resolving conflicting motives related to the adoption of a practice. On the basis of this scrutiny, a consensus is build in the community whether to accept or reject the message.

4. Serial communication

The message will be passed person to person like a chain. Sender pass the message to one person, then that receiver passes information to other and so on.

5. Mechanical communication:

By using mechanical devices the message will be communicated or transferred, e.g. typing, computer assisted like internet, web site.

6. Physiological communication

If a stimulus received by the body immediately the brain receives the information and transmits to the respective organ through the neurons, where it has to be passed.

7. Psychic communication

Extra sensory perception occurs, i.e. something which will occur in future. The person perceives and predicts that in advance is called psychic communication.

8. Verbal communication

Language is the chief vehicle of verbal communication. Through it, one can interact with other and exchange of ideas and thoughts will take place and information can be passed through. Most persuasive. "When we communicate verbally with others, in a conversation or in a presentation our goal is, to make people/listeners to understand what we are trying to say. Keep it short, simple and careful in selection of words. It requires a common spoken and written language with consistent messages. It is our responsibility to make sure our message gets across to our audience. When we communicate, we need to put ourselves in our listener's shoes. The tone of voice can communicate feelings and emotions that are as significant as the words being spoken. Accordingly, it is important to choose words that do not offend in any way and that are easily understood. One should avoid using trigger words, jargon, medical or other sophisticated terms. The use of particular languages may be important in reaching all sections of a community, e.g. Housewives/Home makers may speak fewer languages than men due to less exposure to out side.

9. Non-verbal communication

In non-verbal communication, body position, gestures, posture and facial expression, often referred to as "body language", can communicate as much as words. It is often through such body language that we express our attitudes towards an issue, a person or a person's behavior, the ideas or the processes will be communicated. Service providers must become skilled in interpreting the body language of users as this may assist them in understanding users' needs and concerns more fully. Service providers must also be aware of their own body language and the signals they may be unknowingly sending to users (e.g. movements or expressions that indicate fatigue, boredom, fear, frustration, indecision). It is important that the attitude conveyed by the service provider be compassionate and non-judgmental through gestures, body movements, posture, facial expressions etc.

10. Formal communication

- Officially organized channels of communication like line of authority, vertical transmission of information. For example: Principal will transmit his/her directions through faculty to a group of students in educational institutions
- Chances for delay in communication

11. Informal communication

- Communication is very faster here. For example: Family, friends, interest groups, like-minded people and casual groups.

12. Mass communication

Mass Communication technique helps in providing information to large audience in a short time. The communication process is information centered and for awareness creation. In certain cases, it results in change in cognitive level but change of attitude for expected behavioral change can not be achieved through mass communication. The Sender will use one or more channels for communicating message to a group of larger population. Audience are free and uncontrolled in nature. Sender will use mass media like TV, Radio, LCD, Projected aids, printed media etc. to reach group. The feed back mechanisms are poorly organized or it takes some time to receive feedback. This method of communication is impersonal in nature and difficult to change the established behavior. The channel is mainly used for creating awareness and transferring knowledge, e.g. Electronic Media, Films; Film Quickies; Video, Tapes; Video Quickies; Radio Programmes; Radio Spots; Audio Tapes; TV Programme; TV Quickies/Spot, Slides, Print Media, Books; Booklets; Folders and Leaflets; Handbills; Letters; Newspapers, Advertisements, Press release; Posters, Kiosks; Photographs; Hoardings; Magazines; Newsletters; Journals, Folk and Traditional Media, Song; Dance; Drama; Kirtan/Bhajan; Puppet Show; Nagada, Wall Writing, Alternate Media, Street Play; Nukkad Natak, Nautanki; Multimedia Campaigns, Publicity Campaigns /Awareness Campaigns; Exhibitions etc. Channel is mainly helps in changing attitudes and practices and bringing about behavioral change. It enhances effectiveness of mass and group communication, provides personal reinforcement, is resource effective and is well accepted in rural and tribal areas, e.g. Home visits, Counselling, Negotiation, Motivation and Persuasion.

13. Group Communication

In Group Communication channel is used for reaching out the selected or smaller group of people for motivating and influencing them usage of normal aids, e.g. usage of visual aids like Flip Book, Flannel Graph, Flash Cards, Charts, Bulletin Board etc. In Teachings groups by specific teaching methods, e.g. Lecture; Group by Meetings; Demonstration; Camps; Field Visit and Role Play

14. Written Communication

Sender will write and print the message content or the scientific information, which is useful to a larger population or to a group of learners, e.g. Teaching materials, Text Books, Published or unpublished articles etc. it ownot be so persuasive like spoken words or teaching by lecture or demonstration method but effective among interested literates.

15. Visual Communication

With the help of visual aids, e.g. Charts, Printed materials, Posters, Flash cards, diagrams, pictures, graphic aids etc. the information will be transmitted to the group of learners or the audience helps in enriching their knowledge in field of interest.

16. Telecommunication

With the help of electromagnetic instruments the message will be communicated globally, e.g. through Satellite, internet, TV, Radio (Channels of Mass Communication), the interested self motivated group will be getting benefitted and they will obtain the information as per their own schedules or at their convenience.

17. Point to point Communication system

It is closer to interpersonal communication, e.g. Telephone, Telex, Telegraph, Postal services. In this type of communication both the encoder and decoder are specific and predetermined.

18. Electronic Communication

The need for electronic communication requires a common 'health language' covering all the basic elements of health and health care: hence the need for the development of controlled terminologies. Each entry incorporates sufficient elements to differentiate one individual entity from another. The essential characteristic of a terminology is that of discrimination.

Techniques

1. Be interested and focus on the student.
2. Share the desk with the student.
3. Listen. Do not interrupt. Re-state what the student has told you. Keep the student on track.
4. Allow for silence. Read body language.
5. Suggest alternatives and discuss consequences. Do not tell the student what he/she should do. Do not assure the student that things will be OK. Work for solutions.
6. Do not be judgmental: be a helper!

Qualities of a Good Communicator

1. She/He knows
   - Objectives (clear, specific)
   - Her/His audience–their needs, attitudes, perception, interests, abilities and predispositions
   - Her/His messages–content, validity, usefulness, meaningful and importance
   - The channels–that will reach the audience and their usefulness
   - How to organize and treat her/his message
   - Her/His own professional abilities and limitations.
2. She/He is interested in his/her audience and their welfare
   - Her/His message and how it can help the people
   - The results of communication and their evaluation
   - The communication process
   - The communication channels, their proper use and limitations
   - How to improve his/her communication skill.
3. She/He prepares
   - Plan for communication
   - Communication material and equipment
   - A plan for evaluation of results
   - She/he has skill in selecting message, treating message, expressing message, selection and use of channels understanding her/his audience and collecting the results.

Principles of Communication
- Based on objectives and purpose which is appropriate to situation
  - Promotes total achievement of purpose
  - Represent the personality and individuality of the communicator
  - It involves special preparation
  - By personal contact
  - Has to be oriented to the interest and needs of the receiver
  - Familiar
  - It has to seek attention
  - Credibility is vital for communication
- Communication programme should make use of existing facilities to the great extent possible and should avoid challenging them unnecessarily, e.g. Organizing IEC programme

Facilitators in Communication Process
Facilitation is the art of leadership in Group communication. A facilitator is one who fulfills this leadership role. The term "Facilitation" is often employed interchangeably with "moderating" and "Facilitator" as "Moderator".

The process of Facilitation aims to promote a congenial social atmosphere and a lively exchange of views. As a Nurse Educator, it is Professional's responsibility to assess the understanding and back ground capacities of receiver/learner/decoder and communicate the content of the message with them in ways, they can understand by utilizing good communication skills. The educator in teaching sessions must demonstrate and performs educational practices with a scientific basis.

Classification of facilitating activities
Zane Berge (1995) has proposed a classification of facilitating activities under four categories:
1. The Pedagogical Role:
   Concerns the teacher's contribution of specialized knowledge and insights to the discussion, using questions and probes to encourage student responses and to focus discussion on critical concepts. In addition, by modeling such behavior, the teacher prepares the students to lead the pedagogical activities by themselves.
2. The Social Role:
   Teaching requires a friendly social environment. The social role of the teacher includes promoting human relationships, affirming and recognizing students' inputs, providing opportunities for students to develop a sense of group cohesiveness, maintaining the group as a unit and helping students to work together in a mutual cause.
3. The Managerial Role
   Concerns organizational, procedural and administrative activities. It involves providing objectives, setting timetables, procedural rules and decision-making norms.
4. The Technical Role
   The Teacher's responsibility for ensuring participant's comfort and ease in using the Communication system and the related literature. It requires the facilitator to be proficient with the technology associated with the Profession.

Facilitation and Teaching
In Educational institutions, skillful facilitation and skillful teaching are essential. A Teacher with adequate knowledge and efficient teaching skills are the backbone for the progress of any educational organization. Sometimes the facilitator will face certain problem, due to inherent limitations of the medium of instruction. In a classroom, the teacher can encourage interaction by remaining open to comments and questions while lecturing. Reading assignments may be helpful along with a classroom experience. Teacher has to correct the reading assignments submitted by the students early to the teaching class. Teacher has to monitor and guide the students on study materials, which they have to possess, as they are interested in students' progress and welfare like a parental role. Interactive/counseling sessions between teacher and students are needed in all educational institutions. In a face-to-face class, facilitation of discussion offers the teacher many opportunities to advance student's understanding, It facilitates the delivery of educational content in a meaningful purposeful,

goal oriented manner. Many of the social and pedagogical activities are best carried out in the course by performing the communicative functions, e.g. maintaining a friendly environment requires recognizing individual contributions promptly so that no one feels left out. Similarly, concepts are often explained in the context of opening discussions with topic raisers.

As a communicative function, weaving enables the group to take stock of agreements and disagreements and to mark its place on its agenda. This is accomplished by grasping in one text the pattern found in a number of previous comments. To write weaving comments, it is necessary to review the discussion archive carefully, refreshing the memory of earlier contributions, clarifying confused expressions, identifying the themes and making connections. It is always good to end the session with a reflective means by asking feedback and starting the next session with reviewing of last session in brief, if continuation of topic for the present class. If new topic of a chapter has to be done, start by reviewing the study guide, terminology and reading assignments

Every learner has some creative talent. Teachers has to promote creativity, Collaboration is a condition for creativity. Innovate appropriate educational policies and extrinsic motivations to achieve/maintain or meet the requirements and to attain grades in an educational Programme. In order to raise the standards the facilitator has to implement activities like; extending time for learning, the measures to improve intellectual skills of the learners, collaboration and cooperation among the groups of learners is needed to build or enhance stronger social community that can strengthen trust, enables interaction between teachers and students to lead enriching communities or environments where each individual through interaction with others will create more novelty than they would do alone and the intrinsic motives emerges more in the course of the interaction. Facilitation works with strong positive motivations by awakening the student's curiosity and a desire to shine by keeping the students attentive till it is satisfied. Surprising facts or concepts excite interest and provoke comments to maintain participation in classes, Similarly, recognizing student's contributions and the tacit responses is essential is to stimulate the desire to contribute again, frequent reassurance from the teacher is needed. Every teacher is aware of these dynamics and plays on them in facilitating classroom discussion.

Misunderstandings can be rapidly corrected in the classroom. Clarity of expression is thus required of everyone and of the facilitator above all. Despite the problems, students enjoy well in facilitated discussions and learn a great deal from the practice of writing and learning the concepts of their field of study. Looking for the messages, which may include responses to one's own comments and new perspectives introduced by the teacher. Participation discussion can acquire an "addictive" quality that keeps the students coming back for more day after day throughout the course of study and after the course also, some times throughout the life also it keeps on continuation.

Facilitation: Communicative Functions

Contextualizing functions

Opening Discussions
The moderator must provide an opening comment that states the theme of the discussion and establishes a communication model. The moderator may periodically contribute "topic raisers" or "prompts" that open further discussions within the framework of the general theme.

Setting the norms
Suggesting rules of procedure for the discussion. Some norms are modeled by the form and style of the moderator's opening comments. Others are explicitly formulated in comments that set the stage for the discussion.

Setting the agenda
Managing the forum over time, selecting an order and flow of themes and topics of discussion. The moderator generally shares part or all of the agenda with participants at the outset.

Referring
The content may be contextualized by referring to materials available in the textbooks, journals, Unpublished Research findings and online resources via Internet by hyperlinking or Web sites.

Monitoring functions

Recognition
Referring explicitly to participant's comments to assure them that their contribution is valued and welcome or to correct misapprehensions about the context of the discussion.

Prompting
Addressing requests for comments to individuals or the group. Prompting includes asking questions and may formalize as "assignments" or tasks. Prompting may be carried out through public requests in the forum or by private messages.

Assessing
Participant accomplishment may be assessed by tests, review sessions, Quiz or other formal competitive procedures.

Meta functions

Meta-commenting
Remarks directed at such things as the context, norms or agenda or at solving problems such as lack of clarity, irrelevance and information under load or over load. Meta-comments play an important role in maintaining the conditions of successful communication.

Weaving
Summarizing the state of the discussion and finding threads of unity in the comments of participants.

Delegating
Certain moderating functions such as weaving can be assigned to individual participants to perform for a shorter or longer period.

Communication Model

Facilitators make an explicit choice for the group they lead, they have to formulate and explain the organizational pattern, roles, responsibilities, norms and expectations of receiver. In face-to-face settings and in Class room teaching, the facilitator's challenge is establishment of contextual cues and tacit signs by insuring everyone a chance to speak through the skillful management of turn taking. The facilitator must outline the norms of the expected behavior early in the life of the group. These contextualizing functions are important in relieving some of the anxiety participants experience in a communication setting. Once a communication model has been chosen, the facilitator must play the specific leadership role it implies, such as chairperson, host, teacher, or entertainer. In part, this role consist in monitoring conformity with the communication model and reassuring participants that their contributions to the discussion are appropriate or where they are not, gently guiding them toward a better understanding of the model. To keep the conversation on track the facilitator must also occasionally offer explicit "meta-comments" which broach communication problems encountered by the group as a whole. Facilitator will use problem solving strategies.

Barriers in Effective Communication

Any difficulty/obstacles/hindrances/hurdles/Problems/breakdowns, which partly or fully affect/blocks the meaning or the transmission or free flowing of message from the sender to receiver in communication process is called as " barriers in communication". It hampers the ways in achieving communication goals. Communication becomes ineffective due to many hurdles, i.e. 'Barriers of Communication'. A good communicator should be aware of the Communication barriers and should try to overcome them to avoid problems.

Barriers in Communication Process may arrive at any level
Sender's Level—For Example Less or more knowledge in related fields, using excess of words, unnecessary repetitions, incomplete sentences, no clarifications, preoccupied with thoughts, poor vocabulary, usage of jargons, slanting, inadequate explanation, rushing, abstract or brief, Poor planning attitude and practices of community, failure to understand cultural differences, poor communication skills of communicator, poor presentation, selection of inappropriate channels and medium, selection of messages contradicting existing beliefs and practices, Inadequate communication material and Inappropriate language.

- Receiver's Level, e.g. Interrupting speaker, asking too many questions, for the sake of Probing, Inaccessibility of relevant literature and emotional factors etc.
- Transmission's Level, e.g. Vague and unclear messages, Irrelevant matter in the expression, Inaccurate translations
- Feedback Level, e.g. Negative returns, unable to comprehend due to low intellectual levels, personality complexes, filtering, Various forms of external noise, insufficient feedback, Technical errors.

Classification of Barriers

1. Semantic barriers

The study of word choice is called "Semantics" and the block that arise from word choice, it's symbols or signs are called "Semantic blocks or Semantic barriers"

For example;

- The difference between inexpensive and cheap. Cheap has a more negative impression or aura associated with it
- Confusion between the symbol and content
- Poor Pronunciation
- Over use of abstractions.

    Words cannot have precisely the same meaning for everyone. Since the same word can mean different things in different languages and may block communication

Remedies/Methods to overcome the semantic barrier

- Educator has to be cautious in selecting the words—Use direct, simple, easy language appropriate to the receiver at specific level. He/she has to make sure to speak in the language that is understood/conveyed the same meaning to the words and going to use by the receiver, proper care has to be taken in selection of medium and communication channel, encoding and decoding of message and feed back
- Be sensitive to receiver's point of view.

2. Physical barriers

- Distance: Physical distance like near or far away from the source or sender
- Time: More information has to be dealt in Limited time or If message gets delayed, it becomes useless and creates confusion or Insufficient time to implement new ideas
- Environmental factors: strange surroundings, loud noise—Disturbance with music and public announcements makes difficult to have concentration for both(learner and sender), Invisibility, congestion

    Effects of natural calamities: Floods, Tornado etc.

    Man made disasters/acquired problems: Stress due to strikes, public processions, political parties influence
- Defects in Channel
- Large working areas making physically separated from others
- Defects in material: Unclear photocopies, unreadable print out or messy corrections.

Remedies/Methods to overcome the Physical barrier

- Adequate distance has to be maintained between teacher and learner, comfortable seating arrangements with adequate facilities is needed
- Session has to be arranged only for 45 to 50 minutes, give a break of 10 to 15 minutes, if it has to be continued, in order to maintain attention span of learners and teacher also may need rest to their vocal cord and to refresh the minds of both teacher and students
- Provide the information/message content at right time in a right way, whereby the learner can understand the subject effectively
- Conduct the teaching sessions in a conducive physical environment with adequate ventilation and silent i.e., free from noise, music or annoyed sound disturbances
- Adequate protective facilities against calamities has to be considered while constructing class rooms for teaching sessions.

3. Physiological Barrier

- Physical ill health of encoder or decoder: sender may have inability to transfer the message or decoder may not be able to receive the message properly, poor listening and poor retention may occur, when she/he is not feeling well
- Defects in the medium: Defects in the devices which are being used, e.g. Poor hearing power, vision defects, Expression difficulties.

Remedies/Methods to overcome Physiological barrier
- Teacher and learner has to be healthy, as sickness affects all aspects of an individual, either to deliver the lecture competently and understand the session effectively
- The needed functional aids, e.g. eye glasses, hearing aids etc. has to be used either by the learners or the teachers in class room interactions to transfer or to understand the content.

4. Mechanical Barriers

For example: Audio-visual aids—Functional defects in the machines, Projected aids, electricity failure, interruptions while projecting, inadequate facilities to arrange the Instructional media.

Remedies/Methods to overcome mechanical barrier
- Teacher has to select suitable and appropriate, good functioning audio-visual aids, specific to the lesson/topic, e.g. To teach Anatomy and Physiology—based on topic, models, specimens, charts, posters, slides, projectors etc., has to be selected
- Assess the working/functioning condition of equipment prior to class/presentation/educational session and if any defects noticed, correct it, to avoid unnecessary interruptions/barrier in the flow of teaching
- The information related to power failure timings has to be gathered, arrange for alternative facilities like generator.
  Check the plug points, if needed, repair it.

5. Psychological Barriers

Barriers related to mind are known as "psychological barriers". Ninty percent of the total barriers in communication are psychological barriers.

a. Emotional barriers
- If receiver is engrossed in emotions for some reason tend to have trouble listening to others or understanding the message conveyed, e.g. Emotional disturbances
- If the receiver has low level of intelligence, comprehension difficulties, language understanding difficulties also unable to understand the message in a correct manner
- If the sender is excited, worried, tense or nervous, his thinking will be confused and he/she will not be able to organize and transmit his message adequately.

b. Perceptual barriers
   Each stimuli will have varied responses, people perceives things differently based on varied factors like their previous experiences and observing others or surroundings, precisely the same data, people see, interpret or respond to them differently. When people fill-in information without checking its accuracy or lack of knowledge

c. Selectivity barrier
   We cannot absorb all the information which is flowing in our way, hence we will screen it selectively. One factor in the way people select and react to stimuli is timing and attention. Some messages that may be effective at one time might be blocked or even detrimental at another time, e.g. a letter of condolence sent out immediately after the event is more effective than one sent later.

d. Inattention or lack of concentration: The receiver is distracted and not paying attention to the sender or the messages conveyed

e. Distrust: Distrust on the part of the sender for the receiver or the receiver towards the sender can give rise to misunderstanding the content

f. Premature evaluation: Immediately framing judgment and replies, even before the message is completed

g. Lack of creativity, goal conflicts, offensive style or confused thinking, negative attitudes, bias and prejudice, impatience, lack of hope and inhibition, non-acceptance, judgmental, closed mind, effect of fear, misunderstandings, halo Effect, Inattentiveness, negative opinions.

Remedies against Psychological barrier
- Develop good listening skills

Rules for Good Listening
Rule - Reasoning Behind the Rule
- Stop talking—You cannot listen if you are talking
- Put the person at ease—Help a person feel free to talk; create a permissive environment. Listen to understand
- Show the person you Look and act interested -show interest when listening, understand, not to oppose
- Remove distractions—Do not doodle, tap, or shuffle papers; shut the door, if necessary to achieve quiet
- Empathize—Try to see the other person's point of view
- Be patient—Allow plenty of time; do not interrupt; do not start for the door or walk away, listen completely and patiently
- Hold your temper—An angry person takes the wrong meaning from words
  Go easy on argument, Don't put people on the defensive and criticism and cause them to "clam up" or become angry
- Do not argue even if you win or you lose
- Ask questions—This encourages a person and shows that you are listening; it helps to develop points further
- Stop talking—This is first and last, because all other guides depend on it; you cannot listen effectively while you are talking.

Other Measures
Develop trust and confidence between the persons who are under interaction
- Learn to use feedback well
- Feel a sense of responsibility
- Learn to use supportive communication not defensive communication
- Provide conducive environment for listening with adequate facilities
- Try to concentrate and understand the situation
- Minimise/avoid distractions, stay calm
- Have open Mind and develop positive attitude in things which you have to do compulsorily
- Eliminate/avoid fear, tension, nervous, have balanced mind, maturity in thinking and analyze the situation effectively, try to understand cues, signs, subject in comprehension
- Use Positive Reinforcement techniques.

6. Socio-Psychological Barrier

Social status and social consciousness, social differences, strained or discomfort in interpersonal relationships, rumors, educational difference/illiteracy.

Remedies/Protective measures
- Have the goals in reachable terms and means
- Utilize the opportunities and improve educational status
- Maintain harmonious interpersonal relationships both in family or in working/living environments
- Steps has to be taken to raise the status of individuals in society
- Improve morale, work right to the conscious.

7. Cultural barriers

Racism, influence of ethnic, religion, caste, traditions, customs, beliefs, language variations, social distance (vary from culture to culture like intimate, personal public) etc.

Remedies/Protective measures
- Maintain the standards of communities and good interpersonal relationships through effective interaction
- Steps to raise the concepts of Equality, Commonness, Fellow being nature, Humanitarian approach
- Develop healthy habits, good beliefs
- Measures to learn the local languages, conduct training programs, group cohesiveness, group dynamics.

8. Organizational Barriers

Hierarchical barriers, Specialization of Workforce, Wrong choice of medium, Communication load, Organization Policy.

Remedies/Protective Measures

- Develop Organizational Policies
- Advancement of Communication pattern among all categories in the organization
- Provide opportunities to specialize work forces like in service education, Continuing Education programmes, on duty facilities, extra privileges like leaves, scholarships/stipend/fellowships for the personal and professional development
- As per the abilities and intellectual capacities of the individual, select the choice of Instructional medium
- Select suitable Educational Technology and communication techniques to enrich the knowledge of learners, information should neither overload or under load
- Tougher test-based accountability—Schools have been boosted by educational accountability movement by holding schools and teachers accountable for student's learning like testing and measuring the performance of individuals (both students and teachers). The key criterion in this accountability process is the test results determined by external standardized assessments and often multiple-choice tests SOCE (Standardized Objective Continuous Evaluation) in order to develop trust, risk-taking and creativity skills among learners. School accountability is linked to consequences in the form of rewards such as higher teacher pay or promotion or in the form of other sanctions/benefits like on duty or leave facilities to upgrade the teachers viz. attending workshops, inservice education, supporting with salary for their higher education and encouraging the teachers to take necessary steps to improve performance of students like revising by extra tutoring the subject, giving additional unit tests to evaluate and the percentage of marks and communicate to the learners and their parents to improve student test scores, thus school's performance and promote creativity among both teachers and learners. Collaboration and cooperation harmonization of structures and processes in school is commonly seen as a condition for creativity and innovation, builds stronger social community by strengthening trust, enriches interaction between teachers and students, develops mutual trust, respect and honesty. Communication, cooperation and respecting others are the most effective means of building trust in a community. Rewarding effort and ideas is essential for promoting creativity and innovation in teams and organizations. In education, the introduction of standards for teaching, curriculum, expected learning outcomes, school facilities, technologies, uniformity is required to have globally recognition.

Enablers/Gate Ways/Methods/Remedies to overcome barriers in Communication Process

The path or the gate ways, provides the guidelines how to deal with the miscommunication and overcome the barriers that are occurred between the receiver and sender. The Nurse Educator with advanced education plays a pivotal position to decrease the barriers in Communication Process. The remedies were explained in detail under each category of barrier.

Health Communication

Health is Wealth, everyone has the right to possess their health, Information on health has to be delivered through health education messages by the health professionals, they will help people to achieve health by their own efforts and actions. Health Communication is essential in transforming health information. Health communication can contribute to all aspects of health maintenance, health promotion and disease prevention. Health communication encompasses the study and use of communication strategies to inform and influence individual and community decisions that enhance health.

Functions

- Provides scientific health information on health maintenance, health promotion, perceiving health needs and demands and disease prevention
- Promotes health development by assisting to enhance or diffuse the knowledge on health
- Prepares the people for their expected role performance effectively
- Motivates the persons to practice healthy life style
- Develops positive value, desirable way of living by maintaining standards and qualitative life

- Raises awareness of health risks and solutions
- Provides the motivation and skills needed to reduce health risks, help them to find support from other people and other resources and agencies
- Affects or reinforces positive attitudes towards healthy behavior
- Increases demand for appropriate health services and decrease demand for inappropriate health services
- Assists in making complex choices such as selecting health plans, care providers, and treatments
- For the community, health communication can be used to influence the public agenda, advocate for policies and programs, promotes positive changes in the socioeconomic and physical environments
- Improves the delivery of public health and health care services and encourage social norms that benefit health and provide qualitative life
- Improves interpersonal and group interactions in clinical situations (e.g. provider-patient, provider-provider, and among members of a health care team)
- The training of focused societal groups in enhancing knowledge levels of health and attaining effective communication skills
- Collaborative relationships are enhanced when all parties are capable of communicating with each other
- Disseminates health messages through public education campaigns that seek to change the social climate to encourage healthy behaviors, create awareness, change attitudes, and motivate individuals to adopt recommended behaviors and practice healthy life styles
- Provides Counseling services to understand and deal with the problems by taking necessary precautions or steps to reduce or resolve their problems
- Attempts to raise the morale of group of people
- Communication in any organization flows in vertical and horizontal directions, whereby people in all directions getting the information and benefitted with the messages
- Promotes intra and intersectoral coordination in the organization.

Attributes of effective health communication

Accurate: Factual and valid health information will be communicated

Acceptance: Easy to understand, clear terminology in local language will be used for the beneficiary groups to accept and apply, self explanatory

Attitude: Focuses on bringing change in specific individual's/targeted /focused group behavior content will be framed

Availability: Health Education materials will be kept in common places, available to the focus groups

Accessible: Content related to health will be reachable to all sectors of population at any time

Adequate: The content represents total aspects of the topic in a comprehensive manner, meaningful, meets the felt needs and demand needs of the specific groups

Balanced: Potential benefits, adverse effects of a specific content will be briefed

Credibility: Maintains internal consistency, reliable, credible information will be delivered

Cultural competency: All cultural variables, educational competency will be taken into consideration in framing the content

Evidence based: Special issues for selected population on specific topics, scientifically proved validated data/ information will be delivered

Reinforced: To bring effective change, to motivate the people to practice, message will be informed repeatedly in varied dimensions

Timeliness: Based on the felt need and health demands of society the information will be communicated in timely manner.

Communication Material

Use of Communication material/Aids help in better understanding of messages being communicated. Communication material should be of good quality and has to be pretested before its use. While preparing or procuring communication material remember that communication material should be

- Attractive and appealing
- Clear and precise

- Pretested with correct messages
- Durable
- Easy to use
- Easy to carry and store
- Cost effective

Communication Materials are: Audio-visual aids like Leaflets/Booklets/Pamphlets, Posters, Charts, Flipbooks, Flannel Graph, Flash Cards, Flip Charts, Slides, Film, Radio and Drama Scripts, Audio Tapes, Puppets and Folk Songs.

THERAPEUTIC COMMUNICATION

Introduction

Therapeutic interaction is a learning experience for both the client and to the Nurse. It is a corrective emotional experience to the client to modify his/her behavior. Repeated human contacts are essential to develop trust, love, tenderness, concern and unconditional acceptance from both the Clients and their families, It occurs when the Nurse exhibits empathy, utilizes effective communication skills and responds to the client's thoughts, needs and concerns; It establishes trusting, protective and corrective relationship by winning the confidentiality in which the client can reveal his/her thoughts and feelings openly. Nurse learns to implement the careful practice with efficient experience and performs many roles such as parent, Counselor, Adviser/Supporter and Role Model for the clients and their families in order to fulfill their needs. Nurses has to accept the client's thoughts, feelings, interests and problems, hence the Nurse's acceptance is unconditional. Nurses has to encourage and support, always expecting the patient's capacity to improve and to excel, yet knowing and making allowances for the shortcomings. Nurse is concerned with all the client's activities Viz. understands the situational support/influencing personalities/care takers(Family and Friends),who are interested in client's welfare, client's learning capabilities, Leisure time activities etc. Total involvement and cooperation of the Nurse is essential. Nurses must be able to communicate effectively with their Clients and their families, Significant others and other Healthcare team members to create conducive environment to the client and their families.

Therapeutic Communication means listening to and understanding the client while promoting clarification and insight. It enables the Nurse to form a working relationship with the Clients and their families, Peers by using both Verbal and Non-Verbal Communication.

Definitions

"Therapeutic/Conscious/Constructive relationship establishes between a helping person/Healthcare Professionals and the client in specific and with their family members in general by meaningful, ongoing communication and interaction with adequate usage of Professional knowledge and skills in an atmosphere of mutual respect and trust, in which each agrees to work with each other collaboratively to alleviate the clients' existing problem or to resolve the health problems by attaining the holistic health of the client, who needs concern and helpful in developing mutual understanding between two individuals."

"It is a process, in which the nurse utilizes a planned approach to learn about the client"—*Potter A, 1997*

Purposes/Goals/Functions

- To achieve Self realization, self acceptance, self respect, self control, Personal identification and Personal integration
- To formulate and maintain good Interpersonal Therapeutic Relationship by encouraging the patient to share her/his feelings with the Nurse
- Responds to the client's feelings in a nonjudgmental, empathetic way, e.g. at the time of Grief or Loss, nurse will provide supportive, by allowing the client to identify feelings and express sadness
- Provides additional opportunity for the nurse to remain with the patient in a supportive capacity, thus enhancing the nurse-client relationship
- Permits the client to express their thoughts truly and openly
- Validate client's experience and feelings by verbally responding to client's feelings

- Validates patient's messages by responding to the patient's behavior, set limits on the behavior, not the patient as a person
- Acknowledges reminiscence is an attempt at healthy interaction for the clients in problems of memory difficulties
- To meet the basic and felt needs of the client
- To formulate and achieve realistic personal goals
- Allows the client to continue to identify and express their concerns, e.g. concerns for hospitalization, surgery or life threatening illness
- Aids in clarification of internal conflicts and frustrations of the client
- Improves client's ego strengths
- Encourages the growth and development of the client and the family by giving accurate explanation of the concerned issues.
- Encourages socialization and family interaction process
- Treats communication problems
- Modifies maladaptive behavior into adaptive behavior
- Motivates the client to utilize new coping strategies
- Helps the Nurse to identify and intervene appropriate nursing approaches
- Assists the client to utilize problem solving skills in dealing with the problems
- Implements Nursing process effectively
- Promotes comfort and well being.

Modes/Types

1. Verbal communication

Factual information can be conveyed through language or words. It is an accurate and effective medium of communication

2. Non–verbal communication

Message or information conveyed through the behavior or body languages or by utilization of five senses it communicates interest, respect, genuineness; checks through feed back.

- Vocal cues/paralinguistic cues, e.g. Noise, Pitch/tone of voice, sounds or extra sounds
- Action cues/Body movements, e.g. posture, facial expression, gestures, mannerisms and other actions
- Object cues, e.g. dressing, furnishings, possessions
- Space, e.g. Nature of relationship between two cues or people
- Touch—provides comfort
- Attitudes
- Appearance
- Uses techniques of validation, clarification, concern towards clients' behavior/welfare by acknowledging and responds to his verbal and non-verbal means, e.g. body language - nodding head, smile or furrow brows in an expression(frown), Eye-to-eye contact in order to exhibit agreement or disagreement while listening.

Therapeutic Communication Techniques

1. *Listening*

   Active process of receiving the information. Complete attention of the Nurse is required. Active listening shows respect towards the person who is speaking and powerful as it reinforces the relationships; allows the client to talk more openly without any inhibitions or bias; It wins the trust or confidentiality; establishes therapeutic nurse patient relationship. Promotes effective communication.

   S–Sit facing the client–It depicts the Nurse is interested in listening to the client

   O–observe an open posture (arms and legs uncrossed)–Nurse is open to client

   L–Lean toward's maintain intermittent eye contact, willingness to listen to what client is saying and involvement

   R–Relax–client will be relaxed and comfortable when the Nurse is actively listening to them.

2. *Broad opening*

   Motivates the client to define the problem or issue select the topic for discussion and indicate that the Nurse is interested in client and encourages the client to talk. Communicates a desire is to begin a meaningful interaction. Allows the client to choose the subject.

3. *Social responding or social interaction*

   First the Nurse engages the client in superficial conversation and no hidden intention for personal disclosures. It helps the client to feel more comfortable, ease and safe, where by she/he can give spontaneous, automatic responses.

4. *Asking relevant questions*

   It is a direct method of getting specific and clear information from the client. Ask the relevant questions in a logical, sequential manner. Questioning is more effective when they are related to the client or subject being discussed in normal socio-cultural context. To get in depth of information or elaborate answer open ended questions can be asked.

5. *Sharing Perceptions*

   Nurse has to share the client's thoughts, ideas and perceptions and clarifies the doubts if client has anything. Nurse has to share empathy, hope and humor. Nurse tries to evaluate whether the interactions are helpful to the client. Nurses will share their observation, helps the client to communicate. Nurse thinks about the client. It is a gesture of warmth and concern towards the client.

6. *Theme Identification*

   Identifying the underlying issues or problems experienced by the client, once the client's problems were identified, it is easy to decide which feelings and thoughts has to be responded and continued.

7. *Using Silence*

   For a therapeutic reason, Nurses has to maintain silence, it prompts the client to think, re-organizes thoughts by reflecting through talk or conversation. It is a safe measure as it promotes insight and allows the client to take a lead in conversation. It requires skills and timing. Provides opportunities to communicate interpersonally. Silence allows the nurse to pay particular attention to non verbal messages which are most accurate reflection of attitude.

   Remaining silence demonstrates the Nurse's patience and willingness to wait for a response, when the client is unable to respond quickly. Silence may be therapeutic during the times of profound distress or grief.

8. *Focusing*

   Concentrate for a particular point. It eliminates vagueness in communication by limiting the area of discussion. Nurse has to focus on particular issue, otherwise the client continues to use vague description. Nurses has to expand discussion on a topic of importance. Client becomes more specific and tries to focus on reality.

9. *Clarification*

   The client's verbalization may not be always clear as she/he is disturbed or confused or feeling very deeply for their illness. So the Nurse needs to clarify their feelings and ideas expressed by the clients. Nurse needs to correlate between the client's feelings and actions. Nurse has to formulate patient's feelings in clearer statements. Nurses will assist the clients to clarify their own understanding by encouraging recall and details of specific feeling or experience.

10. *Pin pointing*

    Nurses pays attention to certain consistent statements made by the client; pinpoints the specifics or differences what the client talks and what he/she does, e.g. In Obsessive Compulsive Neurotic clients are consistent in their actions though they speaks ideally, totally talks were different from activities, so it is the responsibility of the Nurse to pinpoint their behavior, aimed towards the modification of client's behavior as they are interested in client's welfare.

11. *Restating*

    Nurse repeats to the client the main thought what he/she has expressed, indicating that nurse is hastening and focusing to the point what client wants to convey.

12. *Linking*

Nurses try to link the client's feelings or events with their activities or to other persons one to another, to make the client to understand in a better manner the situation.

13. *Encourage the client to formulate a plan*

Nurse will not suggest anything; encourages the client to formulate her/his plan of action with her/his own efforts to solve the problems by utilizing coping strategies.

14. *Testing discrepancies*

Assist the client to become aware of her/his behavior and inconsistencies as it allows gentleness and clarifies issues.

15. *Information*

Nurses will educate the client and her/his family related to problem solving techniques to provide personal, social and therapeutic information; Nurse clarifies doubts; teaches the independent living skills, decision making power, where by the client relieves her/his anxiety, tension and feels safe and secured. The client will attain additional information and insight into the situation. It encourages further responses, promotes healthy living: Nurse will gain and maintain trust and wins the confidentiality in the client. It increases the client's resources. Nurse shares facts with the client.

16. *Suggesting*

Nurse will suggest alternative ideas, new coping strategies and useful communication techniques to enhance the client's choices which she/he can use in day to day life activities.

17. *Reflection or validation*

Directing back to the patient his/her ideas, feelings, questions and content. It consists of responses to the client's feelings about the content. It signifies understanding, empathy, interest and respect for the client. It increases the level of involvement with the patient. Nurses confirms the accuracy of data or information given by the patient during interaction. It helps the client to make additional clarification regarding his/her statements.

18. *Paraphrasing*

Reflects the meaning of client's message in the nurse's words; the client will understand, that the nurse has understood the message what he/she told and allows for clarification, motivates for further communication.

19. *Placing events in time sequence*

Encourage the client to organize thoughts, giving clues for recurring patterns, there by the health care professionals will understand the client's feelings and plans care accordingly.

20. *Voicing doubt*

Encourages, reconsideration of challenges the client's perceptions

For example 1. Really? 2.Do you mean that your siblings will not consider you and your decisions in family decisions? 3. I am not sure, what you mean..................?

21. *Using Assertiveness*

Standing up one's rights without violating those of others. Through assertiveness people express their feelings and emotions confidently, honesty and spontaneously. The persons with assertiveness makes choices and decisions, able to control their lives effectively than non assertive individuals. To promote client's health, Nurses has to inculcate assertiveness among the client. Messages has to be clear, specific and complete.

22. *Offering general leads*

Encourages the client to communicate elaborately the Nurse suggest or gives certain leads so that the client will elaborate it.

23. *Summarizing*

Nurses will highlight the main theme of what has been discussed; specific important things only taken into consideration. It helps the client to focus the issue under the discussion.

Non therapeutic communication techniques

1. Authoritarian

   Choices in which the nurse is telling the client what to do without regard to the client's desires or feelings. For example 1. Insisting that the client follow unit rules, 2. Insisting that the client do what you command, immediately.

2. Eliminate closed-ended questions

   Avoid 'Yes'/'No' or another monosyllabic responses as they discourage the client from sharing thoughts and feelings. For example 1. Are you feeling responsible about what happened? 2. Has the pain increased?

3. Avoid asking 'Why' questions

   The questions that seek reasons or justification. 'Why' questions imply disapproval of the client who may become defensive. A 'why' question can come in many forms and need not always begin with 'why'. Any response that puts the client on the defensive is nontherapeutic. For example 1. 'What makes you think that? 2. 'Why do you feel this way?

4. Avoid 'Lets' explore' questions

   Analyzing /interpreting the clients' feelings or behavior. It is not the nurse's role to focus into the reasons why the client is feeling a particular way. The client must be allowed to verbalize the fact that he or she is sad, angry, fearful, or overwhelmed. For example 1. Let's talk about why you did not take your medications? 2. Tell me why you really injured yourself.

5. 'Do not worry' or giving false assurance

   These responses would discourage communication between nurse and the client by not allowing the client to explore his or her own ideas. False reassurance also discounts what the client is feeling. For example 1. It is going to be Okay. 2. Do not worry. Your Physician will do everything necessary for your care.

6. Nurse-focused responses

   The focus of the comment is on the nurse is to be avoided. It may be empathetic. The focus of therapeutic communication should always be on the client. For example 1. Avoid the responses, such as 'That happened to me once'. 2. 'I experienced it, it is hard for you'. This type of conversation shifts the focus away from the client and their family.

7. Offering advise

   In any given situation, allow the client and their family to analyze and take their decisions by responding their own feelings. For example 'Why don't you wait and see your family's reaction before you get upset'.

8. Avoid 'Passing the buck'

   If it is within the scope of nursing practice, the nurse has to respond to the client's questions. Avoid transferring the clients' question to others. For example 'I will call the doctor, so you can discuss with him'.

9. Disagreeing/Arguing with the client and family members

   The family member wants to discuss the clients' discomfort with the nurse, the nurse instead of explaining/clarifying the concern with necessary interventions, either argues or not allowing the family members to discuss the concern. For example The caretaker of a post-op client wants to discuss the patients' pain level with the nurse-incharge, the nurse-incharge either denies the request or show any concern to address the issue.

   Other techniques like rejection, giving approval, consent, defend, request, changing the subject, Belittling, stereotyped comments, moralizing, interpretation, challenging defending etc. has to be avoided.

Characteristics of Therapeutic Communication

The Nurse has to possess certain characteristics to develop and maintain Therapeutic relationship. Therapeutic responses are based on assessment of the clients' needs which are designed to foster the growth and establish mutually formulated goals.

1. Response dimensions

- Active Listening and Genuineness Openness, honesty, sincerity, active involvement, accepting the client as he is, personal freedom to the client, e.g. The Nurse–asks questions that relate directly to what the client says

Maintains eye to eye contact
- Leans forward in the chair to face the client
- Nods, smiles, frown to show agreement or disagreement
- Understands that Personal feelings, past experiences of the Nurse can either positively or negatively affects the relationships with the clients
- Validates the clients' experience and feelings by responding to the client verbally.
- Respect–Warmth, positive regard self respect, respecting others; caring, concern, liking, valuing, worthfulness; nonjudgmental, maintains confidentiality, Nurse makes the client to feel accepted and respected the client as an individual irrespective of her/his verbal or nonverbal behavior and promotes comfort and well being of client

  For example:
  - Assumes that the clients' behavior is purposeful and meaningful, even though it may not make sense to others
  - Defines limits or boundaries (Physical, Social and Emotional) for client's behavior or set limits for their own behavior and structures time frame work of Nurse–Client relationship
  - Creates a safe and secured environment for the client
  - Formulates contract with the client
  - Accepts dependency needs of the client like movement and supportive system
  - Rejects the behavior of the client but not the client if it is inappropriate
  - Responds to the client
- Empathetic understanding and communicating interest

  Empathy is "the ability to perceive what another person experiences using that person's frame of reference." Nurse's sensitivity to the client's current feelings and responds to it appropriately, concerns of client's families and or staff. Accurate empathy involves more than knowing what the patient means; confirms with the client the accuracy of perceptions and guided responses among the client.

  Allowing client to comfortably communicate concerns and behave in new ways.

  For example
  - Introducing themselves to the client
  - Maintains eye contact
  - Giving verbal responses to the client's conversation
  - Responses focus on strengths and resources of the client
  - Consistent response to patient's non verbal cues
  - Conveying interest, warmth and concern
  - Focuses conversation on the client's feelings
  - Appreciates and understands that clients responds to the behavioral expectations of the staff
  - Responds directly to client clues by analyzing client's behavior, validates client's feelings
  - Anticipates the client's difficulties in advance
  - Help the clients to set appropriate limits on their behavior or set limits for them if they are unable to do so.
- Concreteness

  Using specific terminology when discussing the client's feelings, experience and behavior with other health care professionals. It avoids vagueness and ambiguity. It fosters the accuracy of understanding by the nurse; It encourages the patient to express specific problem areas.

  Gives correct information, encourages the client to talk, e.g. the patient is experiencing memory loss, nurse explains more about the problem details.

  Level of concreteness varies in different phases of therapeutic nurse patient relationship, e.g. orientation phase–High level of empathy and concreteness, Working phase–Low level of empathy and concreteness, Termination phase–High level of empathy and concreteness

2. Action dimension

Confrontation

It is an expression by nurse of perceived discrepancies in the patient's behavior. Three categories in confrontation were identified

  a. Discrepancy between the patient's self concept and self ideal
  b. Discrepancy between the client's verbal expression about himself and his behavior
  c. Discrepancy between the client's expressed experience of himself and the Nurse's experience of him.

The Nurse has to use an active role in modeling; insight and understanding to remove ambiguity and inconsistency; develops deeper insight into the client's problems.

- Immediacy—Focusing on the current interaction of the Nurse and the client. Sensitivity by the nurse to the client's feelings and willingness to deal with these feelings
- Nurse's self disclosure—Nurse reveals information about themselves, e.g. values, feelings, attitudes, It is an index of the closeness of the relationship and develops respect. It determines optimum therapeutic level.
- Patient self disclosure—It is necessary for a successful therapeutic outcome.
- Emotional catharsis—Motivate the client to talk about his views, feelings, experiences openly after gaining confidence and trust, establishing therapeutic relationship
- Role Play—It involves acting out a particular situation, increases the client's insight into human relations and deepens the ability to see and feel the situation. It provides a link between thought and action in a constructive environment. It promotes awareness and experience in the situation. Brings attitudinal change
- Reflection—Communicates to the client that the nurse has heard and understands what the client is trying to communicate, when reflecting feelings, the Nurse focuses on the feelings and not the content of what is said, e.g. You seem very stressed out, tell me how you are feeling now

Barriers in effective therapeutic communication

- Belittling client, family members or staff concerns
- Blaming the external environment for the situation
- Choosing sides with the client, family member or staff member in a conflict
- Defending one's own actions or behavior
- Disagreeing or arguing with the client or family member
- Giving approval
- Giving false reassurance
- Giving one-word responses to the questions
- Ignoring client clues to help the client set appropriate limits on his/her behavior
- Interpreting or analyzing both verbal and nonverbal behavioral clues in the situation to the client
- Invalidating the client's, family member's or staff feelings
- Minimizing concerns
- Offering advice about a situation
- Offering unrealistic hope for the future
- Pressuring the client or family members for an explanation
- Rejecting the person, not the behavior
- Shifting the focus of the conversation away from the client, family members or staff
- Using denial
- Using jargons or medical terminology without explaining the details to the client/family members

Therapeutic Communication skills

Skill is the ability or efficiency of the Nurse to utilize their knowledge systematically and effectively in proficiency manner.

- General abilities, e.g. ability to listen, interpret, speak and express through writing.
- Special abilities, e.g. Observation and its interpretation, Process the therapeutic interaction to attain the goals, ascertain/determining skills, differentiates and follow when to be silent/speak/smile/interact, ability to wait, proceed, speed, participates actively and maintains therapeutic nurse patient relationship.

QUESTIONS

- Barriers of Communication (5M, MGRUHS, Feb, 2010 & 5M Baba Farid UHS, 2009, 5M, RGUHS, Aug, 2010).
- Channels of communication (5M, NTRUHS, Nov, 2010).
- Communication skills (5M, NTRUHS, Dec, 2007).
- Define Communication (2M, MGRUHS, Feb, 2010).
- Define Communication? List down the values of Communication? Explain the Communication process (10M, RGUHS, Nov, 2007)
- Describe the Therapeutic Communication Technique (5M, Baba Farid UHS, 2010; 4M, NIMS, May, 2009 & May, 2010).
- Discuss the barriers of communication. As an educator how will you overcome these barriers while educating a group of mothers? (10M, RGUHS, Feb, 2010).
- Elements of Communication (2M, RGUHS, Aug, 2009 & 2010).
- Enlist the Components of Communication Process (10 M, MGRUHS, Aug, 2008 & 5M, RGUHS, Sept, 2009).
- Explain Communication Process (4M), Explain Facilitators and Barriers of Communication (4M), List any 4 techniques of Communication with suitable examples (4M) (Baba Farid UHS, 2008).
- Explain in detail the Methods and Media for communicating Health Education messages (8M, MGRUHS, Feb, 2010).
- Explain the Process of Communication and elaborate the Channels of Communication (15 M, NTRUHS, JUNE 2009).
- Explain the techniques of therapeutic communication (7M, RGUHS, 2009).
- Explain the various techniques of communication and mention the techniques used in nursing with illustrations (15M, NTRUHS, June, 2010).
- Facilitators of Communication (5M, NIMS, May, 2010).
- List the Barriers to effective Communication, Why it is important to develop Therapeutic relationship between Clients & Health team, Explain one type of Patient record in brief (4+6+5=15M, NTRUHS, July 2008).
- List the communication techniques (2M, NIMS, April, 2009).
- Mention Models of Communication (2M, MGRUHS, Feb, 2010).
- Methods for communicating health messages (5M, RGUHS, Sept, 2009).
- Methods of effective communication (5M, RGUHS, Sept, 2009).
- Non Verbal Communication (5M, NIMS, March, 2008).
- Process of communication (5M, RGUHS, Sept, 2009;5M, NIMS, May, 2008).
- Theory of Communication (5M, RGUHS, 2005; 5M, NTRUHS, 2001).
- What are the Elements of Communication Process? (2M, RGUHS, Sept, 2009) Discuss Therapeutic Communication Techniques (20M, Rajasthan UHS, March, 2010 & 16M, Rajasthan UHS, Feb, 2008).

10

Health Education

INTRODUCTION

"You can lead a horse to the water, but you cannot make him drink, unless he wants to" says the old proverb, but that concept is improved upon and nowadays, "make the horse thirsty, before you take him and show the water". In other words, make the people to realize that health is the most valuable asset/possession which will shape all of their activities, as 'Health is Wealth', the people must desire to attain their health by themselves, with their own efforts. Then, it is easy task for health professionals to enrich the people with health information. Education and health are the two most important investments in human capital individuals make. Their economic values are founded in the effects they have on productivity: both education and health make individuals more productive. Also, education and health have a considerable impact on individual well-being. Behavioral change related health education programs represent a main stay of health care activity.

Health Education is an essential tool of Community health. Health Education in any subject should be sound and built on the correct attitudes and understanding of the people to be educated. Health Education strategies can be evolved and focus on the goals and which can be realized with the capacities and resources and based on varied factors like educational, social, economical, cultural values, needs and wants. It is a collaboration effort of health professionals, developmental agencies, community, friends and influencing personalities which will affect and changes in individual and group behavior. Health Education is one of the most cost effective intervention. If people were sufficiently informed and encouraged to take adequate precautions in time, many diseases can be prevented, knowledge is essential to the fullest attainment of health. It is concerned with promoting health behavior.

Health Education can be taught as a separate subject in the curriculum, it may also be integrated in general subjects like Science, Social Studies, Technology, Physical Education and Home Economics. At present from preschool education, health education is included in their curriculum to enrich the knowledge related to health for the younger generation.

DEFINITIONS

"A process of change within a person in his knowledge, attitude and practices related to development or enhancement of their personal and community health".

"A process that informs, motivates and helps people to adopt and maintain healthy practices and life styles, advocates environmental changes as needed to facilitate this goal and conducts professional training and research to the same end".

"An educational process where the individual and community behavior patterns will be changed into desirable manner, by enhancing the health information through health professionals, Mass Media and by the community itself".

"The process by which the individuals and groups learn healthy practices and behave in a conducive manner to the promotion, maintenance and restoration of health".

"A process aimed at encouraging people to want to be healthy, to know how to stay healthy, to do what they can individually and collectively to maintain health and to seek the help when needed"—Alma -Ata Declaration (1978).

"A Social Science that draws from the Biological, Environmental, Psychological, Physical and Medical Sciences to promote health, to prevent diseases and disability and premature death through education driven voluntary behavior change activities".

"Health Education is the development of individual, group, institutional, community and systematic strategies to improve health knowledge, attitudes, skills and behavior".

Concept

- Translation of Scientific health knowledge into healthy practice which is a desirable behavior pattern
- It is concerned with establishing or inducing changes in knowledge, attitudes, feelings and behavior, promotes healthier living
- It involves Community Participation and Community Involvement
- Reduces Behavior induced disease.

Objectives

- Informing People about
    - Prevention of Disease
    - Promotion of Health
    - To exclude the barriers related to health and disease
    - Create awareness of public their own needs and able to identify their own problems
    - Utilize the effective resources for the solution of problems
    - Curative services, rehabilitative services, restorative services
- Motivating the people
  Providing scientific information is not enough, motivation to use the information and positive reinforcement are essential., the learning experiences and practical sessions has to be organized to change their habits, attitudes and to develop positive healthy practices to modify their life style to promote health pattern and quality of life
- Guiding into action
    - Government has to provide good infrastructural facilities and services, the public has to be aware and effectively utilize those resources without any inhibitions, prejudice, bias or misconceptions
    - Promote effective community participation and community involvement in implementation of national health programs and utilization of those resources in an effective manner
    - Practical self help measures and health tips has to be adopted to improve their own health status with their own efforts.

Aims

- Help the people to understand that health is their fundamental right and community asset
- To develop a sense of responsibility for improvement and enjoy decent health as individuals and families within the communities
- To encourage people to adopt and sustain health promoting life style and practices, habits, positive attitudes and skills through the inculcation of correct health concepts and behavioral patterns, with the ultimate objective of enabling the people to make the best possible choice for his or her optimum health and total well-being
- To provide Healthy Environment by enriching the people with scientific information about health and disease
- Information, Education, Motivation and Communication activities has to be carried out to bring behavioral changes for betterment of their health
- Health Education programs has to aim in bringing change in knowledge, attitude, habits, customs, behavior and healthy practices
- To make people aware of their needs and health problems
- To promote the proper use of health services available to them
- To arouse interest and to provide new knowledge
- To improve skills and change the attitudes in making rational decisions to solve their own problems
- To enhance the role of people in conveying health messages to the community and in giving active support in implementation of National Health Program interventions.

- To stimulate individual and community self-reliance and participation to achieve health development through the individual and community involvement at every step from identifying problems and implementation efforts in solving them
- The focus of Health Education is on people and on actions, to make realistic improvements in the basic quality of life. It influences the behavior and attitudes of people
- To improve cognitive (Health information), Conative (Skills to exhibit), Affective Domains (Attitude towards health and illness) of an individual and Community
- Individuals can look after themselves and take care of others and Protect the environment with the knowledge they obtained by health education
- To positively influence the health behavior of the individuals and communities as well as the living and working conditions that influence their health.

Philosophy

Health education is a unique and separate academic discipline. It influences individual, family and societal development, knowledge, attitudes and behavior. It seeks the improvement of individual, family and community health. The individual is not a composite of separate entities, such as body, mind and spirit, arranged in presumed ascending order of importance. The individual is a multi-dimensional entity, with each component—chemical, physical, spiritual, intellectual or emotional-existing as an element within a complex of interrelationships. Good health requires positive efforts directed toward total well-being. These efforts have larger potential for success when operating in a socio-political system that values individual, family and societal well-being. Individual attempts to enhance one's own well-being should be joined by a commitment to enhance societal well-being. Education in health helps individuals seek that which moves them toward optimal stages of wellness. The ultimate goal of health education is to enable individuals to use knowledge in ways that transform unhealthy habits into healthy habits. It thus is an objective for health education to provide learners with the skills to judge messages received in terms of their potential benefit to self and society. Educators in general or health educators in particular must teach individuals to look beyond health as an end or goal and to utilize health enhancing skills as a means for achieving life's goals. Though health itself may be quantitatively evaluated biochemically, health status can only be used as a qualitative measure of functional ability. Wellness is, in this functional sense, a means, not an end. Thus, the end should involve greater societal well-being.

Health Education can be envisaged on a continuum, suggesting differing approaches and emphasis. One such continuum contrasts emphasizes on the individual and society. A health education program may focus both on the individual and society, however, contemporary approaches to health education recognize the importance of including a concern for the role of society. This perspective recognizes that factors such as income, housing, cultural practices shape a person's health. There are limits to the choices open to individuals – limits imposed by their physical, social and cultural environments and by their financial means. Some physical and social factors which influence our health.

Individual	Society
Improve health by changing their practices, negative attitudes	Improve health by changing personal behaviors, economic, social and environmental factors
Health as Physical fitness	Health as social issues
Medical Treatment of Illness	Broad Preventable Strategies
Mass Media Campaigns	Community Based Action

Physical	Social
Residence	Genetic Inheritance
Individual Behavior/Life Style	Weight
Global Environment (Biosphere)	Income (Money)
Culture	Social Relationships
Family Relationships	Access to Health Care
Age	Sex
Environment/Occupation	Faith/Education

As well as including a social perspective, contemporary approaches to health and health education also emphasize:
- A holistic orientation which values physical, mental, emotional, social, environmental and spiritual dimensions of health and their interrelationships. When a holistic approach is taken, feelings are considered as well as facts
- That someone's health does not remain static or the same but rather that it is dynamic, changing along with changes in the many factors which influence health
- Learning oriented towards people's action, which enables individuals to influence their wider social and physical environment
- A life skills approach which aims to introduce, build and reinforce the knowledge and skills upon which students can make lifelong healthy decisions.

Principles
- Credibility—It is the degree to which the message to be communicated is perceived as trust worthy by the receiver. Health Education has to be based on facts, it must be consistent and compatible with scientific knowledge and also local culture, language, educational system and social goals. The people must have trust, confidence in the educator then only desired action will be ensured
- Interest—Health Educators must identify the felt needs of community and assist them to prioritize, teach them the problem solving techniques, focus from top priority to low priority, help them to develop interest in their own living conditions
- Community Participation and Community involvement, Learning by Doing—It is based on personal involvement and personal acceptance. Encourage the community to participate in promoting their total health with their own efforts. Health Educators has to motivate the public to meet their felt needs and target needs set by the Nation for them. Group Discussions, Work shops, Project methods (Individual and Group) has to be encouraged to disseminate the health related knowledge. Encourage the people to practice healthy living and have healthy life style
- Known to Unknown—For clear understanding and to develop systematic knowledge it is always essential to teach from Known to Unknown, easy to difficult approaches
- Comprehension—Educate the community based on their mental capacity, educational background, quoting examples in their own language such that they can understand easily in a comprehensive manner.
- Motivation—The inborn desires of the individuals has to be recognized and motivate the people to fulfill their healthy desires into action. Incentives and Rewards for exhibition of healthy behavior and healthy living conditions has to be encouraged
- Reinforcement—Motivation will act as a booster dose and reinforcement will act as key factor
- To bring behavioral modification the educators has to reinforce the community, in health education campaigns varied methods and different mass media approaches will be used to reinforce the needed modification of behavior
- Soil, Seed, Sower—The community is the soil, health facts are seeds and the transmitting media are the sower. The Health Educators must carefully observe the customs, habits, taboos, beliefs, health needs of the community and plan health education campaigns. Use the transmitting media must be attractive, palatable and acceptable
- Good Human Relations—Health Educators has to develop good rapport and establish effective human interpersonal relationship, communicate the health related concepts in a clear, understanding manner to facilitate conducive learning
- Leaders—Identify the local leaders within the community, if the leaders are convinced with health education campaigns, they will take active part in convincing people and assist in imparting scientific knowledge, the task of implementing the Health Education program will be easier for health professionals in community. They will understand the needs and demands of the community and provide the guidance and takes initiative actions, assist necessary help for active participation and active implementation of health education activities
- Setting as an example—Health educator should be a role model and an exampler eg: when he is educating about hazards of drug abuse, he should not have that habit

- Feed back—it is one of the key concepts of system approach, The health educator can modify the elements of the system in the light of feed back from his audience
- View health as more than the absence of disease
- Utilize all educational opportunities for health: formal and informal, traditional and alternative; inside and outside the focused areas, harmonize all of the health messages
- Empower focus groups/students /community/individuals to act for healthy living and to promote conditions supportive of health
- Establishes a basis for lifelong learning and promotion of health foster interaction between schools, the community, parents and local services
- Ensure a Healthy Environment.

Content—Content is selected based on Focus Group, Age, Need assessment
- Human Biology, e.g. Functions of body, exercise, Rest and sleep
- Communicable Diseases – Prevention and Control – STD and AIDS, Malaria, Diarrhoeal Diseases, Worm Infestations, ARI, Cholera etc.
- Mental Health and Mental Hygiene
- Prevention of Accidents
- Availability and utilization of Health services
- Nutrition Education–PEM, Dietary requirements, Malnutrition, Breast Feeding, Weaning, Deficiency Disorders etc. and its prevention
- Child Growth and Development/Mile Stones
- Family Planning and Family Welfare
- Healthy Recreation, Healthy Habits and Healthy Practices
- Timing of Births and Safe Motherhood
- Sex Education
- Home economics
- Child rearing practices
- Family formation and Family building
- Hearing and Sight impairments
- Personal Hygiene and Mental Hygiene
- Immunizations
- Safe Water Supply
- Family Education
- Substance Abuse
- Physical Activity and Exercise
- Environment
- First Aid and Treatment of Minor Ailments
- Defence Mechanisms
- Utilization of community resources.

Importance of Health Education Utilization of Community Resources

- It Promotes the Health status and Well-being of individuals, families, communities, states and the Nation
- Enhances quality of life for all people
- It reduces Premature deaths
- Prevents the occurrence of Diseases and illnesses
- Reduces the cost (Economic and Human) that the individuals, families, medical facilities, communities, the state and the Nation would spend on Medical treatment.

Scope of Health Education

Learning related to health is not limited to situation in which actual instruction is given. It results from wide variety of exposures, the various situations and factors that arise within the social settings which affects health related attitudes and practices.

In Home
- Guidance will be given to children in the formation of healthy living habits, Practices related to qualitative life
- The healthy Relationship between family members, Love and bondage
- Family attitude towards health and illness
- Family responsibility in meeting primary needs
- Budgeting
- Situations in Home, e.g. Safe Drinking Water Supply, Adequate Nutrition—The preparation, serving, preservation of nutrients, Proper disposal of liquid and solid wastes, environmental sanitation
- Selection of Play materials as per age
- The Quality of living
- Religious and Cultural Behavior of the family.

In Educational Institutions
- Conducive Environment for teaching and learning
- The standards of cleanliness
- Curriculum content related to health
- Co-curricular and Extra-curricular activities
- Teaching Strategies
- Learners' participation in community projects
- Teacher as a role model
- Influence of Rewards and Punishments on the personality of the learner
- School Health Services
- Handling of health emergencies
- Group Activities, e.g. Association meetings, Formal and Informal meetings.

In the Community
- Experiences that influence health behavior
    - Advises and services received from health professionals
    - Participation in governmental and Voluntary organizations activities
    - Membership and Participation in organized group activities
    - Experiences in the work situations and disasters
    - Leisure time activities
    - Religious ceremonies and observances.

Approaches to Health Education

1. Regulatory Approach/Managed Prevention
   "Any Governmental intervention, direct or indirect, designed to alter human behavior". It seeks change in health behavior and improvement of health through a variety of external control or laws placed on the people. Government can make laws to prevent a person spreading disease in his community, e.g. vaccination, Quarantine and Surveillance, however laws may be helpful in times of emergency or in limited situations, e.g. Control of an epidemics, Management of fairs and festivals.
2. Service Approach
   Aimed at providing the health services needed by the people at their door steps on the assumption that people would use them to improve their own health with their own efforts. As it is not based on the felt needs approach, this is of failure.
3. Health Education Approach
   Many problems can be controlled by this approach. People must be educated through planned learning experiences what to do and be informed, educated and encouraged to make their own choice for a healthy life. The Mass Media and Social Organizations has to be mobilized to introduce new positive attitudes.
4. Primary Health Care Approach
   New approach where community participation and community involvement, intersectoral coordination emphasized in the planning and implementation of Health Education Campaigns. The aim of this approach is to help the people to become self reliant in matters of health.

5. Individual Approach
   Opportunity has to be utilized when educating the individual on matters of his/her interest. Topics for Health Counseling may be selected as per relevance of the situation. Based on this the health educator will be equipping the individual and the family to deal more effectively with the health problems. The educator has to create trust worthy, friendly environment and allow the individual to talk more effectively, encourage him/her to talk more deeply about a particular health problem and the educator will have the opportunity to discuss and persue the individual to change his behavior, provides an opportunity to ask questions in the area of his/her interest.

6. Group Approach
   Society consists of many groups of individuals like school children, women, Adolescent children, Young Adults, Elderly, etc. Group teaching is an effective way of teaching the group, related to the interest of the group topic will be chosen and discussed and solutions will be suggested.

Personnel Providing Health Education
- Trained or certified Health Education Specialists
- Health Care Professionals, e.g. Doctors/Medical Professionals (in all categories), Nurses (in all categories), Physiotherapists, Mass Media Officers, Social Workers, Health Care Workers
- Teachers are trained to teach Health Education as a part of their curriculum to the group of students, they will inturn educate their families directly and the community and the Nation indirect, overall the Nation progress improves.

Placement of Health Educators
Healthcare Settings
Educational Institutions—Schools, Colleges, Universities
Companies—Government and Private sector
Community Organizations—Voluntary organizations (National, International), Governmental agencies, Non Profit Organizations.

Methods and Media for communicating Health Messages /Practice of Health Education
- Through Audio-Visual Aids /Educational Communication Media
- Cooperative Small Group, Class or Video Discussion, Panel Discussion, Symposium, Seminar, Conference, work shop
- Lecture Method
- Brainstorming
- Role Playing and Simulations
- Performing Tasks/Demonstrations
- Conducting Surveys, Interviews, Experiments etc.
- Field trips
- Health Museums, Exhibitions
- Folk Media
- Utilization of Mass Media like TV, Radio, Internet, Newspapers, Printed Materials, Direct Mailing, Posters, Bill Boards and signs
- Visits by the Specialists and Experts' advises that emphasize
  - Focus Group Oriented/Student Centered activities
  - Task-based activities
  - Cooperative Learning
  - Assist the individuals/Families/Community/Focus Groups in setting and acting upon setting goals for themselves
  - Inclusion of health aspects like Physical/Psychological/Social
  - Assigning Home and Community assignments and do follow up
  - Supplement classroom activities by home and community assignments
  - Challenge focus groups by altering the context or conditions for the health practices
  - Involve the expertise the services and resources of the community

- Guide the focus groups in community how they can learn more about a topic by utilizing available learning technologies
- Create a comfortable, supportive and healthy learning environment.

Educators has to remember to reach out to the family and community by
- Show genuine concern for the welfare and opinions of the public
- Build on what the learners know
- Demonstrate the relevance of the topic to the present and future lives
- Employ a variety of teaching strategies by varying modalities
- Consulting with the audience specifically with respect to sensitive issues
- Informing the community what the Nation/State/Social Organizations are attempting to achieve
- Involving parents and families in child learning
- Consulting appropriate personnel from the health field, extending field work by focus groups in the community. In this way, health messages may extend across the community

Therefore, the Educators' role is complex viz.,
- Assisting rather than being the Expert or Director
- Providing the reference materials and resources
- Motivating and Coordinating people progress
- Guiding individuals'/pupils' reflection on their learning process
- Co-ordinating with the community
- Create a comfortable, supportive and healthy environment
- Guide the students towards how they might learn more about the topic.

Methods in Health Communication and Health Education

Individual Approach	Group Approach	Mass Approach
Personal Contact	Lecture Method, Discussion, Demonstration, Guiding and Counseling teachniques	Utilizing Mass Media – TV, Radio, Newspapers, Printed Material, Direct Mailing, Posters, Pamphlets, Hand outs, Leaflets, Museums, Exhibitions, Folk Media and internet
Home Visits	Demonstration	T.V. Demonstration
Personal Letters	Discussion – Group Discussion, Panel Discussion, Symposium, Workshop, Conferences, Seminars, Role Play, Simulation Method	

(Source: Modified from Park's Textbook of Preventive and Social Medicine, 20th Edition, P.766)

Role of Trained Health Educator

A health educator is "a professionally prepared individual who serves in a variety of roles and is specifically trained to use appropriate educational strategies and methods to facilitate the development of policies, procedures, interventions and systems conducive to the health of individuals, groups and communities" (Fig. 10.1).
- Assess the individual and community needs
  - Provides the foundation for program planning
  - Determines what health problems might exist in any given group
  - Includes determination of community resources available to address the problem
  - Community Empowerment encourages the population to take ownership of their health problems
  - Includes careful data collection and analysis
  - Develop, Plan, Implement, Manage, Evaluate and Coordinate Health Education Programs
- Actions are based on the needs assessment done for the community
- Involves the development of goals and objectives which are specific and measurable
- Interventions are developed that will meet the goals and objectives
- According to rule of sufficiency, strategies are implemented which are sufficiently robust, effective enough, and have a reasonable chance of meeting stated objectives

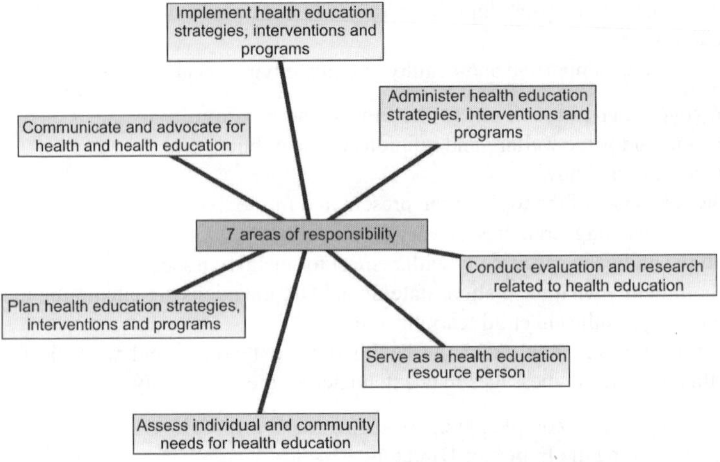

Fig. 10.1: Responsibilities of health educator

- Implementation is based on a thorough understanding of the priority population
- Utilize a wide range of educational methods and techniques
- Depending on the setting, utilize tests, surveys, observations, tracking epidemiological data or other methods of data collection
- Health Educators make use of research to improve their practice
- Administration is generally a function of the more experienced practitioner
- Administer Health education strategies, Interventions and Programs
- Involves facilitating cooperation among personnel, both within and between programs
- Serve as a Health Education Resource Person
- Involves skills to access needed resources and establish effective consultive relationships
- Communicate and Advocate for Health and Health Education
- Translates scientific language into understandable information
- Address diverse audience in diverse settings
- Formulates and support rules, policies and legislation
- Advocate for the profession of health education
- Write Grants
- Build Coalitions
- Identify the resources
- Make Referrals
- Develop Social Marketing and mass media campaigns
- Organize and mobilize communities for action
- Handle controversial health issues and content
- Advocate for health related issues
- Encourage the healthy behavior
- Uses a variety of training/teaching methods
- Develop audio, visual, print and electronic materials
- Conduct Research and write Scholarly article.

Model of Planning and Evaluating Health Education and Health Promotion

Model can be used to gain insight into the quality of the interventions described. Based on the model the quality of an intervention can be divided into three components

- The Quality of the Planning Process
- Evoluation process
  - The Quality of the Formative Evaluation
  - The Quality of the Summative Evaluation

During the planning process five questions has to be asked
1. How serious is the problem?
2. What behaviors is involved? Is behavior related to the problem?
3. What are the determinants of that behavior?
4. Which interventions might change that behavior? How can an intervention be developed and pretested?
5. How can the developed intervention be implemented?

The Evaluative process refers to Formative and Summative process.

Formative Evaluation provides us with an understanding of how people perceive an intervention. Why people reacted the way they do? Why the programs have specific effects? What the unanticipated consequences of that interventions are? By examining why interventions do work or do not work? Useful insights into the conditions characteristics which promote and hinder effectiveness will be gained in order to improve future interventions. Information from formative evaluation can also be very useful to make recommendations for the possible dissemination of the intervention to other settings or to other target groups or for studying the theory or the policy upon which an intervention is based.

The Summative evaluation is concerned with the degree to which the objectives of the program have been met and with the achievement of intended effects.

Standards and Sets of Criteria

- Behavioral objectives should be formulated in measurable terms
- Multidisciplinary care plans should be developed and documented
- Personnel should be qualified and trained
- Evaluation components should be based on measurable objectives and impact on health behavior
- Reinforce positive behavior
- Offer feedback
- Individualize the educational program to provide opportunities for patients to set the pace of their learning and get answers to their personal questions
- Facilitate behavior by providing the means for individuals and families to take action or reduce the barriers to action
- Assure that the content and educational methods are relevant to the learners' interests and circumstances
- Interventions should stress the personal advantages of the targeted behavior because health considerations as such are less important for the people
- Learning practical and social skills has to be emphasized
- A variety of methods should be used within the interventions
- Careful planning is necessary when designing and implementing the interventions.

Information Education and Communication (IEC)

IEC is the process of learning that empowers people to make decisions, modify behaviors and change Social Conditions. IEC activities are developed based upon needs assessment, educational principles and periodic evaluation of using a set of goals and objectives.

Information is, "Telling something to an individual about a person, topic or a subject".

Types of Information

1. Conventional Information—which confirm and change is brought out (Accepting).
2. Progressive Information—Which reform and behavior change is brought about (Adoptation).
3. Liberating Information—Which transform and Social change is brought out.

Health information can be communicated through many channels to increase awareness and assess the knowledge of different population about various issues, products and behaviors.

Education

"A gradual process of learning through which a person gains Knowledge and Understanding Subject".

Communication

"A two way process of giving information or sharing and transmitting the ideas and messages between two or more persons".

Mass Media

"An agency through which communication takes place".

Types of Media

- Electronic Media—Can have a better reach among a particular section of society and can be used for creating awareness and reinforcement of messages, e.g. Films, Film Quickies, Video Tapes, Video Quickies, Radio Programs, Radio Spots, Audio Tapes, TV Programs, TV Quickies, Slides etc.
- Print Media—It has limited use in areas with low literacy levels, e.g. Books, Booklets, Folders, Leaflets, Hand Bills, Letters, Newspapers, Advertisements, Press Release, Posters, Photographs, Magazines, News Letters, Journals
- Folk and Traditional Media—is more popular in tribal and rural areas, e.g. Song, Dance, Drama/Role Play, Bhajan, Kirtan, Show, Wall Writing
- Alternate Media—Street Play, Drama
- Rural Resources—Wall Paintings, Sloagans, Exhibition, Banner display
- Multi Media Campaigns—Publicity Campaigns, Awareness Campaigns, Exhibitions.

Points to Remember While Selecting Mass Media

- Educational level of Target audience
- Habits of Target audience
- Media—Mix approach or use of various media forms at the same time is more effective.

Planning and Organizing a Information, Education and Communication Program

It has to be organized based on the needs of target audience

- Identify the felt needs of the community
- Prioritize community needs and decide subject/topic for communication
- Identify target audience and assess their knowledge, attitude and Practices
- Define Communication goal and Objectives
- Give a name to communication program with specific logo
- Prepare Media Implementation, Plan for each day as for the format
- Identify suitable Channel, media and techniques of Communication
- Develop suitable social messages, materials and aids
- Prepare Communication Material
- Train Communicators
- Prepare budget and ensure its availability
- Decide duration, place, time for organizing communication activities
- Implement the program, assess the impact and reinforce the messages if required.

Name of Activity	Time	Place	Communicator	Target Audience	Channel and Medium	Message	Communication Materials/Aids	Feed Back

The Essentials of IEC

IEC strategies, Approaches, Methods that enable individuals, Families, Groups, Organizations and Community to play active roles in achieving, protecting or sustaining their own health. Health Information can be communicated through many channels to increase awareness and assess the knowledge of different population about various issues, products and behaviors. Good Communication between users and providers of any service is essential. IEC approaches carefully selected and designed. Building trust, communicating effectively within the group and community is also vital. Selection of approach, materials, methods also is essential. Field staff should not ignore informal opportunities to educate the public through casual conversation with people in the community. Good Communication skills are essential, e.g. Active Listening, Rephrasing, asking open ended questions, eye contact, Providing complete Attention, exhibiting positive attitude towards audience, body language and facial expressions etc. Health Educators has to familiarize themselves with the community, Identify individual needs, identify influencing personalities, Provision of clear cut information is needed.

Counseling is a Key component in IEC Program. A good Counselor has to be Compassionate, non judgmental, aware of verbal and non verbal communication approaches, knowledgeable, respectful of the needs and users of the group. Counselor has to provide conducive environment for the implementation of IEC strategies.

Counselor will use GATHER technique in the counselling process.
G–Greet Others
A–Ask Others about themselves
T–Tell about availability of services
H–Help others to choose the available services, whichever they like
E–Explain how to use the services
R–Return for follow up

Quantitative assessment—assess available incidence and prevalence of problems, KABP surveys (Knowledge, Attitude, Behavior and Practices surveys). Qualitative assessment—Individual and Group interviews, focus group discussions, leader questions, Survey for analysis by computer and hand, Checklist.

Steps in Developing IEC Activities

- Conduct a Need Assessment
- Prioritize the Needs
- Set the Goals and Behavioral Objectives (SMART approach—Specific, Measurable, Area specific, Realistic and time bound)
- Develop IEC activities, involve as many as possible
- Identify potential barriers and methods to overcome them
- Identify resources and other supportive services
- Establish an evaluation plan.

IEC Messages

Develop IEC message (Short, accurate and relevant), disseminated in the language of target group of audience, use appropriate vocabulary.

Message tone may be humorous, didactic, authoritative, rational or emotional appealing.

One time appeal or a repetitive reinforcement

Prepare IEC materials

Try Out

Determine suitable methods and Choice of communication channel or medium of channel are inseparable.

HEALTH INFORMATION

Components (Fig. 10.2)

The Health Information broadly divided into three components
- Inputs
- Processes
- Outputs.

Inputs

It includes all Health Information System (HIS) resources. The Physical and structural prerequisites of an HIS. Those include the ability of those responsible to lead and coordinate the process, the existence of necessary Policies, Laws, Procedures, financial resources, skilled personnel and physical facilities like office space, filing system, computer systems with internet connections.

The HMN roadmap to building as integrated HIS

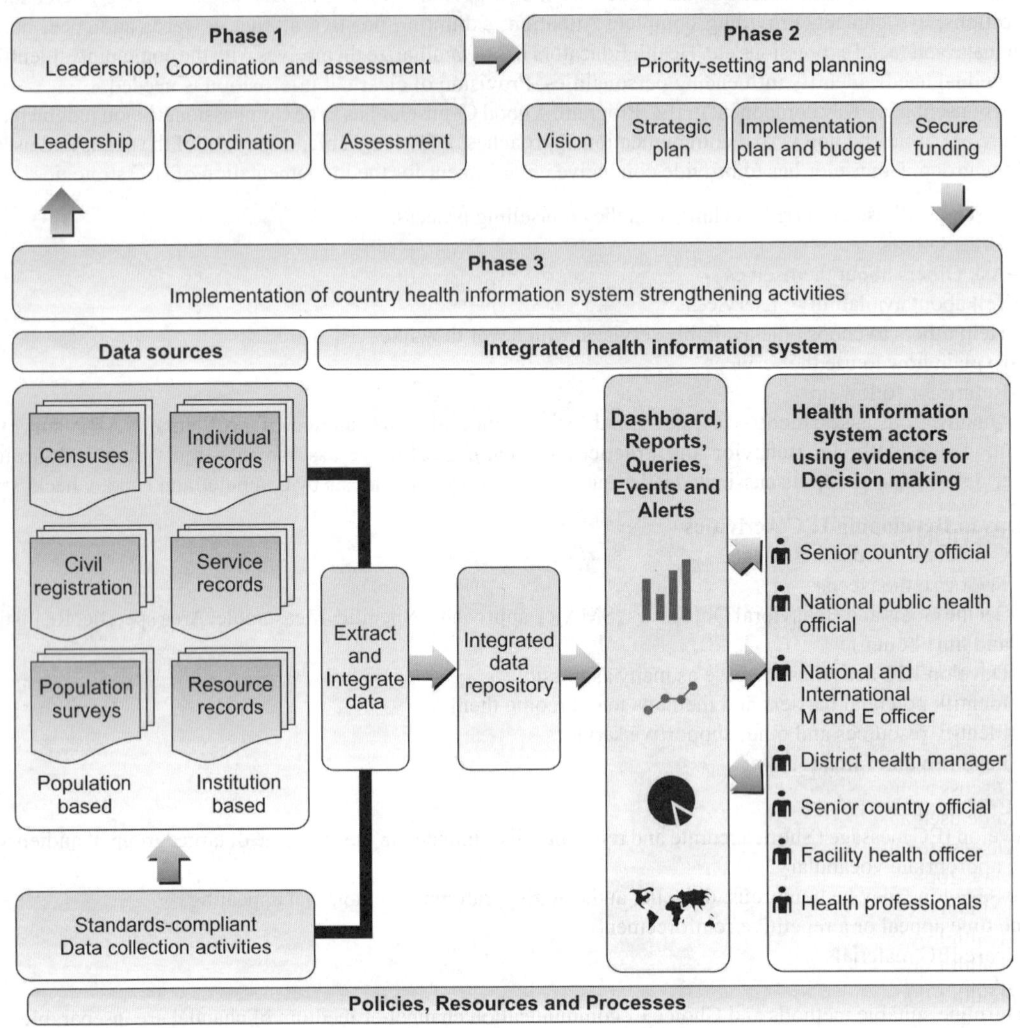

Fig. 10.2: Components of health information

The Processes Include

Indicators

A set of measures that show changes in the country's health profile.

Data Sources—An integrated HIS brings data together from different sources.

Data Management—Easy access to relevant information for those who need it, while protecting the privacy of individual patients (Fig. 10.3).

Outputs

Needs to be relevant, accessible, useful evidence from decision making.

Information Products—collected from varied resources and synthesized into statistics that can be analyzed and compared. HIS provides direct benefit to all those who participate it, providing an ongoing incentives for users to continue and strengthen the system.

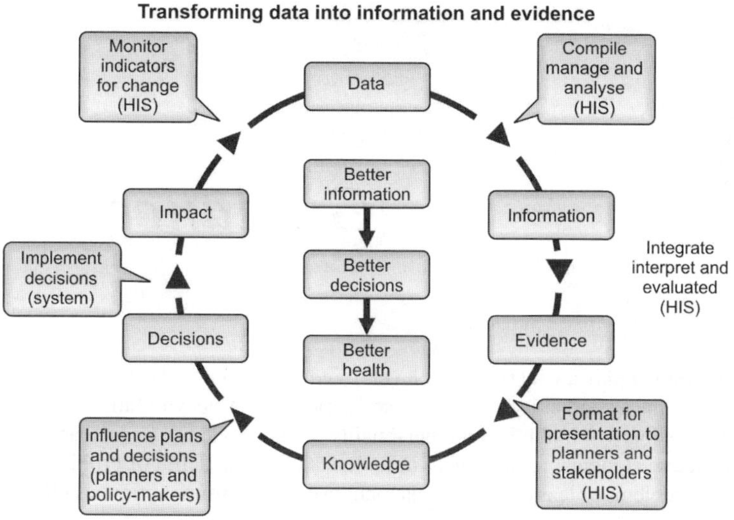

Fig. 10.3: Transforming data into information and evidence

QUESTIONS

- Aims of Health Education (5M, NTRUHS, Dec, 2007).
- Components of Health Education (5M, NTRUHS, June, 2010).
- Define Health Education (2M, NTRUHS, June, 2009 & July, 2008).
- Define Health Education, State the principles of Health Education, Explain the role of Community Health Nurse using A.V. Aids in Health Education (2M +7M+6M=15M, NTRUHS, June 2010).
- Define Health Education, Write the objectives of Health Education (4M), Plan Health Education Programme to a group of antenatal mothers about the importance of balanced diet(6M, NIMS).
- Discuss a blue print to communicate messages on AIDS prevention, specify the target group, type of media to be used and the methods of collecting feedback (10M, NIMS, May, 2008).
- Discuss the importance of Information, Education and Communication in the Indian context (10M, NIMS, May, 2008).
- Explain the principles of Health Education, as a Community Health Nurse, how will you conduct effective Health Education Programme in community (15M, NTRUHS, July, 2008).
- Health Education (5M, NTRUHS, Dec, 2007).
- Health Education Methods (5M, NIMS).
- Importance of Health Education (5M, NTRUHS, Dec, 2007).
- List any four Principles of Health Education (2M, MGRUHS, Feb, 2010).
- List the different types of mass media used in health Education(2M, RGUHS, Feb, 2010).
- Methods for communicating health messages (5M, RGUHS, Aug, 2009).
- Methods of Health Education (7.5M, Baba Farid UHS, 2010).
- Methods of health teaching (5M, RGUHS, Feb, 2010).
- Plan and conduct Health Education session for a group of people in community on the topic "Immunization" (13M, Baba Farid UHS, 2008).
- Plan of Health Education (5M, Rajasthan UHS, Feb, 2008).
- Planning for health education (5M, RGUHS, Sept, 2009).
- Principles of health education (5M, RGUHS, April, 2009 and Principles of Health Education (5M, NTRUHS, July, 2008).
- Uses of Mass Media (2M, RGUHS, Sept, 2009).
- Using Mass Media (5M, NTRUHS, Nov, 2010).

Guidance

INTRODUCTION

Guidance and counseling play a vital role in all levels of education. One of the purposes of education is to help the individual to become a good citizen of society and serve the Nation with full of his/her abilities and talents. Guidance and counseling will mold the total personality of an individual. Good teachers always interested in providing assistance to students, to help them in understanding the depth of problems and adapts necessary steps to overcome problems of learning and adjustment in order to ensure optimum achievement and profitable placement in their career.

"To Guide"—Means

- To indicate
- To point out
- To show the way
- To lead
- To direct
- To seek.

DEFINITIONS

"A process of dynamic interpersonal relationships designed to influence the attitudes and subsequent behavior of a person"—*Good*.

"Assistance made available by qualified and adequately trained personnel to an individual of any age to help an individual to manage his own life activities, to develop his own points of view, make his own decisions and carry his own steps to solve the problems"—*Crow and Crow*.

"A process through which an individual is able to solve their problems and pursue a path suited to their abilities and aspirations"—*JM Brewer*.

"An educational service designed to help students make more effective use of the schools and training program"—*Educational Point of View*.

"A process consists of a group of services to individuals to assist them in securing the knowledge and skills needed in making adequate choices, plans and interpretations essential to satisfactory adjustment in a variety of areas to solve their personal and other problems"—*Smith*.

"A facilitative service, which provides aid to learners:
- To determine the courses most appropriate to their needs and abilities
- To find instructors who will be more sympathetic and assisting in meeting the individual requirements and seek out activities which will help them to realize their potentialities"—*Mc Daniel*.

"A continuous process of helping the individual development in the maximum of their capacity in the direction most beneficial to himself and to society"—*Stoops and Wahlquist*.

"A Continuous process where the teaching faculty will assist the learners individually:
- To formulate or frame their educational goals or Objectives
- To improve their potentialities/strengths/abilities
- To work effectively or to implement focused activities to attain their goals

- To direct the pathways which will be helping the learner to solve their problems or the issues by taking necessary steps
- To adopt measures which will strengthen the coping abilities
- To choose right career which is beneficial and promotes the growth of an individual in a right direction
- To meet the individual and societal needs.

Meaning

- Some form of help or assistance given to an individual to solve their problems by expert in the field or seniors or elderly; Guidance is designed to assist a person in deciding:
  - Where he/she wants to go?
  - What he/she wants to do?
  - How he/she can best accomplish his purposes
- Guidance is the promotion of the growth of an individual in self-direction. The individual attains self-direction in a fast manner, as far as his mental, social and emotional abilities permit
- Guidance of the younger or less mature individual calls for closer direction than does guidance of the older or more mature individual
- It is a Process of learning, helping and effecting changes in an individual: Learning about the individual student, helping him/her to understand herself/himself effecting changes in him and in his environment which will help him/her to grow and develop as much as possible
- Process of helping every individual through their own efforts, to discover and develop their potentialities for their happiness and social usefulness
- Process of assisting an individual to find their place: Guidance seeks to help the individual to discover their talents in comparison to the opportunities of the world and help him/her to prepare himself/herself so that he/she can find or develop a place in which he/she can live a well balanced life and contribute his/her part to the welfare of his/her fellow beings
- Establishing an effective relationship with the learner by mentor to improve educational experiences and thereby meeting personal needs and potentialities in an effective way
- Process of assisting (helping) to adjust: Guidance will be given whenever an important activity has to be learnt and assistance is needed by an individual to adjust himself/herself related to any type of activity like the choice of Professional courses, selection of job, the way for further growth like education or job, leisure time activity or eating habits or any other area of interest to improve their professional efficiencies
- Guidance helps the learner to become adjusted to the situation and to plan his future in line with his interests, abilities and social needs
- Guidance helps the person to adjust to environment
- Educational guidance viewed as encompassing the objectives of:
  - Attaining sound Physical and Emotional health
  - Well-rounded social development
  - Effective utilization of leisure time
  - Mastery of fundamental school processes
  - Curricular, Co-curricular and Extracurricular activities
  - Guidance is essentially an educative process the outcomes of which are mental and educational preparedness for course of action centered round the basic functions of learner especially those pertaining to vocational, recreational and community service field.
- Vocational Guidance—The guidance facilitates the choice of an occupation or way of making a living either semi-skilled, skilled, technical or professional occupations. In this phase, the individual is assisted to make the optimum adjustment to the opportunities whatever he gets and lives happily in it and progress themselves in a right direction
- Guidance covers the whole gamut of youth problems. It helps the students to plan their own future wisely in the full light of all the factors that can be mastered about themselves and about the world in which they are to live and work.
- It is a continuous and pervasive process as a favorable directional influence upon
  - Appropriate social behavior
  - Personal effectiveness in everyday affairs

- Academic competence
- Progress
- Assimilation of right values and attitudes

Thus guidance is
- Orientational
- Developmental
- Remedial
- Guidance as "individualized education"—Each student has to be helped to develop himself to the maximum possible degree in all aspects
  Four-fold functions of a guidance program
  - Where he/she has been?
  - Where he/she is now?
  - Where he/she is going?
  - What he/she has with which to get there?
- Guidance aids in the identification and the development of abilities and interests among the learners
- Guidance is a special training in which an individual discovers his natural endowments so that he makes living to his own best advantage and that of society
- Guidance is a systematic, organized phase of the educational process which helps to improve their powers and gain richer personal experiences while making his own unique contribution to the society in specific and to the Nation in general.

Elements

- It focuses teachers' attention on the individual—their growth and development and not on the problem
- Guidance leads to the discovery of abilities of an individual
- Guidance is based upon the assets and limitations of an individual
- Guidance leads to self-development and self-direction
- Guidance helps the individual to plan wisely for the present and for the future
- Guidance assists the individual to become adjusted to the environment and to achieve success and happiness

It focuses to improve students' capacity related to
- Educational (Curricular and Cocurricular)
- Moral
- Vocational, avocational
- In all aspects of Health—Physical, Psychological, Social, Spiritual and Ethical
- Leisure activity (Extracurricular Activiites).

Nature

- Guidance involves personal help given by someone: It is designed to assist a person to decide where he/she wants to go, what he/she wants to do or how he/she can best accomplish his purpose
- It is an instrument, which helps in the realization of general objectives of education
- Systematic professional process of helping the individual through education and interpretative procedures to gain a better understanding of his/her own characteristics and potentialities and interests
- It is a process or service designed to help the individual to attain total maturity
- To provide service to the society
- Competent experts in the field to provide assistance to an individual of any age
  - To formulate life goals
  - Make their own decisions
  - Direct the activities to accomplish the goals in their own point of view
  - Implement sincere efforts by following specific steps to solve his/her own burdens or problems or issues that will arise in life.
- The Expert in educational program concerned specifically helping individual learner to become adjusted to the present situation and to plan for the future activities, in line with his/her interests, abilities and social needs

- Experts will assist the individual learner to meet satisfactorily to educational and social requirements and explore the available opportunities in accord with social and moral values
- To attain a state of complete and mature self-guidance in a desirable member in order to maintain the social order.

Characteristics

1. It helps every individual to help themselves to recognize and use their inner resources
   - To set goals
   - To make plans
   - To work out his own problems related to his career and Personal development
2. It is a continuous process: Guidance has to be provided throughout life-cycle of an individual, e.g. Childhood, Adolescence, Adulthood and Elderly.
3. Choice and problem points are the distinctive concerns of guidance.
   The individual's unique world of perceptions interacts with the external order of events in the life context.
4. Assistance to the individual in the process of development, e.g. To develop the capacity for:
   - Self-direction
   - Self-guidance
   - Self-improvement.
   Through an increase the understanding of their problems and resources as well as limitations to solve the problem.
5. Guidance is a service meant for all: It is a regular service, which is required at every stage for every student, not only for awkward situations and abnormal students, it is a positive program geared to meet the needs of all students.
6. It is both generalized and a specialized service.
   - Generalized service: Every one, e.g. Teachers, Advisers, Deans and Parents Play part in the guidance program of learners.
   - Specialized service: Specialized qualified personnel like Counselors, Psychiatrists, Psychologists will Join hands to help the individual learner to solve the problem with their own efforts.

Principles

"The sum total of efforts and influences of all those who assists an individual through association, counsel dissemination of facts, utilization of appropriate/special techniques and control of environment to attain optimum development like personal, social, vocational, cultural and spiritual aspects".

1. Guidance services are aimed at bringing desirable adjustment in any particular area of experience must be taken into account the all-round development of the individual.
2. Individual differ in native capacity, ability and interests. Individual differences must be recognized and considered in any efforts aimed at providing help or guidance to a particular individual.
3. To help the person
   - Formulate and accept stimulating, worthwhile, and attainable goals of behavior.
   - Apply the objectives in the conduct of his affairs.
4. Existing social, economic and political unrest is giving rise to many maladjustive factors that require the cooperation of experienced and thoroughly trained guidance counselors and the individual learner with a problem.
5. Life is dynamic: World is fast changing. Individual requires help for the solution of problems; Individual face problems throughout their lives, hence Guidance is a continuous process of service to an individual from young childhood throughout the life.
6. Guidance service should not be limited to the few, who give observable evidence of his need, but should be extended to all persons of all ages who can benefit either directly or indirectly.
7. Curriculum materials and teaching procedures should be based on guidance point of view.
8. Guidance touches every phase of an individual's life pattern, e.g. generally accepted areas of guidance include: concern with the extent to which an individual's physical and mental health interfere with his/her adjustment to home, school, vocational and social demands and relationships or the extent to

which his/her physical and mental health are affected by the conditions to which he/she is subjected in these areas of experience.

9. Parents and teachers have to guide the children with specific responsibilities for all round personality development of the child.

10. Specific guidance problems on any age level should be referred to persons who are trained to deal with particular areas of adjustment.

11. For guidance purpose, the data should be accurately recorded and utilized.
   For example: Cumulative records of progress and achievement
   - Accessibility of records and reports
   - Instruments of evaluation
   - Intellectual capacities
   - Success of achievement
   - Demonstrated interests
   - Personality characteristics.

12. Organized guidance program should be flexible according to individual and community needs.

13. Highly qualified and adequately trained persons should act as chairman or head of the guidance program, who can work cooperatively with his assistants and other community welfare and guidance agencies.

14. Periodic appraisals should be made: The success of curriculum functioning should rest on outcomes that are reflected in the attitudes towards the program of all who are associated with it, guiders has to guide in the displayed behavior of these who have been served through its functioning as a role model.

15. Guidance is a slow process: An individual cannot make wise decisions and adjustments in a day or month or so. It requires a considerable time to make suitable adjustments.
   The counselor needs time to understand the counselee who has a complex personality and who may confronted with an intense problem.

16. Guidance helps in developing the insights of an individual: The counselor should help the individual in such a way that he gains his own insights, accepts responsibility, develops self-confidence and ultimately makes his/her own decisions in dealing with problems and solve the problems with their efforts.

17. Inform all students that the services of the guidance will be available to everyone; whenever the need arises, they can approach the faculty in Guidance department and they will be available to all 24 × 7 days.

18. Counselor must be aware of the difference between symptoms and causes.

19. Personality of an individual is a complex and integrated whole. The individual is a psychobiological organism in constant interaction with a complex array of environmental forces. As an organism he necessarily responds to his environment as a "whole being", i.e. educational, vocational and personal problems are interrelated.

20. Guidance is based on a right code of ethics: Establish and follow a rigid code of ethics by every professional who has access to the confidence of the students.

21. Guidance services must be an integral part of the school organization: Guidance work should not be treated as an isolated work. It should not be left to the counselor to render guidance to the students. All or most of the members of the staff should take a keen interest and active part, in assisting students to solve their problems. Guidance work should be closely integrated with the work done by other agencies engaged in child development work.

22. Guidance is an organized service: Guidance is not an incidental activity of the school. It is a service which is broad base and a definite purpose.

23. Guidance is both a specialized and a generalized service: Guidance requires the help of a specially trained staff for its proper functioning.
   For example: School Counselor, School Psychologist, School Social Worker, School Physician, School Psychiatrist, Curriculum Expert, Placement Worker, Coordinator of school activities.

24. Guidance is universal and meant for all.

25. Guidance is based on educational objective which reflect the aim and purposes of society. Collection of full information about an individual. All members of the guidance service should cooperate whole-heartedly.

26. Guidance services should supplement and complement instructional work.

Need for Guidance

Guidance is based upon the fact that human beings need help. Everyone needs assistance at sometime or other in their lives, some may need it constantly and throughout their entire lives, while others used it only at rare intervals at the time of great crisis. Guidance will be given by experts, older people and experienced associates to youngsters and assist them in meeting their needs during problematic situations.

The need for guidance is universal, as it is not confined to a few individuals or a few countries. Guidance has been there from time immemorial and will continue to be as long as human beings exists.

1. Complex Nature of Society

Changes have taken place in the entire structure of economic, social and political system. The process of:

- Consumption
- Production
- Distribution
- Exchange

Has become very complex and intricate. It has become very difficult for an individual to achieve satisfactory results without the aid of guidance. Various public service agencies have been set up to give assistance to the people.

2. Individual Differences

No two human beings have ever been found to be alike. On the whole world, there are probably no two things exactly alike. They differ physically in size, weight, color, hair texture and skin color, mental (emotional characteristics), social and spiritual life also, personality traits—ability, interest, achievement, etc.

The requirements of various occupations also differ; this makes increasingly necessary to have a definite provision for certain form of guidance.

3. Welfare State and the Individual

Every individual must be helped in certain way and in a definite direction. Give scope for the individual to improve and express himself as a person have flourished. Through guidance services, the individual is aided in self-development and self-realization and a wide use of human resources is made.

4. Changed Societal and educational pattern of the Nation

The needs of society will be ever changing, attempts are being made to change the educational system of country in order to equalize global educational requirements and to meet societal needs, the curriculum has to be revised, the teaching faculty has to provide guidance services in educational program to overcome the problems in selection of subjects and vocations are formidable problems and meet the educational requirements of the learners.

5. Changed Economic Patterns of the Country

The country is in the era of economic planning. We require—scientists, industrialists and bankers, etc. to meet the growing demands of a progressive country. Economy is a basic need and everyone has to fulfill this need. Learners will select varied types of educational programs for their livelihood and to meet their aspirations and interests and to achieve their life goals, guidance is required.

6. Conservation of Human Energy

Well-planned guidance is required to conserve the human energy. Improvement of vocational efficiency is the aim of education. Through educational guidance, education should train their various aptitudes and enable them to take up varied vocational pursuits.

Guidance is needed to assist an individual to make the right use of leisure time and to triumph over social problems. To adjust themselves to the changing needs guidance is required. For development of wholesome relationships, guidance acts as an instrument for the qualitative improvement of education and national development.

For academic growth i.e., development of abilities and skills consistent with varying capacities of the individual and and to overcome difficulties in understanding the subject content.

And getting expertise in knowledge. Vocational maturity i.e., development of technical skills and right attitudes towards work.

Personal—Social Development—Self-understanding and proper adjustment to self and society.

7. Family Life

Guidance is required for better family life i.e., right attitudes towards home and understanding of fundamental relationships, emotional ways and bondages.

8. Guidance for Good Citizenship

Appreciation and understanding of social values, needs, problems, issues together with developing social attitudes and habits.

Guidance is required for conservation and proper utilization of human resources, as it points out for the need of a well-organized vocational guidance service, to meet the dual responsibility of reconciling individual aspirations with social demands on a basis of free individual choice.

Guidance is required for the students in the following areas: Study habits and Adequate Knowledge and Skills, Mental hygiene, Discipline and Confidence, Intellectual and Functional proficiency, Development of aptitudes and abilities, Social and occupational awareness, Development of personality, Family relationship, Sex education and Career choice/vocational choice.

The teacher can help the students to lead a trouble free or problem free life, teacher can help them to resolve their difficulties or if not possible, to live with them.

The response of an understanding and empathetic person and an atmosphere of understanding, faith and sincerity. To meet the varied needs of learners in educational system, administration and students—guidance and counseling is required.

9. Intellectual Development

Faculty has to help students to understand themselves. Teachers has to understand the students' strengths and weaknesses, abilities and aspirations. To produce competent, mature and well-rounded citizens, good teaching is an explode myth. Help the student in making meaningful occupational selection and preparation for an entry into them to have a fulfilling and rewarding career.

The young students in colleges and universities need to be informed about various jobs and opening available to them and work involved in them so that they could measure themselves upto them and develop and crystallize their occupational goals. They need to be helped in making meaningful occupational selection and preparation for an entry into them to have a fulfilling and rewarding career. Majority of students in colleges and universities are the first generation learners. In their family, they have no one with an experience of professional background to guide them in the choice of a career.

With a right to the best education available and a wide range of jobs open to them, these students need mature help by the teaching faculty in personal and professional development and adjustment by making a judicious right choice in all aspects.

10. To Help Students in Vocational Development

The process of vocational development covers almost the entire span of life of an individual. It begins early in one's life and continues till sometimes after retirement. In this process, the individual paves through various stages—Growth, Exploration, Maintenance and Decline.

Guidance and counseling has to help the student, particularly in the stages of growth and exploration of self and world by making it possible for them to gain knowledge about themselves—Their abilities. Interests and needs on one hand and knowledge about the world of work on the other hand; it facilitates their transition from education to work.

11. To develop readiness for choices and changes to face new challenges: On graduating, he/she will be called upon to make use of the kind of person, he/she has become as much, if not more than what he/she has learnt in his/her course of study—Not only to make an initial choice of what he/she is to do on graduating but will be called upon to change his/her occupation several times in a lifetime. Readiness for these choices and changes is essential, not only to the student himself/herself but to the society as a whole, to the extent to which he/she is able to capitalize on his/her experience and face new challenges with a realistic expectation of success, to that extent he/she will benefit society.

If the individual is unable to meet the changing demands, not only of the working world, but also of his/her other roles of his/her life, to that extent he/she will be a liability and will fail to fulfill the expectations which society has for its most able people. Guidance services are needed to develop in the students is the ability to cope with their problems and concerns in such a way that they become more competent to meet the demands which will continue to be made upon them in the future. To minimize the mismatching between education and employment and help in the efficient use of manpower. Most of young graduates have no clear objectives or career targets; they pass through university courses of learning without acquiring much knowledge of preparing themselves for an uncertain future. Guidance facilities can help in reducing the wastage and thus ensure efficient use of manpower. To motivate the youth for self-employment. Arrangement needs to be instituted in the colleges to identify the deserving cases fit to take up employment, educate them on how to proceed about the job of setting up a venture, help them through the cooperation of the concerned agencies in this sphere to prepare technically sound and economically viable sponsor their cases to the banks for loan assistance and guide them to over come the teething troubles through effective follow-up after the commencement of the venture. To help fresher establish proper identity.

Young adolescents are passing through the stage between childhood and adulthood, and between the morality learned as a child and the ethics to be developed as an adult. They find it difficult to establish a satisfactory identity. This crisis in role identity is very acute today. The uncertainties of the future, the conflicts in languages, culture, region are: Achievement in life, Self-reliance, Sense of security, Success in college and university and Understanding about families and friends. Strong, tactile presence of a hand for guiding the anxious and enabling them to develop realistic goals or expectations. To identify and help students in need of special help, e.g. Gifted, Backward and Handicapped—Identify the learners who need special opportunities and provide them with help account to their requirements.

12. Utilization of Leisure time activities

To ensure the proper utilization of time spent outside the classroom. The manner in which students spend their non - class hours clearly affects their success in achieving both academic competence and personal development of all types. Positive direction to students by influencing how they can use those leisure hours.

Guidance is required to tackle the problems arising out of student explosion.

- To check migration
- To minimize the incidence of indiscipline
- To make up for the deficiencies in home and outside the school

Areas of Guidance and Counseling

The student life is getting complex day by day. They have to face varied difficult situations, for example:

- Make a wise curricular and cocurricular choice
- Acquire basic study skills for optimum achievement
- Live with and share facilities with students from varied social and economic backgrounds
- Adjust to the peers and parents, teachers, administrators
- Secure adequate financial aid to carry on the studies
- Utilize leisure time with good skill oriented activities.

The students need expert help for optimum achievement and adequate adjustment in varied life situations.

I. Education

Vocations in many forms are penetrating in colleges, universities. Competitive examinations for entry into institutions and services have become a normal phenomena, expert help is required by the students in making wise choices between their interests and the availabilities of opportunities and be successful in competitive examinations. Students have to be assisted in making decisions and choices involved in planning a future and building a career. Help the students in developing an integrated and adequate picture of themselves and of their role in the world of work. Expert assistance is also required for enabling the students in making proper adjustment in relation to general academic life at college to effect maximum intellectual, emotional and physical development.

A. Pre-admission guidance needs

To be imparted to help the students to make educational plans consistent with their abilities, interests and goals. To select appropriate courses and cocurricular activities which will enable them to join careers of their choice.

B. Post-admission guidance needs

Impart guidance to enable the students to succeed in their educational plans. They need to be guided for developing good study habits, Preparing for examinations adequately with confidence. They need to be guided in selecting subjects for specialization and additional courses of studies. Made familiar with various fellowships, scholarships, competitive examinations, etc. so that their journey ahead becomes smooth and profitable. Special facility of guidance is needed at crisis points, e.g. students find difficulty in following certain subjects, lacks concentration, gets poor grade, Indecisive about a change of subject. He/she has to be guided as to how he could overcome these difficulties and what special efforts he/she has to make in that direction.

Help the students to develop

- An attitude of interrogation
- Dependence on evidence and reasonable explanation of facts
- Efforts need to be made to ensure that his intellectual pursuits and interests which have so far been manifold become focalized, few but stable.

II. Vocation

Every vocation needs guidance in

- Educational
- Professional
- Preparation.

Hence, the need for guidance to the students for a right choice of a vocational arrangement has to be made. Assist the student to have a reasonable estimate of their abilities and limitations, a balance between their aspirations and those of their parents, between their interests and the availability of opportunities. Guidance should be flexible, it should help the students to be able to respond to their changing needs as they grow more mature and as the circumstances and experiences of life pose unpredictable problems, requiring:

- New information
- Fresh thinking
- Revised plans
- Compromise
- Acceptance of socio-economic conditions
- Personal limitations that cannot be changed.

Aims

Promotion of *personal satisfaction* with life as a whole.

Factors considered in provision of vocational guidance.

1. Make the students to discover information about themselves, i.e.
   - Abilities
   - Interests
   - Needs
   - Ambitions
   - Limitations and its causes.
2. Give information about their environment. For example:
   - The advantages and disadvantages of Educational courses and different occupations
   - The qualifications necessary for entry into them
   - Range of opportunities available to them.
3. Providing them with a "Frame of reference" in which to see themselves in relation to these educational and vocational opportunities. To orient them to future decision-making points in their career.
4. Vague notions about certain jobs has to be removed.
5. Providing counseling
   - To promote self-understanding
   - To develop educational and occupational plans.

6. Providing placement service
   - To help them implement those plans.
7. Provide follow-up service
   - To help them for taking future, decision-making situations.
8. The total life of an individual, i.e. working life and non-working life has to be taken into consideration.
9. Assist the learner to develop: The individual's self-concept related to Occupational and extra-occupational.

III. Avocation

Teachers are giving guidance and direction to students' lives i.e., They should be keenly concerned with the nature of day long learning aside from books or lectures, e.g. only 4-6 hours of a 24 hour day the student spends in classes, the rest of the time is the area of student services like Physical activities, Social interaction, Emotional experiences and Cultural programs, Sports and Games, etc. Teachers must realistically recognize where learning is going on; help the students plan for them and actively participate in them.

Avocational guidance will help the student to prevent confusion, doubt, anxiety, aimlessness, exploitation by others or indulging in destructive acts or in unwholesome activities. The students need to be properly guided for effective participation, in varied types of avocational pursuits so that they are able to shape their interpersonal behavior in desirable direction and widen their outlook. Sustained encouragement, systematic coaching and training arrangements should be given for the students to participate in co-curricular activities and to manage them.

For example: Participation in team games, intellectual contests, learning of productive hobbies, organization of small interest groups, developing healthy aims, etc.

IV. Social Guidance

To establish social relationships through effective social interaction, social guidance is essential.
- Students need a structured situation within which to socialize classroom or college atmosphere, an extra-curricular interest, e.g. Picnic
- Students are guided to live as socially well-adjusted individuals, they need to be helped in making friends, improving their style of conversation and know how to become leaders in their own groups. Students can be guided in developing constructive expression of their emotions, an objective interpretation of situations. Assist the students to reduce their excitability to emotional stimulations and facing conflicts. Help the students to acquire the feeling of security and being accepted by the group—In developing a social poise, In becoming tolerant towards the behavior of others and In achieving individuality and freedom.

V. Guidance Related to Health

Society has responsibility in the health and physical well-being of students, rising generation and in whom it has to invest large resources and to whom it looks for the advancement of national interest. The preventive, promotive, curative and restorative measures has to be provided to ensure the achievement of this objective. Health officer will be the incharge of student health center. He should set a tone of acceptance is particularly important in the case of early detection of disorders, since student may be afraid to reveal symptoms like that those of CD. At the commencement of academic year the health officer has to conduct general medical check up for all the students and all the reports may be sent to the parents and a written report of the action taken may be insisted.

A. *To promote the health facilities within the college environment certain measures has to be adopted:*
   1. Healthful conditions within the college has to be maintained and it has to be supervised.
   2. Specific protection against communicable diseases like typhoid, hepatitis-B vaccines can be given to all the students who are predisposed or chances of exposure for a particular disease.
   3. Conduct health education awareness campaigns within the school, arrange orientation training programs and Counseling program for the teachers to look after the students during their illness.

B. *For early diagnosis and treatment of illness*
   1. An adequate physical examination of every student at the beginning of an academic year.
   2. Follow-up treatment of detected disorders.
   3. If necessary, reference of students to other medical resources.
   4. To keep track of mind and body's harmonious functioning confidential records has to be maintained.

C. *For disabled patient*

Remedial and measures has to be planned and collaborated activities has to be taken.

D. *Curative service*

If any student suffers with any disorder whether mild, acute or chronic, treatment and follow-up services can be given.

VI. Moral Guidance

For the students who are having undesirable practices, moral guidance has to be provided to keep them in track and lead noble lives.

VII. Personal Guidance

Students face many health problems related to themselves, their friends, family, teachers, educational achievement, social adjustment, feeling of disappointment, unfavorable atmosphere at home for studies, strained and unhappy interpersonal relationships and progress in study is hampered. Expert guidance has to be provided to those students to face the situations boldly and with confidence; to enable the students to adjust to the situations which they cannot change. Some students may face the problems like lack of friends, loneliness, inadequacy, feeling of insecurity, chaos and despair feelings. They need counsel to overcome their difficulties.

Make students to assess liabilities, assets and identification of their self to achieve desired goals. Students may face adjustment problems help them to understand the normal interaction with the opposite sex and casual acceptance give this information in a scientific manner so that they will be benefited. Some students may have financial crisis guidance services has to be provided related to scholarship, fee concessions, stipends, and fellowships, etc.

VIII. Marital Guidance

Students may need guidance for the right choice of a life partner or for happy marital life.

Types of Guidance

Guidance is a continuous process and deals with all aspects of life.

1. WM Procter's view:
   - Educational guidance
   - Vocational guidance
   - Guidance in social and civic activities
   - Guidance in health and physical activities
   - Guidance in the worthy use of leisure time
   - Guidance in character building activities.
2. John M Brewer in his famous book 'Education as Guidance' described the types of guidance as:
   - Educational guidance
   - Vocational guidance
   - Guidance for home relationship
   - Guidance for citizenship
   - Guidance for leisure and recreation
   - Guidance in personal well-being
   - Guidance in right doing
   - Guidance in thoughtfulness and cooperation
   - Guidance in wholesome and cultural activities.
3. Paterson et al's view:
   - Educational guidance
   - Vocational guidance
   - Personal guidance (includes social, emotional and leisure time guidance)
   - Health guidance
   - Economic guidance

4. Nursing educator's view:
   - Group guidance
   - Individual guidance
   - Personal guidance
   - Marital guidance
   - Professional guidance
   - Clinical guidance

I. Educational Guidance

It is a process concerned between an individual learner with his distinctive characteristics on the one hand, and differing groups of opportunities and requirement in the other, a favorable setting for the individual's development of education—*Myers.*

1. Harmony between the unique potentialities of a learner and the opportunities which are available to him. It deals with the help needed by an individual for his/her educational development with a view to make himself/herself useful in the society.
2. It is concerned with the student's success in his educational career.

   It relates to the students' adjustment to school and to the preparation and carrying out of suitable educational plans in keeping with his educational needs, abilities and career interests.

   It includes the adjustive phase which involves for the student a liking for understanding of and suitable adaptation to school and its purposes.

   It provides suitable information about courses, curriculum, requirement, for education and entrance to institutions that offer advance preparation to the students.

   It gives information to students i.e., helpful in making the desirable choice of courses and desirable educational institutions—*CC Dunsmoor and LM Miller.*
3. It is concerned with assistance given to learners in their choices and adjustments with relation to schools, curriculum, course and school life—*Jones.*
4. It is an aid to the individual in choosing an appropriate program and in making progress in it—*Strang*
5. It is a process of aiding the individual to place wisely his educational program and to put himself/herself in position to carry forward successfully that program along lines that society considers wholesome both for itself and for him—*Myers.*

Objectives
1. The physical, emotional, social, mental and spiritual development of the individual, i.e. it includes all-around personality development of the individual. To help the individual in his educational pursuit so that he/she is able to make right choice keeping in view his/her mental abilities and capacities.
2. Provision of Health
3. Command of fundamental processes
4. Worthy Citizenship
5. Vocation
6. Civic education and responsibility
7. Worthy use of leisure time
8. Ethical Character
9. Development of self-realization
10. Development of human relationship
11. Economic efficiency
12. Select the curriculum that fits his/her abilities, interests and future needs
13. Develop work and study habits that enable him/her to achieve satisfactory success in his/her studies
14. Gain some experience in learning areas outside the particular field of his/her special interests and talents
15. Understand the purpose and the function of the school in relation to his/her needs
16. Plan a program of studies
17. Learn about the purpose and function of the college or school, she/he may wish to attend later
18. Gains insight into learning areas

19. Participate in and out of class activities in which he/she can develop potential leadership qualities.
20. Develop an positive attitude which will stimulate him to continue his/her education in relation to his/her talents and training.
21. Adjust to the curriculum and the life of the school.

Principles

- Standardized tests has to be made keeping in view of prognostic of success
- Selection of a curriculum should be decided in the light of test result, degree of achievement on the precious school level, learner and parent interest
- Follow the learner's achievement in each term and counselor has to help the student when the need arises
- A learner should not be required to repeat more than once with the same teacher any course, which he/she fails as personality differences between the teacher and the learner interfere with learning progress.

Problems in Educational Guidance

- To help the individual to make desirable progress in educational career
- The problem of motivation and morale in the classroom needs the attention of teachers
- The problems of understanding by the learner the aims and values of the study; finding the work interesting or do they attack it with happiness and success
- Attacking the problem
- Understanding of outside assignments
- Preparation and take the examinations
- Information related to additional studies and course are ahead of them.

II. Vocational Guidance

The term 'Vocational' applies to 'all gainful occupations'.

Definition: "It is the process of assisting the individual to choose an occupation, prepare for it enter upon and progress in it." Hence, it is a long continued process.

Meaning: It offers information and assistance which leads to the choice of an occupation and the training which proceeds it; It is required by person in order to select a suitable profession of vocation for himself/herself.

- It is concerned with helping individuals make decisions and choices involved in planning a future and building a career decisions and choices necessary in effecting satisfactory vocational adjustment
- Two sets of differences are involved in vocational guidance:
  - Differences among individuals.
  - Differences among occupations.

Aims

The student will be assisted to:

1. Acquire the knowledge of Characteristics, functions, duties, responsibilities, rewards of the group of occupation that lie within the range of intelligent choice.
2. Discover his own potentialities, abilities, skills and to fit them into the general requirements of the occupation under consideration.
3. To think critically about various types of occupations and to learn a technique for analyzing information about vacations.
4. To evaluate his/her own capabilities and interests with regards to their greatest worth to him/her and to society.
5. It helps the individual to develop an attitude towards work that will dignify whatever type of occupation he/she may wish to enter, the choice is based on personally achieved satisfaction and the service that can be offered.
6. Assist the learner to secure the necessary information about the facilities offered by various educational institutions engaging in vocational training.

7. Provides information related to
   - Admission requirement
   - Length of training
   - Cost of attending to the institution of higher learning
   - Adjustment during the job.
8. Alerting the learners to the long range training needed to become proficient in most lines of endeavor.
9. Helping the learner to learn the realization of the success purchased at the price of effort and the satisfaction on the job derives from doing his work conscientiously and competently.

III. Personal Guidance

Definition: 'The assistance offered to the individual to solve their emotional, social, ethical and moral as well as health problems.'

Nature and Purpose
It will deal with all problems of life. It is concerned with social and civic activities, health and physical activities, worthy use of leisure time and character building activities. It has a major concern for individual and social problems. To help the individual in his physical, social, emotional; moral, spiritual development and adjustment personal guidance has to be organized.
1. *Pre-primary stage:* The learner should be helped in achieving emotional control and developing desirable social relationships.
2. *Elementary stage:* To develop self-discipline and through it they can achieve happiness.
3. *Junior high school stage:* To help pre-adolescents to become adjusted in their new environment.
   To develop a feeling of belongingness and leadership. They must learn to function in a group with the team spirit.
   It covers vocational and educational aspects and interests.
   To stimulate their desire to develop those qualities that are basic to the constructive living.
   To develop an attitude of willingness to seek any needed individual counseling.
4. *High school stage:* Effort should be made to offer personal guidance for adjustment.
   Useful information pertaining to life may be provided.
   It should be offered within the cultural framework of the society.
   It should enable young one's to develop interest in healthy recreation and they should be helped in organizing wholesome recreational activities for themselves.
   It will be provided for social and moral development also, so that it may be able to develop a sense of social responsibility and community service.
5. *College and university stage:* To enable them to have a satisfactory personal and social adjustment in their new environment. For profitable use of leisure time through wholesome recreational activities. Personal Guidance may be provided to solve economic problems. For ethical, moral development and social development, personal guidance is essential. Young adults can be encouraged to study the basic principles of all religious and discover for themselves the underlying fundamental unity. Personal guidance has to be given with a view to helping the students in developing wholesome social, moral and religious attitudes.

IV. Recreational Guidance

The individual needs assistance in choosing recreations which are suited to his/her personal characteristics.

V. Group Guidance

To assist each individual in the group to solve their problems and to make necessary adjustments. To improve students' attitude and behavior. To orient the newly arrived learners to the program of the school. To give training for the students in different aspects of leadership. Counselor may save time by the group approach and is able to pay more attention to more difficult and complex aspects of the situations faced by an individual student. It gives an opportunity to the students to express their anxieties and relieve the pent-up feelings. To convey information to the students in less time than individual counseling; The teacher can utilize his/her time in finding solutions to more difficult and complex aspects of the situation faced by an individual student. It affords opportunities to the counselor to study students in group situations and thus acquaints himself/herself with his social attitudes and behavior. It helps the participants to achieve better balanced judgments by free exchange of opinions and realistic analysis of attitudes. It makes the normal student to more enlightened as he/she learns to manage his/her own affairs in a better way. It prepares the way for individual counseling. It multiplies contacts with students. In group guidance, the problems related to adjustment personality, occupational and economy were solved. The tasks related to hobbies, job finding, leisure time and its usage, social situations, home and school adjustment and educational plans were also discussed. It helps the individual to achieve self-direction, self-knowledge, self-realisation, satisfactory development or adjustment to the life situations.

Principles

It should be regarded as supplement to counseling, not as a substitute for it. Encourages certain members of the group to seek individual counseling help. Group should be homogeneous in various aspects. Appropriate project to the students should be introduced. The person responsible for group guidance should be well-versed with this type of work. It should be considered as one of the means and not the only means of guidance.

Techniques

1. *Talks:* Class talks are one of the effectives means of providing students with educational and vocational information and of developing in them right attitudes to education, learning experiences, social and personal relations; it stimulates the students to give a serious thought in planning their educational and vocational career.

   Types
   - General orientation talks
   - Education orientation talks
   - Vocation orientation talks
   - Personal-social adjustment orientation talks.

2. *Career conferences:* It supplements the information given to a group to explain the vocations in which they work and answer about their jobs.

3. *Audio-visual aids:* It provides a realistic representation and to show the actual operations and processes involved, to give more intelligent understanding; it makes learning vivid and attractive.

4. *Visits:* It provides concrete experiences for learning. It is based on actual and direct experiences. Immediately after the visit, a group conference should be held to discuss that place or occupation.

5. *Group activities:* Vocational, e.g. Drama, costuming, felt work.
   Recreational, e.g. Art club, music group.
   Educational, e.g. School publications, school forum.

6. *Occupational information through school subjects:* It is the simple way of imparting information, teachers should acquaint the students with the occupational possibilities of their subjects. They should prepare the lists of occupations connected with their subjects, they should encourage and assist students to prepare such lists through their own efforts.

7. *Informal discussions.* Should center around desirable objectives, find solutions or conclusions which will help the group as a whole.

8. *Group reports:* Students are divided into groups which have certain specific problem to tackle and later reports are presented in larger groups so that all the members will be aware of problems and its solutions.

9. *Lectures:* By experts on certain problems.

10. *Dramatics:* Certain interested topics should be selected with theme and dramatized and the students can be given guidance in an interesting way, how to solve different problems.

11. *Question box:* It gives the shy and retiring pupil an opportunity to propose a question, i.e. bothering him/her without revealing that is his/her question. So if the question could be proposed in a silent way, the same could be discussed in a group and valuable guidance to the students.

xii. *Case conferences*: Here the problem faced by the majority of the group is started concretely by way of a case. Each group member reviews their own experience in a similar situation. The group is guided for immediate solution of the problem by means of social thinking.

Kinds of Groups for Group Guidance
- Regular subject groups
- Special groups organized for the consideration of special topics
- Tutorial group
- Advises under a special or specific adviser
- Career or educational groups
- Groups with common interest
- Groups with common adjustment problem.

Advantages
- Economical and efficient
- Aids the normal students to give them information and the direction that he/she needs and wants
- Helps in having more contacts with students
- Provides an opportunity to discuss common problems
- Helps to improve students' attitudes and behavior
- Focuses on collective judgment on problems that are common to the group
- Provides an admirable opportunity to observe each student, how he/she behaves and reacts in group situation
- Helps in the development of wholesome personality of individual student
- Brings awareness of unrecognized needs and problems of students.

QUESTIONS

- A Student is repeatedly absenting herself due to fear of internal examination. Basic principles of Guidance and counseling; enumerate (5+10=15M, NTRUHS, June, 2010).
- Define Counseling (2M), What Principles will you apply? (7M), What type of Guidance will you provide (4M), List the Counseling Committee Members (2M) (MGRUHS, Aug, 2007).
- Define Guidance and Counseling (2M, NTRUHS, June, 2010 & RGUHS, Aug, 2009 and 4M, MGRUHS, Feb, 2009 and 5M, RGUHS, Sept, 2009).
- Define Guidance and Counseling, enumerate the problems of counseling(15M, RGUHS, May, 2010).
- Describe the need for counseling of guidance, Explain the steps and techniques of counseling (5+10=15M, NTRUHS, Nov, 2010).
- Differentiate between Guidance—Counseling (5M, MGU, Oct, 2007 and Dec, 2008).
- Discuss the Purposes and the Need for Guidance and Counseling ? (10M, Rajasthan UHS, 8M, Feb, 2008 & March, 2010).
- Guidance and Counseling for employees (15M, NIMS, Oct, 2009).
- Guidance and counseling (10 M, RGUHS, MAY, 2009).
- Importance of Guidance and Counseling for Nursing students (15M, NIMS, Oct, 2008).
- Justify the importance of guidance and counseling services in Nursing educational institutions (10M, RGUHS, Oct, 2008).
- Need for guidance and counseling (2M, RGUHS, Feb, 2010).
- Objectives of Guidance and Counseling services in a College of Nursing (4M, Baba Farid UHS, 2008).
- Organization of guidance and counseling service in Ist year B.Sc nursing students (5M, MGU, Dec, 2006).
- Scope of guidance and counseling in Nursing education (2M, RGUHS, Aug, 2010).
- What is Guidance and Counseling, Discuss the role of Teacher in Guidance and Counseling (5+10M, MGRUHS, Feb, 2009).
- Write differences between Guidance and Counseling (10 M, MGRUHS, Aug, 2008 and 3M, Baba Farid UHS, 2008).
- Write any two purposes of Guidance and Counseling (4M, NIMS, May, 2010).
- Write short notes on Guidance and Counseling (5M, NTRUHS, July, 2008).

Counseling

'Counseling' denotes, "Giving advice". It is a wider procedure concerned with emotion as well as giving information.

DEFINITIONS

"A helping process where one person, explicitly and purposefully gives his/her time, attention and skills to assist a client to explore the situation, identify and act upon solutions within the limitations of their given environment"

"A method that helps the client to use a problem-solving process to recognize and manage stress that facilitates interpersonal relationships among client, family and health care team"

"Consultation, mutual interchange of opinions deliberating together"

"A dynamic and purposeful relationship between two people, who approach a mutually defined problems with mutual consideration of each other to the end that the troubled one or less mature is aided to a self-determined resolution of his/her problem"—*Wren, 1962.*

Concept

- Counseling is the relationship between two persons in which, one of them attempts to assist the other in organizing himself to attain a form of happiness, adjustment to a life situation, i.e. self-actualization
- An accepted, trusting and safe relationship will be formulated in which clients will learn to discuss openly their problems, acquires the social skills, courage, self-confidence to implement desired new behaviors
- The relationship between two personnel or the interaction between the counselor i.e., one a professionally trained professionals and the counselee i.e., the person who seeks the services or who cannot cope up alone, who requires help from the skilled personnel to resolve his/her problems by finding new ways
- Helps the individual to become aware of himself/herself and the ways in which he/she is reacting to the behavioral influences of his/her environment
- To develop a set of goals for future behavior of an individual.

Meaning

Counseling is a specialized service of guidance, it is an enabling process designed to help an individual with his/her life and grow to greater maturity through learning to take responsibility and to make decisions for himself/herself.

It is an helping relationship which includes:

- Someone seeking help
- Someone willing to give help
- Capable or trained to help
- In a setting that permits help to be given and received.

It is an accepting, trusting and safe relationship in which individual/client learn to discuss freely what upset them, to define their goals, to acquire the essential social skills and to develop the courage and selfconfidence to implement desired new behavior.

Patterson (1967) has pointed out certain behaviors that are not synonymous with the process of effective counseling:

Counseling is **not**
- Giving the information, though information may be present
- Giving an advice—Though making suggestions and recommendations
- The behaviors by persuading, threatening or compeling without the use of physical force
- The selection and assignment of individual to job
- Interviewing, though interviewing is involved.

Scope of Counseling Services

The scope of guidance and counseling is extremely comprehensive. As the life is getting complex day by day, the problems in which expert help is required are increasing proportionately.

It helps the students in the selection of educational courses, profitable occupations, job placement, higher education and training, selection of improvement of study skills and study habits formation, maintenance of mental health, help the students to achieve maximum efficiency in meeting their needs.

Individual services will be provided, granting loans and scholarships, handling discipline cases, selection and staying with room-mates, advice on students' activities and programes, helping the students to choose vocational objectives, selecting optional courses to the study, concerns about educational progress, course programe planning, financial and health matters, problems of family, social, educational, vocational, avocational, personal, moral, marital life, etc. are the context of counseling.

Levels of Counseling

It is a face-to-face interview in which the counselor attempts non-coercively to help the client or counselee to make personal decisions.

1. *Informal counseling:* Any helping relationship by a responsible person who may have little or no training for the work.
2. *Non-specialist counseling by professionals:* It is help provided by professional who do a great deal of face-to-face work with psychological problems in the course of their work.
3. *Professional counseling:* It is helping another person with decision and life-plans whether personal or educational or vocational by a person specially trained for this work.

Elements in Counseling Process

Counseling involves two individuals; it is a communication between the counselor and counselee (i.e., Tone of voice, facial expressions, gestures and postures of both play an important role).

Counselor—A professionally trained person who can assist or help the counselee.

Counselee—A person who seeks help or needs assistance. Mutual respect, rapport and satisfactory relationship should be established.

Counselor should be friendly and cooperative with counselee.

Counselee should have trust and confidence over the counselor.

Counselor should have thorough experience and sound knowledge with counseling process.

It concerns itself with attitudes and actions, Information; intellectual attitudes, understanding of emotional feelings also plays a significant role.

It produces change in the individual, improves thinking process whereby the individual will extricate himself from his/her immediate difficulties.

It provides an opportunity for reflection on the impact of the problem on daily life.

Working out ways of learning the impact.

It involves 3 domains of learning
- Cognitive domain—Storing, recalling of new knowledge and information
- Psychomotor domain (Conative)—Physical skill has been learnt
- Affective domain—It changes the attitudes, feelings and values.

It encourages independent decision-making.

Ask the client to get family and friend's support.

Get or refer to consultation, when it is beyond the skills of counselor.

Maintain confidentiality; counseling interview must be structured.

Elements that hinder Counseling Process: (Problems of Counseling Process)

Passing moral judgments on client's behavior or feelings.

Taking more than you can handle.

Stereotype the client.

Increase or slow the pace of process according to your needs.

Make generalization and minimize the issues or compare it to others' situations or problems.

Ask questions for your interest or needs rather than those of the clients.

Need of Counseling

- To help the client to accept actual or impending changes that are resulting from stress. It involves psychological, emotional, intellectual and spiritual support
- To foster cognitive, behavioral, developmental and emotional growth in clients
- To encourage the client to examine the available alternatives
- To decide or directs which choices are appropriate and useful for problem solvation
- To develop a sense of control for better management of stress. It provides an opportunity for emotional release and to discuss the ways of coping with problems. To relieve distress among people who are reacting to difficult circumstances. To change the behavior by reducing the stress or risk
- It helps the counselee to acquire independence and a sense of responsibility
- It helps the client to explore and fully utilize his/her potentialities and actualize himself
- It provides information for the student on matters important to success. Establishes mutual relationship and understanding between counselor (teacher) and counselee (student)
- Helps the students to know him/her better i.e., his/her interests, aptitudes and opportunities
- To encourage and develop special abilities and right attitudes
- To inspire successful endeavor towards attainment
- To assist the students in planning for educational and vocational choices
- To help the student to work out a plan for solving his/her difficulties
- Helps in the total development of the student
- The counselor must expect and accept the difference in the students, understands them and plan the solutions
- It helps in the proper choice of course according to the interest, aptitude and intelligence of the student
- To help the students to grow, explore and maintain or develop their overall personality
- To develop readiness for choices and changes, to face new challenges
- To help for efficient use of manpower
- To motivate the students for self-employment
- The fresher will be helped to establish a proper identity
- To help the students in the period of confusion or turmoil
- To help the students in checking wastage and stagnation
- To help the students in need of special help
- To minimize the incidence of indiscipline which is leading to destructive activity and social damage.

Aspects

- Collection of information and careful analysis of the available facts
- Forecast of the outcome of the counselee's course of action
- Assistance to the counselee in working out of solution of his/her problem
- Follow-up work.

Characteristics

- It is a purposeful learning experience for the counselee

- It is the purposeful oriented and private interview between the counselor and counselee
- Based on mutual confidence satisfactory relationship will be established
- Counseling process is structured around the felt needs of the counselee
- Main emphasis in the counseling process is on the counselee's self-direction and self-acceptance.

Principles

- Tailor-made to the requirement of an individual's problem
- Emphasizes thinking with the individual
- Avoid dictatorial attitude
- Maintains relationship of trust and confidence with the client
- Client's need is to be put first
- Everyone participating in the counseling process must feel comfortable
- The client's family members and significant influencing personnel must be included in counseling process
- Skills of warmth, friendliness, openness and empathy are ingredients of successful counseling process
- Counselor has to listen attentively, answer questions objectively; reinforce important information
- Let the client make voluntary informed decision
- Maintain dignity of individual as individual is primary concern in counseling.

Range of Skills Required for Effective Counseling

- Active listening
- Respecting
- Simple acceptance
- Identification
- Structuring or Prioritization
- Non-directive lead
- Persuasion
- Questioning
- Interpretation
- Paraphrasing
- Advice/Suggestion
- Reassurance of praise (Positive evaluation of the client by the counselor)
- Criticism or negative evaluation
- Confrontation
- Summarizing
- Reflection of feeling.

Differences between Guidance and Counseling

- Guidance and Counseling are not synonymous terms
- Counseling is a part of Guidance, not all of it
- The concept of Counseling as a group of services, which make up the guidance programe is generally accepted
- Guidance is the total programe or all the activities and services engaged in by an educational institution that are aimed at assisting an individual to make and carryout adequate plans and to achieve satisfactory adjustment in all aspects of his/her daily life
- Guidance will be done by teachers; it is an important component in all educational programes. It uses counseling as one of the services
- In counseling two **phases** are available:
  - The adjustive phase—the emphasis is on social, personal and emotional problems of an individual. The adjustive Phase can be considered as Counseling.
  - The distributive Phase—the focus is upon educational, vocational and occupational problems. Distributive Phase can be aptly described as Guidance.

Relationship of Guidance and Counseling

Guidance is an organized service, to identify and develop the potentialities of learners comprehensive information about all the students is collected with the help of different tests, tools, resources recorded and interpreted. This information is communicated to the individual to help them to understand themselves and for their all round personality development.

In counseling, information is given to solve their problems. Although the information is given in both the processes, but two are not the same.

Thus guidance is preventive and developmental, whereas counseling is preventive, developmental and remedial.

Guidance information makes the basis for counseling sessions. Guidance may be done by any guidance professional; whereas counseling requires a high level of skill as well as special professional training, hence may be taken up by persons, who have the training and expertise knowledge.

Guidance may be given at any normal setup, whereas counseling requires a special setup (room to conduct interview).

Guidance is an integral part of education and assists it in fulfilling its aims, whereas counseling is needed in all fields.

In guidance decision making operates at intellectual level, whereas in counseling it operates at emotional level.

Thus guidance and counseling is concerned with the 'whole' individual, developing student's self understanding and self determination, recognizes the existence of individual differences, hence limits and problems of each individual is different from one to another.

It accepts that problems have causes and are interrelated, so a deep knowledge of causes is essential.

Both are continuous and slow process.

Bases of Guidance and Counseling

It has been categorized into

1. Individual base
   a. Academic growth
      - The counselor has to bring all round personality development of the learner
      - Counselor has to understand the needs, abilities and interests of her/his students to develop their potentialities.
   b. Vocational development
      - Development of self-awareness
      - Awareness about the world of work. It helps the learner to formulate right attitude toward the world of work. Guidance provides learner with holistic development.
   c. Personal social development
      - An individual faces many problems in his/her life; the problems may relate to health, academic, teachers, peer groups, family, physical appearance etc. to manage them.
2. Societal bases
   a. **Proper utilization of human resources:** Care is needed for selection of best suited individual in terms of her/his abilities, skills and attitudes for the needed job to meet his/her needs and societal needs.
   b. **Good citizenship:** A developing society faces many new challenges, if the citizens are intellectually developed and also have integrity, honesty, right attitudes, social values, habits, social responsibilities in relation to maintenance of democracy.
   c. **Better family life:** Family is a basic social unit, a better adjustment within it leads to the development of well adjusted individuals. Guidance and counseling helps the pupil to maintain good relationship with their family members.

Attributes and Skills Required for the Counselor

For effective counseling the counselor needs to demonstrate certain attitudes, skills and knowledge.

Pre-training Attributes
- Self-awareness and understanding
- Good psychological health
- Sensitivity about resources, limitations and vulnerability of other persons
- Open-mindedness
- Objectivity
- Trust worthiness
- Approachability.

Inter-training Attributes
1. Interview setting and getting started
   - Physical arrangement—chairs should face each other with leaning facility for both. The closeness of counselor helps in indicating the attentiveness and willingness
   - Greeting—A warm friendly greeting facilitate the helping process
   - Inviting the counselee to participate in counseling process
   - Maintaining eye contact
   - Demonstrating proper body posture.
2. Problem focus
3. Identifying an important theme
4. Focusing on a theme
5. Directing the theme towards a goal
6. Managing interaction with the individual
   - Restatement
   - Interpretation
   - Managing pauses and silence.

Characteristics or the Qualities of a Counselor
1. Interpersonal Relationship
   - Friendly nature
   - Gets along with others
   - Sympathetic understanding
   - Fairness
   - Sincerity
   - Sensitivity to the attitude of People
   - Tactfulness
   - Patience
   - Ability to maintain confidentiality
   - Respects client's abilities and needs
   - Attentive listener
   - Speaks in clients' language, gives responses objectively
   - Shows careful concern, listens the demands and complaints of the client and family, then responding them in an effective and facilitating manner
   - Capacity for being trusted by others
   - Tolerance power, openness, empathy are ingredients of successful counseling
   - Accepts and maintains good interpersonal relationship
   - Caring and meeting the needs of the individual based on humanistic philosophy.
2. Personal Adjustment
   - Shows matured behavior, integrated personality
   - Maintains emotional stability
   - Flexibility and adaptability
   - Aware about one's limitations
   - Mentally sound and healthy in all the aspects, shows unbiased attitude in using coping mechanisms

- Aware of one's limitations
- Possesses a sense of worth and sense of humor
- Freedom from withdrawing tendency
- Able to accept criticism
- Shows self-respect, self-reliance and self-confidence.
- Personal magnitism
- Possess Knowledge of self
- Ability to tolerate ambiguity

3. Scholastic Potentialities and Educational Background
   - Should possess relevant as well as broad knowledge and efficient skills; able to decide the method to be adopted in counseling process
   - Should be motivated and committed
   - Aware of policies, beliefs, misconceptions and rumors existing within the local community
   - Highly cultured social interests
   - Capacity for work
   - Intelligent to tackle the situations effectively
   - Positive interest
   - Scholastic aptitude
   - Respects the facts
   - Possess common sense and uses good judgment when tackling issues
   - He/She will have Master's degree in the essential area of guidance program. The areas in training are: Counseling Process, Understanding the Individual, Educational, Occupational and Vocational Information, Administrative relationship, Research and Evaluation Procedures; Additional training in behavioral sciences (Psychology and Sociology) Economics and Community Health
   - Ability to work with people
   - Experience in teaching and follow-up services

4. Health and Personal Appearance
   - Pleasing voice
   - Pleasing appearance
   - Freedom from annoying mannerism
   - Poise and Neatness
   - Vitality and endurance

5. Leadership
   - Ability to stimulate and lead others
   - Reinforces important information
   - Directs the counselee, the ways to solve the problems and guide him/her to choose appropriate one with his/her own decision (Voluntary manner)

6. Philosophy of life
   - Good character
   - Wholesome/Positive Philosophy of life
   - Civic sense
   - Integrated Personality
   - Possesses an acceptable value system
   - Faith in human values and human nature
   - Shows significant spiritual and religious values
   - Convictions, interests and exhibit positive appreciations

7. Professional dedication
   - Possesses vocational interest and interest in guidance work, professional attitude
   - Shows loyalty, enthusiasm to provide services for the student
   - Had strong sense of professional ethics and professional growth
   - Willingness to work beyond call of duty

- Maintains ' helping relationship'
- Shows interest in research activities
- Uses ' Psychotherapy' in solving clients' problems.

8. Faith in the spiritual quality of the world, respects universal principles of religion.
9. Had a high sense of morality.

Nature and Functions of the Counselor

Counselor plays a vital role in the counseling process. He/she will devote more of his/her time to guidance. Counselor is one who counsels, he/she will meet the following needs during counseling process.
The need for

- An interested interpretation of information adapted to an individual problem
- Listening, checking up and advising process
- Gives needed direction to the counselee to voluntarily choose the decision and initiates, motivates, inspires the counselee to take an appropriate constructive actions to solve his/her own problems; in which the student does not have an easy access
- Arousing awareness of problems existing, but not recognized
- Helping the student to define the problem recognized
- Helps the student to use appropriate coping process in salvation problem
- Teacher or Counselor should know what he/she is and what is his/her purpose in Guidance and Counseling program
- Teacher should possess a well-balanced democratic and ethical, personality or a wellbeing in nature
- Good basic intelligence and knowledge, counselor must possess; he/she obtained it either through experience or formal teaching or from other resources
- Counselor should possess wide knowledge of the world and its ways (especially in his/her own profession and other occupations)
- Counselor should be aware of possibilities of future employment, special intensive information about the roads of education and training that lead to them
- Counselor should have wide knowledge about people and their motives, inhibitions, etc.
- Counselor possesses special skills in employment and technique of finding jobs and placing the people; technique of testing, interviewing
- Feels an urge to help everybody life
- Wholesome, energetic, dedicative, sensitive to the feelings, attitudes of others. He/she should be an extraordinary person
- Counselor's attitude in terms of respect for his/her client
- Respect for the personal autonomy of the client, i.e. right to make decisions; right to seek assistance; right to refuse help
- Builts sense of responsibility, understanding of self and others
- Gives respect for whole person within the client. For example, family life, vocational, financial matters, feelings, attitudes of person (either positive or negative)
- Tolerance and acceptance of the client's difference
- He restrains himself from showing surprise, disapproval or strong approval of the client.
- He requires intensive training in counseling and professionalization
- Provides free educational and vocational counseling to applicants at the social centre or community - supported agency
- Refers cases to appropriate community agency and plans future programs
- Selects and administers appropriate tests to applicants; conducts case conferences with other counselors, interprets findings
- Counsel the clients on the basis of interview, test result and case conference
- Places applicants desiring jobs within limits of agency or advice clients of other agencies for placement
- May recommend agencies for financial, medical, legal, social, welfare employment and for other assistance
- Organizes programs in conjunction with fellow workers as to improvement or enlargement of services

- Conducts, assists research projects and other organizational agencies
- Conducts group guidance for young people regarding problems of adjustment related to vocational, occupational or educational.

Counselor Preparation

a. Education: Master's or Bachelor's degree in Teaching and education. They should have basic course in principles and practice of the guidance program and additional area of training either in Behavior Sciences or Community Health.
b. Experience: 2 years in Teaching or Counseling.
   1 year of cumulative work experience in the field of school program.
   3 to 6 months of supervised counseling experience.
   Significant experience in social activities (e.g. working within the community, volunteer work, participant in community training programs) to reveal interest in working with others and to indicate leadership ability.
c. Personal Fitness: Scholastic, Aptitude, Interests, Activities, Personality Factors.
   He/She should show positive interest and ability to work with people.

Ethical Principles to be considered for Professional Growth of Counselor

Counselor should be responsible to his/her counselee, school and society.

Counselor has to appraise the counselee before starting the process.

Counselor has to maintain confidentiality, develop trust and establishes satisfied relationship with the counselee and his/her family.

Counselor is expected to report the facts (if he/she suspects any problem will arise) to an appropriate responsible authority or takes other emergency measures as the situation demands.

If need arises he/she can consult with other professional competent persons in professional settings for referral services and for the welfare of the counselee.

Counselor will use discretion power and judgment in giving information from a counseling relationship to other professional workers and expects the same from them in their release of information given to them in confidence.

Counselor has to interpret in a constructive manner the psychological information of counselee and his/her family.

Counselor Maintains legal rights of counselee.

A counselor can decide either to initiate or terminate the counseling relationship when he/she cannot be of professional assistance to the counselee either because of lack of competence or personal limitations.

Counselor does not criticise unreasonably.

For Professional Growth

- He/She exerts the influence to foster the development and improvement of his/her profession
- He/She does self-study, professional study; participate in conferences, seminars, workshops organized by professional Institutions
- His/her professional activities must be in accordance with policies, objectives and ethical standards of the school
- He/She does not seek self-enhancement through expressing evaluations or comparisons damaging to other professional workers
- He/She does not accept a private fee or other form of remuneration for his/her professional work
- Provides accurate, appropriate information to the public or other professionals
- He/She refrains from undertaking any activity which are apt to result in inferior professional service
- He/She engages in research activities which are contributing for his/her personal and professional growth
- Recordings of counseling interviews are made and presented only with the counselee's permission
- He/She accepts all who seek his/her assistance regardless of race, caste, creed, color, social or economic status.

Media of Counseling

- Regional centers

- Study centers
- Teleconference
- Face to face contact
- Interview
- Letters
- Phones
- Audio-Video cassette
- Broadcast—Radio and Television
- Computers.

Process of Counseling

- Giving guidance or assisting the client in problem solving. The family members and significant or influencing personalities will be included in counseling session
- Counseling varies with situation to situation
- Everyone participating in the counseling situation must feel comfortable
- It is a process initiated by distressed client or student who is having a problem, it is a two way interaction between provider and the client
- Situational support will be provided for the client
- Correct information will be given, encourages the client the freedom of choice and changes available as it facilitates client to make proper decision
- Helps the counselee to focus and identify themselves for their immediate and long-term needs, propose realistic actions suitable for meeting their needs
- Assist the clients to accept reality
- Help the clients to accept the problem and provide information on all aspects of problem, e.g. technical, social and legal, etc. and its correction.

Steps

G—Greet the clients
A—Ask clients about themselves
T—Tell clients or give the information of strategies of coping mechanisms
H—Help the client to choose a method
E—Explain how to use a method
R—Return for follow-up

Supportive Behavior

Verbal behavior—Uses languages which is understood by the client, Clarifies clients' statements, Explains clearly and adequately, Advising, preaching, moralizing, Directing, demanding, Reassuring, Summarizing, Responds to the needs of client, Encourages the client to speak, Gives needed information, Non-judgmental; does not criticize or censure the clients feelings or thoughts.
C—Clarify
L—Listen
E—Encourage
A—Acknowledge
R—Reflect and Repeat.
Does not speak too quickly or too slowly.

Non -Verbal Behavior

R—Relax
O—Open and Approachable
L—Lean towards client
E—Eye contact
S—Smile and sit comfortably.

Uses tone of voice similar to that of a client

Maintains eye contact; occasionally nods the head; maintains suitable distance.

Process of Student Counseling

Knowledge of self, which the counselee should be able to achieve. He/she should understand his/her abilities, limitations, capacities (inner world).

To develop an attitude of self-acceptance.

To help the individual to attain social harmony.

Principles to be followed in Counseling technique

1. Acceptance: The client should not be hindered in any manner; he/she should be fully encouraged to express his/her feelings freely.
2. Restatement: The Counselor should enable the counselee to realize that he/she is being fully understood and accepted.
3. Clarification: The counselor tries to give correct information, clarifies the doubts of counselee.
4. Reassurance: Confidence in counseling being given to him/her, reassures the client about the effectiveness of counseling.
5. Interpretation: To develop insight by the counselee, he/she understands the unconscious motives that he/she resolves his/her inner conflicts.
6. Advice: Advice should be given only in those causes where it is sought for.
7. Rejection: It reverses the direction of thoughts of counselee.
8. Lead: The client is asked a question in a manner that is helpful to him/her in determining the answer.

Counseling Services Carried out at Institutional Level

By the Faculty

Counseling services are aimed to meet the students needs

To aid the student in the identification of his/her abilities, aptitudes, interests and attitudes.

To help him/her to understand, accepts and utilize his/her traits.

To provide him/her with opportunities for learning the areas of educational and occupational endeavour.

To help him/her in obtaining experiences which will assist in making voluntary, free and own choice.

To assist him/her in developing his/her potential to the optimum so that he/she will become self-directive.

Specific Services

a. Pre-admission Service: To enable the student to get admission in the right course, to ensure him/her the occupational aspirations of the students related to scholastic achievement, family background, subjects selected and their job aspirations, familiarity with the repercussions of choosing a particular course of study. Planning for future by knowing his/her own assets and liabilities.
b. The Admission Service: For the total development of students, admission service is needed to admit the right persons for right course and for their success or achievement in the respective course.
c. The Orientation Service: Heterogeneous population will be admitted; The campus map, Time-table, Calendar of events, students handbook, rules and regulations everything has to be informed to students so that they will accommodate and adjust to the situation.
d. The Student Information Service: Assist the student to obtain a realistic picture of the abilities, interests, personality characteristics, achievement level of aspiration. It Enable the student to know himself/herself, It provides a record of student's progress.
e. The Information Service: To develop a brand and realistic view of life's opportunities and problems at all levels of training. To promote self-defectiveness, To create awareness, the information will be given to the students in the fields of
    i. Educational: Prospectus from different colleges under different universities, Directories, Brochures related to scholarships and loans study habits and skills, Illustrative material regarding educational facilities and processes.
    ii. Occupational Information: Abstracts, briefs, guides, monographs, pamphlets, files, dictionaries, career information manuals, illustrative material regarding jobs.

iii. Personal-Social Information: To increase self-understanding material will be provided, e.g. hygiene (personal, Mental and environmental), adjustment process.
f. Placement Service: To place the student in proper scholastic track in the proper course and university, choice of job-oriented courses; getting admission in professional institutions, getting part-time jobs.
g. The Remedial Service: Training related to study skills for the handicapped persons who seeks higher education the remedial services could be given.
h. Follow-up Service: Systematic evaluation is carried out to review or to find out whether the counseling services (general specific) are satisfying the needs of students or not. The techniques followed are: Interview, Post-card Survey or Questionnaire.
i. Research Service: To examine both the personnel performance and techniques followed by the counselor, To discover strong and weak points of the program.
j. Evaluation Service: To evaluate the use and application of information activities in order to determine their effectiveness or efficiency.

Organizing Guidance and Counseling Program in Nursing Educational Institutions
Purposes of organizing counseling services
- To help adolescents with normal developmental problems
- To help individuals through temporary crisis
- To identify signs of disturbed/problem behavior at the earliest
- To refer cases needing specialist treatment
- To facilitate communication within and between the nursing schools, home, the communities and the resources
- To support teaching faculty who are helping individuals but who themselves want guidance and reassurance

Guidance and Counseling has made an integral part of higher education to make it meaningful and purposeful for the students. The kind of guidance and counseling programs can be:
- Inherent (Unintentional and Unorganised)
- Informal (Intentional but not Coordinated)
- Professional—A well-organised structure covering the three major functions of the program, e.g. adjustmental, oriental and developmental.

The organizational setup
1. For constituent colleges on the campus: If 1000 students on rolls
   - A counseling officer assisted by guidance committee can plan the program according to their needs and implement the same with the cooperation of deputy chief and academic adviser
   - If less than 1000 students, a liaison officer will look after
   - If more than 1000 students an assistant counseling officer /senior may be appointed to assist the counseling officer
2. For affiliated college at a distance
   - If 1000 students—Counseling officer assisted by guidance committee implement the activities with the help of vocational guidance officer.
   - If less than 1000 students—liaison officer will look after.
3. At Universities: Deans are assisted by HOD of Psychology and Education Guidance Committee, Counseling officer can plan the program and implement the activities.

Essential Activities
1. Formation of guidance and counseling committee
To serve in an advisory capacity or a policy making body for the program.
The committee can list out problems requiring group solution, plan, monthly, quarterly and yearly program. Coordinate guidance activities and assess the work done.

Members in the curriculum committee
- Dean
- Counseling/Liaison Officer
- Teachers from different specialties and academic disciplines

- Student representatives
- Parents
- Deputy Chief
- Vocational Guidance officer
- Peer group
- Librarian
- Warden
- Medical staff
- The principal has to specify the roles of each faculty member
- Clerical assistance will be provided for liaison officer.

2. Counseling Center

Every university and a large college should have a counseling center headed by a (trained professional) counseling officer, with Ph.D or Master's degree in Psychology and counseling with considerable experience.

Functions

Gives assistance either or individuals, small groups of students, staff members with special educational, vocational and personal problem.

Develops counseling programs and consultation specially on psychological problems.

Provides psychological testing facility both for individuals and groups.

Carryout research activities on testing procedures and experimental programs.

Helps in the training of P.G. students in counseling and testing.

Conducts special clinics for developing study skills and reading improvement.

Maintains integrity and confidentiality of the students and groups, faculty will refer the students to it and students too would like to visit and get help from center.

Orientation talks to students and parents to give information regarding

The courses of studies

Facilities available in the institution like library, workshops, labs, playgrounds, fee concessions etc.

Career Talks—Information about a particular job, e.g. themes avenues open to graduates, PG, self-employment schemes, govt jobs, abroad jobs.

Career Conferences—Providing occupational information for the group of students.

Plan Tours—e.g. visits to research institutions, professional colleges, etc. provide the students with direct and first hand experience of the work done and the physical, social environment in which it is done.

Starting the cumulative record of students.

Identification of students with problems.

Arranging personality counseling for low achievers and students with other problems or sending them to specialists.

Tools for Collecting Information

The information collected through the use of these tools should be cumulative; about the individual as a whole, based on a variety of sources and tools. These tools may be considered under the following categories:

Non-testing Tools

They provide a set of tools for individual assessment without the use of psychological tests. These tools are generally developed by the counselors and teachers themselves.

- Interview— is basic tools of counseling. It is described as a conversation with a definite purpose. Information with the help of interview can be collected from the individual student (counselee) herself/himself or from their family members, friends or teachers. Interview permits flexibility, clarity and an opportunity for observation to the counselor. It also provides the counselor with an opportunity to understand the counselee better. At later stages, the understanding forms the basis of therapeutic interview in the process of counseling. Structuring of these interviews helps in making the information more reliable and valid.

- Observation—is a careful study of counselee with a specific purpose. Counselor makes the observations either by participating observations, i.e. as a member of the group of counselee—participative or as an outsider—Non-participative observations can be made interview or testing or in the classroom or in the community/ward. Sometimes one-way screens are used to make these observations. By structuring and using rating scale/checklist. These observations can be made more reliable and valid
- Anecdotal records—recording important incidents. It is a verbal snapshot of an incident. Case should be taken to record the incident as it has happened. Tutors should be encouraged to participate in it. Decisions should not be made on the basis of a single anecdote
- Cumulative record card—is a method of recording and providing meaningful, significant and comprehensive information about the individual over the years. It is useful in organizing and integrating information collected through the use of different tools. Besides recording attendance and achievement and also it registers learner's social adjustment in the school, behavior with other learners, attitude towards school and teachers. It also contains the counselor's estimate of qualities like hard work, perseverance, tolerance, sociability and such other attributes which make a portrayal of the learner more complete. Cumulative record card can be maintained either in folder form or file form or card form. Tutors should be involved in maintaining it and teacher should be given some training in interpreting the information contained in it
- Problem/interest checklist—is given to identify their expressed problems or interest
- Rating scales—are used to get the assessment of learners' characteristics/trait such as initiative, responsibility, truthfulness, attitude of cooperation, honesty etc., either by others or the learner herself/himself
- Sociometry—is used to measure sociability or social distance amongst the members of a group
  - Autobiography and diaries—maintained by the learners may also provide useful information. Learners should be encouraged to keep their diaries in which they can record notes about themselves in relation to courses and certain situations. This/herself-evaluation will help pupils in developing self-understanding
  - Psychological test—Tests are a set of stimuli to provide sample of behavior of the respondent for different purposes. Psychological tests provides information about an individual's psychological characteristics such as intelligence, aptitudes, interests, abilities and personality, etc. and thus become an essential tool for understanding people. The choice of test should be made by looking at their validity, reliability, usability and practicability aspect.

The following purposes can be served by these tests
- To identify bright and low intelligent students, so that remedial teaching can be arranged for the less mature learner
- To identify the areas of weakness (diagnostic)
- To serve as the basis of counseling (Self-understanding)
- To serve as the basis of vocational guidance
- To serve as the basis of conference with the parents and teachers (supportive)
- To select the individuals from a group of applicants (selective)
- To predict the potentials of individuals (predictive)

A counselor should not give too much stress on the test score but should interpret them cautiously and has to involve all the tutors and administrator in the program of testing.

Counseling Personnel

Any successful counseling program cannot just depend upon a counselor alone but has to involve other members of the school like librarian, medical personnel, etc.
1. Principal/tutor/tutor-in-charge/Medical superintendent—For the counseling program to succeed the support of these persons is essential. These persons should recognize the need of the program, provide facilities, finance, give it, its rightful place in the school timetable, coordinate with other members of the staff, give publicity to the program and evaluate the counseling program.
2. Counselor — Every school will have either a fully trained counselor or some tutors who are trained through inservice/distance education program to take up the role of counselor.
   Specifically the counselor's functions are:
   - learner's appraisal; using appropriate test and non-testing devices
   - learner orientation; involving tutors, wardens, librarians, doctors and other resources

- Helping emotionally disturbed learner; using counseling techniques
- Helping learner to overcome academic and social deficiencies
- Helping learner to overcome their financial, health, sex, residential and mess problems
- Gaining cooperation from other tutors and helping them in gaining understanding of the pupils
- Gaining cooperation from parents and other personnel of the counseling process
- Maintaining up to date records of pupils concerning counseling
- Arranging for referral services for those who need them
- Evaluating and doing the follow-up work
- Giving career talks to potential beginners to the nursing profession
- Disseminating information relating to employment, recreational and professional opportunities.

3. Teaching Faculty are the key professionals in the school setting. Their support and participation is crucial in making the counseling program a success. They have the maximum and important contact with the learners. They act as a source of referral and appraisal to counselor, reinforces the counseling outcomes besides providing conducive environment. They give encouragement and support to the counselor. They also motivate the learners. To utilize the counseling services and help them to develop a positive attitude towards counseling. It is imperative for the counselor to share her/his expertise and orient the tutors for either roles as members of the counseling personnel team.

4. Parents— As the counseling program extends beyond nursing school, parents must be told about the need and scope of counseling program. learner's life, aspirations, adjustments, personality, etc. all will have the influence in home, so parents should be made aware of this impact. Parents also provide information about the child, i.e. his/her life style, reading habits, temperament, her/his interpersonal relationship, style of reaction, his/her emotional adjustment etc. parents also act as support to the counseling process they have a two way role. They need to be oriented about their role by the counselor.

Resources for Counseling

Counseling is an integral part of education, which takes place in a social matter. Hence counseling should take place with greater utilization of community resources. A counselor can refer students or their parents for help on special problems to these agencies or use them as energy resources - agencies willing to spend time/money/ human resources to sponsor certain activities related to counseling program such as funding, the purchase of films, publications, testing materials or visit to place of counseling interest, etc.

- Medical services—A counselor can refer students for special examination or treatment to such agency or special clinics
- Mental health services— A student who needs such help should be referred to psychiatric hospital, psychiatrist or to a special ward attached to a general hospital
- Social welfare agencies—For example: YWCA, Nehru Yuvak Kendra, Youth club, Lion's club, Rotary club, Sports club, Recreational club, etc. learners having financial problems with leisure time, social or employment problems may be referred to these agencies
- Law/Law enforcement agencies—Sometimes the problem faced by the learner is such that it requires taking help of legal/law enforcing agencies
- Employment exchanges—Provides employment information but also provide speakers for orientation/ inservice education programs and testing facilities, etc.
- Parents—Either individually or in the form of group (parent-teacher association) are a great resource. They can render help in the form of: arranging for tips, organizing finances launching social or recreational activities

Phases of Counseling

During the process of counseling in accordance with the nature of the person being helped, narrates different approaches to counseling, it will be useful to identify some common phases of the counseling process.

The phases may overlap each other, e.g. the assessment may begin while the phase of establishing the relationship is still going on or goal setting may start while assessment is still going on. These phases are in progressive movement and collectively describes the counseling process (Fig. 12.1).

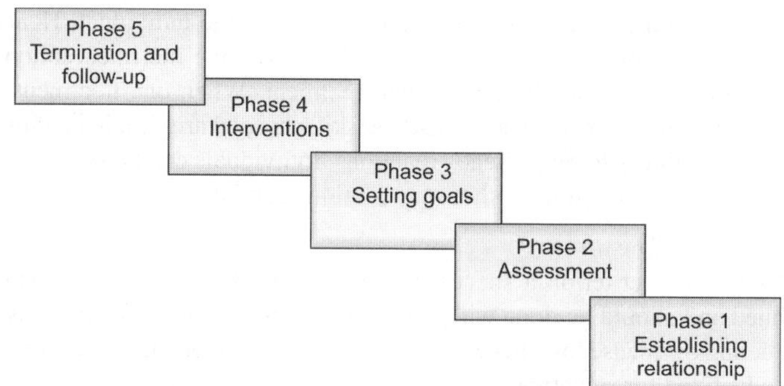

Fig. 12.1: Phases in counseling process

Phase-1: Establishing relationship

Is the core phase in the process of counseling. It affects the progress of the process and acts as a curative agent in itself. It should be recognised that each counselee—counselor relationship is unique and hence it is not possible to have a generalized relationship. It includes factors like: respect, trust and comfort etc.

Begin the phase with adequate social skills

- Introduce yourself
- Listen attentively and remember the client's name
- Always address the individual by his/her preferred name
- Ensure physical comfort
- Do not interrupt the individual while he/she is talking
- Observe non - verbal communications.

The relationship is not established in just a single session but may require several sessions before he/she becomes comfortable with you and accepts you into her/his inner world.

Phase-2: Assessment

It is a phase in which individuals are encouraged to talk about their problems; counselor asks questions, collects information, seeks his/her views, observes and possibly helps the individual to clearly state his/her problem. This is the data collecting phase and involves several specific skills such as:

- Observations
- Enquiry
- Making associations among facts
- Recording
- Making educated guesses
- Recording the information systematically and promptly.

Phase-3: Setting Goals

The purpose of this phase is to provide direction to the individual and counselor. It involves making a commitment to a set of conditions, a course of action or an outcome. Setting goals helps to know how well counseling is working and when counseling may be concluded. Setting goals two types—Immediate and Ultimate.

The process of setting goals is cooperately done by the counselor and the individual. It requires:

- The skills of drawing inference
- Differentiation
- Teaching individuals to think realistically.

It should be emphasized that goals are not fixed for all time to come and can be changed whenever new information is received or new insight is developed.

Phase-4: Intervention

It is a phase which is more influened by the view points a counselor holds about the counseling process. After setting goals the question that follows is 'how shall we accomplish these goals?' the intervention used will depend upon the approach used by the counselor, the problem and the individual. Hence the choice of the intervention is a process of adaption and the counselor should change the intervention when the selected intervention is not working. This is similar to medical treatment. When one treatment does not work that practitioner tries the alternative treatment. The counseling skills needed are skill in handling the interventions, knowledge of its effects and ability to read client's reactions. Individuals can be asked in the beginning about what interventions they have earlier so that other interventions can be used.

Phase-5: Termination and Follow-up

All counseling has its ultimate criterion a successful termination. It must be done without destroying the accomplishments gained and should be done with sensivity, intention and by fading. It is not unusual for the individual to have a feeling of a sense loss, hence termination should be planned over few sessions. Follow-up appointments can also be fixed for sometime.

Types of Counseling

Common *factors* in different approaches of counseling are:

- Interview is the best tool of counseling
- Counselors should accept the importance of satisfying relationship between counselor and counselee
- Counselor should give respect for the counselee
- Honesty, sincerity and openness are common in counseling process
- How the counselee perceives the counselor is more important than the skills and knowledge of the counselor.

1. Directive Counseling or Prescriptive Counseling or Counselor-centered Counseling

To attempt the reconcile and integrate interests of the personnel with the interest of more sophisticated common forces of counseling where the superior understands the problem, formulates correct answer, persuades the worker to perceive the answer in the same ways.

Tools

- Advice
- Warning
- Exhortation
- Praise
- Reassurance

The counselor is the central figure and plays more active role, where he/she directs the counselee to take steps in order to resolve his/her conflicts. It believes in the limited capacity of the client. It emphasizes on cognitive and intellectual aspects of the problem, and therefore efforts are made to solve the problem as such and not to help client in attaining his/her full growth.

The client makes the decision, but the counselor does all that he/she can to get the counselee make a decision in keeping with his/her diagnosis. He/she tries to direct the thinking of the counselee by informing, explaining, interpreting and advising. A considerable use of interpretation and direction by the counselor had led to directive Counseling

Stages

The counselee

- Seeks the help of the counselor
- Gives free expression to the emotionalized attitudes
- Gains insight
- Formulates plans
- Terminates the counseling contract.

Steps

1. Analysis: Collecting from a variety of sources, the data needed for an adequate understanding of the student.
2. Synthesis: Summarizing and organizing the data so that they reveal the students' assets, liabilities, adjustments and maladjustments.

3. Diagnosis: Formulating conclusions regarding the nature and the cause of the problems exhibited by the student.
4. Prognosis: Predicting the future development of the students' problems.
5. Counseling: The counselor takes measures with the student to bring about adjustment and readjustment for the student.
6. Follow up: Helping the student with new problems of with recurrence of the counseling provided to them.

Role of the Counselor

Assists the students to understand their Physical needs, psychological needs.

Helps them to accept their—Aptitudes, abilities, interests, opportunities for self-fulfillment.

Assist them to develop decision-making competency

Helps the other staff members to understand individual students by providing material information and evaluation.

Determines the impact of curricular program on student development and conveying that information to staff members.

Informing the staff members of significant changes in the school and non-school environment which have implications for instruction.

Assists the parents to understand the developmental needs and progress of their children.

Uses community resources for meeting the extreme needs of the students.

2. Non-Directive Counseling or Client-centered Counseling

It rests upon the fundamental respect for the individuals' belief in persons ability to solve personal problems with the aid of a sympathetic listener.

Purposes

To facilitate development of self - insight components.

To release of tensions

Formulation of new choices and plans in friendly atmosphere.

Process

Client , i.e. the counselee is the pivot, he/she takes an active part in the process of therapy. He/she gains insight into his/her problem with the help of the counselor. He/she only decides and takes necessary action.

The counselor's role is passive. This type of counseling is a growth experience. The goal is the independence and integration of the client rather than the problem oriented. The counselor creates an atmosphere in which the client can work out his/her own understanding. The emotional aspects are concentrated more, it leads to a voluntary choice of action.

In this counseling, the client has to be led to a point of self-realization, self-actualization and self-help. This method is useful in solving educational, vocational and marital problems.

The client is inclined to give information needed by the counselor.

Information may be used to classify a choice and to implement a decision.

Information may be used to help the client to discover the real problem.

In this type of counseling, the counselor has the respect for the personal autonomy of the client i.e., the client has to make the final decision. Counselor believes in the ability and capacity of his/her client to adjust and to adopt in terms of the demand of the situation. The counselor has to accept the capacity of the client to make adjustment and adaptation. In this, total personality of the client will be considered.

The principles of tolerance, acceptance are extremely important, hence the counselor is not free to express the difference of his/her opinion. He/she should be remain neutral and try to make the client that he/she is fully accepted and understood by him/her. The counselor has to make the client to develop awareness of himself/herself and his/her poten-tialities. Make the client to realise his/her abilities.

Steps
- The individual comes for help
- The counselor facilitates and encourage the client to think to solve his/her own problems

- The counselor is friendly, interested and encourages free expression of feelings related to problem. He/she accepts the clients' feelings whether it is positive or negative followed by a gradual development of the insight
- As the client recognizes and accepts emotionally as well as intellectually his/her desires and attitudes, he/she perceives the decisions that he/she must make and the possible courses of action open to him/her
- Positive steps towards the solution of the problem situation begins to occur
- The client only decides when to end the contract

3. Short-term Counseling

Used in situational crisis in which disruption of life occurred. It focuses or concern of the client or family. It can be relatively minor concern or a major crisis, but whatever the situation, it needs immediate attention. Counselors will assist the client and guides problem-solving in a systematic way or decision making (logical manner). In crisis situations, the counselor can share problem-solving abilities with the client.

4. Long-term Counseling

It extends over a prolonged period of time. (It varies, daily, weekly or monthly basis). It is focused for the client who experiences developmental crisis may need long-term counseling. (Developmental crisis can occur when a person is going through a developmental stage or passage), e.g. women with menopause; women with breast-feeding. Support groups can be involved in group counseling.

5. Electic Counseling

The counselor will make use of both directive and non - directive counseling which may be considered useful for the purpose of modifying the ideas and attitudes of the counselee. It puts check on the client's emotional expression whenever it is in his/her interest. The techniques are electic in nature because they have been derived from all sources of counseling, selecting the best and leaving out that what is least required. It is possible for the counselor to alternate between directive and non-directive methods even in the same interview without disrupting the non-directive permissive relationship with the client.

Steps
- The counseling starts with interview
- The counselor tries to establish rapport and make the client, what he/she can expect from him
- Counselor studies the personality and needs of the individual. Information may be gathered from different sources and case history
- Tentative diagnosis is made based on case history and a plan for counseling is formulated
- The client needs has to be helped to assimilate this information
- If need arises give information related to educational, vocational and occupational etc
- The client achieves emotional release and insights alter his/her perceptions and attitudes about himself/herself and his/her situations
- During the closing phase, the client makes decisions and plans, modifies behavior, solves his/her problems
- If needed follow-up contacts can be planned.

6. Clinical Counseling
- The diagnosis and treatment of mind functional maladjustments and to find better adjustment and self - expression
- A relationship has to be established primarily between counselor and client (face-to-face) contact
- The study of the individual as a unique whole, specific behaviors are observed and specific traits may be inferred, but the goal is particular individual
- It describes the problem and also suggests the solution or remedies for the problem
- It includes training, actual practice in diagnosis, treatment, prevention and research.

7. Psychological Counseling
They rely simply on conversation between client and therapist. This may take in the form of questions and answers, reconstruction of past history or discussion of current difficulties. It consists of catharsis or an

emotion-laden monologue by the patient or the therapist make an initiative in making the patient to speak out his/her repressed feelings and emotions. The therapist may offer/may give him/her—Encouragement, Give information and advise/ Hope.

8. Psychotherapeutic Counseling

Psychologically trained individual consciously attempts verbally to assist the other persons to modify emotional attitudes which the subject is aware of the personality reorganization through which he/she is undergoing. The person will attain higher level of personal and social development.

9. Student Counseling

It is concerned with helping the student to solve his/her problems pertaining to the choice of educational institutions, courses, methods of study, adjustment, vocational choice, etc. it deals with total personality of the individual, it connects directly to the needs of the individual, in a personal contact situation.

10. Placement Counseling

Counselor will advise to the counselee in regard to jobs and posts which are suitable to the client depend upon his/her abilities, attitudes and interests.

11. Marriage Counseling

Advise and help will be provided in selecting the suitable spouse.

To identify the positive aspects of relationship as well as those cause conflict.

To solve the problems related to their marital problems and marital relationships.

It focuses on the need for each partner to understand the point of view and feelings of the other.

It is directed to helping couples to talk constructively about problems in marital relationships.

It focuses on the need for each partner to understand the point of view and feelings of the other.

To identify positive aspects of the relationship as well as those causing conflict and implement steps to resolve strained inter personal relationships.

12. Vocational Counseling

Procedures centred about the problem of selecting a vocation and preparing for it.

If any problem arises within the specified vocation, necessary steps or advises will be carried out to solve those problems. It gives greater control over his/her own future actions. Counselor will help the client to improve his/her all round personality development and helps the individual to develop skills and efficiency, mastery over the vocation so that the counselee will best among his/her collegues in his/her profession.

13. Individual Counseling

Interview

Counseling may be preceded by an interview; the counselor will try to establish rapport and structuring has to be done so that the client understands what to expect at counseling. Interview consists of: Consultation, Mutual inter-change of opinions and deliberating together. It will be used to get information; To give information and to change behavior.

It involves:

- Gathering all available pertinent facts
- Making a diagnosis on the basis of all available pertinent facts
- Formulating an appropriate plan of action
- To enhance client's self-understanding, information about his/her background or any other related information, e.g. educational, social and occupational; may be gathered from various sources. Counselor will help the client to assimilate the information. The client achieves an insight and a sense of emotional release which alters his/her perception and attitude about himself/herself and his/her situations
- During the closing phase, the client makes decisions and plans, modifies behavior and solves problems. If needed follow-up contacts may be planned.

Types of Interviews

1. Introductory Interview: For mutual acquaintance and building rapport the counselor will introduce himself and state the purpose of interview and advise the subject about the follow up procedures.

2. **Fact-finding Interview:** To discover the intensity of a counselee's attitudes towards persons and situations which he/she cannot or will not reveal either in writing or in response to formalized questions which do not allow for indications of strong feelings. It allows the counselor to determine their strengths, sources, relationships and activities of other persons that are carried out with them.
3. **Informative Interview:** Data will be obtained from different sources to gather the information what is already possessed or available facts will be gathered.
4. **Therapeutic Interview:** It is one type of catharsis where the counselee will have a chance to talk about himself/herself, his/her past, wishes, fears, hopes, aspirations. By this process the counselor brings clarity of thoughts, relief from tensions and a new objectivity.

Procedure for Interview

1. **Preparation:** To eliminate unwanted responses and to achieve definite objective, preparation is essential. Interviewer has to decide what has to be accomplished, formulated goals or objectives for the interview.
   - Know the interviewee
   - Fix an appointment
   - Provide Privacy
   - Interviewer must see the interviewee's point of view
   - The interviewer must know the personality of the interviewee.
2. **The Process**
   - Establish rapport
   - Help the interviewee feel at ease and ready to talk
   - Help the interviewee to obtain and organize into a meaningful pattern of the information
   - The interviewer should ask unambiguous questions, listen to the interviewee's responses and he/she should have control over the interview
   - In the closing phase of interview any additional information is needed, he/she can add in the remarks.
3. **Interpretation:** The counselor has to listen to the clients' conversation and responses, she/he should distinguish between facts and fictions. Interpretation requires skill and great understanding. Interviewer has to interpret carefully the ideas, attitudes and responses of the interviewee.
4. Developing insight into the problems of counselee and put the action into a plan of work.
5. Recording of the total interview process is necessary for follow-up services and to take necessary plan of action.

14. Group Counseling

New way of working to help people, where peer group values are more important, e.g. adolescences. Sometimes it is successful with students who have not responded well to individual counseling. The individual may gain an insight and understanding into his/her own problems through listening to others, who will be discussing their difficulties. Ideas, values may become more understandable and acceptable. The counseling group helps the individual to change desires and gain abilities through their relationship in an accepting and meaningful social situation. The counselor should select the warmth and comfortable room for group counseling. The counselor should encourage team spirit and create a climate of harmony, cooperation, understanding and the acceptance. For homogeneous group (6 to 8 or below 20 members) group counseling will be advised. The counselor should have sound knowledge and sufficient skills, e.g. leadership.

Uses
- The individual will understand himself
- The individual feels that others also had the same problems too
- Feeling of acceptance and understanding of others also
- ' Trust', 'Intimacy' feelings will be developed
- Group counselor must be very clear in his/her mind in regard to the nature of the problem faced by the group, he/she has to identify himself with the group.

Principles of Group Counseling
- It is a function of a group of any individual

- It establishes right climate within the group and understands group problems, finds the way or discover solutions for group problems
- It determines its own way of procedures
- It will be useful for all the members in the group
- It will make them to understand the limitations and potentialities of its members
- It enables its members to tap their own inner psychological resources and gain desirable outcomes.

15. Behavioral Counseling

To change specific behavior and to treat the behavioral disorders. Behavioral Counseling will be effective. It is based on, principle 'learning by conditioning'.

Process of Counseling

The counselor should specify and define the specific inappropriate behavior which has to be changed. Prepare and develop the social history of the problem. Specify the goals of counseling and select the appropriate method.

Techniques used in Behavioral Counseling

1. Operant conditioning: The person will learn to behave in a different way, if the new behavior is rewarded and the old behavior is ignored.
2. Aversive conditioning: To eliminate specific behavior pattern, e.g. alcoholism, homosexuality, obesity and smoking this method is used. The therapist teaches the person to associate pain and discomfort with the response he/she wants to unlearn.
3. Reciprocal inhibition: The therapist establishes a hierarchy from the least to the most anxiety provoking situations; next he/she teaches the client to clear her/his mind, release or relax tensed muscles. Once the client has mastered the deep relaxation technique, he/she will lessen his/her anxiety.

   The therapist asks the person to imagine the least threatening scene and to signal when he/she begins to feel tense. At the signal, the therapist tells him/her to forget the scene and concentrate on relaxing. After a short period, he/she instructs him/her to return to the scene. This process is repeated until he/she feels completely relaxed. Gradually then move up the list until the client is able to imagine the situation he/she most feared without anxiety. The clients will learn to inhibit anxiety responses with incompatible and deep muscle relaxation.
4. Desensitization: To reduce irrational behavior, e.g. phobias related to sex, animals, closed rooms, etc. desensitization technique will be used. The client has anxiety producing situations, ranked interms of disturbances.

   The client will be instructed in relaxation techniques. Each anxious situation is presented starting with the one that produces the least anxiety. As the situation is recalled by the client, he/she is reinforced by the relaxation process, until there is no anxiety.

   The success of behavioral counseling is depended upon the following factors
- Establishing a valid hierarchy by the client and by the therapist.
- Discovering an adequate reinforcer (co-operant conditioning) by the therapist.
- Lack of counter conditioning outside the therapy sessions.

16. Dietary Counseling

Helping the individual to learn more about diet and meeting the nutritional needs.

Helps the person to become more aware of the role of food plays in providing, maintaining and building health and strength. Minimizing some of the discomforts of disease.

It is easier to accept diet modifications, if the person understands the benefits of good nutrition.

If the health team is able to promote acceptance of an appropriate diet within the health care facility; the person may permanently adopt more sensible eating habits at home.

Instruct the person about good nutrition in many ways.

Arrange planned conversations with the individual during which Nutrition expert can discuss dietary issues.

Explore the specific needs of the client and deal with questions related to the workability of a special diet.

When the person makes choices from the hospital menu, provide sound guidance in appropriate meal planning. Discuss comparative food values.

Mealtime itself presents opportunities for teaching.

When serving the individual the meal tray or assisting with eating, point out certain food items, e.g. If the person requires protein to promote wound healing, you can point out the protein containing foods on the tray. Learn to take advantage of all opportunities to assist the individual in acquiring sensible food selection patterns. Educate the client in detail about deficiency disorders and its prevention.

17. Motivational Counseling

It involves discussing feelings and incentives with the client. The counselor can encourage to establish helping relationship to avoid despair feelings and work through the feelings of their motivation, e.g. if the patient is having despair i.e., "I have nothing to live for "encourage the patient to talk about what is generating disinterest in recovery, if a problem is identified, the nurse and client can utilize the problem-solving technique to work toward an acceptable solution. If the client shows unwillingness to participate in learning activities, counselor has to assess any factors from the past or present that might be negatively influencing motivation for learning. Motivational counseling helps the client to work towards health promotion.

18. Interpersonal Counseling

Indications
- Changes in life events
- Sources of persistent distress in the family or place of work
- Current difficulties in relationships
  Patients are encouraged to consider whether there may be better ways of coping with these difficulties

19. Bereavement Counseling

It focuses on working through the stages of grief. It combines an opportunity for emotional release including the expression of despair and anger.
- Develop a therapeutic relationship.
- Clients or families needing counseling include persons who must adjust to changes in lifestyle body image as the disease progresses.
- During life-threatening illnesses, clients and families need counseling to cope with the possibility of death.
- Bereaved people have to be counseled individually.
  The bereaved person needs to talk about the loss, to express feelings of sadness, guilt or anger. To understand the normal course of grieving. It is helpful to warn a bereaved person about unusual experiences. For example, feeling, as if the dead persons were present, illusions and hallucinations, otherwise these experiences may be alarming.

Help may be needed:
- To accept that the loss is real
- To work through the stages of grief
- To adjust to the life without the deceased
- To accept that the loss is real.
- Viewing the dead body.
- Putting away the dead person's belongings, help this transition.
  A bereaved person should be encouraged to perform these actions.
  Practical problems may need to be discussed, e.g. funeral arrangements. Financial difficulties, e.g. young widow may need help in maintenance and caring for young children and in supporting them without inhibiting his/her own grief excessively to time passes, the bereaved person should be encouraged to resume social contacts, to talk to other people about the loss to remember happy and fulfilling experiences that were shared with the deceased and to consider positive activities that the latter would have wanted survivors to undertake.
  Hypnotic or anxiolytic drug may be needed for few days to restore sleep and to relieve any severe anxiety. Antidepressant drugs may be beneficial. Support groups have been developed to help recently bereaved

people, they can share grief, obtain practical advice and discuss way of coping. Psychotherapy may be helpful when the person is at high risk of an abnormal grief reaction.

Avoidant behavior can be reduced by guided mourning, a behavioral treatment in which the bereaved person is helpful to confront memory of dead person and to enter situations that provoke these memories.

20. Problem-solving Counseling

- Suitable for patients with reactions to stress and with minor affective disorder. The patient is helped to identify and list problems that are causing distress
- Consider what practicable courses of action might solve or reduce each problem
- Select one problem and try out the course of action that appears most feasible and to succeed
- Review the results of the attempt to solve the problem and then either choose another problem for solution if the first action has succeeded
- Choose another course of action if the first action has not succeeded, e.g. reactions to stress minor affective disorders, major depressive disorders.

21. Case Study

It is a non-standardised technique of collecting information about individual in all aspects of life.

Definition

1. A comprehensive collection of all available information social, psychological, physiological, biographical, environmental, vocational that promises to explain a single individual or a single social unit , i.e. Family.
2. Case study is a method of exploring and analyzing the life of a social unit — Be that a person, a family, an institution, a cultural group or even an entire community.
3. It is a complete analysis and report of the status of an individual subject with respect, as a rule, to specific phases of his/her total personality.

The team members like Psychologists, Physicians, Social workers and Teachers may cooperate in making case studies of an individual and thus collect useful data which may provide unique information about an individual. It is a detailed study of an individual, conducted for the purpose of bringing about better adjustment of the person, who is the subject of investigation. It serves diagnosis and treatment.

Types of Case Study

1. Formal Case Study
It is made with an outline in which all aspects of individual's life are included.
Outline:
Statement of the problem and state purposes, for case study.
Collection of data
Identification of the individual , i.e. Bio-data.
Family history
Environmental history, e.g. Neighborhood, home
Personality evaluation
Health history and present health status
Educational history and present status, e.g. IQ levels, achievement level, interest, aptitudes, social and emotional adjustment, physical development
Interpretation of data
Selection of therapy or remedial treatment
Follow-up evaluation.

Format
Teacher making study and Date of Investigation:
- Identification of the learner
- Statement of the problem
- Diagnostic test data
- Interview with learner
- Observe physical condition of learner, social and emotional adjustment, IQ levels

- Observation of educational records
- Observation of special interests and attainment of home conditions
- Diagnosis of the case
- Recommendations.

2. The Informal Case Study

It does not require the detailed outline and writing of the case material. In order to make teaching effective and better understanding of students, teachers can use informal case study.

Advantages

A good case study will make use of all possible factors, e.g. Mental, Physical, Social and Emotional etc. which may give clue to the problem behavior.

- It will be used as a tool of evaluation
- Reliable
- It leads teachers to be more aware of the special problems of individual children, thereby helping to weaken the tendency of susceptibility to the problem and steps to resolve it and to teach the same lesson to a whole class
- Reality situations can be used
- Used with regularity as a part of teaching process to find out the cause and effect relationship
- It helps to gain a better concept of normal behavior
- Teachers will become sensitive to behavior symptoms in all the children.

Limitations

- It is time consuming
- It may be too subjective
- The teacher may lack the necessary skills for collecting and interpreting data

3. Descriptive Case Study

The case study is a form of descriptive research. Although it consists of a vigorous, detailed examination of a single case, the underlying assumption is that this case is an example of many other such cases. Consequently by in depth study of a single case, a greater understanding about other similar cases is achieved. The purpose of case studies is to make generalizations. But drawing conclusions from a case study is not justifiable.

4. Historical Case Study

It emphasizes longitudinal or genetic approach, showing development over a period of time. It is concerned with everything that is significant in the history or developmental of the case. The purpose is to understand the life cycle of an individual unit, it may be a person, a family, a group, a social institution or an entire community. it probes deeply and intensively; analysis interaction between factors that produce change or growth.

Case study involves the collection and analysis of many sources of information. It consists of intensive study of a single unit, to develop insight and knowledge of a general nature and improved practices.

You can take an example from the past and use it to help us today that are very practical use of history. A case, historically scientific document, of any institution or individual becomes inevitable. Historical research is an accurate record of how, when and where the event started; how it progressed and when it ceased. The historian explains the event by describing the condition which led unto it and out of which it grew.

Integrated Methodology

The case study is very flexible as to the amount and type of data that are gathered as well as procedures used in gathering the data. hence the steps in the methodology are not distinct of uniform with all case studies. To gather valid and reliable information for a case study, an integrated methodology is adopted. The investigator conducts personal interviews, search through literacy source materials and adopts questionnaire method.

Interview Technique

The interview gathers data from individuals in face to face contacts. The interviewer prepares a structured interview questionnaire clearly outlining the best sequence of questions and stimulating comments, which would systematically bring out the desired responses. A written schedule prepared for the study provides a set plan for the interview, precluding the possibility that would fail to get important and needed data prior to the day of scheduled interview the investigator visits the respondents on several occasions to enhance rapport with the interviewees.

Interviews may be conducted with the case under study and his/her friends, relatives, coaches, administrators, the secondary source of information may be correlated with the recorded information from the case himself/herself and reliability established.

Literacy Source Method

The investigator searches through the primary and secondary sources and documents the available information from books journals, magazines, etc. internal and external criticisms are applied to establish validity and reliability of the data.

Questionnaire Method

A standard questionnaire to record the psychological traits of the case under study is used. Opinion questionnaire are constructed to collect information on the case under study, from his/her friends, relatives, coaches, administrators, ampires, spectators and others. They are standardized by internal consistency statistical technique before application.

22. Educational Counseling

- It helps the learners to get maximum benefit out of education and solve their problems related to education
- To help learners to orient themselves to the new purposes and philosophy of Nursing Education
- To assist the learners to identify the need of educational planning
- To make the students to develop study habits related and appropriate to the study of nursing
- To orient the learners with clinical field and methods of clinical learning
- To orient the learners with library and other facilities which are available to them in and outside of school of nursing
- To help the learners to choose specialization according to their needs and interest
- To give information about higher education and stimulate them to consider them carefully.

23. Vocational Counseling

- Individuals make different demands from different individuals. This function assists the learners to select an occupation most suited to their abilities, interest and aptitude. It helps them to prepare for it, enter it and progress in it. This function is concerned with following:
- To help the student to understand their abilities, interest, values and goals
- To provide information of occupations—rewards, conditions of employment, opportunities for advancement and requirement for success in it
- To help them to know about the various programs of financial assistance—Scholarships, Fellowships; to improve their career. The teachers will act as career counselors.

24. Counseling in Health and Living Conditions

Purposes
- To develop referral services for health guidance-social, mental and physical
- To provide sex education
- To help the authorities in the supervision and maintenance of proper sanitation in and around the hostel, or to help authorities in providing satisfactory living conditions along with the food to the students
- To help students to develop interest in games and other activities which will promote health.

25. Personal Counseling

Every student faces certain problems about which he/she may be very anxious. She/her generally tries to cope up with the problem by himself/herself. Here a counselor helps pupils to understand and solve these problems. Specifically counselor performs the following
- Provides advice on personal problems
- Provides at the right time or suggestions to improve personal appearance
- Helps learners develop interpersonal skills

- Helps learners to accept themselves and others
- Provides marriage counseling.

26. Moral, Religious and Social Counseling

In the moral, religious and social area counseling is undertaken with a view to
- Providing and developing, learning experiences to inculcate right ideals and conduct of living
- Providing training in correct social convictions
- Enabling students to inculcate and priorities their values that would be beneficial to them and the society.

27. Counseling in Leisure Time

Learners need opportunities of self-expression in which they can try out their talents and express themselves. Some students are shy and they need encouragement to make proper use of their potentials and talents. Counseling function in the area was to help the students to find opportunities for creative use of their leisure time. Counseling function in this area: Provides opportunities for extra-curricular activities to develop interest which provide avenues for recreation

28. Self-help group Counseling

It is a process of counseling of people in groups. It involves only minimal or no therapist contact to bring behavioral change. Groups are formed by the individuals suffering from the same problem. Many self-help programs are developed and disseminated through self-help groups. In a self-help group each member of the group shares his/her problems and all participants work together towards their solutions. This provides its members with many valuable experiences and facilitates self-exploration, self understanding and self acceptance. This also eliminates isolation and shyness of the group members and develops within them a feeling or mutual trust. 'Alcoholics anonymous (A.A)' is an example of self-help groups.

29. Peer Group Counseling

Peers are also important members of the team of counseling. Many students would prefer discussing their problems with their fellow members rather than with their tutors or counselors. Students accept their peers as counselors because they share the same problems and communication is at the same level. They also have more trust in them.

Peer counseling can be very useful in Nursing Education. It will be used at the initial stage of the problems and for screening of individuals with problems. The concept of peer counseling does not replace the faculty counselors but supplements their work. It can be used to provide support:
- To solve problems as well as for understanding each other
- Help individuals to adjust to the new setting (school or hostel or clinical field)
- In terms of practical problems it can solve problems such as of housing, transport, study-skills, stipends and loans, providing favourable climate at the beginning of students' studies
- Peer counseling can be made more effective by identifying potential counselors amongst the students and giving them some training.

30. Orientation Service Counseling

Is meant to help the learners become fully aware of himself/ herself and the new environment (nursing school/hospital/community field) so that at the beginning of school/college career, he/ she is oriented to the purpose, history, nature and scope of nursing education and nursing practice, besides being helped to acquaint herself/himself with library and other physical facilities which are available for them in school/college and outside the school/college. After general orientation, sessions should be plan when intensive guidance services are provided.

31. Appraisal Service Counseling

Is meant to gather record, maintain and use adequate information about each student to help each student achieve optimum potential and for helping her/him to develop self-insight as the progress through education and occupation of parents. Information is also collected about pupil's interest, from different sources such as student himself/ herself, family members, friends, teachers his/her previous school through the use of interviews, questionnaire, observation, checklist, anecdotal record, problem checklist, records school/health, psychological tests. The information thus collected is recorded in a cumulative record card (CRC), which is kept confidentially. The CRC is maintained by recording all the up-to-date information/achievement about the pupil in it. All the staff members should be encouraged to participate in this service. Only reliable, usable and accurate information should be collected. The record should be clearly maintained with updating.

32. Information Service Counseling

To serve the individual and society. Here occupational information is given to the individual. A nursing student has already taken a unfortunate consequences arising from maladjustment to his/her job and contributes to his/her well being and efficiency. This service acquaints the nursing students with different types of workers, particularly community helpers; assists them to see and gives them information about higher training/courses available to them. Career talks, newspapers, employment news, pamphlets, charts, occupational guides (job description booklets), audio-visual materials, etc. are used to convey such information to the nursing students. As a nurse educator teaching faculty can act as a career master and give/arrange a career talk in the neighbour-hood, general schools so as to motivate the students to join nursing profession.

33. Counseling Service

Is the pivot of all services available under the banner guidance and counseling in a school of nursing. It aims at developing learners' self-understanding, self-acceptance and self confidence. It is a process by which an individual learns to be independent, to make decisions, to live with a problem situation and to face any crisis situation.

Types

a. Developmental Counseling

Helps individuals to

- Achieve personal growth by making them aware of themselves and their environment
- Set clear goals for future behavior and methods of achieving these goals
- Develop positive attitudes, values and morals.

b. Preventive Counseling

Helps an individual to prepare for future specific concern such as failures in the examinations and shock if not getting a job or admission, or delay in getting married. This type of counseling is specially needed for educating students on the abuse of drugs, suicide and truancy etc.

c. Facilitative Counseling

Referred as remedial or adjustive counseling which means to correct a fault or an undesirable behavior. All individuals will commit some fault or the other and need help of someone who can provide counseling services.

d. Crisis Counseling

Helps an individual to overcome the effects of crisis situation such as loss of a family member, family conflict etc., These situations may affect the normal behavior of an individual and she/he may develop a feeling of anxiety and develop new pattern of behavior.

Ingredients of Counseling Services

a. Planning service—is meant to help learners to overcome their problems of hostel, mess and finance; help is also rendered for enabling the students to adjust to new situations. School can organize programs for securing scholarships for students, getting funds from different sources, arranging for different co-curricular activities, educational tours and cultural programs with the help of student adviser.
b. Placement service—The assistance offered to an individual in taking the next step, whether towards further training or job. A strong emphasis is on placing students in jobs suitable for them. It can be done through coordination with employment exchanges and different employing agencies.
c. Follow-up service—Keeping in touch with students who have qualified from the school as well as the dropouts for some years after they leave the school. This is done to find further opportunities for serving these students and evaluating the program. The common tools used for conducting follow-up services consist of questionnaires, interviews, letters and telephone calls, etc.

d. Research and evaluation—is a service meant to evaluate the school counseling program. A counselor acts as research and conducts surveys follow-up or evaluate (formative summative) the effects of counseling programs.

Problems in Guidance and Counseling

The counselor will face some of the problems in their profession.

1. Resistance to counseling—Either by counselee or by faculty.
2. Counselee with different cultures—The nursing student will come from different cultural backgrounds, they will have their own set of values and expectations. The counselor should be very careful in dealing counselee's with different cultures. He/she should not impose his/her personal values on counselee.
3. Counseling individuals with strong emotions such as anxiety, anger, depression, intimacy, etc. which will hinder counseling process. During strong emotions the counselor should calm and listen to the counselee and encourage him/her to ventilate his/her feelings.
4. Counselor burn out the symptoms such as restlessness, boredom, irritability, lethargy fatigue, negative feelings etc., can be managed by changing work environment, approach taking care of themselves, e.g. enough sleep, rest, diet, play, entertainment and accept others' view.
5. Lack of awareness of value of counseling by public.
6. Inadequate administrative set-up.
7. Lack of physical facilities, non-availability of time and tools, dearth of training facilities for counselors.

QUESTIONS

- Basic principles in Counseling(5M, RGUHS, Aug, 2010 & 10M,RGUHS,April,2007)
- Counseling (5M, NTRUHS, June, 2009)
- Couseling committee (5M, NIMS, May, 2007).
- Define Counseling and write the importance of Counseling in Nursing (3M), Write the principles of Guidance & Counseling (3M), Describe the role of Nurse in Counseling and Guidance (6M)
- Describe the types of Approaches used in Counseling and steps of Counseling Process (10M, Baba Farid UHS, 2010)
- Explain in detail how will you organize counseling services in Nursing Educational Institutions (5M, RGUHS, Sept, 2009)
- Explain the need and significance of guidance and counseling services in a School of Nursing, Describe the role of a principal, School of nursing in organizing counseling services for the students. (6+9 = 15 marks, MGU, Nov,2009)
- Explain the organization of counseling services for first year B.Sc. (N) students(6M, May 2010, NIMS)
- Issues of Counseling of Nursing students (5M, Baba Farid UHS, 2009)
- Issues related to Counseling the Nursing students (5M, NTRUHS, June 2009)
- Mention the Types of Counseling Approach (2M, MGRUHS, Feb, 2010 & 10M, Rajasthan UHS, 8M, Feb, 2008 & March, 2010)
- Steps in Counseling Process (5M, MGRUHS, Feb, 2010 & 6M, Baba Farid UHS, 2008)
- Technique of counseling (10M, RGUHS, April, 2006)
- The Types of Approaches in Counseling (5M, NIMS, May,2008)
- Types of Counseling approaches (5M, RGUHS, Feb, 2010)
- Types of counseling approaches (5M, RGUHS, Feb, 2010)
- What are the issues for counseling in Nursing. Explain the counseling process in detail (10M, NIMS, May, 2008)
- What is counseling? What are the different types of counseling? How will you differentiate the counseling with guidance? (2+5+8 = 15M, NTRUHS, June, 2009)
- Write the Principles of Counseling (7 M) How will you organize Counseling program for your students in your College of Nursing (8M, MGRUHS, Feb, 2009)

Discipline

INTRODUCTION

"To enjoy good health, to bring true happiness to one's family, to bring peace to all, one must first discipline and control one's own mind. If a man can control his mind he can find the way to enlightenment and all wisdom and virtue will naturally come to him"—Buddha

The word 'discipline' comes from the word 'disciple'. A disciple is one who learns and is constantly aware of his/her learning. The importance of discipline is well recognized in every aspect of life. Teachers use discipline strategies for behavior management in the classroom. Character that got us out of bed, commitment that moved us into action and discipline that enabled us to follow through. Effective leadership is putting first things first. Effective management is discipline, carrying it out. Discipline is the bridge between goals and accomplishment. We must all suffer one of two things: the pain of discipline or the pain of regret or disappointment.

DEFINITIONS

"The subject matter of instruction; a branch of knowledge and the treatment suited to a disciple or learner in education; development of the faculties by instruction, exercise and training, whether physical, mental or moral"

"Training to act in accordance with established rules; accustoming to systematic and regular action or to drill"

"Subjection to rule; submissiveness to order and control; habit of obedience".

"Severe training, corrective of faults; instruction by means of misfortune, suffering, punishment, etc."

"The enforcement of methods of correction against one guilty of offenses; reformatory or penal action toward a member who committed mistake"

"Self-inflicted and voluntary corporal punishment, as penance"

"To educate; to develop by instruction and exercise; to train and a system of essential rules and duties"

"To accustom, to regular and systematic action; to bring under control so as to act systematically; to train to act together under order; to teach subordination to; to form a habit of obedience in"

"To improve by corrective and penal methods; to chastise; to correct".

Meaning

Discipline means the willing submission of a person to rules, regulations and instructions to someone recognized by society. It is a willing and polite discharge of one's duty towards others in society. Discipline must be observed by everyone of us in all walks of life. One should be disciplined whether at home, in school on the play ground, on duty or in the office. Discipline is a virtue. It provides mental strength to discriminate good from bad and to defend the right against wrong. The strength and backbone of a nation lies in discipline. No nation can progress unless its citizens are disciplined. Citizens of a disciplined nation work in a spirit of co-operation and unity. Only those nations where people have a sense of discipline can proper in all fields. They even rule other nations. Discipline is a valuable asset at all levels of the society. Chanakya once said, "United we stand, divided we fall".

An educational institution having no discipline does not impart value based education. The indiscipline of the student is reflected on the whole society. The whole group suffers. The students with indiscipline does not make progress.

Discipline should be the first criterion of the family. Parents must bring up their learners in congenial disciplined atmosphere and teach the right values to transform them into balanced adults. Therefore, they can give their best to the country as disciplined citizens.

Discipline is necessary for both the teacher and the taught. A good teacher has a great responsibility of keeping a high image of his personality in the society. He can't do it unless he maintains an intellectual and more discipline of a high order. No student will obey and respect an indiscipline teacher, however high may be his knowledge.

Similarly only a serious and self disciplined student achieves something worth in the life. Indiscipline students just wander here and there, waste away their precious time and energy in useless activities and later on repent in life. They soon learnt that there is no shortcut to success and it is only through consistent hard work and self discipline that they can achieve their objective in life. Discipline is born out of a sense of responsibility towards the society among the people.

Differences between Discipline and Punishment

Discipline	Punishment
Logical consequences that are directly related to misbehavior	Consequences that are unrelated and illogical to the misbehavior
When the learners' behavior negatively affects someone else	When learners' are punished for hurting others
Understanding individual abilities, needs, circumstances and developmental stages	Inappropriate to the learners developmental stage of life, individual abilities, circumstances and needs are not taken into consideration
Teaching learner to internalize self discipline	Teaching leaner to behave well
Listening and modeling	Constantly reprimanding learners for minor infractions causing them to timeout
Using mistakes as learning opportunities	Forcing learners to comply with illogical rules 'Just because you said so'
Directed at learner behavior	Criticizing the learner rather than learner's behavior

Aims

- To follow certain norms of social order
- To make great progress of school and nation
- People must demonstrate a sense of discipline even in small things being responsible is discipline. If every person fulfills the responsibility, then his dreams as well as his country's dreams will come true. Therefore, discipline is necessary for an orderly society
- Ensure the safety of staff and students
- Create an environment conducive to learning
- Promotes personal safety, good behavior and ensures academic growth for students
- Orderly schools, usually balance clearly established and communicated rules with a climate of concern for students as individuals.

Types

1. Classroom Discipline

"The strategies a teacher uses to manage student behaviors and attitudes during instructional time".

Discipline is a key component to effective classroom management. A teacher who uses consistent discipline strategies exhibits more effective classroom management than an inconsistent teacher. Teachers usually will develop their own styles of discipline for their classrooms.

2. Preventative Discipline

"A concise outline about classroom expectations for students as well as for teachers; students need to know what expected of them for the remainder of the class. Such guidelines might include rules regarding talking, homework or language use in the classroom".

It establishes the types of consequences that will follow a forbidden act or behavior. Preventative discipline strategies create a safe, nonconfrontational classroom atmosphere in which students feel that they understand what to come. The most basic component to preventative discipline is a concise outline about classroom expectations for students as well as for teachers.

3. Supportive Discipline

When a teacher offers a verbal warning or a suggestion for correcting behavior while a student is disobeying an established classroom rule, the teacher is using supportive discipline. It provides a student with suggestions and options for correcting a behavior before a consequence is necessary, e.g. if a student is wandering around the class after a teacher has announced it is time to sit down, the teacher may say, "I made the announcement that it is time to sit down. Find your seat so we can get started". The student has been given the option to accept or avoid further punishment; the behavior has been redirected through a teacher's supportive discipline strategy, e.g. reminders, redirection and nonverbal communication. This facet of discipline assists students with self-control by helping them to get back on task often only the student involved knows it has been used.

The following tactics are suggested for supportive discipline:
- Use signals directed to a student needing support
- Learn to catch student's eyes and use head shakes, frowns and hand signals
- Use physical proximity when signals are ineffective
- Show interest in student work. Ask cheerful questions or make favorable comments
- Sometimes provide a light challenge. For example: "Can you complete five more before we stop?"
- Restructure difficult work by changing the activity or providing help
- Give hints, clues or suggestions to help students progress
- Inject humor into lessons that have become tiring. Students appreciate it
- Remove distractive objects, return them later
- Acknowledge good behavior in appropriate ways and at appropriate times
- Use hints and suggestions as students begin to drift toward misbehavior
- Show that teacher can recognize students' discomfort: ask for a few minutes more of focused work.

4. Corrective Discipline

"The set of consequences delivered to students following an infraction". When a student has failed to redirect her/his behavior after repeated attempts at supportive discipline or preventive discipline, a teacher may opt for a corrective discipline strategy. Consistent application of consequences is an essential component of corrective discipline strategies. Engaging in a verbal altercation with a student is a corrective discipline technique, but it may escalate a volatile situation and undermine authority as a teacher and leader. Corrective discipline strategies should be adapted to the students' age or grade level, e.g. placing in a time out may be effective for kindergarten students, for higher grade level, e.g. giving assignments, counseling and guiding them not to repeat the behavior, if the learner is not changing and doing the same mistake repeatedly, reinforce hard behavior in the form of punishments like not allowing them to take the examinations, penalties etc.

When students violate rules, teacher must deal with the misbehavior expeditiously. Corrective discipline should neither intimidate students nor prompt power struggles; but rather should proceed as follows
- Stop disruptive misbehavior. It is usually best not to ignore it
- Talk with the offending student or invoke a consequence appropriate to the misbehavior in accordance with class rules
- Remain calm and speak in a matter-of-fact manner
- Follow through consistently on promised consequences
- Redirect misbehavior in positive directions
- If necessary, talk with students privately about misbehavior. Ask how you can help
- Be ready to invoke an insubordination rule for students who refuse to stop misbehaving.

5. Preventive Discipline

To prevent classroom misbehavior is to provide a stimulating curriculum that involves students so successfully spend most of the time.

Positive Rewards

1. Immediate Rewards: Rewards should be given to learners as soon as possible so that students will identify why they are being rewarded. Behavior is learned more quickly if the reward appears immediately after the desired behavior.
2. Changing the Rewards: Different rewards for different activities, e.g. different awards for the academic excellence, clinical skills, extra curricular activities, Cocurricular activities etc.
3. Giving Cues for the Desired Behaviors: Cues can help to avoid problems that might occur if learners do not understand what is considered proper behavior. Cues can help learners to understand what is expected of them in a positive manner. When students perform properly after they receive cues, they should be properly reinforced (or rewarded) by the teachers in the form of appreciation for their performance.

Tips beneficial to prevent misbehavior among the students
- Make the curriculum as worthwhile and enjoyable as possible
- Remember that students crave fun, belonging, freedom, power and dignity
- Be pleasant and helpful
- Involve and empower the students by asking them for input and help
- Teach the method of appropriate class conduct
- Teach the subject effectively, as it promotes clear understanding for the students
- Discuss and practice behaviors to which you have jointly agreed
- Continually emphasize good manners, self respect and respect for others
- Teacher should act as a role model.

6. Progressive Discipline

Wherever feasible and effective, discipline will be applied progressively. Both Verbal and Written Warnings issued by the school will be noted on the learner's record. Copies of warnings issued will be provided to parents by the school.

Management of Misbehavior or Controlling measures against Indiscipline

- Rules and policies related to discipline and the consequences of breaking them should be clearly specified by discipline committee in the school and communicated to staff, students, parents and community representatives by such means as newsletters, student assemblies like general body meetings, student welfare body meetings and handbooks (Informative booklets or brochures of school indicating rules and regulations that has to be followed by student)
- Each academic year or periodically, the rules has to be restated based on institutional policies and curricular requirements. Once rules have been communicated, fair and consistent enforcement helps to maintain students' respect for the school's discipline system. Consistency will be greater when fewer individuals are responsible for enforcement of school discipline
- Social rewards such as smiling, praising, and complimenting are extremely effective in increasing desirable behavior
- Student input is also desirable
- Making school enjoyable and interesting for as many students as possible, e.g. by changing instructional practices to accommodate a variety of learning styles may dramatically decrease discipline problems
- The principal plays an important leadership role in establishing school discipline, both by effective administration and by personal example. Principals of well-disciplined students are usually highly visible models, describes as "management by walking around". Effective principals are liked and respected, rather than feared and communicate caring for students as well as willingness to impose punishment, if necessary. Principal should be able to create consensus among staff on rules and their enforcement. Teacher input is especially important because their support is crucial to a plan's success
- Good communication and shared values are important elements in maintaining relationship between teachers and principal and contributing factors in maintaining school discipline
- Stable and supportive administrative leadership is essential.

Positive Discipline in the classroom

Remember: Catch students doing the right thing and reward them immediately. This is the core of positive discipline.

Students respond better to positive approaches, including negotiation and systems of rewards, rather than punishment through verbal, physical or emotional abuse.

Seven Principles for Positive Learner's Discipline

1. Respect the learner's dignity.
2. Develop pro-social behavior, self- discipline and character.
3. Maximize the learner's active participation.
4. Respect the learner's developmental needs and quality of life.
5. Respect the learner's motivation and life views.
6. Assure fairness (equity and non-discrimination) and justice.
7. Promote solidarity.

Positive discipline is a four-step process that recognizes and rewards appropriate behavior

1. The appropriate behavior is described verbally to the group of learners.
2. Clear reasons are provided: "We are going to start our mathematics lesson and everyone needs to listen closely". This means that quieting down quickly will show respect for others. It is a good example of treating others as you would like them to treat you.
3. Acknowledgement is requested: "When can we all talk without disrupting others and their opportunity to learn the lesson".
4. The correct behavior is reinforced: Eye contact, a nod, a smile, an extra five minutes of play time at the end of the day, extra credit points, having a success mentioned in front of the class or school (social recognition is the greatest award). When rewards are used, they should always be immediate and small, yet gratifying. Teachers who use positive discipline believe in their students' abilities and communicate affection and respect for their students. When teachers are willing to observe their students and respond in ways that encourage positive behavior, they help their students become responsible for their own behaviors and they reduce the likelihood of misbehavior.

Action Activity: Positive or Negative Discipline

Which disciplinary actions in the table below are positive and which are negative? Place a check mark (✓) in the appropriate column. Next, place a check mark in the last column for each action that you have ever used or might use, to correct a learner's misbehavior.

Sl No	Have you ever used this action?	Positive (✓)	Negative (✓)
1	Getting the student's attention before you begin class		
2	Using direct instruction (tell them exactly what will be happening)		
3	Making assumptions		
4	Making accusations without proof		
5	Getting up and walking around the classroom		
6	Using physical force		
7	Commanding		
8	Acting in the way that you want the learner to act (modelling)		
9	Generalizing about a student's behavior		
10	Publicly comparing one learner to another		
11	Enriching your classroom environment		
12	Anticipating problems		
13	Insisting that you are right and acting superior		
14	Establishing clear and consistently enforced rules		

Answers: Actions numbered 1, 2, 5, 8, 11, 12, and 14 are positive, Actions numbered 3, 4, 6, 7, 9, 10, and 13 are negative. How did you score? How many of the negative and positive methods have you used?

Building Positive Teacher-Student Relationships

Teachers who use positive discipline respect nurture and support their students. They understand why a student behaves – or misbehaves – as he/she does, as well as how the student sees himself/herself, which may cause misbehavior. They also empathize with the learner's abilities and his or her situation in life. The teacher's expectations of the student are realistic, accepting the learner as he/she is and not on what he/she should be. The teacher understands that misbehavior is a constructive learning event, both for the learner and for his or her teacher, and that it is an important, natural part of the learner's development, not a threat to a teacher's authority.

By building such a positive relationship on understanding and empathy, students come to trust their teachers and to value their approval. As students respond to the positive nature of the relationship and consistent discipline, the incidence of misbehavior decreases and the quality of the relationship improves even further. Towards this end, the best teachers are ones who are good role models and about whom learners care enough to want to imitate and please.

Learners learn and behave—as a result of hereditary factors, the environment in which they live and their own personal and psychological needs. Any one cannot change their heredity and they may have limited control over their environment, understanding and communicating with parents and influencing personalities in learners' life. Yet by understanding that each students in making choices about how he/she behaves, teacher can provide with strategic leverage for influencing them. Behavior is understandable and purposeful. Students do what they do with a purpose. When teacher can begin to see the world or just your classroom through their eyes, teacher can respond to them rationally, confidently and effectively.

If the teacher believe that each student is making choices about his or her behavior, teacher must also apply this approach to their own reactions in the classroom and all other dealings with students. Teacher must ask themselves about the choices and actions they are making and then take with greater care about how teacher can express themselves both in voice and gesture.

The ultimate goal of student behavior is to fulfill the need to belong, which is fundamental one and everyone can share it. Each one of us in life continually strives to find and maintain a place of significance, a place to belong. We select beliefs, feelings and behaviors that we feel will gain us significance. Most students spend several hours a day in school, so their ability to find their place in the classroom group and the school at large, is of major importance. Moreover, whatever method each student chooses to use in achieving the goal of belonging—either through proper behavior this method is selected early in life and becomes the lifestyle that characterizes that person.

Students need to satisfy three 'C's in order to experience a sense of belonging.
- They need to feel Capable of completing tasks in a manner that meets the needs of the classroom and school
- They need to feel they can Connect successfully with teachers and classmates
- They need to know they Contribute to the group in a significant way.

The three factors that affect students' abilities to satisfy the three C's and which require action on your part, are: the quality of the teacher-student relationship, one based on trust, mutual respect and understanding, the strength of the classroom climate for success (for instance, all learnerren feel that they are included, that they are valued and that they can work together cooperatively and effectively) the appropriateness of the classroom structure (how it is managed). By finding ways to satisfy these three C's along these three lines, teacher can fulfill students' need to belong and therefore prevent misbehavior that may arise in their search to satisfy this need. Teacher will also be well on way to inspiring both well-behaved and passive students to actively participate in your class. In all cases, one of the strongest tools teachers have is encouragement, without which students cannot develop the tools to succeed and achieve their sense of belonging.

Positive disciplinary actions:
- Every learner demands attention, an important goal of teaching is to provide attention so that students develop healthy self-esteem
- Avoid scolding or bribing which encourages more misbehavior
- Catch them being good; praise them when the students are behaving normally
- Ignore the misbehavior, if it is not troublesome

- Giving the learner positive attention during pleasant times
- Teach them to ask for attention
- Give them a stern "eye" (look) but do not speak
- Stand close by rather than far away target the student by name, identify the behavior to be stopped, tell the student what he is expected to do at that moment, let him make the decision about what he does next and its consequences
- Distract the student, such as ask a direct question, ask a favor, give choices, change the activity
- Never give attention on demand, even for useful behavior. Help students become self-motivated. Give attention in ways they don't expect. Catch them being "good"
- Put the student in a position of responsibility and grant him or her legitimate power
- Try to build a caring, trusting relationship with the student while improving his or her self-esteem. This can be easily done by placing the student in situations in which he/she cannot fail. When a student has a better opinion of himself or herself, they rarely misbehave to seek revenge
- Teach the student how to express their feelings appropriately. Rather than taking revenge for being hurt physically or emotionally, teach the learner to "talk it out" to tell each other how hurt the revenge were and try to determine the cause and how to avoid revenge in the future
- Some students fear failure or feel that they are inadequate and cannot live up to their own, their parent's or their teachers' expectations. This feeling of inadequacy is an escape for the discouraged learner. Start where they are (not what they are supposed to be), develop realistic expectations, eliminate all criticism of their work, encourage their slightest effort, and, above all, don't pity them. You must restore their faith in themselves and encourage them by praising whatever successes they achieve, no matter how small. Intentionally arrange for them to succeed in easy tasks and find opportunities to compliment them on their behavior and positive efforts
- Building a trusting and caring relationship between teacher and students, one that promotes good behavior and prevents misbehavior
- Students' positive achievements reflect how well teacher is performing and how well students can see teacher as a "role model"
- In a respectful environment, all students feel safe and valued. The teacher has a friendly in nature, open rapport, show concern and support to the students
- Giving thoughtful attention to a student's work demonstrates caring and respect
- A teacher needs to know the interests and dreams of each student, talk with students, develop lesson plans and design learning activities
- Set aside 10 to 15 minutes during the day or at least once a week, for students to share in small groups how they are feeling, bad things and good things that are happening in their lives. A group can elect to share information they feel is important with the teacher or the class
- Praise them whenever possible and appropriate
- To guide the learner's behavior in a positive manner, teachers need to understand his or her total learning environment and the factors that may affect his or her behavior at a personal level, a family level, and a community level
- Encourage strong, caring and productive families and communities to be supportive for their growth and development
- Encourage regular "teacher-parent/caregiver" conferences to discuss student's learning progress and how better care giving can improve their learning, self-esteem and behavior.
  - To discuss a specific academic issue requested by the school, such as the learner's learning performance (good or poor) or a request for parental assistance in the classroom or school;
  - To discuss the learner's attendance or disciplinary issues;
  - To discuss an issue brought up by parents, themselves;
  - To hold a regular conference as set in the school calendar;
- Encourage learners work together cooperatively
- Building a positive teacher-student relationship, one that promotes good behavior and also involve parents in their learner's education and achievements

- Maintain "Behavioral Incident Logs" to keep track of incidents of misbehavior and to take necessary steps to correct the behavior
  "Behavioral Incident Logs" contain: (a) the learner's name (b) date and time of incident (c) brief description of behavior observed (d) The action taken (e) Name of the person to whom the incident was reported, as well as the time and method of reporting (written/verbal) (f) name of persons witnessing the behavior (g) name of person completing this log/report and date (h) any contributing factors and/or changes to be made that might have affected the learner's behavior (i) signatures of the principal, witnessing teacher and parent as well as date.

Encouragement Strategies

- Maintaining a positive emotional tone in the classroom
- Providing attention to the student to increase positive behavior
- Providing consistency in the form of regular routines for daily activities and interactions
- Responding consistently to similar behavioral situations
- Being flexible
- Building confidence. Promote positive self-talk
- Focusing on past successes
- Making learning meaningful. Modify instructional methods.

Class Room Management

Definition

"The procedures, strategies and instructional methods that teachers use to create a conducive environment that promotes learning, as well as to develop and manage the behaviors and learning activities of individual students and groups of students within classroom environment".

Advantages

- Effective classroom management is the most important-and the most difficult-skill a new teacher must master. Even experienced teachers often find themselves faced with a student or an entire class-who challenges their longstanding management skills and forces them to find new ways of dealing with classroom situations
- In order to develop good behaviors for students, they must be in a classroom environment that is well-managed and well-organized
- In a well-managed classroom, a positive discipline technique, will take little time and will only slightly break the flow of a lesson
- Effective classroom management, creates an environment that is conducive for teaching and to the learning and behavioral development of all students
- Creating a safe and orderly environment in the classroom where students gather to learn, a survival skill for teachers that optimizes the learning environment for all students
- A well-planned classroom space, therefore, can help us to prevent misbehaviors that might arise. Organize classroom and then ask students if they are comfortable with it
- Teacher must be able to see all students at all times in order to monitor their work and behavior. Teacher will also need to be able to see the door from desk. Students must be able to see teacher and the area from which teacher is teaching without having to turn around or move a lot
- Conducive seating arrangements, creative teaching approach, active interaction session, give a break after 45 minutes of teaching, encourage group work, arrange for reflective session at the end of the class, arrange for field trips where the learner will learn both cognitive skills and gain experiences
- Books and other instructional materials need to be stored so students can be obtain and use them adequately as references
- Student involvement—Students can be very helpful in managing the classroom's physical space and it helps them to develop a sense of responsibility. They can create bulletin boards and put instructional materials at the end of each lesson
- Good discipline and the creation of positive student behaviors is much more likely to occur if classroom and its activities are structured or arranged to enhance cooperative behavior between students and teacher

- When discipline is necessary, it focuses on the student's behavior, not the student. The student's dignity is maintained
- Some of the characteristics students appreciate in a teacher and should form a core part of monitoring teachers' behaviors are:
  - Fairness—It means being fair in activities such as making assignments, settling disputes, giving help and choosing students to be assistants or to participate in special activities
  - Humour—The ability to respond lightheartedly to students
  - Respect—This means showing regard for the rights and feelings of the student
  - Courtesy—This is another sign of respect
  - Openness—Students need to see the teacher as a real person. The teacher needs to explain clearly his/her feelings and the circumstance that caused the feelings
  - Active listening—This means responding when a student speaks. Teacher need to show that he/she heard the student and to give him or her a chance to correct a misunderstanding or interpretation. You might try restating what has been said or a use of body language to show empathy
  - Providing positive reinforcement—Positive discipline is a way to reduce misbehavior by rewarding positive behaviors. Promoting positive social relationship and help them develop a sense of self-discipline that leads to positive self-esteem
  - Give positive statements—Listen carefully and help them to learn to use words to express their feelings, not destructive actions
  - Provide students with opportunities to make choices and help them learn to evaluate the potential consequences of their choices
  - Reinforce emerging desirable behaviors with frequent praise and ignoring minor misdeeds
  - Model orderly, predictable behavior, respectful communication and collaborative conflict resolution strategies
  - Use appropriate body language—Nod, smile and look directly at the student.

Principles of Discipline

Several Educators formulated theories related to Modern Discipline

1. William Glasser—Choice Theory

- The teacher's role in discipline is to help students to make good choices, continually, throughout their life.
- Teacher has to formulate class rules. No excuse for students' misbehavior
- Teachers must see reasonable consequences follow student behavior good or bad
- Voluntary behavior is shaped, when reinforcement done immediately after learner performs an act in a desirable manner
- Behavior modification refers to the overall procedure of shaping student behavior intentionally by the teacher
- Successive approximation refers to a behavior—Shaping progression in which behavior comes closer and closer to a preset goal
- Punishment often has negative effects in behavior modification and hence is not used in the classroom.

2. Jacob Kounin—Discipline and Lesson Management Theory

- Teachers need to know what is going on in all parts of the classroom at all times
- Good lesson momentum helps to keep students on track
- Smoothness in lesson presentation helps keep students involved
- Effective teachers keep students attentive and actively involved—student accountability
- Teachers good in behavior management are able to attend to two or more events simultaneously—overlapping
- Effective teachers see to it that students are not given overexposure to a particular topic—satiation
- Effective teachers make instructional activities enjoyable and challenging.

3. Haim Ginott—Congruent Communication Theory

- The cardinal principle of congruent communication is that it addresses situation – not student's character or personality

- It is harmonious with students' feelings about situations
- Learning is always a personal matter to the student and takes place in the present tense
- Effective teachers invite cooperation from their students by describing the situation and indicating what need to be done
- Teachers have a hidden asset, e.g. "How can I be most helpful to my students right now?"
- Teachers should use appreciative praise when responding to effort or improvement
- Always respect students' privacy
- When correcting students, teachers should provide directions concerning the behavior desired
- Sarcasm is almost always dangerous and should not be used
- Punishment should not be used in the classroom
- Teacher should strive for self-discipline in themselves and their students.

4. Rudolph Driekurs—Discipline through Democracy Theory

- Discipline at its best is defined as self-control, based on social interest
- Good discipline occurs best in a democratic classroom
- Almost all students have a compelling desire to feel they are valued members of the class - that they belong, and they were able to gain sense of belongingness in the class, to overcome the untoward effects of power, revenge and inadequacy
- Teachers should learn how to identify mistaken goals and deal with them
- Punishment should never be used in the classroom.

Disciplinary Procedure

Policy and procedures provide a framework for maintaining good order in the institution to allow all students and staff to study and learn in the most conducive environment. The Policy and Procedures apply to all students enrolled with the Educational Institution.

- A breach of discipline—An 'act of misconduct' i.e., improper interference with the proper functioning or activities of the Educational Institution or those who study or work in or visit the Educational Institution. The Policy and Procedures will also apply to students when they are out of Educational Institution, on organized educational institution events or when it is found that there is a link to the educational institution or its reputation
- Misconduct, e.g. Disrupting any class or any other educational institution activity, whether or not involving staff or other students; Any drunkenness or intoxication on Educational Institution premises; Any activity associated with the Educational Institution which leads to damage
- Serious Misconduct, e.g. deliberately or by serious negligence, causing damage to or defacement of any educational institution buildings, equipment, books or furnishings or any property of others, acts of dishonesty-including theft, fraud, deceit or deception in relation to the Educational Institution, its staff, its students or its visitors, misuse of any drugs (prescribed or otherwise) on educational institution premises or on any activity associated with the educational institution
  - Behavior, which has a significant adverse impact on the Educational Institution's reputation, violent, indecent, disorderly, threatening or offensive behavior or language whilst on educational institution premises or engaged in any Educational Institution activity
- Behavior which constitutes harassment or is racially or sexually offensive or which is offensive to those with learning and/or physical disabilities or impediments. Physical or verbal assault, any possession of offensive weapons
- Suspension—In cases of alleged serious misconduct or because of some other urgent cause it is inappropriate for the student to remain at the educational institution, Head of the institution may consider suspension of the student on receipt of the allegation(s) pending a full investigation or if the nature of the initial allegation(s) is/are amended during the course of the investigation. The Director of Curriculum and Quality or his/her designated nominee should be notified of the suspension as soon as practicable
  - A suspended student will be given written confirmation of the suspension and the reason for the suspension. The student should not return to the educational institution or contact students or members of staff of the educational institution whilst suspended.

- The suspension will be kept under review and time limits will be set for the review to take place, depending on the circumstances of the case and the availability of evidence and witnesses. It is envisaged that apart from the most exceptional cases the suspension would be for no longer than two weeks.
- An *investigation*—After an incident has been reported by an educator/learner/parent to the Head of the institution—an investigation/informal enquiry takes place, wherein the learner has an opportunity to state her/his case
- *Formal Disciplinary Measures*—would include either the issuing of a Formal Written Warning and Contract or the calling of a Formal Disciplinary Hearing. All formal measures will need to be handled by the relevant HOD or the Head
- *Formal Disciplinary Hearing*—In the event of a Formal disciplinary hearing, the learner will be represented by a member of staff (School Counselor, Class Teacher, Grade Head). Parents/Guardians will be allowed to observe the process, should they wish to do so. As a disciplinary hearing is an internal school process, the learner will not be allowed any external representation at all
- *Appeal review*—"A fundamental right in terms of the "Rules of Natural Justice" and thus could be requested by the learner or her/his parent if they do not agree with the outcome of the disciplinary hearing. The bonus would be on the learner/parent/guardian to justify the reasons for the appeal. If the Appeal is successful, another Disciplinary Hearing would be set up.

General Principles

- Discipline in a school/college is necessary to preserve and promote educational excellence and for the protection of the rights of all stakeholders
- Discipline can be initiated by the educator or the school authorities. The school will be entitled to apply corrective action/disciplinary measures that it believes are appropriate to the circumstances. Thus, the discretion to apply disciplinary measures will not be rigidly restricted by the code, but will be guided by the circumstances
- The severity of the action taken will depend upon the circumstances, the seriousness of the infringement, the interests of fellow learners, the school and its employees, the interests of the offending learner and any other mitigating or aggravating factors that are of relevance. Thus, the disciplinary code acts as a guide to promote consistency, but does not remove the necessary discretion of school authorities to apply a lesser or more severe penalty should the circumstances so dictate
- The disciplinary procedure is associated with the Code of Conduct and is applicable to all learners. Corrective action will be taken by the school should expected norms of conduct not be met by a learner
- Supports the principles of fair discipline, the consistent and justified application of appropriate disciplinary measures
- Disciplinary measures may be formal or informal and are designed to prevent further occurrences of unacceptable behavior and to restore the school/learner relationship
- Maintaining discipline and ensuring orderly classroom behavior is an integral part of an educator's job, as is the responsibility for ensuring that disciplinary measures are applied equitably and effectively
- Disciplinary measures may be imposed on learners whose behavior outside of educational institution negatively impacts the school/learner relationship, the reputation/integrity of the school or other learners in the school
- Educators: All educators in the school, Code of Professional Ethics and to the school's own Code of Conduct for staff. Be punctual, well prepared and professional in their approach to education. Manage learner performance effectively and motivate learners to achieve realistic and meaningful personal and educational goals
  - Be sensitive to the needs of their learners and address learning difficulties in a positive manner
  - Praise, encourage, recognize and reward learners who strive to achieve. Create a classroom climate which is based on a learning partnership which makes education relevant and stimulating
  - Set a positive example for their learners to follow
  - Administer discipline correctively and with dignity when necessary

- Parents/Guardians: While parents must expect the school and its educators to provide the best possible education with the resources available to the school, they must also accept responsibility to help the school to achieve this goal. Parents would thus have the responsibility to actively support the efforts of the school and its educators to teach their learner to
  - Involve themselves to the fullest possible extent in School activities
  - Make positive suggestions and contributions to improve the School's education process and learning environment
  - Support the disciplinary structures and procedures of the school and the reasonable efforts by the school to apply discipline effectively and fairly
  - Encourage their learner to participate fully in school and extra activities
  - Participate in the learning process and assist their learner with homework, provide encouragement, check results and communicate fully with the school
  - Not expect the school to meet their learner's every need
  - Ensure that their learner is at all compulsory attendance events
  - Acknowledge the guidance/expertise of educators
- Learners: Constitutionally, all learners have the right to an education. However, this right must be seen in the context of the responsibilities they have to their parents, the school, their educators and their fellow learners. These responsibilities include:
  - Complying with the rules of the school, its Code of Conduct, its Conditions of Enrolment and the instructions of school officials
  - Behaving responsibly so as to not endanger the safety, welfare and rights of others
  - Showing respect and care for the property of the school and others
  - Maintaining sound relations with others at the school, being courteous and showing respect for the dignity and self worth of others
  - Being punctual and observing the time keeping practices of the school, demonstrating a positive attitude towards the opportunity to learn and being diligent in their efforts to learn
  - Behaving honestly and conducting themselves with integrity, not harassing, not threatening violence nor using force to intimidate, abuse, coerce or interfere with others, with school activities or school property
  - Accepting legitimate disciplinary measures taken against them as necessary
- The Faculty recognizes that in most instances minor in-discipline can and should be dealt with informally and promptly by the class in-charge or subject teacher without recourse to the formal disciplinary procedure. In such instances the student may be issued with a verbal warning. A note of such an active warning will be notified to the head of the institution and kept on the course file
- The Head of the Institution has to call for general body meeting where all the faculty and students will be participating, the administrator will inform the Educational Institution rules and regulations, hostel rules, Disciplinary Committee and their role, if the students are violating the rules the type of disciplinary procedures adopted, line of authority, rewards for appreciation of services, etc.
- All matters relating to the application of disciplinary procedures will be kept confidential
- No student will be permanently excluded from the Educational Institution for a first breach of indiscipline except in the case of serious misconduct
- No formal disciplinary sanction will be imposed without a disciplinary hearing. A student will have the right of appeal against any written disciplinary sanction imposed
- At all stages, the student may be accompanied by a friend, student representative or relative (but not by a legal or other professional adviser) at the interview and will be entitled to state his/her case (including any mitigating factors) before any decision is taken
- All appeals against actions/decisions taken in accordance with this procedure will be address within this procedure

- Students will be notified in writing of any disciplinary sanction, a copy of this letter shall be placed on the course file, and a copy will be sent to parents or care givers, when such warnings reach their time limits, the letter notifying the student of the disciplinary sanction shall be removed from the course file and destroyed, subject to the student's conduct having been satisfactory throughout the period.

Policy Review

The effectiveness of present policy will be monitored annually and reviewed every five years in light of experience and best practice. This mechanism recognizes that changes to legislation may prompt a review of the policy before the five years stipulated.

QUESTIONS

- Aim of discipline in Education (5 M, MGU, Dec, 2008).
- Disciplinary procedure (5 M, MGU, Oct, 2007).
- Discipline of students in School of Nursing (5 M, MGRUHS, Nov, 2010).
- Ideal classroom environment (2 M, RGUHS, Aug, 2010).
- Influence of punishment on learning (2 M, RGUHS, Feb, 2010).
- Preventive Discipline(5 M, MGU, Nov, 2009).
- Students indiscipline (10 M, RGUHS, May, 2009 and 5 M, MG, Dec, 2008).
- Three principles of discipline (3 M, MGU, Oct, 2007).

Individual and Social Groups

DEFINITIONS

Individualization is the process by which, an individual is made independent of his/her group.
'It is the process of attaining to one's own self. It makes him/her independent and self-determining'.
It is carried out by the individual himself/herself and it is mainly a mental process, which is spread through the prevailing ideas. Socialization brings man in relation with others.

ASPECTS

- Independent, Individualized
- The process of becoming different from other people
- Democratization
- Free competition
- Social mobility
- Aware of one's own specific character
- A new kind of evaluation
- The individual will consider himself/herself superior to others and evaluates himself/herself in high terms
- A feeling of self-glorification
- It is the wishes through objects
- Social mobility may also bind the individual to specific wishes
- Family conditions
- The feeling of loneliness may lead the individual to introspect and take independent decisions.

In big cities, the community or neighborhood does not have much influence on the individual and so he/she develops a feeling of privacy and partial isolation. It leads to individualization.

Relationship between Individual and Society

Individual is a core of society. Lot of individuals is present in galaxy of society.

Historical Evidences
Earlier sociologists have made an attempt to understand the relationship of individual and society. Basing on their intuitions, theories have been formulated, however these theories, some criticism is lying. They attempted to understand the social phenomenon existed in the society.

By means of human touch, the living organism is made into social beings. He/she undergoes the process of socialization to survive in the society.

Individual has certain biological, anatomical, physiological features with he/she cannot satisfy the needs of society; he/she should form social relationship through social interaction.

The earlier thoughts of former sociologists were

I. Divine Origin theory
Human beings are born to enjoy the relationship between male and female. God has created them and also created the society, e.g. Conjugal union of Adam and Eve. God has created the rights for individuals, but no script was available this theory is not fully explaining, the various social phenomenon, societal relationship that exists in the society, e.g. Polyandry, sex ratio.

II. Social Contract theory

T. Hobhouse, Locke explained how the individual is preceding the society. All the individuals are born free and equal to fulfill the needs, which he/she cannot fulfill by alone. Through socialization process he/she is performing his/her functions in the society. The individuals formed several groups, they have created the norms and laws.

III. Organic theory

Plato in ancient period and Herbert Spencer were explained, according to this theory, The individual is a living organism, the various systems has to coordinate to maintain his/her living functions. Individual is a part of social system, various social systems has to coordinate to meet the societal needs. Cell cannot survive or existence on its own; but the individual can survive apart from the society.

The cell cannot think on its own, whereas the individual can stay alone, forms new groups, new communities, can adopt themselves, to stay in different social structures. In the society, if one system fails, the individual can survive in another area.

In physiological systems, the cells join together to form as an organ and fulfill its function just like that, even in the society, each individual has to function cooperatively for effective functioning as a member in the society. if an individual fails to perform their function other individual may come and occupy and fulfill those functions, but it is not so with the cells, each system has its own function, one cannot replace the other. In the social system, several specialized systems, structured organisations are present.

IV. Group Mind theory

Maciver and Page described this theory. Collective thinking, cohesiveness among the group members and cooperativeness are main features of this theory. Individuals in the society develop rules, regulations and norms in the social system. Group mind facilitates collective thinking, collective acting, each group exhibits their own goals, needs which have emerged out of interaction of group, within the society, vested interests, different needs of individuals formed into different outlook. To some extent, collective thinking does not exist in India, e.g. different castes, cultures, identity, affinity was developed. Universality among diversity is observed. Individual and society are not separate entities. Individual neither precedes society nor society precedes the individual. They are interdependent, leading symbiotic life, mutually dependent on each other; they are interrelated. People will cohesively interact with each other to solve their problems.

V. Evolution theory

From single cell to homosapiens, the individual is evolved. We cannot conduct tests in labs. Individual and society are mutually interdependent. Individual needs society for socialization.

Example 1, Ferral cases in anthropological studies.

Children were brought out in different environment; one was placed in jungle in the midst of animals. No single social factor was observed in this individual. Child behaves like an animal. After the child's death, postmortem studies revealed that the brain was not developed. This case proves that the individual needs society.

Example 2, Two sisters were placed in jungle were brought out by wolfs. After sometime, these two children were brought into the society, one dies and the other was crawling like the wolf. It indicates that individual needs society to be socialized.

Example 3, 6 months old child is placed in a room after her mother's death. The child was found like a creature without any sign of social being.

These ferral cases have amply throw light that society is a must to precede the individual. Man is social by nature, they like to live in company of others and they are gregarious in nature, crave for other's company and interact with others and establish relationship. They do not like to live alone. Man likes to share the values, feelings with others. Socialization is unending. Individual precedes the society, the necessity compels us to be within the society. We acquire many traits from the society.

Society determines the personality of an individual. Individual is the product of society in which individual is socialized and cannot survive independently without society. Society teaches where and how to behave. It makes the individuals to be as a member of society and compliment each other.

Role of Nurse in Indian Society

The health care services (preventive, promotive, curative, rehabilitative and restorative) bringing closure to the doorstep of the community, who require the services at most, more particularly to the weaker, deprived sections of the interior corners of society. The Public Health Nurse has to shoulder the responsibilities especially for the provision of first level care in the community, thus acting as a changing agents in bringing good quality of life to the people at large.

1. Direct Health Care Provider to the Community

Nursing professionals who are working in the community will conduct domiciliary visits, observes the pattern of living, practices of the families. There by they can able to identify family health problems and meet the health needs of the members in the family by adopting principles of Community Health Nursing process and by implementing nursing models. Nurses should orient the community the importance of health maintenance and qualitative living. Nurse should be sensitive to the individual health needs in the context of broader social changes. Nurse will act as a direct health care provider in meeting the health needs of the community by implementing appropriate and suitable nursing interventions.

2. As a Health Educator

To achieve 'Health For All' and to attain holistic health and development, nurses will organize the health awareness campaigns to educate the community to understand the importance of health by practicing healthy life styles and by developing healthy behavior. Nurses has to focus the social consequences of illness and its effects and motivates the community to actively participate and involve in planning and implementing the health care programs for the attainment of qualitative life. Nurse has to educate the public to identify and fulfill their health needs with their own efforts.

3. Manager and Supervisor

The nurses will perform community organizer role and motivates the leaders in planning, organizing and implementing health care services through community participation. He/she supervises the activities of health care professional in rendering health care services.

4. Planner

Identifies beliefs, practices, customs which are affecting the health and illness of the community.

Formulate the community diagnosis by identifying the sociocultural barriers and promotes activities related to treatment, prevention of diseases and promotion of health.

Identifies the various community resources who are interested in community developmental activities.

Selects suitable health education methods

Develops plan of operation by involving local people and others who are engaged in community development activities.

Plan for supportive supervisory activities

Researcher: Nurses has to conduct research projects in the clinical settings, e.g. In community by identifying the social problems and needs of societal members, for the solvation of the existing problems, identifying incidence and prevalence of health problems, assesses the risk factors in causation of diseases, etc. and in educational institutions like Implementation of newer teaching methods, Curriculum revision, Teacher and learner interaction pattern analysis, teaching learning process and performance appraisal, etc. Nurses will communicate research findings to the Nursing Fraternity by publishing the research reports or abstracts in nursing journals and create awareness to obtain "Health For All".

SOCIAL GROUPS

Social group is a basic social unit when two or more persons interacting with each other, interrelationships are directed towards fulfillment of certain common goals or purposes. Inter-stimulation and response are the key factors in the process of social interaction.

Definitions

"A social group grows out of a situation which permits meaningful inter-stimulation and response between the individuals, focusing of attention on common situations or interest, the development of certain common drives, motivation or emotions"—*Gillin and Gillin*

"It is a system of social interaction"—*HM Johnson*

"Any collection of human beings who are establishing human relationships with one to another"—*Maciver RM and Page*

"Two or more individuals come together and influence one another"—*Ogburn and Nimkoff*

"Two or more individuals who have common objects of attention, stimulating to each other, who have common loyalty and participate in similar activities—*ES Bogardus*

Characteristics of Group Life

- The members of the group are known to each other and possess a sense of 'we' feeling
- Group involves a sense of unity
- The interests, ideals, values of the group members are common
- Similarity of behavior among the group members is observed
- There are certain norms, customs and procedures which are acceptable and everyone in the group has to obey the norms, rules and regulations of their own group
- The members of the group are affected by its characteristics
- Homogenous
- Good interpersonal and interactional relationship
- Collective perception of their identity and unity
- Shares certain goals, values and beliefs
- Emerges social control over the behavior
- Cooperation
- Power relations
- Members behave in a natural and relaxed manner
- Membership is by voluntary, automatic in informal groups, with some purpose in formal groups
- Joining in a group may be motivated by a variety of personal needs
- Individuals who has similar values and beliefs will join together.

Classification of Groups

Sociologists classified groups into several categories
- Charles Cooley:	Primary group, e.g. Family, friends
	Secondary group, e.g. Social institutions or Social organization
- WB Sumner and Kellerr:	In group and Out group
- Miller and PA Sorokins:	Vertical group and Horizontal group
- Gidden's:	Public and Private
- Elwood:	Sanctioned and Unsanctioned
- Gillin and Gillin:	Based on blood relationship, Based on Physical traits, Based on cultural interests and Based on situation proximity
- Charles Elwoods:	Voluntary and Involuntary.

a. WB Sumner and Keller Classification
In group
- The members in the group will have 'we' feeling and a common attitude and treats the group members as one, e.g. family, group of friends
- Based on ethnocentrism
- People exhibit good behavior with one to another.

Out group

People will develop a sort of hatred feeling on a particular group and treat the group completely away from them.

b. Cooley's Classification

Charles Cooley has classified social groups on the basis of importance and the form of relationships among the group members.

Primary group

Characteristics

- People will have intimate face-to-face, close, cooperative relationship
- Play fundamental role in forming the social nature and ideals of an individual
- Participation in primary group will lead to a fusion of individualities in a common whole
- Wholeness involves the sympathy and natural identification for which 'we' is the proper expression
- People will have close intimacy and nearness in relationship
- It meets the needs and mould the holistic personality of an individual
- Physical proximity: the relationship among the group members is close and they will have intimate contact with each other. Exchange of their ideas and opinions will take place
- Small in size (to develop intimate and personal relationship, the group will be small)
- Stability in nature (to promote closeness)
- Continuity in relationship (by meeting frequently and by exchanging thoughts the intimacy increases. When this chain is broken, the relationship does not remain the same)
- Common aims among the members (every member will share pleasure, pain, worthy for common interests. Relations are ends in themselves. The relationship between members will have mutual pleasure and contentment)
- Spontaneous, personal and inclusive relationship (every member of the group feels intimacy for others in a natural way, there is nothing like compulsion or pressure between them)
- Maximum control over group members in the family affairs.

Importance

- To develop the personality in total
- The efficiency of the members will be increased and persons of the group get help, inspiration and cooperation from one another
- Satisfaction of total needs (physical, emotional, psychological, social and spiritual) of the individual
- Group members will provide love, security, belongingness to the persons and satisfy their desires of loving and beloved, a person gets the benefits of companionship, sympathy, exchange of thoughts and satisfies most of their psychological needs
- Socialization process will take its origin within the family and maintain the control. Family teaches the person to work in the society according to their roles. The primary groups are the foundation of the whole society, basic social unit the individual acquire the basic attitudes towards people, social institutions and the world around them
- The individual acquires the attitudes of kindness, tolerance, love, generosity, mutual concern and affection.

Secondary group

Characteristics

- Groups are constituted for some specific aims, after achieving the goal the members will not maintain required relations within the group. The relationships are indirect, short and formal. They are representatives of a cold world
- Individuals do not have any interest in the pleasure and pain
- Relations among them are competitive, casual and impersonal
- Demands of person receive segments of their time and attention
- Position of a member depends upon their role and status
- Individuality develops in the persons because their relations are based on self-interest
- Self-dependence among members

- Large in size
- No physical closeness
- Lack of intimate relationships or associations
- Formed for some purpose after attaining the goal or purpose, group lapses when they are no more required.
- Group cannot exercise control to that extent due to large size
- Lacks stability and personal relationships. The group covers wide area, but not formed on the basis of identical, common ends. Status is determined by the function
- Has the limited acquaintance and responsibility
- Group form with definite objective, its function is not spontaneous
- Members play active and passive role based on the need
- Possibility of development in individualism.

Importance
- The needs are satisfied in the group with the advance of technology and associated with social change. This group will satisfy the changing needs of society and individual. The growth of social group has created some problems and many benefits
- Rules and responsibilities formed by the group head or the committee or head authority
- Rules will increase the efficiency of the work
- Delegation of authority, coordination and planning of the activities which will be implemented
- Channels of opportunity is wide, individuals can develop themselves by using their talents
- Wider outlook: it has to accommodate large number of members/localities which widens the outlook of its group
- It breaks the barriers of class, caste and province
- Must articulate with primary group.

Differences between Primary and Secondary group

Primary group	Secondary group
Size—small	Large
Relations—direct, personal, face-to-face, intimate, inclusive, spontaneous.	Indirect, impersonal, formal, exclusive.
Natural situation	Artificial situation
Aims, purpose, interest, values are same for the group members	Individual interest is dominant
Foundations of relations are important	Relations are not important
Found mostly in traditional societies	More commonly seen in urban society
Concern with total personality development and maturity of group members	Concern with only one aspect of personality
Warm relation	Cold relation
Qualities of love, affection, sympathy will flourish	Self interest will flourish
Control by elderly persons or head of the family	Control is exercised by designated persons, laws, norms
Good social control exist	Less social control
Permanent relation	Temporary relation
Groups are complete, good deal of cooperation among its members	Partial cooperation exist
Are misery of socialization based on culture or blood relationship	Are born after socialization and they don't have any common bond of culture or blood.

GROUP DYNAMICS

"Never doubt that a small group of thoughtful citizens can change the world. Indeed, it is the only thing that ever has"—Margaret Mead Kurt Lewin, Social Psychologist is the founder of Group Dynamics.

Group dynamics is a critical factor in group performance. Understanding how the group works and if and how it is developing will help the team leader to lead the team better. In organizational development context, the need for managing or improving the group dynamics will lead to an intervention based consulting project, where tools such as team building or Sociomapping are used.

Key theorists

Gustave Le Bon was a French social psychologist in their study, The Crowd: A Study of the Popular Mind (1896) led to the development of Group Psychology.

Sigmund Freud's Group Psychology and the Analysis of the Ego, (1922) based on a critique of Le Bon's work, led to further development in theories of group behavior in the latter half of the twentieth century.

Kurt Lewin (1951) is commonly identified as the founder of the movement to study groups scientifically. He/she coined the term group dynamics to describe the way groups and individuals act and react to changing circumstances.

William Schutz (1966) looked at interpersonal relations from the perspective of three dimensions: inclusion, control, and affection. This became the basis for a theory of group behavior that sees groups as resolving issues in each of these stages in order to be able to develop to the next stage. Conversely, a group may also develop to an earlier stage if unable to resolve outstanding issues in a particular stage.

Wilfred Bion (1961) studied group dynamics from a psychoanalytic perspective, Ernest Jones, key figure in the Psychoanalytic movement discovered several mass group processes which involved the group as a whole adopting an orientation which, in his/her opinion, interfered with the ability of a group to accomplish the work it was nominally engaged in. his/her experiences are reported in his/her published books, especially Experiences in Groups.

Bruce Tuckman (1965) proposed the four-stage model called Tuckman's Stages for a group. Tuckman's model states that the ideal group decision making process should occur in four stages:
- Forming (pretending to get on or get along with others)
- Storming (letting down the politeness barrier and trying to get down to the issues even if tempers flare up)
- Norming (getting used to each other and developing trust and productivity)
- Performing (working in a group to a common goal on a highly efficient and cooperative basis)
  Tuckman later added a fifth stage for the dissolution of a group called adjourning. ('Adjourning' may also be referred to as 'mourning', i.e. mourning the adjournment of the group). It should be noted that this model refers to the overall pattern of the group, but of course individuals within a group work in different ways. If distrust persists, a group may never even get to the norming stage.

Definitions

"The social process by which people interact and behave in a group environment".

"The study of groups and also a general term for group processes".

"The study of the forces or social processes that are responsible for various group phenomenon".

"Study of group behavior".

"The interacting forces within groups as they organize and operate to achieve their objectives".

"Political ideology concerning the ways in which group should be organized and managed, this ideology emphasizes democratic leadership, the participation of members in decisions and the gains both to society and to individuals to be obtained through cooperative activities in groups".

"A set of techniques, e.g. role playing, buzz sessions, observation and feed back of group process and group decision, which have been employed to improve skills in human relations in the management of conferences and committees".

"A field of enquiry dedicated to achieving knowledge about the nature of groups, the laws of their development and their interrelations with individuals, other groups and large institutions".

Group

In the fields of Psychology, Sociology and Communication studies, a group is "two or more individuals who are connected to each other by social relationships". Because they interact and influence each other, groups develop a number of dynamic processes that separate them from a random collection of individuals. These processes include norms, roles, relations, development, need to belong, social and effects on behavior. The field of group dynamics is primarily concerned with small group behavior. Group influences individual behavior in many ways, individual follower will have influencing tendency over the group, thus mutually dependent groups appear to satisfy many needs, but they often lead to performance or decision making.

Group Processes

"Understanding of the behavior of people in groups", e.g. task groups, that are trying to solve a problem or make a decision.

"Two or more people working together on some need or problem toward some end or goal".

"The actions and interactions used by a group to develop and maintain its identity as a group and its effects upon individuals who compose group".

Aspects/Dimensions of Group Process
- Patterns of communication and coordination
- Patterns of influence
- Roles/relationship
- Patterns of dominance (e.g. who leads, who defers)
- Balance of task focus vs social focus
- Level of group effectiveness
- How conflict is handled?

Emotional State of the Group as a Whole

In social behavior the movement is largely from individual to individual, whereas in group behavior there is a tangible qualitative interdependence of each upon others which cooperates in three ways: Individual to individual, individual to whole and whole to individual. This quality in the relationship of individuals is the group and the way they work together to produce is the process., It is the way people work together to release an emergent quality, called 'Psychological climate, group morale, spirit de corps or cooperative units' through which each discovers and develops inner capacities, realizes better the nature of his/her self, releases more of his/her past experience and learns how to create this emergent quality in all life situations.

Group processes are continuous, dynamic and directional in movement. An individual with expertise in group process, such as a trained facilitator, can assist a group in accomplishing its objective by diagnosing how well the group is functioning as a problemsolving or decisionmaking entity and intervening to alter the group's operating behavior. Because people gather in groups for reasons other than task accomplishment, group process occurs in other types of groups such as personal growth groups (e.g. encounter groups, study groups, prayer groups). In such cases, an individual with expertise in group process can be helpful in the role of facilitator.

Group dynamics will develop group cohesiveness and problem solving skills and encourage collaboration and creativity. Group dynamics involves the influence of personality, power and behavior on the group process. Is the relationship between individuals conducive to achieve the groups goals?

Is the structure and size of the group an asset in pursuing both the task and maintenance functions of the group? How is formal and informal power used to build consensus or reach decisions? Does the combination of individuals produce the right culture? How these individuals, cultures and internal forces interact and allows to analyze and better understand group effectiveness?

The focus of group dynamics is the study of forces within the group that produce group productivity or the ways and means that members invest themselves in problem solving. To intricate group processes and procedures and the roles enacted within a group. A number of individuals have developed techniques that facilitate group control and group problem solving, e.g. the utilization of an observer whose task is to organize group meeting, in an effort to discover why things go well or why they bog down?

There are two types of groups: 1. Formal groups/Secondary Groups—who are structured to pursue a specific task, 2. Informal groups/Primary Groups—who emerge naturally in response to organizational or member interests. These interests may include anything from a research group charged with the responsibility to develop a new product to a group of workers who spontaneously come together to improve social or member activities. While we can learn a lot from informal groups in terms of leadership and motivation, we will concentrate mostly on formal groups, characterized by member appointment and delegated authority and responsibility.

Group Size

Effective group performance depends to a large extent, on the size and composition of the group. A group may consist of as few as two people (giving credibility to the statement that "two heads are better than one") or as many as three to four hundred. In order to be effective, group size should be kept to a minimum without jeopardizing workload and goal achievement. Larger groups increase the possibility of conflict due to the variety of viewpoints, few opportunities for the development of social relationships, a decrease in participation levels and lack of opportunity for individual recognition. Individual skills and performance must be a consideration in forming a group. Diversification is a factor in both group development and skill requirement. While the former group may be better able to communicate, set standards and grow as a cohesive unit, it may not be diverse enough to meet all the community or organizational needs. A more diverse group may take longer to reach peak performance due to the number of cultures, language differences and interpretation of the task to be completed, but once they do develop, diverse groups are equally productive and may even be more creative in problem solving because members have access to a broader base of ideas for solutions.

Group Structure

Is based on stability and becomes structured. Group norms and standards, positions/authority and responsibilities are developed to regulate the actions of its group members. The group power (expert power, legitimate power, assumed power) is the ability to control some aspect of the behavior of others by giving some rewards or punishments. Group structure may be based on communication, as communication is essential in transforming information and coordinating the activities of individuals in groups. Stabilization of particular line of communication is essential, e.g. two-way communication in family and in students and teacher relationship. The sociometric structure is the pattern of personal attractions (interaction, social relationship) within the group among members. It tends to lengthen the channels of vertical communication, increases the difficulty of upward communication in large organization. Group structure has an impact over the quality of employees' relations; flat structure increases the group morale by decreasing the length of vertical communication. Self-actualization, self-realization, independent activities and effective thinking raise the morale of an individual.

Group Formation, Membership and Development

Persons who are bound together by specific relationships, which set them apart from others and work together to achieve certain common goals or aims. Groups vary in size from two persons to millions-related to their degree or organization and the degree to which the members function together in a coordinated way, e.g. Organized groups like family, school or any social institution. Needs of the individuals are the basis for the formation of groups. Group formation provides security for their members to carry specific responsibility and perform defined, scheduled activities. It provides social experiences where an individual enjoys cohesiveness and feels protected.

Groups form more or less spontaneously by the mutual agreement of people, who share common interest or are facing with a common threat. For continuation and to meet changing needs, it may expand in size and organization, sometimes, it may be formed largely through the activities and persuasive powers of a particular articulate person. New groups may also be formed by elections or appointment by larger groups already in existence. The way the group is formed will strongly influence the role expectations and activities.

For example, members in appointed group would have their goals and functions laid out by the organization.

- Leader formed group, the main initiative of activities may be held on group leader
- Members of group formed by mutual agreement will feel more personal responsibility in determining the goals and activities of the group.

Individuals attain group membership by birth (ascribed status); by choice, by invitation and by mutual consent (achieved status), e.g. Political parties, marriages. The groups formed by achieved status, the extent to which the member perceives the group as related to the meeting of his/her needs is likely to be a key consideration in membership decisions. In determining the performance and effectiveness of the group, the composition of the group is essential (e.g. in terms of age, sex, interests, capabilities, values).

Group Attractiveness to the Individual

- Commonality of interests, values, goals
  The individual tends to join and participate in groups whose purposes and values are congruent with his/her own success and status of the group
- Individuals tends to be attracted to groups which have a demonstrated record of competence and success, which have high status among their peer group
- Difficulty of gaining entrance in the group
  Individuals often place a high value on membership in a group to which it is difficult to gain entry
- Measures of security or anxiety reduction
  To avoid loneliness, confused, alienation, the individual joins the group as it provides him/her with readymade purposes, values and norms.

Group Participation

Improves members morale; when the leader recognizes individual's efficiencies whatever the leader decides the activities for effective functioning of the group, members has to give respect and actively participate in implementation of group welfare activities at the same time, the leader has to give respect, exhibit concern, identify their efficiencies and utilize their services. Participation is a natural way of management by means of integration and self-control. Managerial actions, suitable degree of participation in situations like the nature of problems involved, individual responsibilities and their nature also has to be cited.

Job Enrichment

Provides opportunity to overcome monotony, fatigue, disinterest and create the environment to satisfy high order needs resulting in high morale enriched job satisfaction.

Group Development

The appointment of individuals to a group based on their compatibility, diversity or expertise does not assure effectiveness in achieving group goals. A group is initially a collection of personalities with different characteristics, needs and influences. To be effective, these individuals must spend time acclimatizing themselves to their environment, the task, and to each other.

Stages

Organizational experts and practitioners have observed that new groups go through a number of stages before they achieve maximum performance. Each stage presents the members with different challenges that must overcome before they can move on to the next stage. These stages are

1. Forming: At this first stage of development, members are pre-occupied with familiarizing themselves with the task and to other members of the group. This is sometimes referred to as the dependent stage, as members tend to depend on outside expertise for guidance, job definition, and task analysis.
2. Storming: At this stage, the group encounters conflict as members confront and criticize each other and the approach the group is taking to their task. Issues that arise include identification of roles and responsibilities, operational rules and procedures and the individual need for recognition of his/her or her skills and abilities. This stage is also referred to as the "Counter dependent stage" where members tend to "flex their muscles" in search of identity. In some cases, the group may have problems getting through this stage. This may occur if the group encounters difficulty clarifying their task, agreeing on their mission or mandate or deciding how they will proceed. Lack of skills, ability or aptitude can also contribute to their inability to get beyond this stage.

3. Norming: At this point, members start to resolve the issues that are creating the conflict and begin to develop their social agreements. The members begin to recognize their interdependence, develop cohesion and agree on the group norms that will help them to function effectively in the future.
4. Performing: When the group has sorted out its social structure and understands its goals and individual roles, it will move toward accomplishing its task. Mutual assistance and creativity become prominent themes at this stage. The group, sensing its growth and maturity, becomes independent, relying on its own resources.
5. Adjourning: During this phase, the group will resort to some form of closure that includes rites and rituals suitable to the event. These may include social parties or ceremonies that exhibit emotional support or celebration of their success.

Group Functions

Three functions that influence the effectiveness and productivity of groups are:

1. Task Functions

This is the primary reason for the establishment of a group. To achieve the task, they must have members that fulfill some or all of the following roles:
a. Initiating: by proposing tasks or goals, defining problems and suggesting procedures for a solution.
b. Information seeking: by requesting facts, seeking relevant information and asking for suggestions or ideas.
c. Information giving: by offering facts, providing information, stating beliefs and giving suggestions or ideas.
d. Clarifying ideas: by interpreting and clarifying input, indicating alternatives and giving examples.
e. Bringing closure: by summarizing, restating and offering solutions.
f. Consensus testing: by checking for agreements and sending up 'trial balloons'.

2. Maintenance Functions

Each group needs social emotional support to be effective. Some members of the group will take the lead in providing this support which consists of the following:
a. Encouraging: by showing regard for other members and providing positive response to their contributions.
b. Improving group by expressing group feelings, sensing moods and relationships, atmosphere and sharing feelings.
c. Harmonizing: by reconciling differences and reducing group tension.
d. Compromising: by admitting errors and looking for alternatives.
e. Gate-keeping: by attempting to keep communications flowing, facilitating the participation of others and suggesting procedures for sharing discussion.
f. Standard setting: by reminding members of group norms, rules and roles.

3. Self-interest Functions

This third function displayed by some individuals, members generally take away from group performance and affects task achievement at the expense of the group. Activities that identify self-interest behavior are as follows:
a. Dominating and by displaying lack of respect for others, cutting them off, controlling: not listening and restating other members' suggestions with a different meaning.
b. Blocking: by stifling a line of thought and changing the topic either away from the point of view or back to his/her or her own interest.
c. Manipulating: by providing self-serving information or a single point of view designed to achieve a decision that is consistent with their position.
d. Belittling: through put-downs, sneering at other's point of view or making jokes about another member's contribution.
e. Splitting hairs: by nitpicking, searching for insignificant details that delay a solution or undermining another person's point of view.

Phase	Task Functions	Personal Relations Functions
1	Orientation	Testing and Dependence
2	Organizing to Get Work Done	Intragroup Conflict
3	Information-flow	Group Cohesion
4	Problem-solving	Interdependence

GROUP NORMS

In the early stages of group development, a substantial amount of time is spent on setting social standards and acceptable group behavior. These standards are referred to as group norms and can be both formal and informal.

Norms are not individual behaviors, but are collectively held expectations of how a group will function, e.g. a new member who joins a group may initially search for clues about what type of behavior is acceptable. What are the dress codes? How do I address my supervisors? What is proper etiquette? What topics or discussions are acceptable or avoided?

Recognition of these norms is important, since they provide regularity and predictability to individual and group behavior. Bosses are more likely to insist on norms regarding work performance or attendance, whereas other norms might address the acceptability of rearranging personal space or assisting co-workers.

Definitions

"Standards of behavior and performance expected of group members".

"Represents group's shared beliefs and ideas about proper conduct and behavior of its members in important areas of group activity"

"Blue prints for behavior setting limits within which individuals may seek alternative ways to achieve their goals".

Types

Group norms may include
1. Loyalty norms—Such as the belief that managers have to work on weekends and holidays or accept transfers to prove their loyalty to the company.
2. Dress norms—May include anything from uniforms to shirt and ties to sarees or chudidars, depending on the establishment or business.
3. Reward norms—Includes perks or benefits that come as a result of individual or group performance. Criteria may include productivity levels, loyalty, equality (everyone gets the same reward) or social responsibility (those who need it most).

Meaning and Nature

- Norms relate to both interpersonal behavior, task performance, conduct and behavior
- In primary group—norms are unwritten and informal; in secondary group—norms are written and formal
- Based on social values which are justified by moral standards and esthetic judgment
- Members will conform to group norms to retain their group membership and to strengthen their associations with the group and to avoid penalties
- There are also social pressures in the group which force the members to conform to norms
- It incorporates value judgments
- Norms are related to factual world.

Purposes

- Established norms on members' behavior and performance are needed for group survival, credibility and effectiveness
- To ensure that the members will behave in a consistent, predictable and proper manner, maintains good interpersonal relationship

- To serve as rules of conduct, e.g. do's and dont's which members are expected to observe in their action behavior within and outside of the group
- Conformity to norms by members is an important aspect of group functioning, group cohesiveness
- Provides structure, balance and discipline to the activities of group members
- Man needs a normative order to live in society
- Determines and guides intuitive judgments of others.

Conformity of Norms

- Norms are formed in matters of consequence to a particular groups goals or objectives
- Social norm operative in one social system may not be operative in another. Conformity to norms is always qualified in view of the socially defined situations in which they apply
- Violators of norms suffer with loss of prestige, ridicule, fines and imprisonment
- Higher the status of man the more likely he/she is to conform to the norms
- A norm need not to be carried out in order to influence the behavior.

Group Roles

There are two kinds of roles present in groups.
1. Assigned roles: These include titles, e.g. chairperson, secretary, manager, treasurer etc.
2. Emergent roles: Arise as a result of group social or emotional needs, e.g. confident, group clown, gossip, mentor or scapegoat.

Two factors that impact the effectiveness of organizational roles are: role ambiguity and role conflict.

Role ambiguity occurs when a person is unclear of what is expected of him/her or her, instructions about performance are not clear, tasks are assigned without context or if a supervisor's actions and instructions send contradictory messages.

Role conflict occurs when a group member feels his/her or her job overlaps with others or if the job description is unclear.

Status

Most organizations have ways of giving status or rank to members depending on many factors. In many cases, these status symbols reinforce the authority, hierarchy and reward system within the group. For example, the move from a cubicle to an inner office to a window office and finally, to a corner office, and as an individual moves through this progression, authority, decision making, and prestige also increases. These symbols are meant to increase motivation (Maslow's esteem needs), as a reward for loyal and productive service and as an acknowledgment of the level of decision making accorded the individual. The group leader (or facilitator) will usually have a strong influence on the group due to his/her or her role of shaping the group's outcomes. This influence will also be affected by the leader's sex, race, relative age, income, appearance and personality, as well as organizational structures and many other factors.

Group cohesiveness

One of the primary factors in group performance involves group cohesion. The ultimate role of groups is to come together as a unit and perform with professionalism and dedication. A group that can work as a unit, share tasks and recognize the contributions of its members will meet with more success than a group mixed in conflict, role ambiguity and lack of motivation. Group cohesion makes it attractive for members to belong, attracts high performers and provides opportunities for individual recognition within a group setting. Cohesion may result from internal successes, high social emotional support or external threats.

Group size can also affect cohesion. A group that is too large may find that members cannot get the recognition they are looking for. This can lead to the formation of subgroups or cliques which further causes members to withdraw or withhold input. It is an act of protest because he/she or she may feel that their achievement is being used to raise the credibility of the whole group or because there is a feeling that members are not pulling their weight. As we have seen earlier, this self-interest approach distracts from group performance and cohesion.

Group Support

Any team or group will need support if it is to be effective. While the successful sports team requires training camps, coaching and team discipline, other work teams have the same needs. First, there must be a recognition of the need for training. Members bring individual skills to the group that may need to be adapted to maximize their contribution to the group task. How are the skills complimenting each other? Is there an overlap and duplication? Is there a skills gap that must be addressed? Second, there may be a need for team-building skills. Is there a need for adaptation from a former environment? For example, a nurse who enters a new institution will need to familiar with new procedures being used in that environment and the members of the unit that he/she or she will interact with. All groups need to be able to identify their successes. This usually takes the form of rewards that recognize accomplishments. Group members should know what is expected and what the rewards are. Are there opportunities for individual recognition? What are the group rewards, what are their performance requirements for achieving these rewards and how will performance be measured?

Management plays a major role in group performance. Is the group self-managed and what is the impact on formal managers? Attempts at new and innovative approaches may threaten "old school" managers and their comfort levels with more traditional approaches. Managers should approach their roles as coaches who ensure that all necessary skills are included, systems and procedures are outlined and that goals and visions are clearly understood, rather than play the role of "boss knows best".

There is often a tendency to have people with similar skill sets on the same team. There is an argument that teams may perform better, if people from all parts of the organization are in the group. This brings diversity and allows the group to take into account all aspects of the job and to include the needs of other parts of the organization which may be affected by the work of the group. It also helps members to identify the need for and importance of other organizational functions in achieving the overall organizational goals.

Transactional Analysis

"Participation in groups is a social transaction between individuals is called "transactional analysis". These interactions were identified by Eric Berne in the 1950s as ego states. There are three ego states which Berne identified, they are parent, adult and child.

1. Parent: Individuals who operate from a parent state may display a protective, nurturing, controlling, critical or guiding role. They may refer to policies or standards by stating "You know the rules, now follow them".
2. Adult: Individuals displaying this approach will appear to be rational, calculating, factual and unemotional. Decision making relies on research, facts, data processing, and estimating probabilities.
3. Child: Individuals displaying this behavior reflect emotions similar to those of childhood. It may be rebellious, spontaneous, dependant or creative and is often recognized by its emotional tone. Like a child, this state looks for approval and immediate rewards.

We can usually recognize the behavior not only by the tone, but by postures, gestures and facial expressions. We can also see that conversations can be complimentary or contradictory. A conversation between two individuals using an adult-to-adult state will be very rational and reasonable. Both see themselves as equals and therefore, will try and find the best solutions to problems.

Interactions may be contradictory or complimentary. Contradictory behaviors may be a parent-to-child, adult-to-child or adult-to-parent interaction. In a conversation between a supervisor and an employee displaying a parent-to-child pattern, the employee may assume the behavior of a child and thus respond to the reward and punishment systems that exemplifies such behavior. On the other hand, a parent-to-adult interaction can result in conflict and dissension due to the unacceptable approach of each participant. While complimentary interactions such as adult-to-adult, child-to-child or parent-to-parent are the most desirable, other interactions can be positive. Should both parties accept the parent-to-child or adult-to-child relationships, there may be good relationships without conflict. For example, the supervisor and employee are comfortable with the parent-to-child arrangement, they may continue to work together in harmony. Unfortunately, the employee fails to grow and mature and may learn only to contribute to the extent that will meet with the supervisor's approval.

These behaviors have led to the following statements about individual interactions. Aggressive people may view a relationship as "I'm OK-you're not OK", while a passive person may view the relationship as

" I'm not OK- you're OK" or "I'm not OK-you're not OK". In both cases, the passive person starts from the assumption that "I'm not OK". The most desirable and the one that presents the greatest possibility for adult-to-adult relationships is "I'm OK-you're OK". It shows a healthy acceptance of both yourself and others.

Whether a person is passive, assertive or aggressive affects the performance of individuals in a group. The passive person is compliant, submissive and nonresistant. He/she may appear to be comfortable with the situation that they find themselves in, but may be building up stress and anxiety as a result of being "pushed around". The aggressive person on the other hand, may be hostile, forceful and may find him/herself in conflict because they either push ahead without regard for others or "blow-up" at the first sign of control. The assertive person is self-assured, positive and will protect his/her or her own rights, respect the rights of others and act with confidence and honesty.

Effective Teams

Effective teams do not just happen, they are meticulously put together consisting of a group of highly skilled, highly motivated individuals who have a clear picture of their goals and can receive clear and tangible evidence of their achievements. A highly charged environment will attract high performers who are looking for success. Success builds on success, therefore, a group's reputation is also a major selling point. There must be an opportunity for individual success within the framework of the group's goals. There must be recognition of professionalism from co-workers, peers and the outside world. These are the factors that contribute to winning sports teams and there is no reason to think that other groups will respond any differently.

Aspects of Group Discipline

- Structure of group
- Group activities
- Composition of group
- Interaction among the group members
- Working Pattern
- Growth and resolution of the group
- Decline and dissolution of the group
- Pattern of achieving unity and handling of conflict situation
- Meeting needs of the group members
- Task performance
- Measures adopted for group members satisfaction.

Group Morale

Every individual in the group will possess certain attitudes that range over the entire spectrum of human behavior. The group leader has concerned for their group morale, which they lead, job satisfaction is an individual phenomena whereas morale is a group phenomena. Group morale increases the work satisfaction of the individual in job area. When individual needs are satisfied and the degree to which the individual desires satisfaction from his/her total job situation. Group morale emphasizes social reaction and concentrate on attitudes towards group values, e.g. cohesiveness, interest, optimistic views, etc. It describes the attitude levels (favorable or unfavorable) collectively to all aspects of their work, i.e. tasks, activities, working environment towards colleagues, superiors. It also describes the thinking capacity and feeling of the personnel about their functions. It denotes the strong emotional elements associated with values. Higher the group morale, higher will be the productivity, if leadership is effective along with proper production facilities and individual's ability that organization will be benefited.

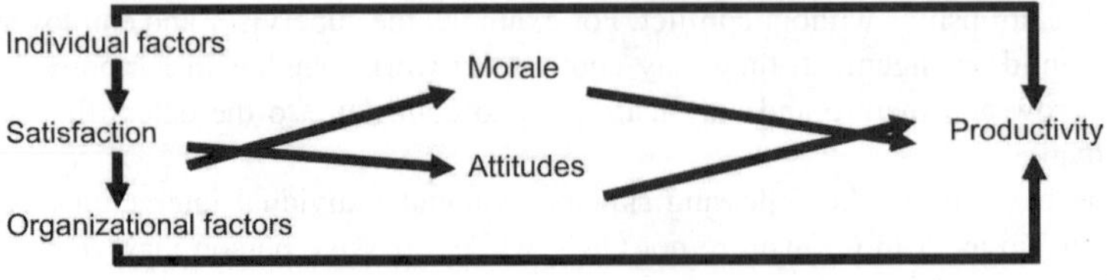

Productivity and satisfaction of individual's results with the interaction of several factors like individual factors, organizational factors. The successful leader recognizes that behavioral management requires a positive integration of goals so that people working together will achieve the desirable high morale with high productivity. If the members in the group show their resistance, dissatisfaction and limited interaction leads to low productivity.

Morale Measurement

Information will be gathered by conducting public opinion, attitude, survey and observation of set of values.

1. Surveys

   Objective, projective and descriptive types of questionnaires will be used to collect the information related to morale.

   For example, objective questionnaire viz., multiple choice, yes/no, fill up the blanks, rating scale, checklist.

   Descriptive questionnaire: open-ended questions, essay type

   Projective questionnaire: the respondent is given situation and he/she is asked to comment on the situation. by observation of comments, morale can be measured indirectly, e.g. Thematic Apperception Test.

2. Indices of morale
   - Turnover, absenteeism, withdrawal
   - Productivity
   - Tardiness
   - Fatigue, monotony
   - Grievances
   - Discipline
   - Wastage
   - Quality control.

3. Other source of information
   - Counseling reports
   - Exit interviews
   - Accident reports
   - Training records
   - Medical records
   - Suggestion system
   - Complaint box system.

Uses of Morale

- To take decisions related to group
- Morale is one of the basic ingredients of the conducive organizational climate which will influence the people to behave in a particular manner
- To introduce or modify group practices, which are conducive to the people in organization
- To control the difficult situations
- Ensures group communication in upward direction. Through group morale people can convey their actual feelings, the leader can make especial action to ensure the free flow of communication
- Provides opportunity to the group members to interact with higher authority. Individuals will feel their importance and motivated, both the parties shows real interest and expresses their feeling outwardly to relieve their tensions
- To assess the needs of people as a whole, i.e. social functioning of the individuals in group activities
- Identifies gaps; wherever assistance is required, provides training to fill up the gaps
- Creates an awareness on morale consciousness.

Morale Building

Is a continuous process and responsibility of group leader. He/she should possess sound management skills, periodic information on the status of individual's morale in the particular direction has to be collected.

LEADERSHIP

Introduction

A leader's job is to look into the future and see the organization not as it is, but as it should be—*Jaack Welch*.

Leadership is a common phenomena seen everywhere in the social organization in one or other form. Leadership is the process of influencing the behavior of followers by inspiring and motivating to work willingly and enthusiastically for achieving predetermined goals. It is a continuous process of behavior, where the followers and leader work together cooperatively. Leadership deals with insight, effectiveness and results; focuses on top; emphasizes transformational; activity oriented. Leader should possess a sense of capacity for and comfort with risk and change leads to an understanding of the role, collaborative style, understanding of multiple cultures; emotional competence; identifying the followers strengths and weaknesses; and greater balance and reflection in life leads to energized work force. Leader has to present model behavior for others and shows the way of life. The individuals in society are generally divided into leader and followers. Emergence of leadership is the result of social process, a bipolar process or behavior.

Definitions

"A behavior that affects the behavior of other people more than their behavior affects that of the leader"—*LaPiere and Fransworth*

"Leader is one who has power and authority"—*H T Mazumdar*

"Activity of persuading people to cooperate in the achievement of a common objective"—*Allen*

"The activity of influencing people to strive willingly for mutual objectives, it affects the behavior of followers in a situation"—*Terry*

"It is the interpersonal influence exercised in a situation and directed through communication process, towards the attainment of a specified goals"—*Temenbaum et al*

"It is the process of influencing and supporting others to work enthusiastically toward achieving objectives".

"The art of process influencing people, so that they will strive willingly and enthusiastically towards the achievement of group goals"—*Harold Koontz and Heinz Weihrich*

"It is the process of situation or reciprocal reinforcement which by the successful interplay of relevant individual differences controls human energy in the pursuit of a common cause"—*Britt*

"To keep, to persuade or to direct man, that comes from personal qualities apart from face"—*Maciver and Page*

"Leadership is in terms of dominance"—*Kimball Young*

"Leadership acts or present which influence other persons in shared direction"—*Seeman and Morris*.

Meaning

- 'To lead'—To excel, to be in advance, to be prominent. The ability to lead effectively the group
- To be head of an organization
- To hold command
- Leadership depends on 4 things: The individual, followers conditions and power/authority
- Leadership is a continuous process
- Leadership may be seen in terms of relationship between a leader and his/her followers, which arises out of their functioning for common goals
- Leader tries to influence the behavior of individuals or group members to achieve common goals
- Followers work willingly and enthusiastically to achieve the goals
- There is no coercive force which induces the followers to work, to shape the groups
- Leaders feel the importance of followers. Gives them recognition and conveys them about the importance of activities performed by them
- Leadership styles may be different under different situations
- Leaders shows the way to solve the problems in working situation and to overcome the obstacles
- Leaders are concerned with bringing together resource, developing strategies, organizing and controlling activities in order to achieve the agreed objectives.

Nature

- Traitist—Superior individuals who would lead in whatever situation or time they might find themselves
- Situationist—Leadership is specific to each situation. It is a way of behaving exhibited by individuals in differing degrees in different situations
- Leader is necessarily a part of the groups and leadership is status and role in that group
- Leadership can occur only in relation to other people, none can be a leader all by himself/herself
- Leader establishes reciprocal relationships with the group members
- Leadership facilitates group life.

Elements in Leadership

- Mutual behavior between the leader and his/her followers
- Two-way affair, the followers influences the behavior of the leader as well as the leader behavior influences the followers
- Without followers, no leader can exist
- The element of willingness, voluntary obedience by the followers, leadership is based on cooperation and goodwill
- It is specific to specific situation, a person cannot be a leader for all situations
- The ability to use power (to control a person possesses—six types of power—coercive, reward, legitimate, expert, referent and information) effectively and in a responsible manner
- The ability to comprehend that people are motivated by different factors at different times and in different situations
- The ability to inspire
- The ability to act in a manner that will develop a conducive climate to respond and arouse motivation
- Dominance—An attempt to guide the others
- Leader influences the feelings, experiences, behaviors and activities of others
- Process of multistimulation; leader is influenced by others, he/she has to model his/her behavior according to the aspirations and desires of the followers
- Authority—The suggestions and the directions as given by the leader are accepted by followers and they accept the superiority of the leadership.

POWER ORIENTATION

Definition

"The influence of an individual who exercises control over others"—*Goldhamer*

Types

1. Physical force/coerciveness
2. Domination
3. Manipulation
4. Legitimate
5. Illegitimate

Power orientation of leadership style depends upon the degree of authority given to the leaders. Power orientation means the authority given by the top management to the leader in order to exercise power in controlling his/her followers. With power orientation leaders are able to use their authority in influencing the behavior of their subordinates. However all the leaders do not use their authority to control the followers to the fullest extent due to various factors based on power orientation.

The leaders degree of use of power can be classified into three categories:

1. Autocratic leadership
2. Participative leadership
3. Free run leadership

Principles of Leadership

The art of war

- Learn to fight
- Do it right
- Expect the worst
- Burn the bridges
- Pull together
- Show the way
- Know the facts
- Seize the day
- Do it better
- Keep them guessing

Sensitive leadership

- 'Eyes and ears—on; hands-off'
- Enabling, facilitating, catalyzing—to develop self-confidence and responsibility to other.
- Exemplary leadership
- Monitor the group's progress against norms and objectives
- Credibility, enduring, competence, courage, effective performance
- Strengthening others and building on their strengths
- Fostering collaboration
- Modeling the way
- Path finding
- Recognizes people's contributions
- Sets high expectations for themselves and for others
- Enable others to act effectively, they make things happen
- Reaffirms norms, standards, values
- Keep the team on track
- Logical thinking
- Relies upon conventional wisdom
- Inspirational leadership
- Exceeds limit
- Demonstrating superiority, pre-eminence in skills
- Achievement or excellence
- Awareness in all the spheres where work has to be completed
- Eccentric
- Creative
- Innovative thinking
- Provocative stimulating
- Challenging
- Effective skills in decision making
- Productive results
- Introduces new ways of doing things
- Holistic thinker
- Uses intuition
- Initiates change
- Supportive followers
- High functional maturity
- Takes ownership of a role, accountability and performance
- Gives out, demonstrable support to the achievement of the team's goals and needs
- Positive, constructive, collaborative
- Alert to changing demands, needs, priorities flexibility and adjusts accordingly.

Origin and Development of Leadership

- Psychoanalysis-Good family, healthy psychological traits, desire to succeed, inspirative, enthusiastic in nature are some of the traits required for the development of leadership
- Heredity—Innate qualities are gifts of heredity

- Social stimulation—Social environment stimulates the individual to acquire certain leadership abilities
- Personality—Individuals with type A personality will have attractive and pleasing in nature.

Emergence of a Leader

A person who emerges as a leader among the group is a very unique task. The emerging of leadership depends upon a number of factors. There are several means and techniques for acquiring the ability to do the special jobs. The following are the most important aspects, which help the person to become group leader.

1. Leadership training

Training programs are offered manages to several or varied leadership situations and teach them how to tackle them. The situations are partly real. The trainers create the situation. Varying the managers undergoing leadership training are provided opportunities to diagnose the problems and think some ways and means in tackling them, which partly involve testing all various types of leadership against relatives. Leadership training gives deep insight and experiences to managers and an appropriate attitudes and behaviors, which they have to adopt in tackling diverse situations on how to gain an initiative and come over a situation. How to inspire and motivate people and the measures in the development of the leader and the group.

2. Internal organizational exposure

Another important reason, which help the person to emerge as a leader is the internal organizational exposure. The critical situations call for application of leadership abilities by the administrators to overcome the situation to see that a leader emerges from the person they have to be put incharge of committees, task of project implementations, coordination, control and employee grievances, which gives an opportunity for the manager or the administrator to develop into a very good leader on emerge as a leader in the group.

3. Autonomy and accountability

Administrators may be able to sharpen their leadership abilities and emerge as a leader in the group under conditions of relative freedom. They should be allowed a large amount of freedom to evolve their own methods or tackling situations calling for critical leadership abilities. This is possible only organizational support in the form of authority (position power), status, top management support and adequate description in dispensing rewards and penalties for their subordinates within the framework of certain norms and rules are given.

4. Opportunities for interaction

Administrator should also have opportunities to interact with their subordinates in amore intense and continuous manner so that they can talk or listen to their subordinates to understand their view points and enable them to acquire qualities like sociability tolerance, nonprovocation, resolution of conflict, verbal ability and supporting a truth to guide them successfully and emerge as a leader for the problem solving and growth and development of one and all.

5. Setting challenging but realistic goals

Administrators have to work very hard to achieve the objectives the in-born leadership ability to emerge as a leader for the group. If the appropriate goals are set which are challenging but realistic.

6. Job rotation

Administrators may also emerge as a leader if they help the followers, colleagues and juniors to develop leadership skills by a process of systematic rotation of their roles. They should be exposed to a variety of superior subordinate relations and job environments, so that they emerge as a leader by developing the ability of coping with situation, which do not permit them to adopt stereotyped styles on approaches, e.g. the role and responsibilities of a Dean in a department will be given on rotation; every qualified member (a set of designation and experience) will get an opportunity to work on rotation basis, a functional role as a leader in the department.

Spotting of a Leader

Organization has to strive hard consistently and continuously to achieve the objectives of the organization. The growth and development of the organization entirely depends upon the people in the organization. If the people or human resources are hard working, talented and able, they will be able to achieve their objectives as well as the objectives of the organization.

In the organization people work in groups and every group has its own culture, people in the group are unique and different from one another in some respects. It becomes necessary to manage these groups effectively and efficiently by the management in order to achieve the objectives that they have to depend on the leaders of the group, department, division and organization. Management has to spot new leaders to enable the organization to grow at good pace.

Spotting leader is a very difficult task in the context of modern organizations. But it is necessary to do so, to survive exist, grow and develop. Spotting of leader is a process of identifying the leader from the members of the group. The identification of the leader has to be done by keeping in mind various factors.

The following are important in spotting a leader:
- Some people in the group are somewhat more intelligent than the other members. The person whose is more intelligent has to be given preference. Because of his/her intelligence and capacity will have a overall view of the problems of the group and the organization
- Persons who have well rounded from the stand point of interest, aptitude, attitude must be selected and given training to become a good leadership
- The persons who have the ability to express their ideas in clear terms to others and explain their position and gain support of other members can be considered as leader
- People are mentally and emotionally matured and able to devote their full attention to the affairs of the group in general and not influenced by their own occupations can be a good leader
- Persons with powerful inner drive, the impulse motivates them to strive hard for accomplishment who are ambitious and willing to work long hours to realize their ambitions can be good leader
- Persons who have the ability to think innovatively, understand the importance and cooperative effort, practice social skills and good human relations are capable of becoming a good leader. Thus, by using above methods, the management or the authorities can identify and spot potential people as leaders in the group.

Leader as Mentor

Agree the topic for development
- Identify specific areas for improvement
- Decide delegation of authority and responsibility for the group members
- Give orientation to the group members towards their job performance and expectations
- Identify short-term, long-term goals and objectives

Promote discovery
- Active listener
- Analyzes systematically
- Push for options and alternatives
- Share experiences
- Promote learning and ownership

Set the parameters
- Establish deadlines
- Monitor the entire process
- Review progress
- Record the events in dairy
- Identify task boundaries and measures

Authorize to empower
- Delegation of authority and responsibility
- Take decisions
- Ensure financial, administrative responsibility and controls

Recap and review
- Get feedback
- Note down action points

* Agree to start date
* Key milestones

Follow-up and follow-through
* Monitor progress with the individual
* Check on target and maintain standard
* Agree remedial and exploitive action
* Judge and plan effectively for modification, if needed
* Fix the review dates and attend it sincerely
* Submit regular reports, update the issues.

Theories Related to Leadership

Leadership styles, which leaders may adopt to influence the followers.

1. Charismatic leadership/Great man theory

'A leader is born and is not made'. A leader has some 'charisma' which acts as influencer. 'Charisma' is a Greek word means 'a person', which makes him as a leader irrespective of the situations, where he/she works. They inspire followers and broaden their vision and energy. They catch public consciousness. These leaders have high levels of referent power, self-confidence, dominance ability to convince the followers and the ability to capture the commitment and energy of followers. Leadership qualities cannot be enhanced through education and training, these are inborn and personal in nature, others cannot share these. Situational factors do not have any influence over the leader.

Limitations
* If the leadership qualities are inborn, it implies that nothing can be done to develop leaders in the organization
* Situations will not have influence over the charismatic leader but situational variables play their own role in determining leadership effectiveness.

2. Trait theory

Leadership traits are not completely inborn, but cannot be acquired through learning and experience. Trait is 'an enduring quality of an individual'. Trait theory approach seeks to determine,' what makes a successful leader' from the leader's own personal characteristics. The individual was successful because of his/her certain qualities or characteristics. The ingredients for effective leaders are:
* Self confidence
* Sociability
* Will (initiative, persistence and ambition)
* Dominance
* Surgency (talkative, cheerfulness, enthusiasm, expressiveness, alertness and originality)
* Supervisory ability
* Self actualization
* Self assurance
* Positive attitude
* Charisma, anticipates opportunity
* Creates shared vision
* Demonstrates personal mastery
* Respects social values
* Innate qualities—personality, physical and constitutional factors like height, weight, physique, energy, healthy appearance
* Acquired qualities—emotional stability (free from bias), consistent in action, refrains from anger, well adjusted
* Human relations-Initiate voluntary cooperation for achieving work goals; establish good interpersonal relationship, develops conducive family environment in working area

- Empathy—Ability to look at things objectively understanding them from others point of view, empathy requires respect for other persons, rights, beliefs, values and feelings
- Objectivity in thinking (without any bias or prejudice)
- Self motivating skills and motivating others for high work performance
- Technical skills
- Communicative skills
- Social skills.

Implications
- A leader requires some traits and qualities to be effective
- Many qualities may be developed through training and education development programs.

Limitations
- Generalization of traits
  Problems in identification and measuring the traits, which may be relevant for a leader to be effective in all situations
- Applicability of traits
  Leadership is a process of influence reflects in leader's behavior and not in his/her traits. Persons have specified characteristics of a leader but not become effective leaders, as the reason for this phenomenon is that, there are no direct cause and effect relationship between a trait of a person and his/her behavior. Traits are necessary for shaping the behavior but other situational factors are also important.

3. Behavior theory

Leadership is shown by a person's acts more than by his/her traits. Groups need some one to perform 'task related functions or problem solving functions'—to solve problems faced by groups in performing their activities.

Group maintenance functions or social functions—actions related to mediate disputes and ensure the individuals feel valued by the group. An individual who is able to perform both roles successfully (by means of effective leadership styles) would be an effective leader.

Leadership behavior views in two ways:
a. Functional behavior
   It influences followers positively, e.g. forming clear goals, motivational employees for effectively work to achieve the goals. Raising the group morale, building team spirit, effective two-way communication.
b. Dysfunctional behavior
   Is unfavourable to the followers and denotes ineffective leadership, inability to accept employee's ideas, poor human relations, display of emotional immaturity.

Implications
Leaders can shape the group member's behavior and discards the dysfunctional behavior.

Limitations
- A particular behavior may be functional at a point of time, but may be dysfunctional at another point of time. Thus, time element will be a decider of the effectiveness of the behavior and not the behavior
- Nature of followers and the situations under which the leader's behavior takes place.

4. Situational trait theory/Contingency theory

Effectiveness of leadership will be affected by the factors (e.g. group characteristics, organizational factors) associated with the leaders and the situation. This theory has a dual focus, the leader and the situation in which the leader works. How the leader's traits interact with situational factors in determining team effectiveness in task performance. Effective group performance can be achieved only by matching the leader to the situation or by changing the situation to fit the leader. Leader's behavior is influenced by their characteristics and hierarchical position.

Situational Factors
Subordinates characteristics, leader's situation, position power, group factors and organizational factors.

Implications
Effective leadership will vary with situation to situation; leader has to adapt management practices along with situational variable.

Limitations
Quite complex in practice due to varied contingent factors.

Situational-Behavior Theories
Identifying the specific leader behavior that are most effective in specific leader situations. The behavioral contingencies of the leader that yield the most effective performance by the followers.

a. Path-goal theory
It attempts to explain how leader behavior can positively influence the motivation and job satisfaction of subordinates. Effectiveness leadership is dependent on clearly defining the paths for subordinates to goal attainment and the degree to which the leader is able to improve the chances that subordinates will achieve their goals. The leader clarifies and set goals for subordinates, helps them to find the best path for achieving the goals and to remove the obstacles.

b. The Expectancy theory
Employees' motivation is dependent on leader's behavior that influences goal paths and the relative attractiveness of the goals involved. A person's perception of achieving or prized reward or goal through effective job performance will motivate the individual. However the individual must see clearly the relationship between the individual's efforts and effective job performance will lead to the desired objective.

Elements
Effort—Performance expectancy (successful efforts will leads to better performance).
- Performance—Outcome expectancy (successful performance will leads to better results or rewards or outcomes)
- Valence—The anticipated value of the outcomes or rewards.
  The path goal theory suggests that 4 leadership styles can be used to affect subordinate perceptions of paths and goals.

c. **Theory of Balance**
The leader should possess balanced personality and coordination of contradictory qualities, integrated in nature.
Theory of flash insight
Leader should have flashes of insight and should be able to see the difficulties that face him/her and ways to solve the problem. Knowledge, intelligence, experience and hard work are the essential qualities of a leader.
Theory of marginal uniqueness
Leader should possess unique qualities, capabilities, extraordinary qualities. It creates personal magnetism, earns respect
Theory of ability and disability
Leaders may have limitations, even with that, the abilities he/she has will to be a good leader
Group process theory
To solve the bigger problems, individuals work in a group more efficiently, cooperatively and by selfless service

5. Direct leadership
Leader should orient the followers about their tasks, expectations, work methods, developing work schedules, identifying work evaluation standards.

6. Supportive leadership behavior
Concern for the well-being and needs of subordinates, creating a pleasant organizational climate by being friendly, approachable, considerate behavior. It has great impact on subordinates' performance when they are frustrated and dissatisfied.

7. Participative leadership behavior

Consulting with subordinates, encouraging them by suggestions and carefully considering their ideas when making decisions, which results in increased motivation. The characteristics of subordinates are needs, confidence, abilities, work environment-task, reward system and relationship with coworkers are involved.

8. Achievement oriented behavior

Leader sets challenging goals-seeks improvement of performance by displaying confidence in the abilities of followers.

The competencies of leadership

- Ability to create and sustain excellence
- Capacity for anticipatory thinking, envisioning and action
- Interested in group work and works for group interest and group welfare
- Skill to tap the available resources
- Good judgment and decision making skills
- Transformational competence
- Marked capacity to generate alternative ideas
- Integrative competence: focus on shared visions, aspirations and legitimate role expectations
- Exemplary behavior
- Ability to define visions and goals with a clear sense of purpose and direction
- Moral sensitivity
- Shows confidence and with whom they work
- Sympathy and dependability
- Readiness to demonstrate personal sacrifice, resolve, determination
- Delegation of responsibility and authority
- Ability to built effective relationship
- Autonomy
- Intuition
- Enthusiastic
- Social adaptability
- Reflector—reflecting ideas related to past
- Theorist—logically analyzing the situations
- Pragmatist—trying out ideas, techniques, tools to see the work in practice
- High social intimacy, sociability, friendliness
- Ability to mediate across disciplines and functions
- Ability to recognize and manage paradox
- Non-interference
- Sympathetic nature, empathy skills.

Coach style

- Directive
- Participative
- Negotiative
- Culture custodian
- Enthusiast
- Delegative
- Consultative
- Confident communicator
- Bureaucrat

Receiving style

- Receptive
- Empowered
- Informative
- Good listener
- Self-reliant
- Collaborative
- Reciprocating

Physical qualities

- Sound health
- Endurance
- Vitality
- Enthusiastic

Intellectual qualities

- Ability to make sound judgment
- Scientific approach
- Prominence, positive interest

Moral qualities

- Honesty
- Integrity
- Moral courage
- Purpose oriented/broad vision
- Achievement drive
- Sincerity
- Fair play
- Will power
- Objectivity

Social qualities

- Initiative
- Empathy
- Trust worthy
- Expressiveness

Guidelines for effective leadership

- Leaders and organization should appreciate the unique attributes, predispositions and talents of each leadership organizational preferences in terms of style—leader should challenge the organizational culture, when necessary without destroying it
- Participative, considerate leader behavior—that should concern for the people to enhance the health and well-being of followers in the work environment.

Types of leadership

I. EB Godwin's
- Intellectuals, e.g. scientists, authors, artists, philosophers
- Executive, e.g. corporation presidents, governors, priests, trade union officials.

II. OL Schwarz
- Men of thought
- Men of action.

III. Sir Martin M Conway
- Group originator
- Crowd representative
- Crowd compeller
- Crowd exponent.

IV. E Jeming
- Princess
- Heroes
- Superman.

V. HD Lasswell
- The bureaucrat
- The boss
- The agitator
- The theorist

VI. HT Mazumdar.
- Traditional leader, e.g. Brahmin
- Bureaucratic, e.g. elected leader
- Charismatic, e.g. creates his/her own authority, viz. party leader, religious leader.

VII. Bogardus
- Direct and indirect leadership
- Social, executive and mentor leadership
- Partisan and scientific leadership
- Prophets, saints, experts, boss
- Autocratic, charismatic, paternal and democratic leadership.

VIII. Bartlett
- Institutional
- Dominant leader
- Persuasive leader

IX. Nafe
- State leadership
- Dynamic leadership

X.
- Formal leadership
- Informal leadership

Importance of Leadership

Leadership is essential factor, for success of any organization to function efficiently and effectively. A leader should function as an executive, planner, policy maker, expert, representative, controller, arbitrator, mediator, exampler, purveyor or reward and punishment, establishes good interpersonal relationships. Leader should have versatile personality. The members' activities in and organization need to be directed in certain manner to attain the objectives.

- Motivation of employers for effective work performance
- Creating confidence in his/her followers by guiding them and getting through good results in the organization
- Building morale—Developing positive attitude of employees towards organization, management and voluntary cooperation to offer their ability to the organization. High morale leads to high productivity and organizational stability
- As an executive—Guiding, directing the behavior of followers to discharge their duties effectively
- Policy maker—The objectives, values will be maintained when certain policies have been framed. When the leader imposes his/her own policies, he/she has to take his/her followers into confidence
- Planner—To meet the policies and objectives of organization, leader has to plan effectively, it reflects his/her imagination and capability
- Expert—Leader should have the knowledge of all the things around him
- Controller of interpersonal relationship—Leader has to control, guide and direct internal relationship of the group, he/she should be aware of the qualities of followers and advocates the group thereby he/she can direct the internal relationship as a successful manner
- Arbitrator and mediator—To keep social relationship intact, to relieve societal tensions or group problems, leader has to mediate the situation and solve the problem
- Ideologist—Leader lays down ideology of the group, which guides the actions of the group
- Parent—Leader plays the role of parent for the group, protects the interests of his/her followers, provides conducive environment for better group performance; listens to the problems, provides efforts and guide the followers to solve the problem whereby the group members feels a sense of responsibility, sharing and security
- Scape goat—When the group, which he/she leads, does not succeed, all the blame is put on the shoulders of the leader. The leader holds responsible for everything, i.e., good or bad.

Functions of Leader

Leadership is a highly complex phenomenon, the functions/responsibilities of the leader vary from one group to the other or depend upon the nature.

- Structure the situation/Surrogator for individual responsibility
  Leader creates the working environment to his/her members such that they work effectively, without any conflict, inhibition or bias. He/she has to formulate and define line of authority, delegation of responsibility and orient the duties, so that every one are aware of their functions and responsibilities.

- Controlling group behavior
  Leader has to prevent individuals from exploiting the group, and the group from exploiting the individuals. it enforces the rules that have been established.
- Speaking for the group/group representative
  Leader is responsible for translating the group feelings into words and actions. Leader is the spokes-person for the group; helping to articulate to the members and interpret outsiders the groups' objectives and desires.
- Helping the group to achieve the goals and potentials
  Planning, coordinating, decision making and mobilizing the energy of group members, ensures active participation of all group members and utilization of their diverse capabilities and resources effectively. Making suggestions for actions, evaluating movement towards goal, preventing activities to the goals. Encouraging the members in relieving tensions, gives chances to explore themselves.

Bernard described the functions of the leader as
- The determination of objectives
- The manipulation of means
- The control of the instrument of action
- The stimulation of coordinated action

LEADERSHIP STYLES

1. Autocratic Leadership/Authoritarian Leadership/Directive Leadership/Monothetic Style

To meet immediate and temporary crisis situations autocratic leadership may be useful. It reduces initiativeness, potentiality of the group. The leader determines the policy, procedures and activities in the group and sets the group goals, controlled group activities with step-by-step directions. The performance of group members is very good, but motivation was low, group members will work only when the leader is present to direct them. Group members are more dependent, submissive, shows less individuality, less friendly, praise to each other; marked intermember irritability, aggressiveness, insecurity, dissatisfaction among group members is observed.

Categories
- Strict autocrat
  The leader influences subordinate behavior through negative motivation, i.e. by criticizing subordinates, imposing penalty etc.
- Benevolent autocrat
  Centralizes decision making power in him/her, but his/her motivation style is positive. He/she can be effective in getting efficiency in many situations
- Incompetent autocrat
  Superior adopts autocratic leadership style just to hide their incompetence.

Advantages
- Many subordinates likes to work under centralized authority structure and strict discipline
- Provides strong motivation and reward to a manager exercising this style
- It permits very quick decisions as single person takes it
- Less competent subordinates have scope to work as they do negligible planning, organising and decision making.

Disadvantages
- People don't like to work, when it is strict and negative motivation or lack of motivation
- Low morale, frustration and conflict develops among employees
- More dependency and less individuality in the organisation observed

2. Democratic Leadership/Participative Leadership/Consultative Leadership
Emotional involvement of a person in a group situation, which encourages him/her to contribute to group goals and share responsibility in them. Leader decentralizes his/her decision making process. It elicits member's active involvement and places minimum restraints on their initiative and creativity, promoting the adaptability

to meet changing conditions and demands. The leader discusses, determines policies and assignments together. Group members' shows more interest in their work and originality and keep on working. Cohesiveness was highest among group members; the leader encourages participation by members in deciding group matters and behaves in a friendly, helpful manner to the members. Giving techniques and suggesting alternative procedures, low dependency on group leader, low incidence of irritability, aggressiveness, high frequency of suggestions is observed, high quality and group satisfaction, e.g. family.

Advantages
- Highly motivating technique to employees as they feel elevated when their ideas and suggestions are given weight in decision making
- Productivity is high as they are partly involved in decisions, thus implement decisions whole heartedly
- Provides organizational stability by raising morale and attitudes of employees high and favorable.

Limitations
- Complex nature of organization requirement needs through understanding of its problems, which low level employees may not be able to do. Thus participation does not remain meaningful
- Some people in the organization wants minimum interaction with their superiors or associates, so this technique is discouraging
- It can be used covertly to manipulate employees.

3. Laissez-faire Leadership
The leader simply stood by and answered when spoken to the groups were entirely on their own in planning and assigning work. Moral and cohesiveness was lowest among group members. The leader allows complete freedom for decisions and activity keeping his/her initiative and suggestions to a minimum. Group shows little dependency on the leader, irritability, aggressiveness, suggestions for group action and group policy, e.g. neighborhood.

- Decision making in leadership
  It is the core activity in the process of leadership and management. As a decision maker, the leader's role is to create relevant order, coherence, committed synergy through others. Awareness, integrity, courage and competence are the crucial determinants of the decisions. The traditional leader concerns with power, rank and status, which are common in positional authority.
- Decision making behavior (Logical/Cognitive responses)
- Inquiry: Searching, Examining, Probing, Defining, Classifying and Analyzing
- Diagnosis: Assessing, Weighing, Clarifying, Crystallizing, Simplifying and Prioritizing
- Planning: Foreseeing, Predicting, Preparing, Over-viewing, Progressing, Follow-up
- Decision process (Stages in making decisions)
- Awareness: (situational analysis), Concerns, Information and Scope
- Direction: Problems and obstacles, Priorities and objectives, Strengths and weaknesses
- Action: (Execution), Opportunities, Threats, Consequences, Outcomes
- Decision making behavior (Emotional/Intuitive responses)
- Insight: Intuiting, Generating ideas, Exploring, Synthesizing, Scanning, Creating options
- Drive: Insisting, Persisting, Resisting, Being resolute, Building purpose, Being determined
- Pace: Sense of timing, Varying speed, Adjusting response, pre-emptying, Recognizing the right conditions and taking appropriate action.

Approaches in Decision Making
- Awareness about a problem and identify the problem
- Define the problem
- Establish goals and priorities
- Explanation of possible courses of action and their respective consequences
- Deliberation of decision on course of action
- Thorough follow-up, with revision if necessary.

Process of Decision Making

1. How we obtain information?

a. Sensing
- Look for specific parts, bits and pieces
- Live in and Live with the present
- Prefer handling practical and tangible matters
- Define the activities in a measurable manner
- Have a start
- Work incrementally and take one step at a time
- Work 'hands on'
- Set procedures and establish routines

b. Intuition
- Look for overall context and patterns
- Concerned with possibilities and the future
- Anticipate and speculate about what might be
- Prefer imagining the possibilities
- Like opportunities to be creative and inventive
- Jump in anywhere-leap around and miss out steps and sequences
- Work out overall plan or design
- Like change and variety

2. How we make decisions?

a. Thinking
- Decide with 'head'
- Go by logic
- Work by truth, justice and objectivity
- See the things as an 'on-looker' i.e., detached
- Take the longer-term view
- Automatically find flaws and criticize
- Analyse ideas, plan and strategies.

b. Feeling
- Decide with 'heart'
- Go by personal convictions (what I feel is ….)
- Work by personal rapport and harmony
- See the things as a participant
- Immediate and personal or subjective view
- Appreciate spontaneously.

3. Degree of Order we Need?

a. Judging
- Formulate an organised life style with definite structure and order
- Like to be in control
- Decisive
- Define clear goals, parameters, limits and categories
- Feel comfortable with definite ends and closures
- Plan in advance.

4. Handle deadlines

a. Perceiving
- Prefer a flexible life style
- Enjoy freedom, autonomy, flexibility, curiosity, discovery and surprise

- Prefer freedom to explore with no limits
- Like open endedness and chance
- Meet deadlines with last minute rush.

Leader's Style in Decision Making Process

The extent to which leaders are developed and integrated into the care goals and direction of organization.

- As Master leader: Transforms, Integrates, Mobilizes
- As Operator: Follows instructions, Works 'hands on' and perform 'how'
- As Custodian: Protects, Preserves and Conserves
- As Maverick: Irritant, Initiator, Changing agent.

Leader is aligned with vision, mission and core goals and is integrated into the organizational structure. Operates appropriate level of competence, confidence and managerial maturity.

i. Master leader

Integrated, aligned and functionally mature manager as, 'master leader'. He/she is capable of envisioning future in realistic, strategic, appropriate and operational terms. Identifies appropriate routes to achieve the associated goals and objectives, generates necessary willing synergy (dynamic, adaptive, organization, renewal)

ii. Operator

Primarily focused on 'doer', follows instructions, works on 'hands-on' and whose time frame is largely 'here and now'. Perception of leaders' role is based on contribution is governed by 'personal experience, common sense empiricism, uncritical and uninformed observation'.

iii. Custodian

Focuses on preservation of the status quo and is more concerned with conservation than transformation.

iv. Maverick leader

Highly intelligent, clever people whose restless intellectual energy and sense of dissatisfaction provides the stimulus for their need to change the established order. Powerful change agent and may use both 'vinegar' and 'honey' according to the situation in order to bring about what he/she considers to have necessary change.

Nurse as an Effective Leader

Nurses are functioning in various settings, viz. educational institutes, hospitals and community settings. They will play different roles, in varying capacities as a team leader; whatever the settings, nurses has to function as an effective leader, by shouldering responsibility to fulfill organizational policies and goals.

- Team leader should have sound knowledge, efficient administrative skills in the area of working
- Keep efforts to understand thoroughly the policies and objectives of an organization
- Prepares master plan in advance, to carry out the activities in a smooth manner within scheduled time
- Develops good interpersonal relationships by establishing adequate rapport with all followers
- Wins the confidence of followers
- Incorporates principles of administration and management (planning, organizing, staffing, decision making, directing, delegating, coordination, cooperation, command, reporting and budgeting) in implementing the activities
- Formulates the job recruitment policies; selects the candidates for varied positions by following organization's policies
- Prepares job charts/responsibilities for all the cadres
- Delegates the responsibilities, encourages group work, team spirit, inspires the members for cohesiveness
- Coordinates interdepartmental and intradepartmental activities
- Conducts counseling sessions with the affected employees, during problematic situations, helps them to cope up with traumatic experiences
- Motivates the employees to conduct staff developmental programs, inservice training programs, etc. for upgradation of knowledge and attaining higher qualification.

TEAM WORK

Introduction

Teamwork has become an important part of the working culture. One of the major responsibility of supervisor Leader/Administrator is to build effective teams for their organization. Productivity, quality of products and services, dealing with crisis, etc. require effective team work. Strong and cohesive teams will influence individual employees. All the team efforts are directed towards the goals, promotes good communication among team members. The most effective teamwork is produced when all the individuals involved harmonize their contributions and work towards a common goal.

T — Togetherness
E — Efficiency
A — Positive Attitude
M — Motivated Spirit
W — Working Cooperatively
O — Organized Way of dealing issues
R — Rational way of Thinking
K — Knowledgeable

Definitions

"A joint action by a group of people, in which each person subordinates his/her or her individual interests and opinions to the unity and efficiency of the group"—Webster's New World Dictionary

Differences between Group functions and Team functions

Groups	Teams
• Members work independently • Members often are not working towards the same goal	• Members work interdependently and work towards both personal and team goals, and they understand these goals are accomplished best by mutual support
• Members focus mostly on themselves because they are not involved in the planning of their group's objectives and goals	• Members feel a sense of ownership towards their role in the group as they committed themselves to goals they helped to create
• Members are given their tasks or told what their duty/job is and suggestions are rarely welcomed	• Members collaborate together and use their talent and experience to contribute to the success of the team's objectives. Suggestions by the group members always welcome by the Manager or Team Leader
• Members are very cautious about what they say and are afraid to ask questions. They may not fully understand what is taking place in their group	• Members base their success on trust and encourage all members to express their opinions, varying views, and questions
• Members do not trust each other's motives because they do not fully understand the role each member plays in their group	• Members make a conscious effort to be honest, respectful and listen to every person's point of view
• Members may have a lot to contribute but are held back because of a closed relationship with each member	• Members are encouraged to offer their skills and knowledge, and in turn each member is able to contribute the group's success
• Members are bothered by differing opinions or disagreements because they consider it as a threat. There is no group support to help in resolving problems	• Members see conflict as a part of human nature and they react to it by treating it as an opportunity to hear about new ideas and opinions. Everybody wants to resolve problems constructively
• Members may or may not participate in group decision-making and conformity is valued more than positive results	• Members participate equally in decision making, but each member understands that the leader might need to make the final decision if the team cannot come to a consensus agreement

"The actions of individuals, brought together for a common purpose or goal, which subordinate the needs of the individual to the needs of the group. In essence, each person on the team puts aside his/her or her individual needs to work towards the larger group objective. The interactions among the members and the work they complete is called as teamwork".

"Cooperative or coordinated effort on the part of a group of persons acting together as a team or in the interests of a common cause".

"A team is a collection of individuals who get together or are assigned to achieve a common goal. In this case, teamwork simply means the process through which they could achieve the expressed common goal".

Characteristics

Larson and LaFasto (1989) described Characteristics of Team Work

1. The team must have a clear goal—Team goals should call for a specific performance objective, expressed concisely that everyone knows when the objective has been met.
2. The team must have a results—driven structure. The team should be allowed to operate in a manner that produces results. It is often best to allow the team to develop the structure.
3. The team must have competent team members.
4. The team must have unified commitment—This doesn't mean that team members must agree on everything. It means that all individuals must be directing their efforts towards the goal. If an individual's efforts is going purely towards personal goals, then the team will confront this and resolve the problem.
5. The team must have a collaborative climate—It is a climate of trust produced by honest, open, consistent and respectful behavior. With this climate teams perform well without it, they fail.
6. The team must have high standards that are understood by all—Team members must know what is expected of them individually and collectively. Vague statements such as "positive attitude" and "demonstrated effort" are not good enough.
7. The team must receive external support and encouragement—Encouragement and praise or appreciation towards the efforts or work accomplished motivates teams as it does with individuals.
8. The team must have principled leadership—Teams usually need someone to lead the effort. Team members must know that the team leader has the position because they have good leadership skills and are working for the good of the team. The team members will be less supportive if they feel that the team leader is putting him/herself above the team, achieving personal recognition or otherwise benefiting from the position.

Stages of Team Growth

It is important for teacher and students (the team members) to know that teams don't just form and immediately start working together to accomplish great things. There are actually stages of team growth and teams must be given time to work through the stages and become effective.

1. **Forming**—When a team is forming, members cautiously explore the boundaries of acceptable group behavior. They search for their position within the group and observe the leader's guidance.
2. **Storming**—Storming is probably the most difficult stage for the group. Members often become impatient about the lack of progress, but are still inexperienced with working as a team. Members may argue about the actions they should take because they faced with ideas that are unfamiliar to them and put them outside their comfort zones. Much of their energy is focused on each other instead of achieving the goal.
3. **Norming**—During this stage team members accept the team and begin to reconcile differences. Emotional conflict is reduced as relationships become more cooperative. The team is able to concentrate more on their work and start to make significant progress.
4. **Performing**—By this stage the team members have discovered and accepted each other's strengths and weaknesses, and learned what their roles are. Members are open and trusting and many good ideas are produced because they are not afraid to offer ideas and suggestions. They are comfortable using decision making tools to evaluate the ideas, prioritize tasks and solve problems. Much is accomplished and team satisfaction and loyalty is high.

Since working as part of a team can improve learning and is a much needed skill in today's workplace, a team exercise should be included in the classroom. With well planned out tasks, careful guidance and close observation, instructors can encourage team exercises which are extremely valuable learning experiences for the group of learners.

Tips for Team Building

- Team goals are totally clear and completely understood and accepted by all team members and team efforts are totally directed towards the common goals, work with consensus and commitment
- Team effectiveness is the diversity of the skills and personalities, people use their personalities in total
- Team leader will build trust by one on one meeting with all team members in an atmoshphere of honesty and openness
- Team leader will try to involve all group members in decision making process
- Team leader will be very careful with interpersonal issues, recognize them early and deal with them in complete
- Supervisor will not miss the opportunities to empower the employees, show appreciation of an individual team player's or employees work
- Team leader should not limit for negative feedback. Be fare. Whenever opportunity comes, appreciates and give positive feedback for the work accomplished and the efforts made by employees
- Team work and team building can offer many challenges, the pay off from a high performance team is well worth it.

Uses

- If Supervisors use teams in a number of situations, the culture of team work is strengthened, e.g. whenever a special problem arises, instead of solving the problem by the specific employee by himself/herself or by a competent employee, the supervisor may set up a special team to work out detailed action plan
- Task forces are very useful in dealing with special issues. These forces contribute to collaborative culture in the organization
- Improvement of quality of products and services is usually done through a team
- Productive teams should be rewarded
- Most of the Organizational Developmental Programs require team building, supervisor may learn process skills and may provide such help to team members to learn from time to time which is helpful for Process analysis
- Team building skills are critical for effectiveness of a manager or entrepreneur
- Team can accomplish something much bigger and work more effectively.

Phases in Team Work

Grid approach

In Organizational Developmental Program intervention will be dealt with step by step. The dimensional concepts of this approach are: "Concern for people and Concern for Production". The most effective manager or supervisor is the one whose rating is high on both dimensions. Grid approach is a combination of Behavioral Science and rigorous business logic.

Pre-Phase: Selected Managers or faculty in the organization attend a grid seminar. In this experience the managers are exposed to the two dimensional grid Philosophy – they are aided in improving their communication skill, they are exposed to the analysis of the own organizational culture and various conceptual inputs.

Purposes

1. The Administrators/Supervisors/Nurse Educators learn how to conduct a grid O.D. Program
2. They are able to evaluate the pros and cons of O.D. approach, either implement it or not into their own organization. If the organization decides to implement the grid approach then Phase-1 is introduced. If this result of this pilot phase is a green signal then the program is initiated.

Phase 1—Attention is focused on each individual's managerial style, his/her problem solving techniques, communication skills, etc. In this phase the trainers are trained to become, in the language of Grid approach.

Phase 2—Team Work Development: Projecting team work in the organization through the analysis of team culture. It involves the development of planning and problem solving skills, the additional aspects of this phase are team behavior and feedback effectiveness. Team work is developed through a face to face encounter with actual problems. Individuals learn how to study and manage the culture of their work teams.

Phase 3—Inter-group development: Inter-group effectiveness will occur, to move groups from ineffective intergroup relationships to more effective and hence productive modes of relationship will result. The dynamics of intergroup cooperation and competition are explored. Each group discusses what an "ideal" relationship is and the information shared between two groups. Steps are then taken to move towards the ideal by assigning tasks to individuals. This phase consists of teams of two or three who meet and discuss on the above stated issues. Only selected members of the team, who are closely related with the work of other teams will take part in these exercises and activities.

Phase 4—Developing an ideal strategic corporate model: The focus is shifted to strategic corporate planning. The attention is shifted from lower level of management to higher officials or top level executives, as these people will engages in the strategy—the plans and ideas are tested and evaluated in conjunction with other corporate members. Top level executives designs an ideal strategic corporate model that would define what is ideal and excellent. All persons in the organization contribute by the way of facts and technical inputs.

Phase 5—Implementing the ideal Strategic Model: Through a gradual phase of conversation, the organizm tries to attain corporate excellence.

BIOLOGICAL BASIS OF INTRINSIC MOTIVATION

Arrested curiosity stays on the plane of interest in local gossip and prying inquisitiveness into other peoples' business". (John Dewey)

Frontal lobes play an important part in the development of balanced personality. Frontal lobe development is a function of the unique human capacity for 'motivation'. As a unique feature of human personality development, motivation is the characteristically human capacity to perform actions which produce delayed responses and rewards. Motivation is the expression of the capacity for initiative and sustained attention and concentration of one's attention on a goal. As a capacity related to causes of action and motives for behavior, the human capacity for motivation is required for adaptive behavior and for survival.

The extreme front part of the frontal lobes—The prefontal lobes—is responsible for motivation. Motivation is an intrinsic function of the development of the prefontal lobes. The prefrontal lobes are responsible for initiative and the maintenance of the proper balance between actions and restraint—sustained attention and the resulting delayed responses and rewards. The proper functioning of the prefrontal lobes is the biological basis for the ability to concentrate for long periods on demanding tasks. It is the basis for the characteristically human ability for productivity or 'work'.

Motivation is a characteristically human capacity which is necessary for adaptive behavior and survival of the human organism as a social organism. Human survival depends on the human capacity for motivation. The human organism is intrinsically motivated for behavior which is adaptive to its environment. The human organism as a social organism is similarly motivated for behavior which is adaptive to its social environment. Adaptive behavior depends on the accuracy of the individual's perception of the social environment and on the way in which the individual thinks about it. Accuracy of the individual's knowledge and understanding depends on the unconscious motivations and thought patterns 'cognitive structures'. The individual's thought patterns determine the accuracy of evaluation which in turn determines the degree of adaptability of behavior. Human survival depends on the capacity for adaptation to a changing social environment and social adaptability depends on the capacity for motivation and work. Intrinsic motivation is a function of the individual's unconscious or 'intrinsic' motives for behavior, i.e. 'human needs'. The key to motivation is recognition of needs. "Human evolution is rooted in man's adaptability and in certain indestructible qualities of his nature which compel him never to cease his search for conditions better adjusted to his intrinsic needs" (source : Man For Himself, 23). The hierarchy of human needs in terms or urgency or 'prepotency' Human needs are human motives for behavior or 'motivations'. Human motivations lie at the subconscious level of brain functioning Unconscious motivations and give rise to emotional forces known as 'deep meanings' or 'drives' of human behavior, i.e. the 'learning emotions'. Deep meanings and drives are at the core of intrinsic motives for behavior. The subconscious emotions determine the nature of the individual's thinking or 'cognition'. Depending on the nature of the individual's motivation, cognitive activity leads to interpetation and evaluation of the environment and subsequent behavior or 'action' which can be creative and 'adaptive' or destructive and 'non-adaptive'. Learning emotions provide the sense of direction and the energy required for learning and adapting to changes in the social environment. There is a hierarchy of needs in terms of urgency or 'prepotency'. The range of human needs includes the most prepotent physiological 'survival needs' for physical security—Food, water, shelter and so on; the so-called 'basic psychological needs' or 'ego-needs' for psychological security and belongingness or 'self-esteem—Care and affection; the 'higher psychological needs' or 'growth needs'—The 'spiritual needs' (spiritual love, lovingkindness or 'compassion') for 'ego or self-transcendance' i.e., 'metaneeds', for mature growth or 'self-actualization'.

Self-actualization is not the end of growth—Not the path to maturity but the path of maturity.

Mature growth or 'self-actualization' involves the harmonization of psychic forces (such as the 'digestion of memory' as 'storytelling') which frees the individual from the limitations of the 'ego-life' and allows them to live in the spiritual realm of human existence, i.e. the realm of 'self-transcendance' or 'being'. Self-actualisation is a function of the unfolding of human 'values for living'—The 'social values' or 'morals' of 'morality'—The moral faculty for accurate evaluation of the social environment and leads to effective decision-making and successful adaptation, i.e. 'social intelligence' depends on motivation by the metaneeds i.e., 'metamotivation' is functional in the process of self-actualization as mature growth and development of 'moral consciousness' or 'conscience'. Development of conscience or 'character'—The human 'soul'—Depends on creativity and productivity or 'work'. Through meaningful work, the growth motivated or 'mature' individual is 'self-actualised' or 'self-actualizing'.

The self-actualizing individual is motivated by the growth needs and lives in the realm of being values of morality or 'ethics' Motivated by the growth needs, their motivation is synonymous with self-actualisation. Their whole being is motivated. Their productivity results from the effects of Metamotivation is a function of communion with what transcends the ego and makes it easily possible to live in the realm of the Being-needs of growth. They naturally make choices within the framework of the intrinsic system of human values which are equivalent to the B-needs i.e., the 'Being-values' or B-values—The 'higher' spiritual values or metaneeds which satisfy the human longing for freedom, love, certainty wholeness, perfection, truth, justice, aliveness, richness, simplicity, beauty, goodness, uniqueness, self-sufficiency and so on. Living in the realm of the metaneeds self-actualizing individuals lead ethical lives. They live by a rational ethical value system—Rational ethics'. They are responsible to themselves making decisions in their own true interest and at the same time responsible to others making decisions in the interest of society. They have a genuine desire to be responsible to others, to help others 'altruism' 'being-motivation' or 'metamotivation'. If personality development is encouraged then the individual is motivated by the 'positive learning emotions' characteristic of self-actualization - curiosity, wonder and reverential fear or 'awe'.

Natural curiosity is the source of 'intrinsic motivation' for learning—It is in fact nothing short of a miracle that the modern methods of instruction have not yet entirely strangled the holy curiosity of inquiry. Human needs must be met during development: role of 'education' During development, each set of needs becomes apparent as the more urgent needs are met (sensitive periods) and motivations for behavior shift from a strong expression of motivation of deficiency—To the subtle expression of motivation of sufficiency—'Growth motivation'. The well developed or 'balanced' personality is motivated by the metaneeds. 'Metamotivation'—The most effective type of motivation for adaptation to rapidly changing social conditions.

Human adaptability depends on effective learning driven by 'curiosity', accurate interpretation or 'perception' and correct evaluation or 'critical thought'. Whatever the motivational state, intrinsic motivation is driven by the instinctive need to make meaning of the environment or 'learn'. Learning is the capacity for observation and inquiry (curiosity) which is necessary for the organism to acquire the information, knowledge and understanding upon which it depends for accurate interpretation or 'perception' of the social reality. Curiosity is a function of the attention on the environment for the knowledge which can be derived from it—An instinctive emotion because it is rooted in the instinct for 'self-preservation'.

"Motivation would also be a significant dimension of health. The most widely accepted transpersonal model of motivation owes a great deal to Abraham Maslow. Human capacity for reason depends on brain development or 'intelligence Human adaptability depends on development of the human organ specialised for processing of information and creation of meaning or 'learning'. Learning is a natural function of the 'brain'. The human brain is a social brain with the potential capacity for development of the intelligence required for adaptation to changing social conditions i.e., 'social intelligence'. The human capacity for social intelligence depends on optimal functioning of the brain or 'optimalearning'—A function of 'creative intelligence'.

MOTIVATION

Introduction

Behavioral changes can be expected in individuals with motivation. The influential personalities like parents, teachers, spiritual leaders, friends and well wishers will influence learners' life and play a vital role in motivating the learner to perform the activity or task in a specified way. Positive motivation is often more successful than negative motivation. It is contagious, as it spreads from one person to another person, e.g. a person who accomplished the specified task will become as an exemplary or role model for the forthcoming followers. Teacher is a positive motivational force for the students to shape their behavior, whatever age may be (even if you consider from a kindergarten student to adulthood the child/learner imitates and follow teacher in dealing with the problems, many times teacher will act as a role model). We make use of motives, incentives, rewards, needs, wants, desires, urges, etc. are all used, these terms are interrelated and interdependent. We make use of motives, incentives in health field, motivation is required to enlist people's participation in utilization of health care services.

Motivation comprises important elements such as the need or content, search and choice of strategies, goal directed behavior, social comparison of rewards, reinforcement and performance satisfaction. Motivated individuals will come out with new ways of doing the tasks, they are quality oriented, more productive, adopts technology for successful implementation. For example,

1. A satisfied beneficiary or user will become an exemplary to utilize the type of service in a better way like a child who is vaccinated against a specific disease will be free from the antigens and healthy, protective, is a model for other parents to follow or utilize the same health care benefits.
2. Motivation of eligible couple for small family norm is an important contribution in implementation of National Family Welfare Program.
3. Parents and Teachers will be motivational forces for young children to develop certain characteristics and achievements in their life.

"Performance of an individual depends on his/her or her ability backed by motivation".

Performance = f (ability x motivation)—'Ability' is 'the skill and competence of the person to complete a given task', however the ability itself is not enough, the person's desire to accomplish the task is necessary. Success is based on abilities and desire to accomplish the assigned or given tasks. 'Motivation' is 'the set of forces that cause individuals to behave in certain ways'.

Definitions

"The inner force that directs the individual to perform and accomplish the task in a predetermined way".

"The result of processes, internal or external to the individual, that arouse enthusiasm and persistence to persue a certain course of action".

"A process governing choices made by persons among alternative forms of voluntary activity".

"A process that starts with a physiological or psychological deficiency or need that activates behavior or drive that is aimed at a goal or an incentive".

Nature of Motivation/Process of Motivation

It begins with the individual's needs. Needs are felt deprivations which the individual experiences at a given time and act as energizers. These needs may be Psychological, e.g. the need for recognition; Social needs, e.g.

friendship, recognition, education; Biological needs/Survival needs/Physiological needs, e.g. water, air, food, Sex, Sleep, Rest, Recreation; Economical needs, e.g. Money; Ego-integrative needs, e.g. desire for prestige, power and self-respect. These deprivations or deficiencies force the individual to search for the ways to reduce or eliminate them. Motivation is goal directed. A goal is a specific result that the individual wants to achieve. Driving forces and accomplishing goals can significantly reduce needs. Such needs and expectations often create uncomfortable tension within the individuals. Positive rewards, e.g. appreciation for the efforts by higher officials, promotions and raises are ways that organizations seek to maintain desirable behaviors. Once the individuals have received rewards or punishments they reassess their needs. Motives can only be inferred, but not seen. Every individual at any given time will have their own needs, desires, expectations and things to do. It is the responsibility of well wisher to motivate them to give a push or acts like a catalyst to shoulder responsibility to accomplish the tasks (Fig. 14.1).

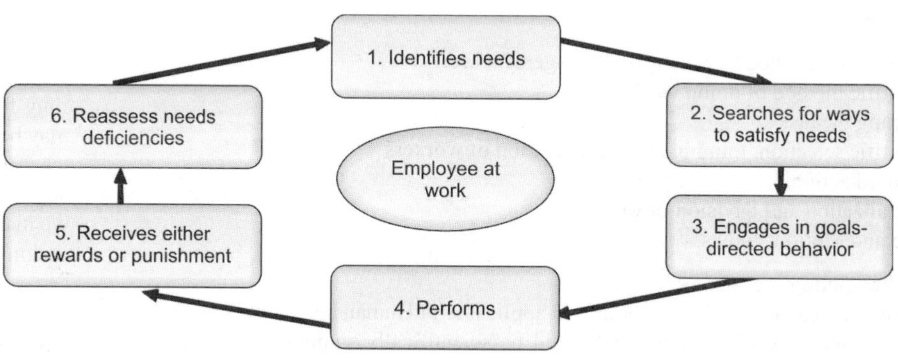

Fig. 14.1: Nature of motivation

Importance of Motivation

Teachers have to motivate their students to progress their efficiency, When people actively seek new ways of doing things, they usually able to achieve them. It is the responsibility of an educator to make their students to look for better ways of performing their scheduled tasks more skillfully and efficiently. A motivated person is more quality oriented. A clear understanding of the way, motivation helps an educator makes his/her students quality oriented. Highly motivated individuals are more productive. An appreciation, the nature of motivation is highly useful for Nurse Educators, Nurse Administrators, Clinical Nurse specialists even for ordinary fellow-being. With stronger motivation greater achievements will be resulted.

Every Educational Institution requires human resources, three behavioral dimensions of HR are significant, professionals must be attracted not only to join the organization, but also to remain in it. Professionals must perform their scheduled tasks efficiently, they have to go beyond this dependable role performance and engage in some form of creative, spontaneous and innovative behavior at work. In other words, for any organization to be effective, it must come to grip with the motivational problems of stimulating both—The decision to participate and decision to produce the younger generation with productive, efficient skills.

Motivation as a concept represents a highly complex phenomenon that affects and is affected by a multitude of factors in the organizational milieu. An understanding of motivation is essential to comprehend totally as they relate to performance and satisfaction.

Theories of Motivation

Theories will assist the individual to understand the nature of motivation in a better way.

I. Early Theories
- Scientific Management
- Human relations model
- Contemporary theories.

II. Content Theories
- Maslow's need hierarchy theory

- Herzberg's two factor theory
- Alderfer's ERG and Achievement motivation theory.

III a. Process Theories
- Vroom's expectancy model
- Adam's equity theory
- Porter and Lawler's performance and Satisfaction model.

  b. Reinforcement Theory

Early Theory
Scientific Management
The theory was developed by FW Taylor, "Father of Scientific Management". A Philosophy and set of methods and techniques stressing the scientific study and organization of work at the operational level for the purpose of increasing efficiency.

Techniques contributed by Scientific Management are:
- Scientific method of doing work
- Planning the task
- Scientific selection, training and remuneration of workers
- Standardization
- Specialization and Division of work
- Time and Motion studies.

Mental Revolution
- Taylor's logical and rational approach is applicable in Human behavior.
- Physical activities of an individual could be scientifically studied to determine the optimal method of performing the task
- Rules and responsibilities of learners will be specified, so that they were able to follow
- Learners and faculty will adhere to the rules and regulations specified. They will try to perform their activities in a systematic way by adopting the specified responsibilities
- The individuals has to meet certain needs in working conditions like need for security, social fulfillment, challenging activities, positive rewards for the accomplishment of activities like appreciation, prize, recognition, etc.

Human Relations Model
Elton Mayo and other human relation researchers found that the social contacts are necessary in the working environment to improve work performance and efficiency.

Fulfillment of social needs is essential for progress of any achievement in the social life of an individual. Freedom to make decisions and implement certain activities is recommended for the fulfillment of specified tasks, though they have to follow stipulated rules and responsibilities.

Content theories: Emphasize the importance of inner needs in motivation. The theories assume that all employees, all situations are alike and there is one way best to motivate the persons.

1. Maslow's need hierarchy theory
The need hierarchy of motivation, propounded by Abraham Harold Maslow his/her approach to human behavior is based on Existential Philosophy i.e., man is a healthy, good and creative being, capable of working out his/her own destiny. Theory deserves appreciation for its simplicity, commonness, humaneness and intuitiveness and directly applicable to work motivation. It is dynamic. It presents motivation as a constantly changing force, expressing itself through the constant striving for fulfillment of lower and higher needs. Instead of resting on his/her or her laurels when one goal is reached or a need is satisfied, the individual is typically redirect his/her or her efforts and capacities towards the attainment of still higher level needs.

The Essence of this Theory
Human beings have wants and desires which can influence their behavior. Only unsatisfied needs can influence behavior, satisfied need do not act as motivators.

Needs are many, arranged in the order of their importance or hierarchy from basic to complex.

The person advances to the next level of hierarchy only when the lower level need is fulfilled.

The person is able to go in the hierarchy, the more individuality, humaneness and psychological health he/she or she will display.

Educators have to uplift learners for the fulfillment of their lower level to higher level needs. Maslow classified needs into five levels. Each level comprises group of needs.

a. Physiological needs—These needs are essential to the understanding and fulfilment of basic needs related to of human behavior. The most basic, powerful and obvious of all human needs for the need of Physical survival, e.g. Food, Air, Hunger, Sex, Thirst, Rest, Sleep. Protection from extreme temperature and sensory stimulation. These needs are directly concerned with the biological maintenance of organizm. The individual who fails to fulfill this basic level of needs, unable to attempt satisfaction of higher need levels. In the educational institution organizational context, physiological needs are represented by educators' concern to meet the basic needs of learners like conducive facilities in classroom minimum facilities like provision of seating facilities, ventilation, lighting, blackboard, podium for teacher, bulletin board, etc. It is the responsibility of teachers to ensure that these needs of learners are met, so that they can be motivated to strive for the gratification of higher level.

b. Safety and security needs—To ensure a reasonable degree of continuity, order, structure and predictability in one's environment. The preference for secured environment , the acquisition of new skills. Religions and philosophies help a person to organize the world and the people in it into a coherent and meaningful whole, thus making the person to organize the world and the people in it into a coherent and meaningful whole, thus making the person feel safe.

Security needs in the educational organizational context correlate to such factors like job security, positive rewards, safe working conditions for protective environment. To satisfy the safety needs of learners include positive rewards, safe working conditions, grievance procedure, etc. create a feeling of security in the student's mind.

c. Love and belonging needs—After fulfilling or satisfaction of physiological and safety and security needs constitute the third level. Group membership becomes a dominant goal for the individual. Maslow believed that love involves a healthy, loving relationship between two people, which includes mutual respect, admiration and trust. Maslow also stressed that love needs involve both giving and receiving love. Being loved and accepted is instrumental to healthy feelings of worth. Not being loved to feelings of futility, emptiness and hostility. Social needs represent the need for a compatible work group, peer acceptance, professional friendship and friendly supervision. Educators has to encourage informal groups, besides, supervision requires to be effective.

d. Self esteem needs/Egoistic needs—Self Respect and esteem from others, e.g. desire for competence, confidence, personal strength, adequacy, achievement, independence and freedom. An individual needs to know that he/she or she is competent and capable of mastering tasks and challenges in life. Esteem from others, e.g. prestige, recognition, acceptance, attention, status, reputation and appreciation. In this case individuals need to be appreciated for what they can do i.e., they must experience feelings of worth because their competence is recognized and valued by others. Satisfaction of the self-esteem needs generates feelings and attitudes of self-confidence, worth, strength, capability and of being useful and necessary in the world. Maslow emphasized that the most healthy self esteem is based on respect earned from others rather than on fame, status or adulation. Esteem is the result of effort—It is earned. Hence there is a real psychological danger of basing one's esteem needs on the opinions of others rather than on real ability, achievement and adequacy. Once a person relies exclusively upon the opinions of others for his/her or her own self-esteem, he/she or she places himself/herself or herself in psychological jeopardy. To be solid, self-esteem must be founded on one's actual worth rather than on external factors beyond one's control.

In the work place, self esteem needs correspond to job responsibilities, peer/supervisory recognition, challenging work, responsibility and publicity in educational institution publications. Educator practices to fulfill these needs include challenging work assignments, performance appraisal, recognition, feedback, personal encouragement and involving all teaching faculty in setting up of goals and decision making.

e. Self-actualization needs: after attaining four needs, the fifth group will come to the force. Self-actualization is the desire to become everything that one is capable of becoming. The person who has achieved this highest level presses towards the full use and exploitation of his/her or her talents, capacities and potentialities. In other words, to self-actualize is to become the total kind of person that one wants to become, to reach The peak of one's potential—The more apparent satisfaction of it a person obtains, the more important the need for more seems to become. People are invariably blind to their own potentialities, the social environment often stifles development towards self fulfillment. Courage is required to fulfill the need, it logically follows that anything that increases the individual's fear and anxiety also increases his/her or her tendency to regress towards safety and security.

In an educational institution, self-actualization needs correlate with the desire for excelling in one's job. Educators can use a variety of approaches to enable them to achieve personal as well as organizational goals. Higher level needs like esteem and actualization needs are important to the 'content of work motivation'.

Evaluation of theory

Administrators have to think about motivating their faculty. As they are familiar with this model, they have to identify the individual specific needs of Teaching faculty and Nonteaching faculty (Ministerial staff) and students, as it accounts for interpersonal variations in human behavior. Offer satisfaction for the particular needs and realize that giving more of same reward may have a diminishing impact on motivation.

2. Two Factor Theory/Dual Factor Theory/Motivation—Hygiene theory

Herzberg and his/her associates Mausner, Peterson and Capwell began their work on factors affecting work motivation in the mid 1950s. There are two distinct aspects, first aspect represents a formally stated theory of work behavior, the second aspect of Herzberg's work has focused upon the behavioral consequences of job enrichment and job realization programs. Intrinsic factors, e.g. achievement, recognition, the work itself, responsibility, advancement and growth related to job satisfaction. These factors are known as Motivators/satisfiers/job content factors. When employees dissatisfied, they tended to attribute these characteristics to themselves to extrinsic factors, e.g. organization policy and administration, supervision, working conditions, salary, maintenance factors or job context factors. According to Herzberg satisfaction and dissatisfaction are two separate dimensions, the key idea of Herzberg is—Satisfaction is affected by motivators and dissatisfaction by hygiene factors and it has important implications for Administrators and Supervisors. To achieve motivation, administrators or teachers have to cope with both satisfiers and dissatisfiers, improve hygiene factors—dissatisfaction is removed from the minds if the staff and students. Provide satisfiers and beneficiaries show some extent act as motivators. Supervisors should be realistic and should not expect motivation by only improving the 'hygienic' work environment.

Evaluation of theory

- The procedure Herzberg adopted is limited by its methodology, when things are going well, people claim credit for themselves
- The reliability of Herzberg's methodology is questioned, since raters have to make interpretations, it is possible that they may contaminate the findings by interpreting one response in one particular manner, while treating a similar response differently
- The theory is valid as it provides an explanation of job satisfaction
- The motivation—Hygiene theory ignores situational variables
- Herzberg assumes that there is a relationship between satisfaction and productivity
- Motivators and hygiene factors contribute to satisfaction as well as dissatisfaction
- There has been an emphasis on motivators, the importance of hygiene factors were ignored.

Merits

- Impact on stimulating thought, Research and experimentation on the topic of motivation at work
- Specific action recommendations for administrators to improve motivational levels of all employees and students
- Content factors primarily related to work motivation
- Job design technique of job enrichment

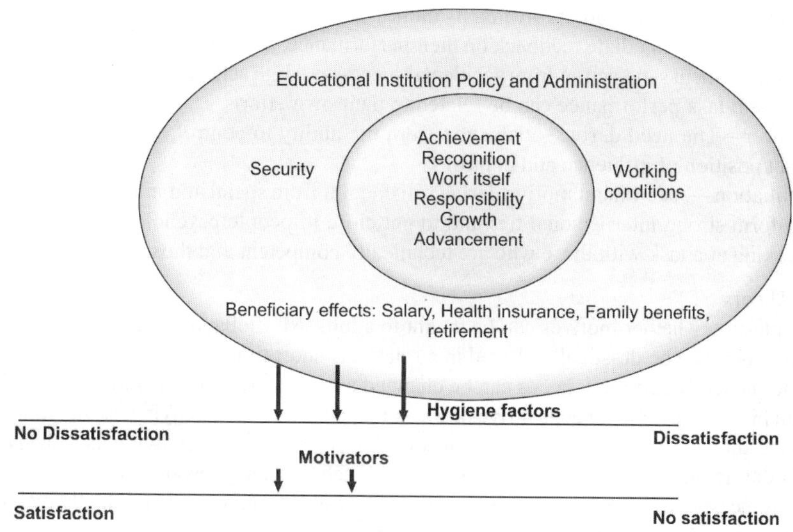

Fig. 14.2: Dual factor theory

Contrasting Views of Satisfaction and Dissatisfaction (Fig. 14.2)

Existence, relatedness and growth theory (ERG Theory)

Alderfer developed ERG theory. The three sets of needs which are the focus of ERG theory of human needs in organizations. More than one need may be operative at the same time. ERG theory postulates a rigid step—like progression. More than one need may be operative at the same time, in other words, Alderfer suggests that there does not exist a rigid hierarchy where a lower level need must be substantially gratified before one can move on. A person can be working on growth eventhough existence or relatedness needs are unsatisfied. When a higher level need is frustrating, the individual's desire to increase a lower level need takes place. Inability to satisfy the need for social interaction, e.g. might increase the desire for more money or for better working conditions. Thus the ERG theory contains a frustration—Regression dimension, frustration at a higher level need can lead to regression to a lower level need.

Evaluation of ERG Theory

It is more consistent with our knowledge of individual differences among people. Variables like Education, Family Background, Cultural environment can alter the importance or driving force that a group of needs holds for a particular individual.

Disadvantages of the theory

• The ERG Model implies that individuals will be motivated to engage in a behavior which will satisfy one of the three set of needs postulated by the theory. In order to predict what behavior any given person will be motivated to engage in, an assessment of that person would be required, to determine which of the three needs were most salient and most important to that person. The individual would then be predicted to engage in a specific behavior, which would lead to the attainment of outcomes, which have the capacity for fulfilling these salient needs

• Too early to pass a judgment on the overall validity of the theory.

3. Achievement Motivation Theory

David C McClelland and his/her associates advocated this theory. The three needs—Power, Affiliation and achievement, motivate human behavior.

• Need for achievement—This need can be learned. Students with a high need for achievement derive satisfaction from reaching their set goals. Succeeding at a task is important to the high achiever. These people are wealthy, their wealth comes from their ability to achieve goals. Goal achievement is rewarded financially, high achievers are not motivated by money per se, money is the indicator of their achievement. High achievers prefer immediate feedback on their performance. They dislike tasks with high risks because they get no achievement satisfaction from accidental successes. High achievers prefer to work independently, so that successful task performance can be related to their own efforts

- Need for power—The need derive satisfaction from the ability to control others. Satisfaction is derived from being in position of influence and control
- Need for affiliation—A dominant motive derive satisfaction from social and interpersonal activities. There is a need to form strong interpersonal ties and to get close to people psychologically. If asked to choose between working at a task with those who are technically competent and those who are their friends.

Evaluation of Theory
- The critics question whether motives can be taught to adults, McClelland however counters and indicated that adult behavior can be drastically altered in a relatively short time
- Needs are permanently acquired, needs can be changed socially through education and training
- Persons with high achievement needs thrive on work i.e., challenging, satisfying, stimulating and complex. They welcome autonomy, variety and frequent feedback from supervisors. Individuals with low achievement needs prefer the situations of stability, security and predictability. They respond better to the persons than to impersonal. A measure of independence, increasing responsibility, autonomy, gradually making tasks more challenging, praising, rewarding and high performance.

Individual + Responsive work   can   ⟶   Work motivation and job satisfaction
Needs   environment   create

Process Theories

1. Expectancy Model/Instrumentality Theory/Path – Goal Theory/Valence Instrumentality Expectancy (VIE) Theory

Victor H. Vroom formulated first expectancy theory (Fig. 14.3). The expectancy theory has its roots in the cognitive concepts of Kurt Lewin and Edward Tolman. This theory is based on the idea that work effort is directed towards behaviors that people believe will lead to desired outcomes, as per this theory the individuals are rational and not impulsive. Through experience, one will develop expectations about whether performance will lead to desired outcomes, and they will direct their efforts towards outcomes that help them to fulfill their needs.

First Level Outcome—Performance achieved as a result of efforts and is reflected through productivity, absenteeism and quality of work.

Second Level Outcomes—The rewards (Positive or Negative) that the first level outcomes are likely to produce. It includes Peer acceptance, increased performance levels, achieving high scores in subjects.

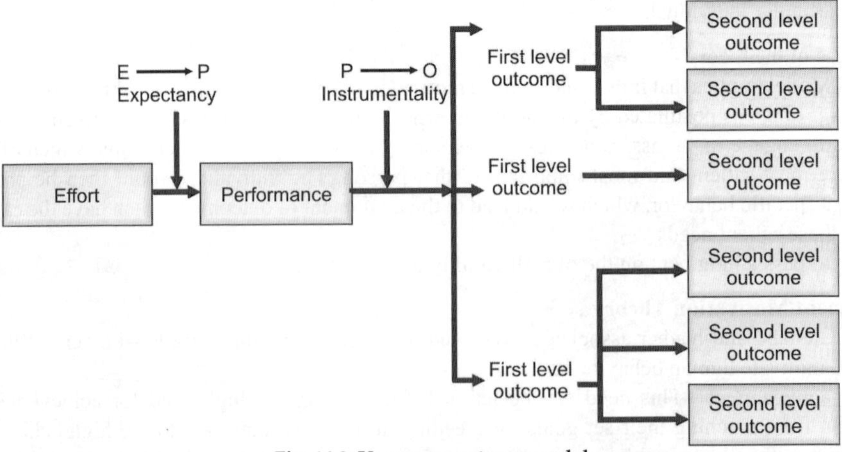

Fig. 14.3: Vroom expectancy model

Expectancy—A particular level of effort will be followed by a specific level of performance.

Effort-to-Performance (E → P)

Instrumentality—Perception by an individual that first level outcomes are associated with second level outcomes. Instrumentality is the relationship between the first level outcomes and the second level outcomes. The values ranging from -1 to +1. If there is no relationship between the first level outcome and the second level outcome the instrumentality is said to be zero.

Performance to Outcome (P→ O)

Valence-An individual's preference for a second level outcome, valence values range from negative to positive. Outcomes having a positive valence includes peer acceptance, respected by friends and educators, performing meaningful tasks, earning enough grades. Outcomes have negative valence includes failures, having disrespect within the group.

Expectancy × Instrumentality × Valence

Educators of successful institutions strive to ensure that student's level of expectancy, instrumentality and valence are high so that they will be highly motivated.

Application of expectancy theory

Variable	Objective	Applications
E → P expectancies	To increase the belief that students are capable of performing professional tasks successfully and fulfill their responsibilities	• Select students with required skills and knowledge • Provide required training and clarify job requirement • Assign simpler or fewer tasks until students can master them • Provide examples of role models who have successfully performed the tasks • Provide counseling and coaching to students who lack self-confidence.
P → O instrumentalities	To increase the belief that good performance will result in valued outcomes	• Measure task performance accurately • Clearly explain the outcomes that will result from successful performance • Provide examples of other exemplars' whose good performance has resulted in higher rewards.
Valence of outcomes	To increase the expected value of outcomes resulting from desired performance	• Distribute rewards that educators value • Individualize rewards • Minimize the presence of countervalent outcomes.

Evaluation of Expectancy Theory

- It provides clear guidelines for increasing persons' motivation by altering the person's expectancies, Instrumentalities and outcome valences
- It is a Cognitive theory, individuals are viewed as thinking, reasoning beings who have beliefs and anticipations concerning future events in their lives. They do not simply act impulsively. It is a model which values human dignity
- Motivation to work can only occur when work can satisfy unsatisfied needs. It is necessary to build and maintain a climate of expectancies that will support requisite levels of motivation to work
- The expectancy model is useful as it serves as a heuristic decision tool to guide managers in dealing with the complexity of motivation in organizations. Motivation principles such as encouraging student performance and matching rewards to performance can be drawn from theory. These Principles can be used to guide educators in designing organizational rewards, work systems, management by objective and goal setting.

2. Equity Theory/Social Comparison Theory/Inequity Theory

Adams' formulation of the equity theory is the most highly developed theory. The equity theory is based on the assumption that individuals are motivated by their desire to be equitably treated in their work relationships. When educators work for an organization, they basically exchange their services for their salary and other remuneration and other benefits. The equity theory proposes that individuals attempt to reduce any inequity they may perceive as a result of this exchange relationship, e.g. if employees perceive that they are either over paid or under paid, they will be motivated to restore equity. The theory proposes that motivation to act develops after the person compares inputs/outcomes with the identical ratio of the comparison other. Inequity is the perception that person's job inputs/outcomes ratio of the comparison other.

Four terms are vital
- Person—The individual for whom an equity or an inequity exists
- Inputs—Characteristics which individuals bring with them to the job, these are subjectively perceived by a person, e.g. Age, Attendance, Interpersonal skills, Communication skills, Level of Education, skills, experiences, job effort, past experience, Performance, personal appearance, seniority, social status, technical skills, training etc
- Outcomes—These are also subjectively perceived by a person, e.g. pay, remuneration, promotion, benefits, challenging job assignments, job requisites, job security, Monotony, Promotion, Recognition, Responsibility, salary, seniority benefits, status symbols, working conditions etc
- Comparison other—Any group or an individual used by a person as a reference regarding inputs and outcomes

The basic equity proposal assumes that, upon feeling inequity, the person is motivated to reduce it. Further, the greater the felt inequity, the greater the motivation to reduce it. Thus inequity as a motivation force will act as follows.

Individual perceives inequity → Individual experiences tension → individual wants to reduce tension — Individual takes action.

When attempting to reduce inequity, the person may try a number of alternatives
- Person altering his/her or her inputs
- Person altering his/her or her outcomes
- Person distorting their inputs and outcomes cognitively
- Person leaving the field
- Person trying to alter or cognitively distort input and outcomes of the comparison other, which force him/her or her to leave the field
- Person changing the comparison other
- It is not that the person feeling inequity alone gets motivated to restore equity. The person with a feeling of equity also gets motivated but to maintain the current situation.

Evaluation of the Theory
- The theory has generated extensive research, with many of the results being supportive
- The theory recognizes the influence of social comparison processes on motivation., inputs and outcomes and their comparison
- It adopts a realistic approach to motivation, it is the perceived equity of the situation that stimulates motivation and satisfaction.

3. Performance Satisfaction Model

Porter and Lawler came out with a comprehensive theory of motivation. They posit that motivation, performance and satisfaction are all separate variables and relate in ways different from what was traditionally assumed. Performance is mediated by abilities, traits and role perceptions. The rewards that follow and how they are perceived will determine the satisfaction.

Evaluation of the Theory
The Porter and Lawler model is of great significance to organizers since it offers guidelines to motivate their employees
- Place the right person on the right job (match abilities and traits of individuals to the requirement of the job)
- Carefully explain to the employees what their roles are, and make sure that they understand their roles
- Prescribe in concrete terms the actual performance levels expected of the individuals
- Make sure that the rewards dispersed are valued by the employees.

The Porter and Lawler model has definitely made a significant contribution to the better understanding of work motivation and the relationship between performance and satisfaction.

ATTITUDE

An attitude represents an individual's degree of like or dislike for an item. Attitudes are learned "predispositions to respond" held by individuals that make them likely to act in certain ways. Attitudes are not observable, but they do serve to help produce observable actions in people. Attitudes are judgments. They develop on the *ABC* model (affect, behavior and cognition). The affective response is an emotional response that expresses an individual's degree of preference for an entity. The behavioral intention is a verbal indication or typical behavioral tendency of an individual. The cognitive response is a cognitive evaluation of the entity that constitutes an individual's beliefs about the object. Most attitudes are the result of either direct experience or observational learning from the environment.

Definitions

"Readiness of the psyche to act or react in a certain way"—*Jung, 1921*

"A mental and neutral state of readiness, organized through experience exerting directive or dynamic influence upon the individuals' response to all objects or situations with which it is related"—*Allport*

"A Readiness to respond in a favorable or an unfavorable manner, to a particular object or class of objects i.e. the attitudes have topic, judgmental or evaluative and are relatively long lasting (The readiness to respond)—*Oskamp, 1977.*

"Attitude is an enduring system that includes a cognitive, conative and affective/feeling components".

Types

Attitudes very often come in pairs

- Attitudes are generally positive (e.g. A positive attitude toward people with mental illnesses is a necessary dimension of psychiatric nursing practice) or negative views of a person, place, thing or event—this is often referred to as the attitude object
- One conscious and the other unconscious. Consciousness has a constellation of contents different from that of the unconscious, a duality particularly evident in neurosis
- Extraversion and introversion. This pair is so elementary to Jung's theory of types that he/she labeled them the "attitude-types"
- Rational and irrational attitudes, e.g. "I conceive reason as an attitude". The rational attitude subdivides into the thinking and feeling psychological functions, each with its attitude
- The irrational attitude subdivides into the sensing and intuition psychological functions, each with its attitude. "Thus a typical thinking, feeling, sensation and intuitive attitude exists"
- Individual and social attitudes. Many of the latter are "isms"
- Abstract attitude—Abstraction is contrasted with concretism—By this I mean a peculiarity of thinking and feeling which is the antithesis of abstraction, e.g. "I hate his/her attitude for being Sarcastic".

Formation of Attitudes

Situational stimuli or events in the environment directly influence behavior. Attitudes are expected to change as a function of experience, values, beliefs and hereditary variables. A change in attitude or beliefs occurs as a result of actions that have been influenced by reinforcers. Social learning theory expands this principle. According to social-learning theorists, it is not essential to learn behaviors directly through action and reinforcement, as traditional behavioral psychologists would propose. Indirect learning through observing a model and receiving verbal instruction has a powerful impact on behavior and attitude formation. Situations that include a change in the behavioral component of attitude lead to changes in attitudes. But there is also a reciprocal action. Since the components of attitude systems are interrelated, a change in liking (affect) may result in a change in behaviors, e.g. the currently popular concept of the cognitive apprenticeship is based on the idea of learners participating as apprentices in real-world activities with those who are more knowledgeable than they. If designed correctly, these situations are perceived by learners as important and realistic and learners come to value them.

The overt activities of cognitive apprenticeships produce in students favorable dispositions (i.e., affects), which in turn promote a sense of value and often a desire to learn more.

Attitude Systems

Attitude positions are the summary aggregation of four components. These four components of attitude form an attitude system. The components are not isolated but are interrelated and produce an organizing framework or mental representation of the attitude construct: (a) affective responses, (b) cognitions, (c) behaviors, (d) behavioral intentions.

- The affective component of attitude is said to consist of a person's evaluation of, liking of or emotional response to some situation, object or person. Affective responses reflect one's attitude with sensations of pleasure, sadness or other levels of physical arousal, e.g. for the attitude construct of computer anxiety, a topic of current interest, the affective component would be a person's liking of the computer and his/her feeling of excitement or dread, when she or he/she used one
- The cognitive component of an attitude is conceptualized as a person's factual knowledge of the situation, object or person, including oneself. In other words, the cognitive component refers to how much a person knows about a topic, such as computers. The cognitive component of computer anxiety would be based on how much a person knows about computers and her/his level of understanding of computer operation
- Since attitudes involve emotional component, the resistance to change occurs and it does not generally respond to new facts. People can have attitudes about almost anything. In each instance the individual is predisposed to respond an object, issue or group, where the object may be a social object, i.e. a person or creation of a person or a social event
- The behavioral component of an attitude involves the person's overt behavior directed toward a situation, object or person, e.g. the behavioral component of computer anxiety would be related to how often a person had used a computer and what kind of experience he/she had. Persons who routinely use computers, especially if they choose to use them freely, would be more likely to have positive attitudes toward computers and be less anxious, than would others who have fewer experiences with computers
- Finally, the behavioral intention component involves the person's plans to perform in a certain way, even if sometimes these plans are never acted upon. For example, Computer anxiety is defined by Maurer and Simonson (1994) as "the fear or apprehension felt by an individual when considering the implications of utilizing computer technology or when actually using computer technology". The behavioral intention component of this attitude construct would be the "apprehension felt by an individual when considering the implications of utilizing computer technology". In other words, if people knew that they were going to have to use computers in an upcoming class, this would partially shape their level of computer anxiety. If the class were to be a difficult one, say in statistics, then computer anxiety would be likely to be increased.

Attitude Change

- Genetic factors influence attitudes in general disposition, e.g. the tendency to experience positive or negative effect—To be in a positive or negative mood. Such tendencies in turn could influence evaluation of many factors in the social world, e.g. an individual who experiences positive mood all the time, might tend to express a high level of job satisfaction, no matter where the person works. Similarly if the person is of negative in nature will express negativity in all the situations; Mate selection, Aggressive nature, Neurotic behavior etc
- Attitudes are acquired through other persons, i.e. social learning, social comparison, e.g. Attraction, Relationships, Perceptions of fairness etc
- The attitude do not always predict behavior uncovered
- A set of tendencies or predispositions to behave in a certain ways in social situations. Thus attitudes were exhibited by individuals' overt behavior
- There is often a sizable gap between what the individuals say and what exactly or actually do. So actual behavior is not just verbally reported as attitudes
- Specificity, Strength, Accessibility, Aspects of situations, e.g. in certain religions, abortion is considered as a sin. Polygamy is followed in Muslims, People choose situations where they can engage in consistent behaviors with their attitudes, the attitudes themselves are strengthened and predicted the behaviors, certain

other situations that allowed them to express their attitudes on several issues, e.g. affirmative action, religion. In addition the same persons performed the tasks in which they were indicated as quickly as possible, whether they agreed or disagreed with statements relating to these attitudes, the stronger the attitudes, people will respond very quickly and predictions of behavior is expected or observed, Situational pressure shape the extent to which the attitudes are expressed in overt actions, but in addition, attitudes determine whether individuals choose to enter into various situations, time factor or time pressure, e.g. the individuals react quickly when pressure is there and other factors will influence attitudes and individuals' behavior

- Attitudes are formed on the basis of direct experience often exert stronger effects on behavior, apparently attitudes formed on the basis of direct experience are easier to bring to mind, and this magnifies their impact on behavior
- The strength of attitudes—The stronger the attitudes, the greater the effect or impact on behavior, they are also resistant to change, are more stable over a period of time and have a greater impact on several aspects of social cognition. The extremity or intensity of an attitude, its importance, which individual cares deeply about and is personally affected by attitudes, how much the individual knows the intensity of the object and how easily the attitudes comes to mind in various situations all these components play a role in strength of an attitudes
- Self interest—The greater the impact of individuals' self interest, the more importance of an attitude
- Identification—The greater the extent to which an attitude is held by with which an individual identifies, the greater its' importance
- Value relevance—The more closely an attitude is connected to an individual's personal values, the greater its' importance
- Attitude accessibility—The strength of attitude object—Evaluation link in memory. The stronger this link, the more quickly or readily an attitude can come to mind—The thought, decision and action
- Attitude specificity—The extent to which the attitudes are focused on specific objects or situations, rather than general ones, e.g. A person may have an attitude about religion, as it is important for everyone to have some religious convictions, but much more specific attitudes about the importance attending services in a week or its' important or unimportant not go every week or wearing religious symbols as dollar for chain, on the face applying Vibhudi or Kumkum, etc. It is something like to do or do not want to do., the attitude behavior link is stronger, when attitudes and behavior are measured at the same level of specificity. We would probably be more accurate in predicting willingness, to take action to protect religious freedom from genera; attitude toward religion, than from attitude about wearing religious jewelry so attitude specificity, is an important
- Aspects of individuals—Some persons use their attitude to guide their behavior, they look inward in their behavior before taking certain decisions in their life situations, i.e. self monitoring. Others in contrast focus their attention outward—They see what others are doing or saying and try to behave in the manner that will be viewed most favorably by the people around them
- Strength of attitude—Behavior link does seem to differ, for persons with high and low ends, high and low self-monitors, respectively. Individuals do differ in the extent to which their attitudes predict the behavior, and self-monitoring appears to play an important role in such differences
- To operate in situations where we give careful, deliberate thought to attitudes and their implications on their behavior
- Attitudes seem to influence the behavior in a more direct and seemingly automatic manner. Some activity motivates the attitude and activated, influences our perceptions of the attitude object
- When we have time to engage in careful, reasoned thought, we can weigh all alternatives and decide, quite deliberately how to act, under the hectic conditions of everyday of social life, however, we offer don't have time for this kind of deliberate weighing of alternatives, in such cases our attitudes seem to shape our perception of various events and hence our immediate behavioral reactions towards them
- Attitudes can be changed through-persuasion and we should understand attitude change as a response to communication
- Intelligence—More intelligent people are less easily persuaded by one-sided messages

- Self-esteem—Higher in self-esteem are less easily persuaded, there is some evidence that the relationship between self-esteem and persuasibility is actually curvilinear, with people of moderate self-esteem being more easily persuaded than both those of high and low self-esteem levels
- Source Characteristics—Like, expertise, trustworthiness and interpersonal attraction or attractiveness. The credibility of a perceived message has been found to be a key variable
- The nature of the message plays a role in persuasion
- A message can appeal to an individual's cognitive evaluation to help change an attitude
- Emotion is a common component in persuasion, social influence and attitude change. Emotion works hand-in-hand with the cognitive process or the way we think, about an issue or situation. Emotional appeals are commonly found in advertising, health campaigns and political messages. For example, no smoking health campaigns, political campaign advertising emphasizing the fear of terrorism
- Attitudes are part of the brain's associative networks, the spider—like, structures residing in long-term memory that consist of affective and cognitive nodes
- By activating an affective or emotion node, attitude change may be possible, though affective and cognitive components tend to be intertwined. In primarily affective networks, it is more difficult to produce cognitive counterarguments in the resistance to persuasion and attitude change
- Affective forecasting, otherwise known as intuition or the prediction of emotion, also impacts attitude change. Predicting emotions is an important component of decision making, in addition to the cognitive processes. How we feel about an outcome may override purely cognitive rationales.
- Emotions perceived as negative or containing threat are often studied more than perceived positive emotions like humor, it appeals may work by creating incongruities in the mind. actors that influence the impact of emotion appeals include self efficacy, attitude accessibility, issue involvement, and message/source features. Self-efficacy is a perception of one's own human agency; it is the perception of our own ability to deal with a situation. It is an important variable in emotion appeal messages because it dictates a person's ability to deal with both the emotion and the situation. For example, if a person is not self-efficacious about their ability to impact the global environment, they are not likely to change their attitude or behavior about global warming
- Message features such as source nonverbal communication, message content, and receiver differences can impact the emotion impact of fear appeals. The characteristics of a message are important because one message can elicit different levels of emotion for different people
- Attitude accessibility refers to the activation of an attitude from memory in other words, how readily available is an attitude about an object, issue or situation
- Issue involvement is the relevance and salience of an issue or situation to an individual. Issue involvement has been correlated with both attitude access and attitude strength
- Implicit and explicit attitudes seem to affect people's behavior, though in different ways. They tend not to be strongly associated with each other, although in some cases they are.
- Implicit attitudes, which are generally unacknowledged or outside of awareness, but have effects that are measurable through sophisticated methods using people's response times to stimuli
- Cognitive schemata provide structure to interrelated attitudes and guide the information processes of attending, interpreting, and reconstructing.

Importance of Attitudes

Traditionally when instruction is designed, there are two categories of outcomes in mind: Those directed toward cognitive goals and those related to the attitudes of the learner. Achievement is the paramount objective of most instructional activities. However, it may also be important to recognize the need for establishing attitudinal goals and for planning activities designed to facilitate affective outcomes in learners as a consequence of an instructional situation. As a matter of fact, it has become increasingly apparent to those involved in educational technology research that one of the major, and possibly unique, consequences of instructional situations involving media is the likelihood of the development of positive attitudinal positions in students. The most powerful rationale for the need to promote attitude positions in learners would be to demonstrate a direct relationship between attitudes and achievement or liking and learning. There are too many intervening forces likely to influence the relationship between how a person feels and how he/she or she behaves. Attitudes are thought to "predispose" persons to act positive attitudes toward a topic are felt to orient the person in a positive manner toward that idea, but not to predict actions directly. The impact of attitude on learning is only one reason for interest in attitudes.

Most educators would agree that there are times when it is legitimate, and important, for learners to accept the truth of certain ideas-in other words, to accept an attitudinal position. The importance of voting is an attitude position that most would agree is important.

While the strength of the relationship between attitudes and achievement is unclear, it seems logical that students are more likely to remember information, seek new ideas and continue studying when they react favorably to an instructional situation or like a certain content area. Learners tend to do what they like, not what they do not like. They gravitate toward their interests.

There are some instances when influencing student's attitudes is not desirable, so educators should be aware of which techniques affect attitudes. In this way, possible bias can be recognized and eliminated. The gender biases found in textbooks are considered partially responsible for gender biases in people. For example, the use of the generic—He/She was long considered appropriate by textbook authors and publishers.

Student attitudes toward a situation can tell the teacher a great deal about the impact of that situation on the learning process. Obviously, attitudes need to be measured in order to know if they have been influenced. As a result of quantitatively and qualitatively assessing the opinions of students toward the learning activities in which they are participating, it may be possible to improve the quality of procedures. One of the most important techniques of evaluation is to ascertain attitudes toward some event, object or person. End-of-course evaluations of attitude toward courses and course content are a standard activity in schools and training centers.

CRISIS

Introduction

Human being has to maintain balance in life; whenever he/she is exposed to stressor or stressful situations he/she will try to overcome it by his/her own way of dealing with problems, by adopting adequate coping strategies and with the help of situational support. 'Eustress' is always essential for the individual to lead qualitative life; but when he/she exposed to many stressors at a time, even with the utilization of balance factors adequately also or if one or more absence of balancing factors results in disequilibrium and it may lead to crisis. A Psychological crisis results when an individual is unable to resolve the problem. As a result tension, anxiety, prolonged period of emotional upset he/she feels helpless and unable to take action to resolve the problem, disorganized behavior will result. The outcome is governed by the kind of interaction between the individual and the key persons or situational support (family and friends) in his/her emotional milieu or appropriate help in right time. Crisis is usually lasts for few hours to 4 to 6 weeks. It may be an integral component of everyday life situations. If proper guidance will be provided at correct time, the victim will be able to solve the problem and will be able to handle future problems in life, in a better manner. Thus crisis is a challenge, an opportunity for learning and growth, it is a sporadic phenomenon that punctuates our existence dramatically.

Definitions

"It is a stressor which, focus an individual to respond and to adopt in some way"—*Psychological terms*

"Any temporary situation that threatens the person's self-concept, necessitates reorganization of the psychological structure and behavior, causes a sudden alteration in the person's expectation of self and can not be handled with the person's usual coping mechanisms"—*Caplan, 1964*

"A state of disequilibrium resulting from the interaction of an event with the individual's or family's coping mechanisms, which are inadequate to meet the demands of the situation, combined with the individual's or family's perception of the meaning of the event"—*Taylor, 1982*

"A sudden event that occurs in one's life, which disturbs the individual homeostasis and usual coping mechanisms will not resolve the problem"—*Largerquist, 2001*

"An internal disturbance results from stressful event or a perceived threat to self precipitatory events"—*Dr. BT Basavanthappa, 2007*

"Crisis is a subjective experience in which old ways of doing things no longer assure success and survival".

"A crisis situation is the result of a person's perception and emotional response to a loss or threat of loss of self-esteem from events".

"When an individual is failing to respond adequately by utilizing efficient coping mechanisms to the stressors/painful stimulus/repeated exposure to stressful events and unable to meet the demands and the needs, a state of internal imbalance will result, known as "crisis".

Crisis Proneness

- Dissatisfaction in life may be with employment or lack of employment
- History of unresolved crisis
- History of substance abuse
- Loss of loved one
- Lack of support systems, e.g. family, social, religious, economic, employment and supportive systems
- Severe family disorder
- Poor self-esteem, unworthiness
- Lack of communication skills or inability to ask for help
- Lack of intimate relationships with others
- Difficulty in using coping mechanisms in everyday situations or inadequate coping skills
- Under utilization or of resources, support systems
- Aloofness, lack of loved ones for showing concern; emotional isolation
- Perceived loss, e.g. death of a significant family member, divorce, loss of job, loss of a body part threat of loss, e.g. illness of family member, conflicts with partner or attempted rape or challenges, e.g. change in responsibilities change in different line of work
- Rapid encountering of one stressful situation after another stressful situation
- Spouse or child abuse
- Accidents.

Characteristics of Crisis

- Individual is totally involved, get hurt in all heightened feeling of stress, i.e. disorganization of
  - Biological
  - Cognitive ⎫ Experience indicating unpleasant emotional feelings
  - Emotional
  - Behavioral
- Unable to interpret and perceive the circumstances of crisis event
- Precipitating by specific identifiable event of actual or perceived losses, threats of losses or challenges
- It occurs in all the individuals at one time or other
- Crisis are personal by nature
- Crisis are acute, will be solved by one or another within a brief period
- It is self-limiting, lasts for 4 to 6 weeks
- Crisis situation may have the potential for psychological growth or retardation or dangerous to person (may harm to self or other); unable to function effectively
- Individual is most open for intervention: Client will develop willingness to learn new coping strategies feels it as an opportunity and ways of attacking problem, hence their personality growth and positive change in attitudes reduces the incidence and severity of mental illness if the crisis is overwhelming nature it may affect any potential growth leads to maladaptive or dysfunctional behavior or deterioration
- Universal experience
- Almost all crises will develop in a predictable fashion.

Developmental Phases of Crisis

Crisis results from certain distinct biopsychosocial phases, it follows relatively predictable course.

Caplan in 1964, described four specific phases, through which individual progresses into crisis in response to a precipitating stressor.

Phase 1: Whenever an individual is exposed to precipitating stressor, it results into anxiety; to overcome it, if individual uses effective problem solving techniques and situational support, then the problem will be resolved and no crisis occurs.

Phase 2: When coping mechanisms are ineffective, anxiety, discomfort, helplessness further increases, person's ability to overcome the stressor will decreases; confusion, personal disorganization prevails.

Phase 3: Individual feels more pressure, unable to respond, anxiety still increases; in this phase all external and internal resources will be tried to resolve the crisis and to relieve discomfort, i.e. the individual uses every means like cognitive emotional and physiological, counseling, etc. as a last resort; if it fails the premorbid functioning will results.

Phase 4: If problem was not solved, tension reaches to its peak, as time passes burden increases over time. Panic state will result and the manifestations includes: labile emotional state, psychotic thinking, depression, distorted cognitive process, unproductive behavior, short attention span, apprehension, distress and impaired relationship will results; They feel they are 'loosing their mind' and 'going crazy'. Extensive treatment is necessary if negative outcomes are apparent.

Tyhurst described the stages in crisis as:
- A period of impact, when an individual realizes the event
- A period of recoil when distress becomes over whelming and the individual struggles to cope up
- A Posttraumatic Period the individual experiences disruption in normal functioning.
  Phase—I: Anxiety
  Phase—II: Tension continues
  Phase—III: Painful state of anxiety
  Phase—IV: When inner resources, situational support, coping strategies failure results into actual crisis leads to anxiety, panic state and personal disorganization.
  The effect of balancing factors in a stressful event (see Fig. 14.4).

Crisis is the turning point or crucial point in the life of an individual, a decisive stage in the progress of anything. It is an emotional reaction to an event or respond to the unexpected. An individual strives to maintain a constant state of emotional equilibrium, if any overwhelming threat occurs, if he/she is unable to cope up, crisis will results.

Types of Crisis

1. Situational Crisis/External Crisis/Coincidental Crisis

If biopsychosocial equilibrium upsets because of external event or due to environmental influence. It is sudden, unexpected onset; majority of times it is singular facet in origin. For example, Death of a loved one, an accident, a sexual assault, divorce, change in geographical areas, loss of employment, loss of valued object, loss of status, an acute illness or admission into hospital. Situational crisis centers around losses that impact on the individual.

Each transition from one developmental stage to another leads to termination of previous life structure; each transition is an ending process involving separation or loss. It is an opportunity to review one's life and separate it from difficult or traumatic events.

An acute response occurs due to an external situational stressor i.e., dispositional crisis.

2. Maturational Crisis/Developmental Crisis/Internal Crisis

In the transitional stage of life, where the individual will move into successive stages often generate disequilibrium. Individuals have to make cognitive and behavioral change to accommodate physical changes that accompany development. It will be dependent on previous experiences, availability of situational support,

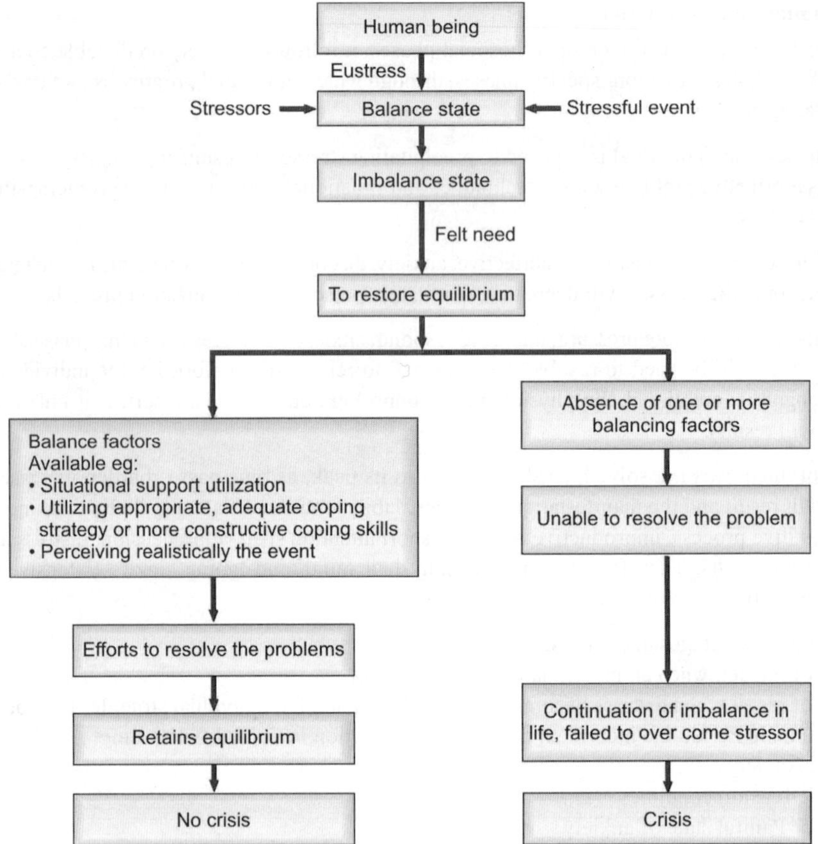

Fig. 14.4: Process of crisis
(Modified paradigm from Aguilera. D.C. and Messick.J.M. Crisis intervention;
Theory and methodology, 1982, 1998 C.V. Mosby Co. St. Louis)

motivation from significant people, acceptability and performance of new role by others. The tasks of each stage must be completed for the individual to grow and move toward maturity. For example, adolescence, marriage, antenatal period, parenthood, retirement, death of spouse or loved one and loss of job, etc.

Maturational crisis involves how an individual will perceive themselves, their role and their status. He/she is unprepared for traumatic occurrences and have negative maturational effects.

Crisis occurs due to situations that trigger emotions related to unresolved conflicts in their life. These crisis are internal in origin, e.g. need for emotional intimacy.

3. **Sociocultural Crisis**

It arises from the cultural values that are embedded in the social structure. For example, discrimination between race; robbery, etc.

4. **Crisis Resulting from Traumatic Stress**

Crisis results when unexpected external stress occur over which the individual has little or no control. For example, Rape; Robbery and Terrorism.

5. **Crisis Resulting from Psychopathology**

Pre-existing psychopathology has been instrumental in precipitating the crisis or in which psychopathology significantly impairs or complicates, e.g. borderline personality, severe Neurosis and Schizophrenia.

6. **Adventitious Crisis/Community Crisis**

   It is accidental, uncommon, unanticipated results in multiple losses may be because of environmental changes. For example, natural disasters like floods, earth quakes; contamination of large areas by toxic waste products, tidal waves, famine, nuclear wars, etc. people believe that the event may occur due to God's anger or fate. The psychological disturbances will occur, e.g. fear, confusion, etc. mental health professionals has to provide counseling services to overcome the problems.

7. **Psychiatric Emergencies**

   Crisis occurs when general functioning is impaired and the individual is incompetent to assume personal responsibility. For example, suicide, addicts.

Crisis Continuum

- Potential crisis state: Whenever any acute problem or serious threat occurs, individuals will become tense and employs emergency problem-solving methods to resolve crisis, but it is ineffective.
- Pre-crisis state: When person has high probability of exposure to stressful events, inadequate support, lack of coping abilities, poor history of handling stress will be more upset and enter into a state of disequilibrium.
- Immediate crisis state: As tensions continue to build, they mobilize all internal and external resources to restore the equilibrium.
- Intermediate crisis state: The problem may be re-evaluated and attacked from a new angle or the problem may be distorted and viewed as unsolvable.
- Advanced crisis state: Persons who has continued to draw all inner resources, has continued failing in attempts to resolve the problems; emotional pressures continue to build and people become completely disorganized or immobilized owing to serve anxiety or depression state.
- Full crisis state: Person who has failed in all attempts to solve the problems, believes that all resources have been used and lack relief from stress.

Clinical Manifestations in Crisis Situation

- Heavy burden or free floating anxiety, e.g. heightened emotional tensions, the drive to act
- Depression or agitated
- Anger, guilt, tension, fear, the drive to act
- Neglects in performing self-care activities and fulfilling responsibilities
- Utilizing unhealthy coping mechanisms
- Irrational and blaming others
- Helplessness, Hopelessness
- Chaos, overwhelmed
- Detached, despair
- Depersonalized
- Panic
- Low self-esteem
- Uncontrollable crying
- Frustration, confused, depressed, immobilized, unable to make decisions
- Lack of confidence and discouragement
- Imperfection, unfamiliarity with self
- Lack of self control
- Altered sensorium
- Disorganized thinking
- Unable to plan, reasoning, logical analysis
- Impaired judgment
- Hallucinations
- Preoccupation with certain ideas
- Somatic distress
- Physical illnesses
- Shortness of breath, choking, hyperventilation fatigue, tremors, anorexia

- Disorganized behavior, unable to think realistically
- Inappropriate relationships
- Apathetic or euphoric
- Avoids thinking about the event, disoriented
- Rigid in nature, Denial
- Withdrawal behavior, aloofness
- Avoids reality with over activity
- Unwilling to initiate new behavior
- Unable to maintain daily routine, work performance or social roles
- Irritable
- Low self-esteem
- Painful feelings, blames others
- Change in life style.

Crisis Therapy

Indications for crisis intervention

- Abstinence
- Pediatric
- Geriatric   }   Maturational crisis
- Adolescent
- People who attempted suicide
- Psychosomatic patients
- Violent behavior, e.g. crime
- Accident victims
- Family crisis
- High risk families, e.g. recent death, H/O difficulty in using coping strategies, chronic illness and bereavement
- Severe depression
- Severe anxiety
- Marital conflicts
- Suicidal thought
- Illicit drug abuse; alcohol abuse
- Traumatic events or traumatic experiences
- Intra group staff issues
- Client management issues.

Settings for crisis intervention

- Hospitals — Out patient
  In patient
  Emergency room settings
- Mental Health Care centers
- Community setting
  - Home visits
  - Out reach centers
  - Deaddiction centers
  - Community Rehab homes.
- Telephonic counseling and Hot line
  - Crisis calls
  - Ventilation calls
  - Information calls.
- Suicide prevention and crisis intervention centers
- Schools, offices and private practice centers.

Principles

Use comfort strategies

- By accepting the person and the problem
- Establishing social relationship by developing rapport and showing positive concern to lessen anxiety and to create a sense of hope and worthfulness
- Let the family understand that coming for help is a good indication and a sign of strength and judgment.

Ventilation or catharsis

- Encourage the client to express openly the facts
- Concern the person's feelings are normal
- Work with feelings of the client
- Help the person to confront with crisis by talking about present denial feelings and recognize denial as a normal reaction to crisis
- Motivate the person to talk about the losses and changes involved in crisis
- Clarify the person's perception of current difficulties
- Explain the relationship between crisis and the present behavior
- Give the person time to experience the feelings and to fully express them
- Avoid giving false reassurance
- Do not encourage the client to blame as, others are responsible for the occurance of crisis situation
- Help the person to confront crisis
- Encourage the person to do what he/she can do for self
- Reinforce previously learned behavior patterns that are effective and useful suggestions
- Involve the client in seeking and accepting help
- Familiarity with community resources needed for additional service.

Tips to be used for successful course of crisis therapy

- Therapist has to establish good rapport, maintains warmth and render care quickly
- Positive attitude
- Constructive use of time in identification of client's response to the event, to plan a course of action; implements steps to resolve the crisis
- Identifying the resources
- Therapist must be open and show acceptance to maintain basic life style and value system.

Techniques of Crisis Intervention

Abreaction

The release of emotional feelings that takes place when the client talks about emotionally charged areas.

The Nurse encourages the client, how he/she feels about a particular incident, recent events and significant people involved in crisis. For example, the Nurse: Tell, how are you feeling, since that incident occurred.

Clarification

Encouraging the client to express more clearly the relationship between certain events in his/her life. It helps the client to understand his/her feelings and the pattern of developing these feelings into crisis. For example, after having an argument, discussion about future in life with spouse: the client became sick. The Nurse encourages the client to understand the relationship between his/her feelings and the development of crisis.

Suggestion

Nurse will suggest the client and it influences him, accepts the idea, and client will feel that the Nurse can help him/her to feel better and optimistic, makes him/her less anxious, For example, show the client, the persons with self-confident, calm, hopeful and who can help, the client also feels optimistic and tries to adapt to situation.

Manipulation

It is a way of influencing the client, using the patient's emotions, wishes or values to benefit the client in the therapeutic process. For example, stronger commitment will have longer and prosperous career.

Reinforcement of behavior

If the client exhibits adaptive behavior give positive response by appreciating it. For example, "I observed, you have done it, you can do it".

Support of defenses

Encourage the client to use healthy and adaptive behavior to cope up stressful situations to maintain ego integrity, at the same time discourage the maladaptive, unhealthy behavior. For example, ask the client, when he/she is angry, over the other, divert it by drinking half glass of cool water and doing other works.

Raising self-esteem

Help the client to regain the feelings of self worth, active participation, communicates effectively, good listening skills, accepts his/her feelings with respect. For example, "You have done so many tasks in your life upto now, I feel you can be able to do this task also".

Exploration of solutions

Examining the alternative ways of solving immediate problem. The Nurse and the client actively explore solutions to solve crisis. For example, you seem to know, many people in your profession and in the area of specialization, you contact them, the availability of jobs and its procedures for better placement.

Disaster work or disaster response

By debriefing method disaster crisis can be resolved. It is an organized planned intervention for larger group of population, Nurses has to go to the places where victims are likely residing after disaster in post disaster period to provide services.

Steps

- Identification of trauma and grief issues
- Assessment of severity and trauma
- Appropriate crisis intervention and support
- IEC strategies.

Problem solving technique

In 1910, John Dewery has suggested certain problem solvation techniques.

- Identify and define the difficulty or problem
- Suggest possible solutions or listing alternatives
- Choosing from among alternatives
- Consider consequences
- Encourage the client to accept and utilize the solution by implementing plan
- Evaluation.

Family work

- Identify the individual and family affected with crisis. Involving the family in client care is essential, Nurses has to have knowledge related to family dynamics
- Provide calm, conducive and comfortable environment to the client, help him/her to establish good rapport and IPR between the client and his/her family identify the stressor and suggest possible attacking of the problem, utilize the best suiting approach to resolve the crisis, follow up visit has to be fixed to evaluate or reassess whether desired outcome achieved or not, if needed modified strategies has to be adopted
- Plan the psycho educational programs for education and support. Self help movement, pragmatic in approach has to be used for effective patient and family functioning. Provide information to family about system of mental health, body and mind relationship and clinical manifestations of mental illness
- Promote skills related to communication, conflict resolution, problem solving, stress management and behavioral management etc.

- Provide opportunity to ventilate, share and mobilize the resources
- Increase use of informal and formal support net works
- To meet a range of needs of the client
- Family interventions consists of educational, supportive, cognitive and behavioral strategies.

Group work

Nurse and Group help the patient to solve the problem and develop new coping strategies. Nurse will be active, focal and present problem oriented. The group and the client will follow the Nurse as a role model and ideal example, uses similar therapeutic techniques. Group acts as a support system for the client. Mostly crisis groups focuses on people who have common traits or exposed to common stressors. Groups facilitate the members to express common concerns and experiences, fosters hope and provides mutual support, e.g. hospitalization of the client.

Patient education

The therapeutic team members will educate and counsel the client and his/her family about problem resolving techniques, alternative adoptive coping strategies; importance of having balance mind and emotional maturity. In evaluation phase of crisis intervention, patient's and their families, anxiety will be reduced and cognitive abilities will be increased, educate the public to identify the crisis situations and victims. Necessary interventions has to be adopted, identify potential available resources in dealing with crisis problems and its solutions, strategies can be discussed.

Process of crisis intervention

The techniques which are used to help the affected individual and his/her family, to understand and cope up with the intense feelings that are typical of a crisis.

Goals

- To return to a precrisis level of functioning
- To provide real perception of the situation by the client
- To assist the individual in managing the intense and overwhelming feelings associated with crisis
- To resolve the crisis situation.

The Role of the Nurse in crisis Intervention

Phase 1: Assessment

- Ability to perceive the problematic situation
- Identification of precipitating event or stressor and when it occurred
- Balancing factors
- Nature and strength of clients. Supporting systems and coping resources, strategies that can be used
- Client's abilities and limitations in dealing with the problem
- Needs of the client, e.g. self-esteem, role mastery, dependency and biological function
- Nature of crisis and its effects on the individual and family
- Associated behavioral problems, e.g. suicidal potentialities
- Physical and mental status of an individual
- H/O previous exposure and adapted coping strategies
- Exploration of problematic situation.

Phase 2: Nursing diagnosis

After analyzing the information gathered through assessment, appropriate Nursing diagnosis can be formulated to solve the immediacy of the crisis situation. Nursing diagnosis may be related to any aspect of the client's life, which can reflect the variety of nursing problems. For example, ineffective individual or family coping

- Disturbed thought processes
- Risk for emergency situation like suicide or violence, post traumatic stress or experiences
- Altered family processes
- Maladaptive crisis responses.

Phase 3: Planning

Based on the assessment and diagnosis, the short-term and long-term goals will be formulated with a specific and appropriate plan of activities. In formulating interventions: client's abilities or strengths, available resources for support, alternative solutions to the problem and steps for achieving the solutions has to be identified.

Phase 4: Implementation of interventions

- Nurses has to use reality oriented approach
- Remain with the individual who is experiencing panic anxiety
- Establish a rapid, positive working relationship by
  - Showing unconditional acceptance
  - Active listening
  - Attending to immediate needs
  - Appropriate communication techniques to make the client to feel more comfortable.
- Discourage lengthy explanation by rationalizing the situation
- Provide adequate situational support and guidance
- Promote conducive atmosphere for ventilation of true or real overwhelming, intense emotional feelings
- Set firm limits (to avoid aggressive or destructive behavior) what is acceptable and not acceptable
- Handle the feelings gently, do not give false reassurance
- Maintain consistency
- Encourage the client not to blame others as it promotes escapism from taking responsibilities
- Clarify the problem; assist the individual to determine precipitating factor of crisis
- Accept the intense emotional feelings, e.g. anger, guiltiness, etc.
- Guide the individual in problem-solving process and to alleviate future crisis by exploring the problematic situations, discussing alternative problem-solving strategies—Its benefits and consequences
- Client should not develop dependency over the counselor
- Utilize external support systems and new social networks to provide assistance and plan of action
- Advise for follow up visit.

Ashields has described four levels of crisis intervention, it will be often helpful to consult with others. When deciding which approach has to be used.

I. Environmental manipulation:

It provides situational support, it will directly change the client's physical or interpersonal situations. For Example, 1. If an individual is facing problem in working environment to avoid stress, he/she may change another job. 2. If the client is feeling difficulty to stay alone, place him/her along with the group or with the siblings for promoting comfort to the client.

II. General support:

Warmth, support, acceptance, empathy, caring, concern and reassurance has to be rendered to provide general support.

III. Generic Approach:

To reach high risk individuals and large groups as early as possible, a specific method will be used to the persons who have similar problem. For example, Grief, disasters.

Debriefing, a therapeutic intervention will be used to recall the traumatic events and to clarify painful experiences and to prevent maladaptive responses.

IV. Individual approach:

Nurse has to understand clients specific psychodynamics that led to the present crisis and must use the intervention to develop an adaptive response to the crisis.

Phase 5: Evaluation of crisis resolution and Anticipatory Planning

The Nurse and client has to evaluate and reassess whether the intervention has resulted in a positive resolution of crisis or not expected outcome; behavioral change has been achieved or not; whether the client returned to the normative level of functioning, if not achieved; modified strategies, e.g. additional treatments have to be planned to resolve crisis is achieved similar strategies has to be reinforced. For example, constructive coping strategies, healthy adoption technique; responses to supporting systems, etc.

Referral in Crisis Situations

India is vulnerable to natural and man-made disasters, prolonged conflicts and other complex situations that impede the country's overall development. Disasters are quite devastating and usually leave a trail of human agony and crisis including loss of human life, livestock, property and physical injuries that have a significant impact on the survivors' quality of life. Along with relief, rehabilitation and care of physical health and injuries, psycho-social and mental health issues are also important that need to be addressed on priority. Apart from logistic and material help, the survivors will require psycho-social and mental health interventions.

Psycho-social support will comprise of general interventions related to the larger issues of relief work needs, social relationships and harmony to promote or protect psycho-social well-being of the survivors. Mental health services will comprise of interventions aimed at prevention or treatment of psychological symptoms or disorders. These interventions help individuals, families and groups to restore social cohesion and infrastructure along with maintaining their independence and dignity.

Psycho-Social Support and Mental Health Services (PSSMHS)—Psycho-social support in the context of disasters and crisis refers to "Comprehensive interventions aimed at addressing a wide range of psycho-social and mental health problems arising in the aftermath of disasters. These interventions help individuals, families and groups to build human capacities, restore social cohesion and infrastructure along with maintaining their independence, dignity and cultural integrity. Psycho-social support helps in reducing the level of actual and perceived stress and in preventing adverse psychological and social consequences amongst disaster-affected community". Psycho-social support has to be provided on a long term basis. Appropriate and timely interventions will determine the victims' adjustment to various changes in lifestyle, caused by the disaster. The interventions have to be community-based and culturally sensitive, taking into account the needs of vulnerable groups like women, children, the elderly, the disabled, etc. Such support can relieve the psychological distress of the affected people to a significant extent.

Aims of Psycho-social Support—To rebuild their shattered life through combined community activity, provided that the diminished capacity and support systems are rebuilt at the earliest and their coping capacity is increased through the simple mechanism of minimal emotional support, combined with a spectrum of care.

Implementation of PSSMHS activities through capacity building, training, service delivery, research, documentation, monitoring and evaluation at the national, state, district and community levels.

The provision of PSSMHS shall be based on the general health programs and will be integrated with National Mental Health Program (NMHP) as well as with District Mental Health Program (DMHP) and it will be delivered through general health care program and district health plan.

Capacity Development

Phase-1

a. Sensitising and training (basic and advanced) on PSSMHS across identified departments, sectors and levels.
b. Strengthening of the national, regional and nodal capacity building institutions and resource centers at state and district levels.
c. Developing PSSMHS needs assessment indicators and templates.
d. Strengthening of District Counselling Centers under the Department of Social Welfare/Women and Child Development.
e. Strengthening the resource base and data management/documentation in PSSMHS.

Education and Training
- Inclusion of Disaster PSSMHS in Post-Graduate Curriculum of Psychiatry, Psychology, Social Work, Disaster Management, Emergency Medicine and Health Education.
- Inclusion of PSSMHS in Under-Graduate Medical studies.
- Integrating with all training programs in the area of Psychology, Social Work, Mental Health, Emergency Medical Response, Hospital Administration, Nursing and Paramedics.

Community-Based Disaster Management (CBDM)
- Training of Panchayati Raj Institution (PRI) members.

- Developing awareness material for the community.
- Evolving a mechanism for community outreach education programs on PSSMHS.

Phase-2
a. Strengthening nodal institutions and hospitals.
b. Developing database management and evidence-based research.
c. Evolving a mechanism for follow-up and response.
d. Establishing a National Accreditation System for quality assurance.
e. Continuation and updating of human resource development activities.

Preparedness
- Creation of a core group of master trainers at district level.
- Strengthening Public-Private Partnership in research and development.
- Formation of National PSSMHS Resource Inventory to be part of National Health Resource Inventory.
- Initiation of distance learning courses for sensitisation across different categories of disaster management stakeholders.
- Development and standardization of uniform training packages for various designated target groups.
  Integration of PSSMHS training in DMHP, district health and hospital plans.

Phase-3
The long-term Action Plan will intensify the areas identified in Phase-1 along with the important issues. A detailed action plan, will be prepared by the National Sub-Committee. The long-term planning will include the following important aspects:
  i. Evolving a mechanism to include disaster-induced psychiatric disorders/physical disability in the disaster insurance and medical/health insurance.
  ii. Intensive Post-Graduate Diploma/Post-Graduate courses in PSSMHS.
  iii. Networking of Institutions and their activities.

The National Crisis Management Committee(NCMC)
It is the apex body of high level officials of the Government of India for dealing with a major crisis which has serious national ramifications. The composition of the committee would be as under:
1. Cabinet Secretary Chairman
2. Secretary of Nodal Ministries Member
3. Secretaries of Support Ministries Member
   An officer of the Cabinet Secretariat has been nominated convenor of the NCMC.
   In addition to these, the Secretary of the Nodal Ministry and/or the Head of the Department directly responsible; for dealing with a particular situation of crisis, are, co opted as member of the NCMC. When a situation is to be handled also by NCMC it gives such directions to the Crisis Group of the nodal Ministry as deemed necessary. The Secretary of the Nodal Ministry is responsible for ensuring that all developments are brought to the notice of the NCMC promptly.

District/State Plans

Most of the actions in a crisis situation are taken at the field/district and state levels for which the District/State Committees has been set up and contingency Plans have been prepared by the State authorities. The Nodal Ministries has issued detailed guidelines to the State Governments for the preparation of local Contingency Plans. State Governments have established a State Crisis Management Committee under the Chief Secretary, with Secretaries and Heads of the Concerned Departments/Organizations, as members.

Natural and State Centers for Disaster Management Program (NCDM) in India
A centrally funded scheme is in operation since 1992-93 to focus on disaster preparedness with emphasis on mitigation measures and to increase level of awareness of community about disasters, prepare them adequately to face the crisis situation. The following activities under the scheme are in progress:
- Human Resources Development
- Research and Consultancy Services

- Documentation of major events
- Operation of Faculty on NCDM in State level training States
- Operation of National Center of Disaster Management
- Public education and community awareness program.

Non-governmental organizations

There are a number of NGOs involved by the State Governments with objective to enhance disaster management capabilities in the field. Most of them are small and work locally. However, Indian Red Cross Society and Ramakrishna Mission are the two organizations, which take very active part in disaster management.

Emergency Medical Preparedness and Response (IEMPRESS)

Under the WHO and GOI collaboration, Initiative for Emergency Medical Preparedness and Response (IEMPRESS) is under implementation the by Rajiv Gandhi University of Health Sciences, Karnataka (RGUHS). This project is aimed at promoting and supporting prompt and essential response to emergencies arising out of natural or man-made calamities. Immediate relevant response, rescue and relief could reduce morbidity, mortality and human suffering and economic loss. The project would be implemented in three phases starting with development of model hospital contingency plan for tertiary hospitals, training of medical and other health professionals, capacity building of hospitals/institutions to meet with management of mass casualties. The expertise so built in the first phase would be extended to district and secondary level hospitals during the second phase and to the primary health care centers in the third phase. The initiative would encourage teaching hospitals in the government as well as private sectors to develop their own individual hospital contingency plans. A networking of hospitals will be established on zonal basis. Professional associations, NGOs and State government health services has been planned to be involved.

The American Counseling Association recommends five ways to help with coping after a crisis situation

- Recognize your own feelings about the situation and talk to others about your fears. Know that these feelings are a normal response to an abnormal situation
- Be willing to listen to family and friends who have been affected and encourage them to seek counseling if necessary
- Be patient with people; fuses are short when dealing with crises and others may be feeling as much stress as you
- Recognize normal crises reactions, such as sleep disturbances and nightmares, withdrawal, reverting to childhood behaviors and trouble focusing on work or school
- Take time with your children, spouse, life-partner, friends and co-workers to do something you enjoy.

Crisis Follow-up

Crisis services provides a follow-up program to assist individuals with support after the initial in-person contact. A crisis worker can offer support in a client's home or the client can come to Crisis Service's office and staff will offer counseling and assist in linking them to community resources necessary to resolving the crisis.

There is no inappropriate referral for Crisis Services. Crisis Services responds to any request according to an established system for prioritization a clinical basis.

The Intervention Priority Code assists Crisis Services staff in responding to those people most at-risk for self-injury or injuring others first, but still assures that every request for service shall be addressed within 24-hours.

Crisis Services are available to anyone regardless of ability to pay. The Dept. of Human Services provides funding for services for people not covered by Medical Assistance. There are no co-payments, monthly liabilities or fees for Crisis Services. Crisis Services is committed to providing a quality customer service approach through collaboration and teamwork at all times, weekly in-services, clinical supervision and 24-hour accessibility to psychiatrists and administrators.

The Counseling and Testing Center's (CTC)

Many students experience a variety of difficulties including stress, depression, anxiety and relationship problems during their college years and find that it is helpful to discuss their personal, educational or career concerns with a professional.

CTC staff of full-time psychologists and supervised graduate intern and practicum students offers students access to a wide range of counseling services and resources. The CTC provides a supportive and confidential environment for students to explore their concerns and learn new skills to deal more effectively with problems that may be interfering with their personal well-being and academic goals. At times, we may decide that a person's questions or concerns would be best addressed by a referral to a professional at the CTC.

Help for Students
Faculty and staff members are in an excellent position to observe students in the classroom or other campus settings and are often the first to notice when a student is experiencing personal or academic problems. If you are concerned about a student's academic or emotional state, you may contact the CTC to consult with a psychologist about your concerns and discuss possible courses of action. You may also refer distressed students directly to the CTC.

Interaction of staff directly with distressed or troubled students and provide suggestions
Listen carefully to the student's concern and try to see the issue from his/her point of view without necessarily agreeing or disagreeing.

1. Attempt to clarify the student's problem and explore alternatives to solve the problem.
2. Ask the student what he/she expects from you and be clear about what you are and are not willing to do in the situation.
3. The CTC offers same-day appointments for students who may be experiencing a crisis situation. The student or anyone referring a student may request a crisis appointment, sometimes it is helpful to offer to accompany a distressed student to their initial appointment at the CTC. Students who are not in crisis may call or stop by the CTC to schedule a regular appointment. Individual appointments are approximately 50 minutes in length. The CTC makes every effort to schedule students as soon as possible. For after-hours crisis intervention, call the CTC and one of the options will be to speak with a crisis counselor or call the nearest hospital emergency room.

Scheduling Appointments
Students may call or stop by the CTC to schedule an appointment. The Counseling and Testing Center makes every effort to schedule students as soon as possible. Emergency (same-day) appointments are also available for students experiencing a crisis that requires immediate attention. The CTC makes every effort to schedule students as soon as possible.

Confidentiality
Counseling sessions are confidential information cannot be released to anyone unless authorized by the student or mandated by law. CTC staff members must report limited information if there is a reasonable suspicion that a minor, handicapped or elderly person is being abused or if a person presents a serious danger of harming themselves or others.

A referral might be indicated when
- Individuals experiencing a personal crisis (relationship problems and family problems, etc.)
- Person under emotional stress or turmoil or severe withdrawn in nature
- Individual is achieving less than indicated abilities would predict
- A student is having little direction or purpose, seems to be just going through the motions of the college experience or is apathetic about his/her college/school work
- An individual is frequently exhibits attention-getting behavior, disruptive behavior or other unusual behaviors
- A student is uncertain about his/her major
- Severe Anxiety Feelings or subjected with Panic
- Learning disability and exhibiting failures in academic or in life
- A student who normally attends class regularly suddenly begins missing classes
- A student makes references to suicide or wishing to be dead or expresses a wish to harm others
- A student who appears to be having difficulties with substance abuse.

How to refer
- Before you refer, let the student know you care about his/her concerns and that you are making a referral because you want to be of help
- Depending upon circumstances, you may wish to obtain the student's permission to call the CTC and make an appointment while he/she is with you in your office. The appointment may be scheduled by telephone at this time
- If there is imminent danger to the student or to others, take an active role in getting immediate help by calling the CTC, walking the student over to the CTC, calling the Office of the Dean of Students or in some cases, the police
- If there are no unusual circumstances or imminent danger, you may suggest the student contact the CTC directly to make an appointment with a counselor.

Crisis Intervention Services
- Individual Counseling
- Group Counseling
- Couples Counseling
- Career Guidance and Counseling
- Alcohol and Substance Abuse Counseling
- Consultation and Outreach
- Self-Help Resource Room
- Biofeedback/Stress Management
- Learning Disabilities/ADHD Assessment
- Testing and Assessment.

Mental Health Center
Free, confidential community information, referrals and crisis line services 24 hours a day.

Behavior Health Reformers Unanimous Addiction Program List
A crisis is defined "anyone experiencing a disturbance of mood, thought, emotions, behavior or social functioning". Examples include: suicide; symptoms of mental illness; bereavement; situational stressors (financial, job loss, homelessness); relationship discord; substance abuse; family discord and parenting concerns. Services will be provided 24-hours-a-day/7-days-a-week, to anyone experiencing a crisis.
- Telephone Crisis Services:
  Crisis staff provide telephone screening to gather information regarding a caller's particular situation, providing crisis counseling and support. This includes outreach to residents of a place, who may be in need of assistance in accessing community resources, referrals and information.
- Walk-In Crisis Services:
  Individuals may come to Crisis Services' office for an in-person assessment of their situation, crisis counseling, information, referrals for ongoing treatment and assistance with hospital admission for voluntary or involuntary evaluation.
- Mobile Crisis Services:
  Crisis staff can provide assessments in the community at the scene of a crisis along with resource and referral information. Options are explored to include continued treatment and assistance to the hospital for voluntary or involuntary evaluation. On-scene support is offered to assist the individual through this process.

Referral to an RTFA (Residential Treatment Facility for Adults)
Person or persons who have a diagnosis of a serious mental illness and are in need of a supportive structured environment to ensure stability, could be referred to a residential treatment facility for adults. RTFA is a structured program to assist clients in identifying their emotional needs. Length of stay is from 1-30 days and is determined by the client's treatment team and RTFA staff.

Substance Abuse/Alcoholism
24 Hour Drug Addiction Hotlines
Drug rehab referral services; includes large list of drug-specific helplines and hotlines.

24 Hour Alcohol Abuse Recovery Hotline
Alcohol rehab referral services; includes state and local hotline information and treatment center facility locator.
The Alcohol and Drug Addiction Resource Center
National Drug Information Treatment and Referral Hotline
Information, support, treatment options and referrals to local rehab centers for any drug or alcohol problem.
Operates 24 hours, seven days a week.

National Cocaine Hotline
Information, crisis intervention, and referrals to local rehab centers for all types of drug dependency.
Operates 24 hours, seven days a week.

Alcohol Abuse and Crisis Intervention
- Al-ateen
- Alcohol and Drug Abuse Helpline and Treatment
- Alcohol Hotline Support and Information Youth.

National Youth Crisis Hotline
Provides counseling and referrals to local drug treatment centers, shelters and counseling services.
Responds to youth dealing with pregnancy, molestation, suicide and child abuse.
Operates 24 hours, seven days a week.

Crisis Intervention/Suicide
Operates 24 hours, seven days a week, provides short-term crisis intervention and counseling and referrals to local community resources. Counsels on parent-child conflicts, marital and family issues, suicide, pregnancy, runaway youth, physical and sexual abuse and other issues.

Child Help National Child Abuse Hotline
Operates 24 hours, seven days a week.
Provides multilingual crisis intervention and professional counseling on child abuse.
Gives referrals to local social service groups offering counseling on child abuse.

Hotline
Crisis line for youth, teens, and families.
Gives callers locally based referrals throughout the Nation.
Operates 24 hours, seven days a week.
Provides help for youth and parents regarding drugs, abuse, homelessness, runaway children, and message relays.

National Domestic Violence/Child Abuse/Sexual Abuse
24-hour-a-day hotline, provides crisis intervention and referrals to local services and shelters for victims of partner or spousal abuse.
Advocates are available 24 hours a day, seven days a week.
Staffed by trained volunteers who are ready to connect people with emergency help in their own communities, including emergency services and shelters.
The staff can also provide information and referrals for a variety of non-emergency services, including counseling for adults and children and assistance in reporting abuse.
They have an extensive database of domestic violence treatment providers in all states and territories. Many staff members speak local languages besides English and they have 24-hour access to translators for all languages. For the hearing impaired, there is a TDD number. This is a great resource for anyone—man, woman or child—who is experiencing or has experienced domestic violence or abuse or who suspects that someone they know is being abused.

Parent Hotline
Parent Hotline is a website dedicated to helping families who are in a crisis situation.
It lists behaviors for parents to be aware of such as drug use and a questionnaire on if a child is in need of intervention. Very resourceful site.

Parent Abduction Hotline
Provides crisis mediation in parental abduction.
Provides prevention information and referrals to local agencies.
Operators available 9 a.m. to 5 p.m. Monday-Friday. Voicemail on evenings and weekends with calls returned.

National Hotline for Missing and Exploited Children
Operates a hotline for reporting missing children and sightings of missing children.
Offers assistance to law enforcement agents.
Hours of operation are 7:30 a.m., 11 p.m.

National Runaway Switchboard
Provides crisis intervention and travel assistance to runaways.
Provides information and local referrals to adolescents and families.
Gives referrals to shelters nationwide relays messages to or sets up conference calls with, parents at the request of the child.
Operates 24 hours, seven days a week.

Child Find Hotline
Looks for missing and abducted children. Operators available 9 a.m. to 5 p.m.
Voicemail on evenings and weekends with calls returned.

Crisis Center
Crisis Intervention Counseling is available 24 hours a day, every day of the year to anyone needing support and assistance. Face-to-face counseling is available from 9 a.m. to 11 p.m. All volunteers are trained on communication skills, management of suicide, domestic violence, grief and loss, mental illness, sexual assault, cultural competency, HIV/AIDS, and substance abuse.

Crisis Child Care
Provides Free, short-term child care to children between 0 and 12 whose families are experiencing a crisis or emergency and lack adequate child care. Provides trained, compassionate telephone counselors 24 hours a day, 365 days a year.

Staff—two crisis counselors both paid staff and volunteers, complete intensive training that prepares them to deal with any issue.

Registered daycare homes or licensed child care centers provide a safe and nurturing environment while parents address the crisis situation.

Behavioral Health Access Provides access to mental health and chemical dependency resources.

Qualified behavioral health professionals help to determine the appropriate level of care for people experiencing an emergent behavioral health crisis.

Registered daycare homes or licensed child care centers
Provide a safe and nurturing environment while parents address the crisis situation crisis intervention services to anyone needing immediate help. These services are available 24 hours a day, seven days a week. Child care can be provided for up to 72 hours per admission, referrals and crisis line services 24 hours a day Staff are trained to handle crisis calls and to make emergency referrals if necessary. The Center's telephone lines are answered around the clock and mental health professionals are on duty to take these calls at all times. Free, confidential community information.

Girls and Boys Town National Hotline
Free phone crisis counseling and resource referral service for children and parents. Counselors will help with any problem like physical or sexual abuse, suicide, drug and alcohol problems, runaways, gangs, family problems.

Child Abuse Hotline-Child help
Trained and experienced crisis counselors respond to any caller in need of assistance, whether the child or adult in an abusive situation, someone concerned that abuse is occurring or someone needing information

about child abuse and neglect. Without making judgements, the Hotline staff promptly counsels or in emergency situations, gets help for the caller.

Children's and Adolescent Programs-Crossroads

These programs interrupt the inter-generational cycle of abuse and provide services to increase the physical and emotional safety of youth victims. Clients are helped to develop healthy ways to express feelings and to learn appropriate anger/conflict management skills. Teens are also helped with issues of abuse in dating relationships and alternative ways to live and love.

Genesis Community Crisis Line

Psychiatric nurses answer this line 24/7 and make referrals for callers.

Crisis Intervention

Provides short-term, 21-day crisis intervention and prevention services to youth, age 0-18, and their families.

Crisis Intervention utilizes the family team meeting concept with goals that include keeping the family intact, connecting them with community-based services, and maintaining the child(ren) in the home. Referrals are accepted from self, schools, provider agencies.

National Youth Crisis Hotline

Provides counseling and referrals to local drug treatment centers, shelters, and counseling services.
Responds to youth dealing with pregnancy, molestation, suicide, and child abuse.
Operates 24 hours, seven days a week.

National AIDS Hotline

Information and referrals to local hotlines, testing centers, and counseling services for patient and family.
Open 24 hours, seven days a week.

Poison Control

Poison control any kind of substance, treatment and counseling services will to provide.

Community Telephone Services Crisis Line for Counseling

Crisis intervention provides short-term, 21-day crisis intervention and prevention services youth, age 0-18 and their families. Crisis intervention utilizes the family team meeting concept with goals that include keeping the family intact, connecting them with community-based services, and maintaining the children in the home. Referrals are accepted from self, schools, provider agencies. Staff are trained to handle crisis calls and to make emergency referrals if necessary. The Center's telephone lines are answered around the clock, and mental health professionals are on duty to take these calls at all times free, confidential community information, referrals and crisis line services 24 hours a Day.

Home Ties Crisis Child Care

Crisis line is answered 24 hours a day. It provides a safe and nurturing place for the young children between the ages of 6 weeks and 5 years to learn and grow, while giving parents the time and help they need to make better lives for themselves and their children. The center provides up to three months of free child care to families in the community who are facing times of crisis and dealing with problems such as homelessness, domestic violence, substance abuse, foster care placement and poverty provides a youth center, transitional living program, and more for youth.

CHILDLINE

It stands for a friendly 'didi' or a sympathetic 'bhaiya' who is always there for vulnerable children 24 hours of the day, 365 days of the year. CHILDLINE is India's first 24-hour, free, emergency phone service for children in need of aid and assistance. We not only respond to the emergency needs of children but also link them to services for their long-term care and rehabilitation. CHILDLINE is a platform bringing together the Ministry for Women and Child Development, Government of India, Department of Telecommunications, street and community youth, non-profit organizations, academic institutions, the corporate sector and concerned individuals.

It will work for the protection of the rights of all children in general. But special focus is on all children in need of care and protection, especially the more vulnerable sections, which include:
* Street children and youth living alone on the streets
* Child labourers working in the unorganized and organized sectors
* Domestic help, especially girl domestics
* Children affected by physical/sexual/emotional abuse in family, schools or institutions.
* Children who need emotional support and guidance
* Children of commercial sex workers
* Child victims of the flesh trade
* Victims of child trafficking
* Children abandoned by parents or guardians
* Missing children
* Run away children
* Children who are victims of substance abuse
* Differently-abled children
* Children in conflict with the law
* Children in institutions
* Mentally challenged children
* HIV/AIDS infected children
* Children affected by conflict and disaster
* Child political refugees
* Children whose families are in crises.

Crisis Intervention
* **Direct assistance**
  Medical, shelter, protection from abuse, repatriation, death, missing children, intensive counselling
* **On phone**
  Emotional support and guidance, information and referral to services for the caller, information about CHILDLINE, silent calls.
* **Long-term rehabilitation**
  After the emergency needs of the child have been addressed, CHILDLINE explores options with the child to study, learn a trade, go back home, etc. Based on the decision of the child, CHILDLINE links, the child to an appropriate organization in the city.

CHILDLINE TODAY

The Government of India has presented CHILDLINE as its response to the Child Rights Convention. It is a one point window, connecting children in need to various NGO's working for child related issues. CHILDLINE works towards ensuring that all children in need of care and protection are aware of and have access to services, that are child friendly, available when they want it and encourage them to participate in decisions that affect them.

The country's first toll-free tele-helpline for street children has grown into a national child protection service that operates in over 83 cities and towns in India. In 12 years, CHILDLINE has received 17 million calls as of Dec. 2009 from children in need of care and protection from across the country.

Nationwide RAINN National Rape Crisis Hotline
Respite Options Program

It is available 24 hours a day, seven days a week to give parents and caregivers temporary relief during critical times. It provides free, short-term respite so parents or guardians can concentrate on decreasing the stress in their home. Families with infants through five-year-old children who are not involved in the court system and who live with family or relatives. The family must have little or no appropriate alternative support system where children can go during a crisis or stressful time Elderly.

To ensure a good, healthy and quality life, the elderly members of the society can move a long way with the support of the family members as well as the other society members. They could play a valuable role in the socialization of young children and it transmitting social and cultural heritage with the help of their vast experience.

QUESTIONS

- Crisis (2 M, RGUHS, 2003, 06)
- Crisis intervention (4 M, NIMS, Dec, 2009, 5 M, RGUHS, 2000, 15 M, MGRU)
- Crisis management (5 M, RGUHS, 2004)
- Define crisis and crisis intervention, how do you assess crisis situation in a community set up (2+4 M, March, 2008)
- Define Crisis, List the types of crisis, discuss the role of nurse in crisis intervention (2+4+5 M, Sep, 2010)
- Describe different types of Leaders (10M, NTRUHS, Dec 2007)
- Define leadership (2 M, MGRUHS, May, 2010)
- Define leadership, its meaning, nature and uses in nursing (10 M, RGUHS, 2002)
- Democratic leader (5M, NTRUHS, July 2008)
- Describe the process of group formation and maintenance (10 M, RGUHS, May, 2010)
- Describe the types of leaders and their personal characteristics (10 M, RGUHS, May, 2010)
- Discuss in detail about leadership and its dimensions (15M, RGUHS, May, 2006)
- Discuss the role of a nurse in crisis intervention (5 M, MGRU, 2002, 10 M, RGUHS, 2001, 5 M, MGRU, 2002)
- Discuss various functions of a leader (6 M, RGUHS, May, 2010)
- Group dynamics (2 M, RGUHS, Aug, 2010; 5 M, NIMS, May, 2010)
- Leaders in groups (2 M, RGUHS, 1997)
- Leaders in nursing profession (2 M, RGUHS, 1997 and SM, NTRUHS, June, 2010)
- Leaders in village (2 M, RGUHS, 1997)
- Leadership abilities of a Nurse Administrator (5M, NTRUHS, June, 2007)
- Leadership styles (2 M, RGUHS, 2002)
- Leadership techniques (5 M, RGUHS, 2002)
- Managing Crisis (5 M, RGUHS, Feb, 2010)
- Maturational crisis (2 M, RGUHS, 2003)
- Motivation (2 M, RGUHS, Aug, 2009)
- Nature of leadership (2 M, RGUHS, 2002)
- Potential qualities of a leader (5 M, RGUHS, 1997)
- Power orientation (5 M, RGUHS, 2002)
- Social behaviour (2 M, MGRUHS, May, 2010; 5 M, NIMS, May, 2008)
- Spotting a leader in group (2 M, RGUHS, 2002)
- Team work (5 M, NTRUHS, Nov, 2010)
- Types of crisis (5 M, GULBARGA, 1995, 5 M, RGUHS, 1998)
- What are the different types of crisis? Describe the its role in each one of them (15 M, RGUHS, 2006)
- What are the important features of leadership? How leaders could be developed (5 M, RGUHS, 2002)
- What are the principles, technique and process of crisis intervention (7 M, NIMS)
- What are the types of crisis? Explain how will you prevent the crisis in the ward (15 M, GULB, 1999)
- What is meant by a social group? How are the groups classified? (15 M, NTRUHS, July, 2008)
- What is Motivation? (2M, NTRUHS, Dec, 2007)
- What is the essence of leadership? How does one acquire such leadership? (5 M, RGUHS, 1997)
- What are the stages of goup development, explain briefly, strategies of improving group functioning (5+5M Baba Farid UHS, 2008)
- Yourself as a leader (2 M, RGUHS, 1997)

Relationship and Behavior

INTRODUCTION

Psychology is "A systematic and scientific study of human behavior". It has its special tools and procedures, which will help in gathering and organizing its subject matter or the essential facts related to human behavior. These procedures will help in understanding of one's behavior in all its forms and expressions. Introspection means 'looking within', looking into the working of our own minds and reporting what we find there means, it is a method of self observation: "observation by an individual of his own mental states directly and by the use of his memory" e.g. an electrician while working, has fallen, a doctor or a nurse may ask him, 'how it happened? To gather the history and assess the situation, what are his present complaints?' the patient will try to look within and recall what happened and how he is feeling now and will accordingly report. In making this report, the patient is making use of introspection method, in which the individual observes, analyzes and reports his own feelings, thoughts or all that possess in his mind during the course of a mental act or experience. It is a transparency condition – Self Knowledge and Self Constitution/'contemplation of one's self /self-reflection'

Definitions

"Looking into our own minds and reporting what we discover there"– *James*

"The self-observation and reporting of *conscious* inner *thoughts*, *desires* and sensations. It is a conscious mental and purposive process relying on thinking, *reasoning* and examining one's own thoughts, *feelings* in more spiritual cases and one's *soul*."

"An art and self description of mind and its activities" – *Ryle*

Nature

Introspection is a process that yields knowledge of one's own current mental state. Introspective knowledge is often held to be more immediate or direct than sensory knowledge. Introspective knowledge can serve as a ground or foundation for other sorts of knowledge. It is philosophy of mind, offer a variety of theories of the nature of introspection and philosophical claims about consciousness, emotion, free will, personal identity, thought, belief, imagery, perception and other mental phenomena are often thought to have introspective consequences or to be susceptible to introspective verification.

One can understand about their own environment and about one's own Psychology is by inner-perception or by introspective awareness. One can understand in a better way is by having faith in themselves and by self confidence. Knowledge of one's own mental states and knowledge of environment. It is peculiar when one compared with knowledge of other's minds. Introspection is an 'inward glance' or observation of one's own behavior.

Moran explained "Inner sense theory" which offers a picture of self knowledge as a kind of mind – reading applied to one self, a faculty that happens to be aimed in one direction rather than the other. Self knowledge or inner observation is required for everyone. "Normal intelligence, rationality and conceptual capacity" are required to understand themselves.

Self Introspection Skills

1. Getting in touch with feelings—When you feel a feeling, ask yourself where in your body that feeling is centered e.g. "recently I felt anxious, and it was centered in my chest. Then, there are four main ways to process and clarify that feeling."

2. Visual—Create a fantasy e.g. "I fantasize in my head that I'm sitting in the control room".
3. Auditory—Give the feeling a voice and listen to what it has to say e.g. "I'm feeling scared. I'm feeling weak and sad, because things are not feel right with my friend"
4. Kinesthetic—Feel into the feeling. Immerse yourself in it like sliding into pool of water. Let it soak through you and soak in it. Let it expand and enlarge until "ah, I feel what it is...."
5. Getting in touch with thoughts—Watch your thoughts. Explore your thoughts. Ask yourself what you think about various things. Use continuous breath to clarify your thoughts.
6. Getting in touch with unconscious motivations—When you want to find out why you do something, hold yourself back from doing it a bit, and see what happens. Your motivations for doing that will come clamoring to the fore. You will notice them as feelings, images and thoughts.
7. Getting in touch with dreams—Train yourself to pause a moment when you first wake up and see if you can remember any dreams, rather than leap into your day. If you can remember any dreams, write them down. Keep a dream journal.

For a process to qualify as "introspective" as the term is ordinarily used in contemporary philosophy of mind, it must minimally meet the following conditions:

a. *The mentality condition*—Introspection is a process that generates knowledge, judgments or beliefs about *mental* events, states or processes and not about affairs outside one's mind. In this respect, it is different from sensory processes that normally deliver information about outward events or about the non - mental aspects of the individual's body. In principle the introspective part of such processes, pertaining to judgments about one's mind.

b. *The first-person condition*—Introspection is a process that generates or aims at generating, knowledge, judgments or beliefs about one's own mind only and no one else's, at least not directly. Any process that generates knowledge equally of one's own and other's minds is by that token is not an introspective process. Of course, introspective self-knowledge may sometimes serve as a *basis* of knowledge of other minds. For example if I learn introspectively that I am angry, I might on that basis conclude that others are angry too. If a certain version of simulation theory is right, much of our knowledge of other's minds depends on, first determining what our own reactions, attitudes or other mental states are or would be, then drawing an implicit or explicit parallel between them and ourselves (Goldman 1995).

c. *The temporal proximity condition*—Introspection is a process that generates knowledge, beliefs or judgments about *one's currently ongoing* mental life only or alternatively (or perhaps in addition), *immediately past* (or even future) mental life. Whether the target of introspection is best thought of as one's current mental life or one's immediately past mental life may depend on one's model of introspection: On self-detection models of introspection, according to which introspection is a causal process involving the detection of a mental state, it is natural to suppose that a brief lapse of time will transpire between the occurrence of the mental state that is the introspective target and the final introspective judgment about that state, which invites (but does not strictly imply) the idea that introspective judgments generally pertain to immediately past states. On self-shaping and self-fulfillment models of introspection, according to which introspective judgments create or embed the very state introspected, it seems more natural to think that the target of introspection is one's current mental life or perhaps even far the immediate future.

d. *The directness condition*—Introspection yields judgments or knowledge about one's own current mental processes relatively *directly* or *immediately and* clear.

e. *The detection condition*—Introspection involves some sort of *attunement to* or *detection of* a *pre-existing* mental state or event, where the introspective judgment or knowledge is (when all goes well) *causally* but *not ontologically* dependent on the target mental state, e.g. a process that involved creating the state of mind that one attributes to oneself would not be introspective, according to this condition, directly, by the means by which I could not know the truth of anyone else's mind.

f. *The effort condition*—Introspection is not *constant, effortless and automatic*. We are not every minute of the day introspecting. Introspection involves some sort of special reflection on one's own mental life that differs from the ordinary un-self-reflective flow of thought and action. The mind may monitor itself regularly and constantly without requiring any special act of reflection by the thinker, e.g. at a non-conscious level certain parts of the brain or certain functional systems may monitor the goings on of other parts of the brain and other functional systems, but this sort of thing is not what philosophers generally have in mind when they talk of introspection. However, this condition, like the directness and detection conditions, is not universally accepted.

The Targets of Introspection

The most commonly cited classes of introspectible mental states are *attitudes*, beliefs, desires, evaluation and intentions and *conscious experiences*—Emotions, images and sensory experiences. While others focus on conscious experiences

The Products of Introspection

Most philosophers hold that introspection yields something like beliefs or judgments about one's own mind, but others prefer to characterize the products of introspection as "thoughts", "representations", "awareness" or the like.

Self Accounts

Symmetrical or self/other parity accounts of self-knowledge treat the processes by which we acquire knowledge of our own minds as essentially the same as the processes by which we acquire knowledge of other people's minds. On such a view, introspection strictly speaking is impossible, since the first-person condition on introspection cannot be met: There is no distinctive process that generates knowledge of one's own mind only. Advocates of parity accounts sometimes characterize our knowledge of our own minds as arising from "theories" that we apply equally to ourselves and others, consequently, this approach to self-knowledge is sometimes called the *theory*.

Behavioral Observation Accounts

We notice how we behave and then we infer the attitudes that would seem to be reflected by those behaviors and we do so even when we actually lack the ascribed attitude, e.g. In classic research, Social Psychology suggested that when induced to perform an action for a small reward, people will attribute to themselves a more positive attitude toward that action than when they are induced by a large reward. When we notice ourselves doing something with minimal compensation, we infer a positive attitude toward that activity, just as we would if we saw someone else perform the same activity with minimal compensation. For example, we might know we like vegetarian food because we have noticed that we sometimes drive all the way across town to get it; we might know that we are happy because we see or feel ourselves smiling. If we are better at discerning our own motives and attitudes, it is primarily because we have observed more of our own behavior than of anyone else's.

Self-Shaping

Although we can seemingly at least sometimes arrive at true self ascriptions through the self-shaping and the self-expression procedures that is, they may depend on the (depending on how they are described and developed) procedures that can yield only knowledge or judgments (or at least self-ascriptions) about one's own currently ongoing or very recently past mental states. It is difficult to find accounts of self-knowledge that stress the self-shaping technique in its purest, forward-looking, causal form perhaps because it is clear that self-knowledge must involve considerably more than this.

Although a number of early modern philosophers had aimed to initiate the scientific study of the mind, it was not until the middle of the 19th century—with the appearance of *quantitative introspective methods*, especially regarding sensory consciousness—that the study of the mind took shape as a progressive, mathematical, laboratory-based science.

Advantages
- It enables us to understand total behavior of an individual
- The method does not need any expenses, laboratory or apparatus. Moreover, we obtain a direct knowledge of the mental experience of an individual.

Limitations

- Children or animals or the mentally challenged individuals cannot introspect, so this method will not be useful
- It is a purely private assessment. Something that is going on in a person's mind is not accessible to another. The introspective results cannot, therefore, be verified by other observers
- Scientific results are always verifiable. Hence, introspection is considered as an unscientific method
- The mental processes changes a little bit. If one does not want to change the mental process, one should study it after the process is complete, rather than during the process. This is called retrospection and requires clear memory, e.g. a sick person may be asked to report how feels. He may report aches and pains which he thinks the doctor or the nurse expects him to feel rather than what he actually feels. Thus the difficulties of really understanding oneself or putting into words one's innermost feelings cannot be overlooked.

SOCIAL BEHAVIOR

Human beings are gregarious in nature, man cannot live alone for long time and are socio-cultural beings. Society is both natural and necessary for man. Human beings have a propensity to organize their behavior in a wide range of groups in order to satisfy their needs and wants to fulfill social functions. The behaviors, thoughts, attitudes of human beings are determined by the quality of the learned ways of interaction in groups. The social interaction is essential in life and in which one person influence the thoughts, attitudes, opinions and behavior of another individual. Interaction pattern occurs within the large social systems in societies, groups, crowds, neighbourhood, community and social Institutions. Through social behavior the social relationships will establishes/formulates and maintains social net work, whereby the individuals will interact continuously or intermittently based on their needs. They formulate social groups, deals with social actions in social systems.

Definition

"Behavior directed towards society or taking place between, members of the same species".

Social behavior is acquired. The existence of society and social processes is possible through socialization. While many social behaviors are *communication* (provoke a response or change in behavior, without acting directly on the receiver). Communication between members of different species is not social behavior.

The term *Behavioral Sciences*, "refer to Sciences that study behavior in general".

Sociology is "the scientific study of patterns of human behavior as they emerge and crystallize out of the interactions of human beings in groups, which comprises society".

Social behavior is followed by *social actions*, which is directed at other people and is designed to induce a response. Further along this ascending scale are *social interaction* and *social relation*. In conclusion, social behavior is a process of communicating.

Socialization is the process of working together, developing group responsibility, being guided by the welfare needs of others. Society is a web of social relationships, which is established through the process of social interaction i.e., mutual influences that individuals and groups have on one another in their attempts to solve problems and in their striving towards goals. Social system is plurality of individuals interacting with each other according to the shared cultural norms and meaning. It is an orderly and systematic arrangement of social interaction.

Social Values are cultural standards which are desirable for organized social life. These are measures of goodness and desirability. Organized social behavior is essential to maintain the social order and social norms, values. It provides social security for the individuals. Every individual in the society occupies a specific status based on their expected and exhibited behavior and maintain specific social roles by fulfilling designated social responsibilities. Satisfaction of value oriented interests through association of individuals grouped together in social organizations or social institutions.

PUBLIC RELATIONS (PR)

Introduction

Public Relations (PR) is a discipline, as an activity PR is very complex and must be consciously designed, planning calls for attention, deliberation, research, anticipation, analysis and consequences. Both Organization and Public has to understand each other, a two-way communication and Sustained effort is needed to maintain PR in logical means. PR is based on moral principles.

Definitions

"The deliberate planned and sustained effort to establish and maintain mutual understanding between an organization and its publics"—British Institute of Public relations

"Public relations is concerned with or devoted to create mutual understanding among groups and institutions". —The Public Relations Society of America

"Management function that identifies, establishes and maintains mutually beneficial relationships between an organization and its publics upon whom its success depends"—Cutlip, Center and Broom

"Public relations consists of all forms of planned communication both inward and outward (Two Way) between an organization and its publics for the purpose of achieving objectives concerning mutual understanding"—Frank Jefkins

"Public relations is the art and social science of analyzing trends, predicting their consequences, counselling organizational leaders as well as planning and implementing a program of action that will serve the interest of not only the organization but also that of its publics"—Public Relations Associations, 1978

Components (Fig 15.1)

* Counselling—Providing advice to management concerning policies, relationships and communication with its various publics
* Research—Determining attitudes and behaviors of publics through research in order to plan public relations strategies. Such research can be used to (1) generate mutual understanding (2) influence and persuade public
* Media Relations—Working with the mass media in seeking publicity or responding to their interest in the organization
* Publicity—Disseminating planned messages through selected media to further the organization's interest.
* Employee/Member Relations: Responding to concerns, informing and motivating and organization's employees or association or club members
* Community Relations—Planned activity with a community to maintain an environment that benefits both the organization and the community
* Public Affairs—Developing effective involvement in public policy and helping an organization adapt to public expectations
* Governmental Affairs—Relating directly with legislature and regulatory agencies on behalf of the organization
* Issues management—Identifying and addressing issues of public concern that affect the organization
* Financial Relations/Investor Relations/Shareholder Relations—It involves creating and maintaining investor confidence and building good relationships with the financial community
* Industry Relations—Relating with other firms in the industry of an organization and with trade associations
* Development/Fund-Raising—Demonstrating the need for and encouraging the public to support an organization, primarily through financial contributions
* Multicultural Relations/Workplace Diversity—Relating with individuals and groups in various cultural settings
* Special Events—Stimulating an interest in a person, product or organization by means of a focused "happening". They are activities designed to interact with publics and listen to them
* Marketing Communications—Combination of activities designed to sell a product, service or idea. These activities may include advertising, collateral materials, publicity, promotion, direct mail, trade shows and special events.

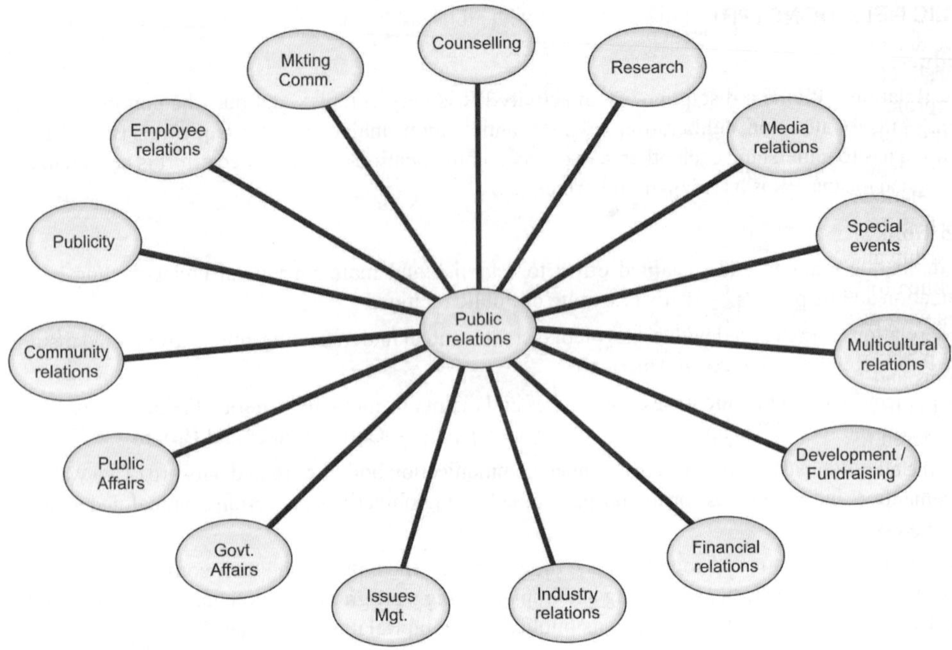

Fig. 15.1: Components in public relation

Public Relations in Context of Nursing

Nurses are the primary providers of direct patient care; Nursing is the largest Health Care Profession; and Nursing is the largest service in a hospital. Health care cannot exist without Nurses. Today nursing has the opportunity to shape the future of health care. Nurses are creating partnerships with physicians and other health care professionals. Nurses are assuming leadership roles in Case Management, Managed Care and Home Health. At present, ratio between Nursing Professionals and Community is inappropriate, to provide health care services and to meet the health needs of community, Poor Working conditions and limited salaries, failure of hospital administrators in meeting the requirements of Nurses and barriers in IPR between Nurses to collaborate the services, Insufficient Public support, apathy, negative attitude on the part of an individual Nurse, etc. all are concerned. A sound Public Relations Program would seem to be a must in any prescribed sector, as Public must know about an organization, a Profession or even a project before it can prefer any real help. Nurses are in the field think of the public not enmasse but as a number of separate entities with distinctive individualities. It is the public, who constitute the audience to be reached and to be motivated to take positive action. As this sequence of behavior is set into motion, a chain of social interaction is established, this will be a powerful force and so effective and proper planning is essential. Only when these public groups know about what the Nursing Profession is doing, what it hopes to do and why with full support, understanding and appreciation to be gained for Nurses.

A Public Relation Program requires careful planning and organization, as there is strength in unanimity, the long range program should be developed on a rational basis with sufficient flexibility to be adapted to meet the local needs. The strength of our Nation lies in the state, in the community and in the individual. It goes without saying that the individual is the important link in this chain. The way in which a Nurse does her/his work is more important, her/his attitude toward her/his work and her/his profession in general influences others and moulds public opinion. Good Public Relations between Nursing Profession and the public depend on varied factors.

Nursing profession depends on many or different kinds of public like Government, Patients, Families, community and specific individuals who ultimately forms as groups. Nurses has to establish good interpersonal relationships through accepted social interaction with all public groups. The relationships may change from time to time, if one nurse gets herself/himself into a sensational situation and the mass media give it wide spread publicity, the public relation of entire profession with all its public may be affected adversely, maladjustments may be due to the fact that the profession actually doesn't meet public needs or due to the public ignorance of the constructive role of the profession. Maladjustments will be found in all phases of life from the family and in all the professions are apt to be less progressive than society demands, sometimes the younger professionals more progressive members of a profession split off and form new groups, sound leadership and prompt action can often lead a profession to meet changing demands by public opinion, by public need., Public opinion, Public relations and profession in general affects each other. Public Relations is the broader inclusive activity which has its roots in human relationships. The goal of Public Relation is to make trouble free, trusting relationship and environment. It is the promotion of good human relationships between Professionals and all the public groups. The relationship may be publicized by friendship and cooperation which may influence the groups with profession is needed.

The best advice on how to build good will for Nurses is, 'be accurate and be positive' both in analyzing problems and finding solutions. There is nothing to be gained by complaining, by blaming others. The best method is to do what you can to help remedy to situation, what should be the remedy and how it has to be administered to promote better understanding, cooperation, positive social interaction and friendly in nature among the co professionals, patients and their families; suggestions in dealing with their social life, their living arrangements, their interest we have to keep in mind when educating them. Invite senior professionals to visit the public on a designated date and to spend couple of hours to interact, assess the situation and analyze the existing problems and guide the professionals and community in taking steps to implement problem solving strategies.

All these changes are how nursing and health care are practiced can enhance the image of nursing. Nursing can be seen as a positive role model, collaborator and integral change agent. How we feel about ourselves as nurses is how we are perceived as a profession, whether by physicians, the public, or prospective nurses. If we feel good about who we are and what we do, we communicate that feeling to others both verbally and nonverbally. The opinion and negative attitudes of the public can be solved, through mass media communicate good things and the services we render, implement necessary steps to change the negative attitude and develop positive consensus among the public. Nursing has the potential both in numbers and through our practice to make the most significant impact on the future of health care.

INTERPERSONAL RELATIONS (IPR)

The relationship is a "hypothetical construct to designate the inferred character of the observable interaction between two individuals". The helping relationship is "the Endeavor, by interaction with another person, to contribute in a facilitating, positive way to his improvement". The intent of promoting the growth, development, maturity, improved functioning, improved coping with life of the other. A unique and dynamic process through which the individual assists another to use his/her inner resources to grow in a positive direction, actualizing the individual's potential for a meaningful life. An interpersonal relationship is a social association, connection or affiliation between two or more people. It varies in differing levels of intimacy and modes of connection, implying discovery or establishment of common ground and may be centered around something shared in common. IPR may be based on limerence, love and liking, regular business interactions, or some other type of social commitment. Interpersonal relationships take place in a great variety of contexts such as family, friends, marriage, associates, work, clubs, neighborhoods and places of worship. They may be regulated by law, custom or mutual agreement and are the basis of social groups and society as a whole. Interpersonal relationships are dynamic systems that change continuously during their existence. Like living organisms, relationships have a beginning, a lifespan and an end. They tend to grow and improve gradually, as people get to know each other and become closer emotionally.

Definitions

"An association between two or more people that may range from fleeting to enduring".

"Reciprocal, social and emotional interactions between two or more persons in the environment".

Types

Based on relational contexts of interaction and the types of expectations that communicators have one another.

1. *Friendship*—A freely chosen association based on like mindedness, which consists of mutual love, trust, respect, unconditional acceptance and usually implies the discovery or establishment of *common ground* between the individuals involved.
2. *Family* and *Kinship* relationships—Being related to someone else by blood (*consanguinity*), e.g. fatherhood, motherhood; or through *marriage* (*affinity*) e.g. father-in-law, mother-in-law, uncle by marriage, aunt by marriage. Communication patterns establish roles, identities and enable the growth of the individuals
3. *Romantic Relationship*—Marriage is a social institution where intimate and committed relationships will be established between two people of opposite sex or gender
4. *Professional—Relationships*—Professional communication encompasses small group communication
5. Formalized *intimate relationships* or *long term relationships*—Through law and public ceremony, e.g. marriage and civil union.
6. *Non-formalized intimate relationships* or *long term relationships*—Such as loving relationships
7. *Soul mates*—Individuals who are intimately drawn to one another through a favorable meeting of the minds and who find mutual acceptance and understanding with one another. Soulmates may feel themselves bonded together for a lifetime and hence, they may be *sexual partners* but not necessarily.
8. *Platonic Love*—Is an affectionate relationship into which the sexual element does not enter, especially in cases where one might easily assume otherwise.
9. *Brotherhood* and *Sisterhood*—Individuals united in a common cause or having a common interest which may involve formal membership in a club, organization, association, society, lodge, sorority, fraternity, the comradeship of fellow soldiers in peace or war.
10. *Partners or co-workers in a profession* business or a common workplace.
11. *Acquaintanceship*—Simply being introduced to someone or knowing who they are by interaction.

Stages of IPR

George Levinger, Psychologist developed IPR Model of relationships.

1. **Acquaintance**—Becoming acquainted depends on previous relationships, physical proximity, first impressions and a variety of other factors. If two people begin to like each other, continued interactions may lead to the next stage, but acquaintance can continue indefinitely.
2. **Buildup**–People begin to trust and care about each other. The need for compatibility and such filtering agents as common background and goals will influence whether or not interaction continues.
3. **Continuation**—This stage follows a mutual commitment to a long term friendship, intimate relationship, romantic relationship resulting into marriage, It is generally a long, relative, stable period. Nevertheless, continued growth and development will occur during this time. Mutual trust is important for sustaining the relationship.
4. **Deterioration**—Not all relationships deteriorate, but those that do, tend to show signs of trouble, boredom, resentment and dissatisfaction may occur and individuals may communicate less and avoid self-disclosure. Loss of trust and betrayals may take place as the downward spiral continues.
5. **Termination**—The final stage marks the end of the relationship, either by death in the case of a healthy relationship or by separation.

Ways to build up good IPR

- Mutual personal respect
- Altruism
- Strong bond of mutual trust
- Friendly relationships
- Closeness
- Cooperation
- Attachment
- Mutual understanding
- The knowledge of each other
- Face-to-face interactive process
- Mutual love
- Equality
- Harmonious relationship
- Affection

- Empathy
- Friendship
- Interpersonal attraction
- Interpersonal compatibility
- Jointness (psychodynamics)
- Communication skills
- Sympathy
- Theology of relational care

- Courtship
- Empowerment
- Human bonding
- Interpersonal communication
- Intimate relationship
- Love
- Social interaction

Phases in IPR

According to Hildegard E Peplau, Nursing is an interpersonal process because it involves interaction between two or more individuals with a common goal. The attainment of goal is achieved through the use of a series of steps following a series of pattern.

Peplau identified four sequential phases in interpersonal relationship.

1. Orientation phase (Fig 15.2)
- Problem defining phase
- Starts when client meets nurse as a stranger
- Defining problem and deciding type of service needed
- Client seeks assistance, conveys needs, asks questions, shares preconceptions and expectations of past experiences
- Nurse responds, explains roles to client, helps to identify problems and to use available resources and services.

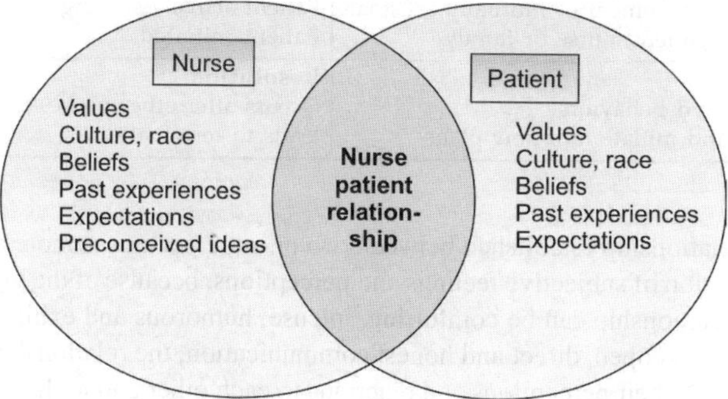

Fig. 15.2: Factors influencing orientation phase

2. Identification phase
- Selection of appropriate professional assistance
- Patient begins to have a feeling of belonging and a capability of dealing with the problem which decreases the feeling of helplessness and hopelessness.

3. Exploitation phase
- Use of professional assistance for problem solving alternatives
- Advantages of services are used is based on the needs and interests of the patients
- Individual feels as an integral part of the helping environment
- They may make minor requests or attention getting techniques
- The principles of interview techniques must be used in order to explore, understand and adequately deal with the underlying problem
- Patient may fluctuates on independence
- Nurse must be aware about the various phases of communication
- Nurse aids the patient in exploiting all avenues of help and progress is made towards the final step.

4. Resolution phase
- Termination of professional relationship
- The patients needs have already been met by the collaborative effect of patient and nurse
- Now they need to terminate their therapeutic relationship and dissolve the links between them
- Sometimes may be difficult for both as psychological dependence persists
- Patient drifts away and breaks bond with nurse and healthier emotional balance is demonstrated and both becomes mature individuals.

Interpersonal theory and nursing process (Table 15.1)
- Both are sequential and focus on therapeutic relationship
- Both use problem solving techniques for the nurse and patient to collaborate on, with the end purpose of meeting the patients needs
- Both use observation communication and recording as basic tools utilized by nursing.

Table 15.1: Nursing Process and Interpersonal theory

Nursing Process	Interpersonal Theory
Assessment **Data collection and analysis [continuous]** May not be a felt need	Orientation **Non continuous data collection** Felt need Define needs
Nursing diagnosis Planning Mutually set goals	**Identification** Interdependent goal setting
Implementation Plans initiated towards achievement of mutually set goals may be accomplished by patient, nurse or family	**Exploitation** Patient actively seeking and drawing help Patient initiated
Evaluation Based on mutually expected behaviors May led to termination and initiation of new plans	**Resolution** Occurs after other phases are completed successfully leads to termination

Characteristics of IPR

- Affectiveness–The relationship established between two or more persons is more affective than cognitive. It involves the exploration of subjective feelings and perceptions, because of the highly personal content of the discussions, the relationship can be comforting, intense, humorous and exhilarating
- Intensity–As it is based on open, direct and honest communication, the relationship can be intense. All are expected to share openly their perceptions and reactions to each other and to the process, this can result in intense communication
- Growth and Change–The relationship is dynamic, it is constantly changing as the persons are interacting, thus the growth and change takes place
- Privacy–All disclosures during interaction are kept confidential. The persons are obligated not to share what inspires in the interaction with others, unless the person has given permission to do so. This protective aspect of the relationship is unique and frequently encourages person's self disclosure
- Support–through IPR, communicator provide support to others, that often provides the necessary stability for taking risks and changing behavior
- Honesty–IPR is based on honest and open, direct communication between two or more persons.

INTERPERSONAL COMMUNICATION

Interpersonal Communication is the interaction between two persons, e.g. in counseling the transaction involves between the counselor and counselee. It takes place within a social context includes all the symbols and cues used to give and receive meaning, as meaning resides in persons and not in words. Meaningful interpersonal communication results in exchange of ideas, problem solving, expression of feelings, decision-making, goal accomplishment, team building and personal growth. Communication is an ongoing, dynamic and multi dimensional process. Through interpersonal communication effective IPR will establish, which means getting best out of people by winning and maintaining their whole hearted collaboration, when the person is working with people requires to possess high degree of interpersonal skills which will be promoted through effective interpersonal communication. The person with highly developed effective skills will have positive attitude, emotions, beliefs and values and be able to communicate efficiently with the other person with mutual respect and maintains human dignity and motivate the person to perform their job effectively increases productivity and attains organizational objectives. Human experience involves interaction and friendly relationships with effective interpersonal relationships, it determines how a person behaves. In the professional role, the counselor must use critical thinking to focus on each aspect of communication so that interactions can be purposeful and effective.

Definition

"Interpersonal communication, is a dynamic process involving continual adaptation and adjustments between two or more human beings engaged in face-to-face interactions during which each person is continually aware of the other(s)".

Basic elements in the process of Interpersonal communication process

1. Referent—It motivates the person to communicate with another person. In health care setting, e.g. sights, sounds, odours, time schedules, objects, emotions, sensations, perceptions, ideas and other cues initiate communication. The health professional who knows what stimuli initiated communication can develop and organize messages more efficiently and better perceive meaning in another's message.
2. Sender—is the person who encodes and delivers the message, he/she puts ideas or feelings into a form that can be transmitted and is responsible for the accuracy of its content and emotional tone.
3. Receiver—The sender's message acts as a referent for the receiver, who is responsible for attending to, translating and responding to the sender's message.
   Sender and receiver role are fluid and change back and forth as two persons interact, sending and receiving may occur simultaneously. The more they have common and the closer the relationship. The more likely , they will accurately perceive one another's meaning and respond accordingly.
4. Messages—It is the content of communication. It may contain verbal, non verbal and symbolic language. Messages are interpreted by those who receive them through personal perceptions that may or may not distort the meaning intended by sender. Sender has to communicate clearly, directly and in a familiar way, whereby the receiver will understand the message clearly. Communication can be difficult when participants have varied levels of education and experience.
5. Channels—These are means of conveying and receiving messages through visual, auditory and tactile senses. Facial expressions send visual messages, spoken words travel through auditory channels and touch uses tactile channels. The more channels the sender uses, the more clearly he/she will understand. Eg: When teaching relaxation technique, the counsellor demonstrates the technique, gives pamphlet i.e., written procedure to follow and assists the client to practice.
6. Feed Back—It is the message returned by the receiver., the sender and receiver both has to be sensitive and open to each other's messages. They have to clarify the messages and modify the behavior accordingly,
7. Interpersonal variables—These are the factors within both (Receiver & Sender) that influence communication, eg: Perception, educational level, developmental level, socio-cultural backgrounds, values, beliefs, emotions, gender, physical health, roles and responsibilities etc.,
8. Environment—It is the setting for the sender-receiver interaction. For effective communication conducive environment should meet the participant needs for physical and emotional comfort and safety. The factors like noise, temperature variations, distractions, lack of privacy etc., will distract and interfere the communication process and messages may not be communicated effectively.

Interpersonal Skills

"Skills that a person uses to interact with other people." communicating with respect for other people or professionals, will enable the person to reduce conflict and increase participation or assisting in, obtaining information or completing tasks. It is how well you communicate with someone and how well you behave or carry the activities by yourself. Having positive interpersonal skills increases the productivity in the organization and the number of conflicts is reduced. These skills are acquired, learned from watching parents, peers and media like the television etc. children imitate in an attempt to learn. Healthy interpersonal skills reduce stress and conflicts, improve communication, enhance intimacy, increase understanding and promote joy. Interpersonal skills are stressed on to help a person to build a network, be it personal, professional or for some other purpose. Communicating in the right way will help the person to build a professional as well as personal network. One has to interact sensibly without severing any relationships.

Interpersonal Skills include—Greeting the individuals, active listening skills, tone of voice, attentive and have a great emotional quotient when comes to dealing with people, respect and care about the people working around, approachable, cheerful, smile, humor, delegation, leadership, assertive, diplomatic, attentive and network to the best of one's own ability with the people that come across, etc.

Definitions

"Mental and communicative algorithms applied during social communications and interaction to reach certain effects or results".

"A person's ability to operate within organizations through social communication and interactions".

"All the behaviors and feelings that exist within that influence our interactions with others".

Ways to improve interpersonal skills

- Think positively and enter the mindset to work well with others and maintain good relationships
- Do not criticize others or yourself
- Be patient
- Develop active listening skills
- Be sensitive to others, do not gossip
- Have a sense of humor, appropriate to the situation. Many people benefit from a good joke
- Treat others and their experience with respect
- Praise and compliment people when they deserve it
- When someone is telling a story, do not interrupt or try to upstage them with a story of your own
- Smile—even when you do not feel like smiling
- Be cheerful and try to make others smile
- Look for solutions
- When someone compliments you, don't disagree or boast about it – simply say thank - you with a smile and move on
- Do not complain
- When you are unhappy, try your best to act happy anyway. You will end up feeling better and your mood influence the people around you.
- Fake it 'till you make it'. If you are not naturally confident or happy, fake it until you generally possess the desired characteristics
- Learn to appreciate, be helpful and not demotivate your team members. Work as a team, not as an individual. This will achieve better results
- Treat your team members and colleagues as friends and not as strangers or subordinates.

Beatrice Vincent once said, "The people with whom you work reflect your own attitude. If you are suspicious, unfriendly and condescending, you will find these unlovely traits echoed all about you. But if you are on your best behavior, you will bring out the best in the persons with whom you are going to spend most of your working hours".

Interpersonal model

Significant contributions in the Interpersonal Model are made by Harry Stack Sullivan (Fig. 15.3) originator of the theory; Adolf Meyer & Eric Berne.

Basic assumptions

Human being is a social being. His behavior grows out of his attempts to establish a meaningful social relationship with others. Human beings are having the capacity to live effectively in relationship with others.

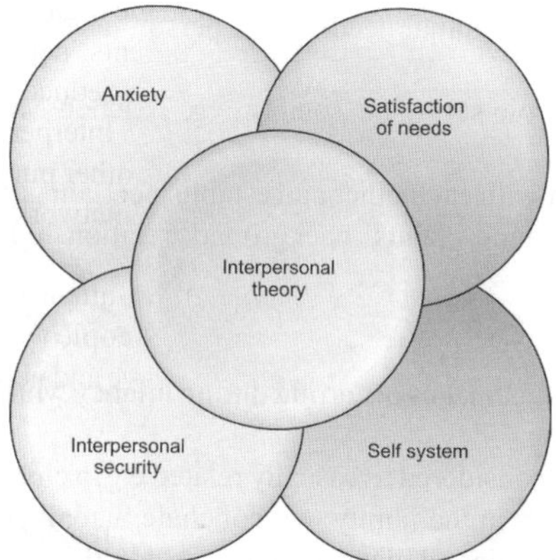

Fig. 15.3: Interpersonal Model

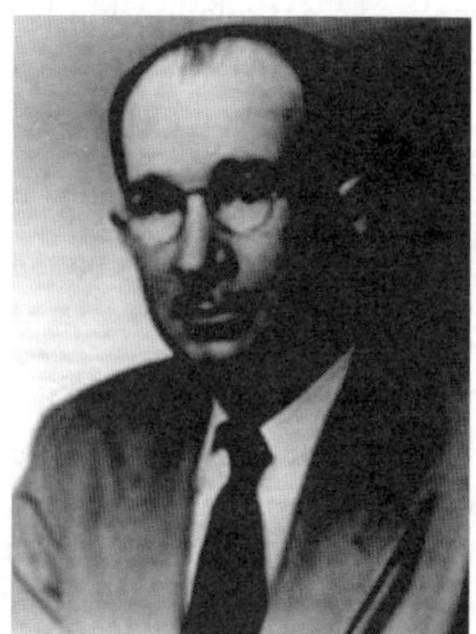

Stack Sullivan (1953)

Personality development is determined in the context of social interactions with others and is influenced by both biological and social factors.

Anxiety is a primary motivator in human personality formation and exhibition of human behavior. Anxiety is important in building self esteem and enabling a person to learn from their life experiences. Interpersonal experiences determine the personality organization achieved by human beings. Security mechanisms are used to overcome or avoid or reduce the anxiety.

Sublimation—It is an unconscious process whereby socially acceptable behavioral patterns are substituted to satisfy partially the need for a behavioral pattern that would result in increased anxiety.

Selective inattention—It is an unconscious substitute process, occurs when many details causes anxiety go unnoticed by the individual.

Dissociation—It will be used by an individual unconsciously to minimize parts of the individual's experiences to avoid anxiety.

Basic principles

a. Development proceeds through various stages, in each stage there is involvement of different patterns of relationship. For example in infancy–need for contact was fulfilled by the parents.
   - In childhood—Active participation in activities and interaction with adults will be observed
   - In preadolescent and adolescent detachment from parents and attachment with peer group increases
   - In early adulthood—Intimate relationship with heterosexual groups resulting into marriage and family formation
   - If any failure to make progress satisfactorily through various stages may result into maladaptive behavior.
b. Anxiety has direct relationship in the personality formation. For example: For fulfillment of basic needs an infant will depend on caretaker, lack of any of these needs will lead to develop mistrust or anxious or insecure and may prone for maladjustment.
c. Early life experiences (attachment with caretakers to the infant especially mother) will influence individual's development throughout his life. This lasting effect is produced by personifications, feelings, attitudes and ideas, forms as the result of experiences with anxiety and needs satisfaction with the mothering one.
   - Personifications of the self arise from infancy as the result of care given by the parents
   - Socialization causes a lot of pressure on children, e.g. appreciation and praise by others, experiences of approval and tenderness is associated with good feelings about the self 'Good me'.

Experiences associated with criticism, high anxiety situations results into 'Bad me' and are associated with feelings of shame, guilt and low self esteem.

'Not I' develops in reaction to overwhelming anxiety arising from situations that provoke feelings of 'horror or dread'. Cover a period an individual develops a 'self system' and 'self esteem' by using coping mechanisms to reduce anxiety of socialization pressures.

d. Social exchange—Social relationship is established to meet the mutual needs. Each person needs mutual help, recognition from others for self identification.
e. Social roles: Every individual has to perform specific social role set by the society, e.g. Teacher, Mother, Priest, etc.
f. Interpersonal accommodation—Two or more persons interact with each other and establish certain goals to build a satisfying relationship. It enables the nurse to understand clients' background, relationship with significant people etc.

Modes in cognitive processes

Prototaxic mode: Characterised by sensations, feelings and fleeting images occurring during infancy which are primitive and illogical.

Parataxic mode: It is illogical in nature. Simultaneous events are considered as casually related e.g. a child who has experienced the amount of loss of several significant members in the family will conclude that all people entering in the hospital will die. It is commonly observed in early childhood, if it continues into adulthood it may predispose into racial, sexual and ethnic stereotype and prejudices.

Syntaxic mode: It is developed form, characterised by logical thinking emerges in the juvenile stage. Individual develops the ability to relate effectively through this mode. It develops when young person engages in the process of consensual validation i.e., the process by which people come to agreement about the meaning and significance of specific symbols.

Human development proceeds through stages of development from infancy to old age. According to Peplau, nursing is an interpersonal process which meets the basic needs of an individual and maintains health status. Processes will progress in the direction of creative, productive, constructive, personal and community living. The components of health are: Physiological demands and Interpersonal conditions. It may be viewed as parallel to the drives of satisfaction and security.

Interpersonal therapeutic process

The crux of the therapeutic process (Fig. 15.4A) is the corrective interpersonal experience and establishing therapeutic relationship with the client in a satisfying manner. The therapist actively encourages trust by relating authentically to the client and shares the feelings and reactions with the client. The interpersonal therapist will explore the client's life history. It focuses on the person's progress through the developmental stages of learning to relate productively to other people. The process of therapy is essentially a process of reeducation, the therapist will help the client to identify interpersonal problems and then encourages him to try out more successful styles of relating closeness within the therapeutic relationship which builds trust, facilitates empathy, enhances self esteem and fosters growth towards healthy behavior. Peplau describes 'Psychological mothering process' in which:

- The patient is accepted unconditionally as a participant in a relationship that fully satisfies his needs
- Recognition and response to the client's readiness for growth initiated by the client
- Power in relationship shifts to the client as he is able to delay gratification and to invest energy in goal achievement.

Therapy is terminated when the client is able to establish satisfying relationship and meets his basic needs. The client learns that leaving a significant member or individual involves pain and an opportunity for growth. Termination will be experienced and shared by both therapist and the client.

- The client and therapist dyad is viewed as a partnership by practitioners of interpersonal therapy. In this model, the therapist acts as 'participant observer'. His/her role is to actively engage the patient, establishes trust and to empathize the role of therapy. There is an effective effort to provide the patient with consensual validation thereby helping him to realize that his/her perception and concerns are in many ways similar to those of others. uncritical acceptance climate was produced to encourage the client to speak out openly
- The therapist will have beliefs, values, thoughts and feelings and interacts as a real person
- The clients' role is to share his concern by ventilating his feelings openly and to participate actively in the relationship with the best of his ability. As the client matures in his ability to relate, he can improve and broader his other life experience with the people outside the therapeutic situation

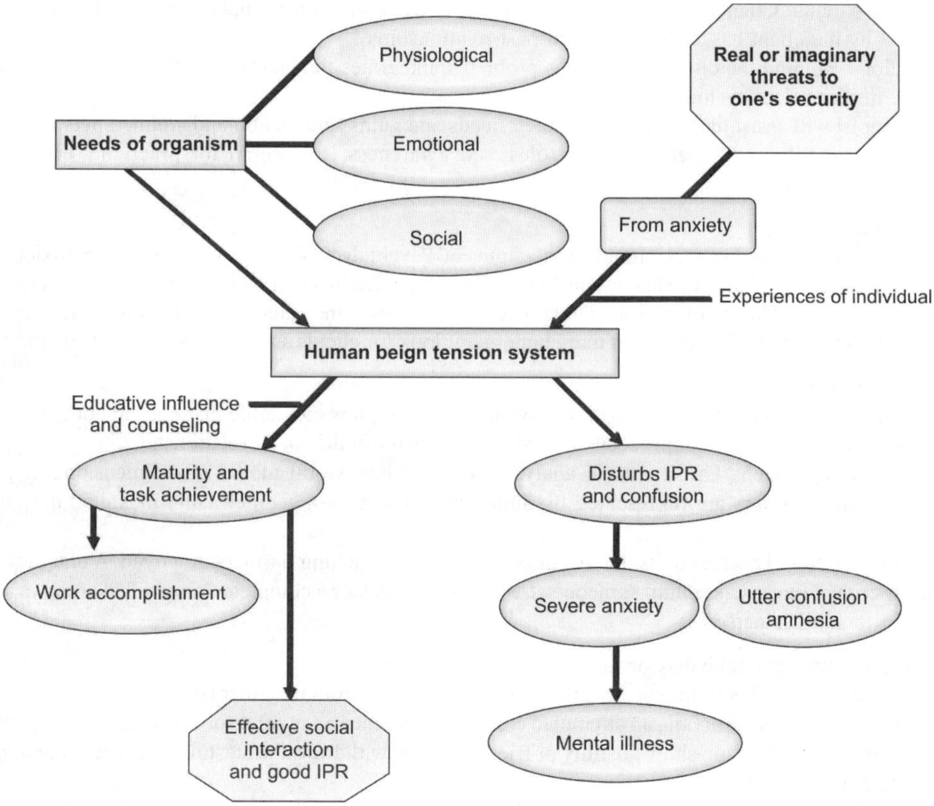

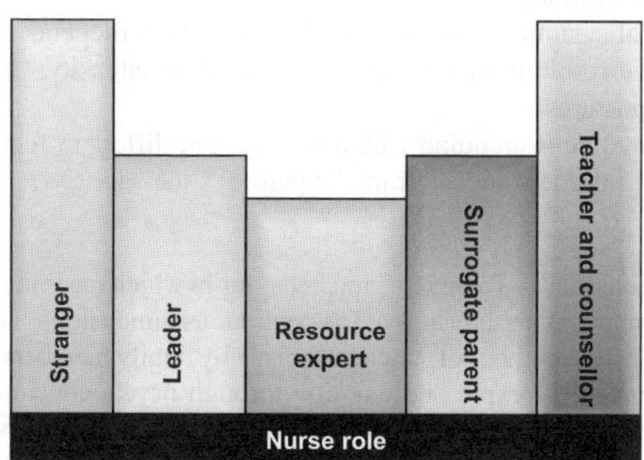

Fig. 15.4A: Therapeutic influence

Fig. 15.4B: Interpersonal Nursing Roles

The Nurse will perform varied roles such as (Fig. 15.4B):
- Stranger—When nurse and client will meet for the first time
- Resource person—Provides the health information to the client who plays consumer role
- Teacher—Assists the client in learning about his disease condition and makes the client to learn from experiences with the health care system
- Leader— Leads the client to actively participate in meeting his own needs by his own efforts

- Surrogate parent—Client transfers his feelings to the health care professionals; they assume different roles assigned by the client based on significant past relationships
- Counselor—Helping the client to solve his problems, integrates the facts and feelings associated with an episode of illness into his total life experience
- The therapist will assist the client to meet their needs and gains satisfaction and attained personal growth. Therapist will effectively perform their roles; self awareness is essential for practicing effectively in interpersonal model.

Application to Nursing

Interpersonal theory has been occupied cornerstone in Psychiatric Nursing. Concepts like anxiety, trust, security, self-esteem and nurse-client relationship etc. were included in nursing curriculums, which were derived from Sullivan's work. The use of interpersonal process recordings in the clinical aspect of mental health nursing practice. It is deterministic in nature and more hopeful outlook for clients and practitioners in using this theory.

Interpersonal behavior

Man cannot live alone for a long time without social interaction; it is inevitable that one cannot choose not to interact or behave. Two major approaches will be used to quantify the social relationships.

1. Dimensional approach: The structural analysis of social behavioral model is a dimensional approach. Interpersonal behaviors are represented by dimensions that have a geometrically meaningful relation in each other.
2. Unit of interaction: Discrete units that occur between two interacting partners or a dyad. A unit may be the entire speech of one speaker until someone else begins to speak or a complete thought that conveys a single message to another person.

Dimensions of interpersonal behavior:
- Focus: The individual is initiating an action towards an action from the other (focus on self).
- Interdependence: It is the action, an attempt to control or influence or an offer for autonomy or independence.
- Affiliation: Does the action show hostility or friendliness or withdrawal protesting a hostile act or approach enjoying a friendly act.
- Patterns of dyadic interaction: It tends to stabilize into a characteristic pattern of interpersonal behavior.
- Complementary postures: involve similar degrees of affiliation and interdependence but differing focus. They are usually stable over time.
- Symmetric postures: involve similar degrees of affiliation and interdependence as well as the same focus. They are usually unstable resulting in interaction of escalating intensity. Over time they typically move toward complementary postures.
- Anti-thetical postures: involve responding with a posture that differs in focus and is directly opposite in degrees of affiliation and interdependence from the partner's message.

Categorical Approach

1. The expressed emotion construct—To quantifying behavior in which meaningful categories of behavior are clustered into discrete groups rather than arrayed as continuous dimensions. The level of expressed emotion in a family is determined by the number of statements made by family members towards the patient that show hostility at reducing the level of expressed emotion through psychoeducational therapy to decrease the level of criticism, hostility or emotional over involvement, both lower the level of expressed emotion and extend the intervals between relapses. Expressed emotion may be a categorical construct that can identify chronically ill patients who are at higher risk for a more difficult clinical course because of familial interactional patterns. The level of expressed emotion decreases in some families after the patients' symptoms improve. Treatment of any family is most effective when health care providers use a non-blaming approach and recognize the burden placed on families with all members.

   A vulnerability stress coping model is used to explain the effect of environmental variables on conditions with clear genetic propensity, e.g. in the case of level of expressed emotion and schizophrenia, patterns are assumed to have an underlying psychobiologic vulnerability that prevents them from coping with the stress of over stimulating social interaction. The vulnerability intensifies the effects of illness.

2. Attachment style—Attachment is a crucial developmental need in human. It starts from infancy onwards, infants attaches more to their significant caregivers. The quality, infant attachment at 12 months is predictive of the child's subsequent progress.

For example: Cognitive development, problem solving, attention to tasks and social functioning in preschool with teachers and peers. Insecure attachment with parents has been observed in child abuse and neglected cases. Healthy functioning is associated with secure attachment.

For example 1: The child is confident that situational support will be available and parents are responsive and helpful, if he/she encounters adverse or frightening experiences. With this assurance the child feels bold enough to explore the world and self confident that he can handle challenges.

For example 2: A child with insecure or avoidant attachment expects that when she/he seeks help, she/he will not receive a helpful response; she acts compulsively self-reliant or in severe cases delinquent.

For example 3: A child with insecure/resistant attachment is unsure whether the parent will be available or responsive. Thus he is prone to separation anxiety, clingy and anxious about exploring the world. Attachments styles are remain stable overtime. Stressful family events can change a secure attachment relationship to an insecure attachment style.

Symptoms indicate barriers in interpersonal relationship

Communication between partners is difficult or non-existent

Frequent fighting or arguing

Loyalty and fidelity begin to be tested.

Appearance of Jealousy

Competition for meeting the needs.

Problems and disagreements go unresolved.

Insistence on doing things together (never alone).

Partners feel chained to the relationship.

People outside the relationship know about the problems.

One person controls problem solving, rules of conduct and planning.

Competition to see who is stronger.

Sense of nonproductivity.

An enabler covers for the other.

Confusion and disappointment is evident.

Talk is about how it "should" be, not about accepting the way it is.

Comparison of partner to previous partners, parents, or other family members begins.

Constant negativity exists.

Problems with intimacy exist.

Each other's feelings and rights begin to be ignored.

Partners are unable to express their feelings to each other.

Relating is at an immature or basic level.

One partner clings to the other.

Partner(s) act disconnected, like "free agents".

Depression becomes evident.

Partner(s) are unable to make a commitment.

Fun goes out of the relationship.

Partner(s) are unwilling to get outside "help".

Stubborn and bull headed behavior is exhibited.

Denial of having problems exists.

Partners ignore and/or run away from offers of help.

Barriers in interpersonal relationships in families

1. Withdrawal—An absence of interpersonal contact. It is both refusal to be in touch and time alone.
2. Rituals—Meaningless, repetitive routines devoid of real contact.
3. Pastimes—Fill up time with others in social but superficial activities.

4. Working Activities—Tasks which follow the rules and procedures of contact but no more.
5. Games—Subtle, manipulative interactions which are about winning and losing.
6. Mistrust—Lack of trust in your partner liking and accepting who you are rather than how she/he wants you to be. You are always on guard, vigilant, waiting to be taken advantage of in the relationship.
7. Fear of rejection—Belief that your partner couldn't possibly like or accept you for who you are and that she/he will probably reject you sooner or later, so you are on the lookout for the slightest signs of rejection.
8. Need for approval—Belief that you need ongoing approval from your partner. You remain cautious about the way you act, believe, feel or behave so as not to offend or lose the approval of your partner.
9. Insecurity—Belief that you cannot rely on yourself or on your partner to take care of you. You are continually anxious about how your personal needs will be met.
10. Inflexibility—Belief that your way is the only or the best way for you and your partner to relate, act, interact, communicate and problem solve. You hold to a rigid, structured, absolutist belief in the way things must be in your relationship.
11. Lack of autonomy—Belief that your partner must act, believe, think, feel, behave, and relate like you do, spending all free time with you. This does not allow the two of you to behave as independent, functioning human beings.
12. Lack of communication—Where active listening, effective, helpful responses, and open, free problem-solving is absent in your relationship. It is either closed (one way) or parallel (talking side by side with no listening) communication.
13. Avoidance of conflict—Belief that if you two never argue, fight, or disagree, the chance of having a lasting relationship is better.
14. Lack of respect for the rights of the other—Conscious or subconscious belief that your rights are the only ones that count in the relationship; therefore, acting in such a way that your partner's rights are ignored, negated, discounted or offended.
15. Fear of intimacy—Belief that if your partner gets too close, somehow she/he will know about the real, feeling, sensitive and human you. This knowledge will make you very vulnerable to being hurt, thus you shy away from getting too close.
16. Need for control—Belief that you can only enjoy a relationship with your partner if you are in complete control. If you are not in control, you will somehow be smothered, taken advantage of or ignored
17. Need for power—Belief that you must be the most powerful or exert the most strength of will in the relationship. You believe that otherwise you will be consumed, become a wimp, be ignored, be powerless, and therefore ineffectual in the relationship.
18. Irresponsible—Belief that you have little or no responsibility for the relationship or for your partner. You do nothing to nurture the relationship or to help your partner cope with life.
19. Over-responsible—Belief that you are solely responsible for the welfare and well-being of both the relationship and your partner; therefore, you do things to improve the relationship and to cover for your partner's lack of responsibility.
20. Low self-esteem—Belief that you are worthless, of no value, with nothing to offer in a relationship. You either take no initiative in the relationship or you continually feel and act inferior, defensive, tentative or resistant.
21. Fantasy or idealized image of what a relationship should be and how those in it should interact: idealistic and unrealistic standards, often unobtainable, yet their lack of attainment leads to depression and dissatisfaction with the relationship, your partner, or yourself.
22. Lack of healthy role models—Lack of an appropriate example (role model) of a healthy relationship, not knowing what "normal" is. Children from dysfunctional families often feel that somehow things are not "right" but seldom can pinpoint the problem of having unhealthy role models.
23. Chronic hostility—Chronic anger due to high-stress background. This may lead to resentment and hostility toward yourself and others. You cannot hide hostility, therefore, your partner might misread it, take it personally and thus be hurt.

24. Hiding feelings—Belief that you should never let your partner know your feelings, especially if they are negative or self-deprecating. The result of not revealing your feelings, be they positive or negative, is that your partner is left in the dark and must always guess at what is really going on with you.
25. Lack of positive reinforcement—Belief that you do not have to reinforce your partner for the good she/he does, says or relates. Without the support of positive verbal or physical feedback regarding sensitivity and kindness, your partner develops a sense of apathy, lethargy or lack of desire to please in the relationship.
26. Over-dependence—Belief that without your partner you are nothing, incompetent, meaningless. It means clinging to your partner in such a way that you never act independently, requiring and expecting full support for the majority of your thinking, believing and problem-solving.
27. Too independent—Belief that you cannot afford to risk depending on anyone except yourself for fear of becoming vulnerable to being hurt, let down, rejected or disappointed if your partner does not respond fully to any request for assistance, support or help. Your behavior, therefore, keeps you and your partner separate and unconnected.
28. Chronic depression—Chronic state of melancholy about yourself and life in general. This interferes with complete appreciation of your relationship with your partner. Your behavior and emotional state can give the message that your partner is the cause for your depression, upsetting the relationship.
29. Avoidance of risk taking—Belief that it is better never to take a risk than to take a risk and fail. In order for a relationship to begin or to grow, active risk taking by each partner is essential. In the absence of healthy risk taking, relationships are usually a dead-end.
30. Absence of fun—Belief that having fun is frivolous and unnecessary in nurturing a relationship. Such a belief can lead to the partners taking themselves and their relationship too seriously and becoming "problem focused" in their interactions.

Steps in handling problems for growth of healthy relationship

Working on improving your communications is a broad-brush activity. One has to change their thoughts, feelings and physical connections. That way, one can break down the barriers that get in way and start building relationships that really work.

Step 1—Admit you have a problem in your relationship. Use the symptoms list to help you identify the symptoms of the problem. In your journal, write down the problem. Then write how you know it is a problem by listing symptoms present in your relationship.

Step 2—Based on your open admission in Step 1 of the problem in your relationship, decide which of the barriers listed are present in this problem. List them in your journal.

Step 3—Once you have listed the problem and symptoms in Step 1 and the barriers in Step 2, share this list with your partner, and ask your partner to read your descriptions in Step 1 and Step 2.

Step 4—Based on your partner's responses in Step 3, you both can compare your responses to the three questions. You are ready for an analysis of your different and similar points of view. Write down on which points you agree or disagree concerning the problem, its symptoms and the barriers present.

Step 5—You and your partner are ready to develop a plan of action to address those barriers (problems) that you agree exist in your specific relationship.

Take each barrier one at a time and decide
a. For whom is this barrier more active?
b. Is the barrier a blocking or irrational belief?
c. Can the belief be refuted?
d. Can the party with the barrier handle it with assistance in the relationship or is outside help needed?
e. How long will it take to overcome this barrier?
f. What behavior can each of us develop to help overcome this barrier?
g. How will we know if we have been successful in overcoming this barrier?
h. What preventive action can we take to ensure that this barrier is no longer an obstacle in our relationship?
i. What replacement behavior is needed to ensure that this barrier does not recur?

j. Are we both in agreement with the remedial course of action needed? If yes, then we need to commit to working on it.

Step 6—Answer the 10 questions in Step 5 for each of the barriers you agree exist in your relationship. Once you have completed this, you have developed a plan of action to address each of these barriers. Now you and your partner need to work on the barriers. Remember, barriers existed on which you two did not agree. If over a period of time you still have barriers in your relationship, return to Step 1 and begin again

	Known to Self	Not known to Self
Known to Others	**1** Open	**2** Blind Unknown
Not Known to Others	Hidden 3	Unknown 4

Fig. 15.5: A model of Johari window

The Johari Window (Fig. 15.5), named after the first names of its inventors, Joseph Luft and Harry Ingham, A Johari window is a cognitive psychological tool created by Joseph Luft and Harry Ingham in 1955 in the United States, used to help people better understand their interpersonal communication and relationships. It is used primarily in self-help groups and corporate settings as a heuristic exercise, is one of the most useful models describing the process of human interaction.

When performing the exercise, the subject is given a list of 55 adjectives and picks five or six that they feel describe their own personality. Peers of the subject are then given the same list, and each pick five or six adjectives that describe the subject. These adjectives are then mapped onto a grid.

Charles Handy calls this concept the Johari House with four rooms. Room 1 is the part of ourselves that we see and others see. Room 2 is the aspect that others see but we are not aware of. Room 3 is the most mysterious room in that the unconscious or subconscious bit of us is seen by neither ourselves nor others. Room 4 is our private space, which we know but keep from others.

Quadrants

In this model, each person is represented by their own window. Adjectives that are selected by both the participant and his or her peers are placed into the **Open** quadrant. This quadrant represents traits of the participant of which both they and their peers are aware.

The "open" quadrant represents things that both I know about myself, and that you know about me. For example, I know my name, and so do you, The knowledge that the window represents, can include not only factual information, but my feelings, motives, behaviors, wants, needs and desires... indeed, any information describing who I am. When I first meet a new person, the size of the opening of this first quadrant is not very large, since there has been little time to exchange information. As the process of getting to know one another continues, the window shades move down or to the right, placing more information into the open window.

The process of enlarging the open quadrant is called self-disclosure, a give and take process between me and the people I interact with. Typically, as I share something about myself (moving information from my hidden quadrant into the open) and if the other party is interested in getting to know me, they will reciprocate, by similarly disclosing information in their hidden quadrant. Thus, an interaction between two parties can be modelled dynamically as two active Johari windows.

Adjectives selected only by the participant, but not by any of their peers, are placed into the **Hidden** quadrant, representing information about the participant of which their peers are unaware. It is then upto the participant whether or not to disclose this information. The "hidden" quadrant represents things that I know about myself, that you do not know.

Adjectives that are not selected by the participant but only by their peers are placed into the **Blind Spot** quadrant. These represent information of which the participant is not aware, but others are, and they can decide whether and how to inform the individual about these "**blind spots**".

The "blind" quadrant represents things that you know about me, but that I am unaware of. So, for example, we could be eating at a restaurant, and I may have unknowingly got some food on my face. This information is in my blind quadrant because you can see it, but I cannot. If you now tell me that I have something on my face, then the window shade moves to the right, enlarging the open quadrant's area. Now, I may also have blindspots with respect to many other much more complex things. For example, perhaps in our ongoing conversation, you may notice that eye contact seems to be lacking. You may not say anything, since you may not want to embarrass me or you may draw your own inferences that perhaps I am being insincere. Then the problem is, how can I get this information out in the open, since it may be affecting the level of trust that is developing between us? How can I learn more about myself? Unfortunately, there is no readily available answer. I may notice a slight hesitation on your part, and perhaps this may lead to a question. But who knows if I will pick this up, or if your answer will be on the mark.

As ones level of confidence and self esteem develops, one may actively invite others to comment on one's blind spots. A teacher may seek feedback from students on the quality of a particular lecture, with the desire of improving the presentation. *Active listening* skills are helpful in this endeavour. On the other hand, we all have defences, protecting the parts of ourselves that we feel vulnerable. Remember, the blind quadrant contains behavior, feelings and motivations not accessible to the person, but which others can see. Feelings of inadequacy, incompetence, impotence, unworthiness, rejection, guilt, dependency, ambivalence for loved ones, needs to control and manipulate, are all difficult to face, and yet can be seen by others. To forcibly reveal what another wishes not to see, is "psychological rape," and can be traumatic. Fortunately, nature has provided us with a variety of defence mechanisms to cope with such events, such as denial, ignoring, rationalizing etc.

Adjectives which were not selected by either the participant or their peers remain in the **Unknown** quadrant, representing the participant's behaviors or motives which were not recognized by anyone participating. This may be because they do not apply, or because there is collective ignorance of the existence of said trait.

The "unknown" quadrant represents things that neither I know about myself, nor you know about me. For example, I may disclose a dream that I had, and as we both attempt to understand its significance, a new awareness may emerge, known to neither of us before the conversation took place. Being placed in new situations often reveal new information not previously known to self or others.

Johari adjectives: A Johari Window consists of the following 56 adjectives used as possible descriptions of the participant are

• Able	• Dependable	• Intelligent	• Patient	• Sensible
• Accepting	• Dignified	• Introverted	• Powerful	• Sentimental
• Adaptable	• Energetic	• Kind	• Proud	• Shy
• Bold	• Extroverted	• Knowledgeable	• Quiet	• Silly
• Brave	• Friendly	• Logical	• Reflective	• Smart
• Calm	• Giving	• Loving	• Relaxed	• Spontaneous
• Caring	• Happy	• Mature	• Religious	• Sympathetic
• Cheerful	• Helpful	• Modest	• Responsive	• Tense
• Clever	• Idealistic	• Nervous	• Searching	• Trustworthy
• Complex	• Independent	• Observant	• Self-assertive	• Warm
• Confident	• Ingenious	• Organized	• Self-conscious	• Wise
				• Witty

The Johari window, essentially being a model for communication, can also reveal difficulties in this area. In Johari terms, two people attempt to communicate via the open quadrants. On the simplest level, difficulties may arise due to a lack of clarity in the interaction, such as poor grammar or choice of words, unorganized thoughts, faulty logic etc. This induces the receiver to criticize you, the sender, by revealing something that was in your blind quadrant. Then, if the feedback works, you correct it immediately, or perhaps on a more long term approach take a course in reading and writing. On a deeper level, you may be in a group meeting, and while you secretly sympathize with the minority viewpoint, you voted with the majority. However, blind to you, you actually may be communicating this information via body language, in conflict with your verbal message. On an even deeper level, you in an interaction with others, may always put on a smiling, happy face, hiding all negative feelings. By withholding negative feelings, you may be signaling to your friends to withhold also, and keep their distance. Thus, your communication style may seem bland or distant.

HUMAN RELATIONS

Introduction

"Humanism is a philosophical approach that suited for Nursing. As a philosophy it is particularly appealing because its basic tenets are not esoteric. They are easy to comprehend and can easily incorporate beliefs about clients, students and nursing education". Human relations covers all types of interactions among people— their conflicts, cooperative efforts and group relationships. It is the study of why our beliefs, attitudes and behaviors sometimes cause interpersonal conflict in our personal lives and in work-related situations. Human relations will have considerable impact on organizational productivity, the focus was mainly on improving efficiency, motivation and productivity.

Human Relation is an institution, a complex form of human association. It is a Discipline in itself. Human Relation is an applied Art and Science. Human beings are the product of the world and its environment. Human behavior is trained on selected policies and regulations. Man's action is shaped by feelings, judgments, action, motivation, determines satisfaction. Individual effectiveness depends to a considerable extent upon the physical and mental effects and abilities to those who manage and perform the productive operations with human energies, skill and knowledge.

Human Relations as a Field of Study—Human relation is an interdisciplinary field as it studies the human behavior in organizational settings, draws in the fields of Communication, Management, Psychology and Sociology. It is an important field of study because all employees engage in human relations activities. Several trends have given new importance to human relations due to the changing workplace and their work activities.

Understanding Human Behavior—Perceptions are influenced by everything that has passed through an individual's mind. This includes all of a person's experiences, knowledge, biases, emotions, values and attitudes. No two people have identical perceptions because no two people have precisely have the same experiences. Mental perceptions may sometimes lead to conflict. Each person has formed mental perceptions relating to a number of controversial issues. People reveal their attitudes through their personality. An attitude is a mental position one possesses with regard to a fact, issue or a belief. Attitudes that often present problems in the workplace are those that concern biased and prejudiced viewpoints. Generally, employees who possess positive attitudes and who are open-minded are judged to have more desirable personalities than those with negative attitudes who hold biased viewpoints.

The social dimension of behavior is determined by a person's personality, attitudes, needs and wants. An individual's personality is the totality of complex characteristics, including behavior and emotional tendencies, personal and social traits, self-concept and social skills. The objective of many training sessions for employees and supervisors is to improve a person's ability to get along with others. A person's personality has a major impact on human relation skills.

Ethics also play a role in interpersonal conflict. Ethics refer to moral rules or values governing the conduct of a person or a group. Perhaps more than anything else, an individual's adherence to values related to what is morally right determines the respect than others that hold for that person. Lack of respect for one individual by another is likely lead to poor human relations between the two.

Today's complex organizations depend on dividing the work among many formalized groups. Informal groups will also emerge, either positively or negatively affecting organizational outcomes. The relationship between organizations and groups must also be considered when quotas or standards are established. The acceptance or rejection of such standards illustrates the interaction between the organization and the group.

Managers and supervisors achieve results through people. Therefore, today's complex organizations require managers and supervisors to display a concern for people. The successful leader creates an effective balance between people and productivity and recognizes human relations as the key ingredient transforming organizational plans into organizational results. Effective human relations will lead to success.

A human relation is not limited to supervisors—it applies to every employee in an organization. Statistics indicate that successful people competently practice interpersonal skills. Good relationships must be built among individuals and within groups of an organization. Although this is not an easy task, success without good human relations is not possible. Every individual must be prepared to meet the challenge.

HUMAN RELATION IN CONTEXT OF NURSING

There is a great need in the health care profession to provide holistic care i.e., body, mind and spirit to all clients, regardless of religious, ethnic or cultural characteristics in a humane manner (non-judgmental and compassionate). Efficiency, accuracy and economy have become core concepts of health care delivery. In the present health care, the professional nurse traditionally has the closest and longest interpersonal contact with patients, particularly when hospitalized, than any other health care provider. Health care providers in general and nursing as a discipline and practice profession in particular are basically considered humanitarian approach concerned i.e., with and focused on the well-being of people. Nursing is a significant, therapeutic interpersonal process, It functions cooperatively with other human processes to have optimum health for all individuals in communities. In specific situations in which a professional health team offers health care services, nurses participate in the organization of conditions that facilitate natural tendencies in the human organisms. Nursing is an educative instrument , a maturing force that aims to promote forward movement of personality in the direction of creative, constructive, productive, personal and community living. Effective communication occurs when the receiver interprets the sender's message in the same way the sender intended it (Patton and Giffin, 1977). Effective interpersonal communication, is the key to humanizing relationships between people. To humanize means to recognize the individual's human characteristics and to address the presented health care issues with dignity and respect. A concerted effort is needed by health care educators, especially nurse educators, to guide students in a careful exploration of interpersonal communication processes that are known to promote humanizing relationships not only between the nurse and client but also between health care colleagues. The importance of effective communication as a fundamental element of nursing has been acknowledged and regarded as integral to the provision of high quality patient focused nursing care. Interpersonal communication and nursing are in the hope of establishing and promoting a benchmark of holistic and humanizing theoretical orientation for interpersonal communication between nurses, clients and others which is appropriate in all areas of nursing practice. The core of holism is that living matter or reality is made up of organic or unified wholes that are greater than the simple sum of their parts. Humanizing, primarily means to be aware of the unique characteristics of being human and relating to the person with compassion and kindness. The use of Humanizing Nursing Communication Theory (HNCT) by Duldt (1984) as a benchmark for effective nurse - client interpersonal communication in all nursing contexts. This theory is perceived as fitting into the philosophical perspective of existentialism, the systems model, and holistic paradigm. This theory is further classified as a symbolic inter actionist theory and as a humanistic theory for nursing communication, human capabilities and potential are shared experiences that superceded by religion, culture, economics, politics, race, and so forth. In addition, the quality of life humans experience is valued.

The Human Relations Dimension—In Education Process, The Human Relations Dimension includes learner, teacher, administrator, group of learners, Patient, Nursing service Professionals, Allied health personnel and their interactions. The interaction of human relations of these individuals in the educational settings both in the school and outside the school exerts an important influence on the effectiveness of the educative process.

Human Relation Model—It is based on assumption that employees are motivated by satisfactory treatment . The social context of work life has become increasingly relevant to the motivation of workers. More attention has been given to Group Dynamics and interpersonal relations in the work place. The concept of Simulation training developed, to help leaders to develop sensitivity and skills in managing people in groups, obtains personal insight into their own and other's reactions and feelings about events in group. Improve both interpersonal skills of the manager and overall performance of the group.

Definitions

"Relationships between people, It can be formal or informal, close or distant, emotional or unemotional".

"Fitting people into work situations so as to motivate them to work together harmoniously. The process of fitting together should achieve higher levels of productivity for the organization, while also bringing employees economic, psychological and social satisfaction."

"A course or A Study or A Program designed to develop better interpersonal and intergroup adjustments".

"The study of group behavior for the purpose of improving interpersonal relationships, among employees".

" A study of human problems arising from Organizational and interpersonal relations".

"Integration of people into work situation that motivate them to work together productively, cooperatively to provide economic, psychological and social satisfaction".

"The Interaction of people in any organization where people are found together in some sort of formal structure to achieve an objective".

"Human relations is the development of producing and satisfying group efforts".

In health care, workers use many kinds of relationships with different people must be considered. As an employee at a health care facility one has a relationship with (1) Self (2) Co-workers (in the unit/department) (3) Departmental Supervisor (4) The patient (5) Patient's family/visitors (6) Physicians,(7) Other health care workers. Nursing is an experience lived between human beings. Each nursing situation reciprocally evokes and affects the expression and manifestations of these human beings' capacity for and condition of existence.

"Humanism is an approach to life based on reason and common humanity, excluding god or higher beings. Certain characteristics of interpersonal communication are of particular relevance to being human and establishing satisfying, warm, personal relationships with others. These characters are as follows:

- Interpersonal communication is a process that is essential in nature.
- Interpersonal communication involves the generation and exchange of meaning, that is a sense of, what is important and what has implications for one's future?
- Interpersonal communication provides information about "outside the skin" reality or facts and about emotions aroused "inside the skin" or feelings
- Interpersonal communication is a dialogic or two-directional process in the sense that one alternately sends and receives messages.

The role interpersonal communication plays in our growth and development is to humanize. Through interpersonal communication processes with significant people, an individual, from infancy, becomes oriented to the physical and social world.

Aims
- To ensure the fundamental rights
- To considerate the human being needs for existence as a respectable citizen of the Nation
- To motivate the people to provide the services
- To promote cooperation among group members through mutual trust and interest
- To gain satisfaction by maintaining group relationship
- To broaden and sharpen sensitivity to the feelings of others.

Factors involved in self-understanding
- Self-acceptance
- Self-image
- Values
- Self-confidence—A belief in oneself and in one's powers and abilities
- Relations with others—The qualities that make a person likable
- Genuineness—Means being oneself; genuine people do not put up false fronts to try to look good; genuine people do not put on an act and are comfortable with themselves
- Trustworthiness—The key to building trusting relationships with others is to be trustworthy; when others take risks with you, you must prove their risks are worth taking.

Factors that affect Human Relations with Employers
- Competence—The ability to perform a required task; as a rule competent employees get along with their employers
- Cooperation—Working with others to reach a given goal; the employer has a right to expect your cooperation
- Loyalty—A feeling of obligation and devotion to one's employer or job; includes not complaining to others about your working conditions
- Initiative—Recognizing what jobs need to be done and doing them without being reminded
- Trustworthiness—The quality that makes one dependable; the employer knows the trustworthy employee will do what is expected and often even more
- Honesty—Qualities of trustfulness, honor, and integrity; free of fraud and deception
- Dependability—Being on the job everyday, arriving on time and notifying the employer if one cannot be at work.

Factors influencing Human Relations
- Development in Science, Business and Finance, Management and Technological Advancement
- Increase in size of organization
- Greater Specializations in respective fields
- High standards of living
- Maturity
- Emotions, impulses, deep feelings
- Possessions.

Effective tools of Human Relations
- Personality Development
- Sound, specific, clear stated objectives and well formulated objectives with well developed Organizational structure
- Adequate Salaries
- Conducive Working Environment
- Sound Policies of an organization and laws related to health field and orienting all staff in advance if any changes has been made
- Opportunity for promotion and monitory benefits like Increase in salaries
- Establishment of Suitable policies related to old age benefits, medical insurance facilities, family benefits, incremental plans, rewards if employee exhibits expected behavior or appreciation of the employees efficiency, activities to improve staff morale and clear information on policies like demotion, cutting up of benefits if the employee misbehaves or not performing the work in an expected manner
- Encourage Two way communication between Organizational authorities and Administrator, with Administrator to employees, among employees
- Upgrading of Employees, e.g. training and rise in salaries
- Flexible links within the organization and opportunities to utilize them for the benefit of institutional activities.
- Promote group work/Team Work and Provision of equal opportunities for all employees
- Framing and informing job responsibilities of each cadre of employees in the organization
- Orientation of employees about the organization and it's objectives and policies, job responsibilities
- Managers/supervisor should know the strengths/capabilities/potentialities and weaknesses of each employee and has to keep efforts to improve strengths to improve work pattern among group members
- Employment security
- Adequate Opportunities and training of employees through Staff development program, Faculty Development Programs, In service and Continuing Education Programs
- Motivating all employees in all levels, in respective fields to attend workshops, seminars, conferences and training programs. Provision of facilities like on job or on duty facility or additional leave facility, supporting their professional growth with monitory benefits.

Techniques for being accepted by Fellow Employees

- Try to get along with co-workers
- Seek acceptance by co-workers in a job
- Accept others' life styles—Everyone should learn to respect another person's right to be different
- Avoid incorrect assumptions to avoid offending others before all facts are known
- Maintain a good appearance because a good first impression will help one on the way to being accepted
- Develop a good attitude—One of the most important factors that determine one's acceptance by others in any environment is attitude
- Observe rules—There is usually a set of rules to be followed at the workplace, but there are also unwritten rules that workers are expected to observe.

Basic ways of getting along with People

- Think before you speak; always say less than you think
- Make promises sparingly and keep them faithfully, no matter what it costs
- Be interested in others—In their pursuits, their welfare, their homes, and families; let everyone you meet, however humble, feel that you regard them as a person of importance
- Never let an opportunity pass to say a kind and encouraging thing to or about somebody
- Be cheerful; keep a pleasant smile on your face
- Reserve an open mind on all debatable questions; discuss but do not argue—It is a mark of a superior mind to disagree yet be friendly
- Discourage gossip and make a rule to say nothing of another unless it is something good
- Be careful of others' feelings—wit and humor at the other fellow's expense are rarely worth the effort
- Reasons why people work and set goals:
  - To achieve satisfaction
  - To support family
  - To attain acceptance of peers
  - To gain power
  - To accumulate wealth.

Establishing Human Relations with Patients

- Learn to know, understand relate to the patient in any situation
- Show sympathy for the patient by being eager to serve and by having a gentle touch
- Realize and understand sick people are sensitive, both emotionally and physically; sickness causes strain and patients are not always on their best behavior
- Remember to be kind and tolerant when patients are irritable and demanding
- Realize much of the satisfaction, assistants derive from their work is due to the relationship they develop with the patient.

Human Relations Skills/ Management skills

- Employees will be selected based on their educational background, technical skills and human relation skills they possess in the specific field, exposure to specific field and previous employment history etc.
- The skills include leadership, communication, decision making and work efficiency, human relation skills are important at all levels of management, which will facilitate effective interaction with personnel. Human skills means how to communicate, tackle people, how to use their skills, how to work within a team, The most important human skill is to be able to communicate with anyone, no matter what the subject, Good human relation skills help others to demonstrate good work ethics.

Human Relations in Communication

- Good attitudes enhance communication
- Good communication eliminates misunderstanding and lowers employee turnover
- Communication implies two important things—sharing means that communication involves the action of more than one person; there must be one to send the message and another to react to it

- Understanding means that both the sender and receiver of the message share the same meaning of what is said, this part of communication is the most difficult because people tend to give different meanings to the same words, and problems in human relations develop because of the failure of people to share and understand messages

In order to develop good IPR and Effective human relations wherever the person exists like within the family or in the work area, if they possess good human relation skills, he will exhibit good humanitarian approach and conducive environment to live happy manner and exhibit satisfied relationship which promote work efficiency.

Tips to develop good Human Relations
- Sensitive to one's attitude—Focus, dedicated, consistent, and disciplined behavior one has to exhibit
- Role Model—One has to set as a role model, exemplary for fellow beings both in personal and professional, to win the confidence of people
- One should possess a sense of humor and exhibit smile on their faces
- Possess and exhibit emotional maturity—Every individual will be exposed for several painful stimuli, no two individuals will not respond in a similar way when they exposed to stimuli within the environment, one has to cool down, control emotional imbalances, do not express your anger to outside, calm down, divert your mind by meditation, prayer, reading interested materials, listening to music etc., after calmness only speak to the people, if it is inevitable, speak in brief. Think thrice before speaking anything to out side including to your own family, once the word comes out you can never take it back, one has to keep it in his/her mind.
- Self Confidence—Awareness about one's own self-worth and will power. As you grow in life ego, jealousy, ill feelings has to be dropped. One should have mastery over the subject and learn required skills and acquire the experiences, efficiency, meet all the requirements of a specific jobs then automatically one's own self confidence which is essential for one's own efficiency in performing the tasks efficiently
- Determination—One has to be determined in his/her goals, then only one can put sincere efforts in achieving the aims in life by putting sincere efforts. Determination is the way to attain higher ends of the sky
- Absence of frictions—An individual has to establish and maintain good IPR & HR both in personal and professional environment , avoid frictions in the environment in order to maintain good working and personal relationships among team members
- Greet the individual—Approach the individual with warm smile and approaching manner, greet the individual, it is the first gate way to approach any one either younger or older, superior authority or co-worker. It maintains smooth relationship and a way or initial step to reach the goal or work to complete
- Address the person by his/her name—Start the interaction by addressing their name, you should not call the person by their designation or physical appearance. It gives an idea, that you know the person and easy for developing IPR
- Show love, concern but do not develop attachments with any one in life, do not live in other's thoughts, follow your inner conscious direction, do not be influenced totally by the people, have emotional maturity in dealing the tasks and handling the situations
- Introduce your friends and family based on situation, occasion and in the environment, do not bring your family matter in the working situations
- Count on your people—When the person in the group will be going on leave and come back to the work, try to express how his/her absence created vacuum or how the work was affected, how you felt for his/her absence to create bondage and develop an association
- Respect one's opinions and convictions—If the opinion or convictions are valuable give respect and welcome the person's ideas or the thoughts, give appreciation for the positive feelings which promote work efficiency, condemn negative ideas or thoughts, do not encourage the people to exhibit their weaknesses or super imposing on you and disturbing your Psychodynamics
- Social engagements—Visit the friends and their families after informing them, and spend some personal time that will fetch the relationships

- Be benevolent—show courtesy when the employee or colleague is sick, sanction the leave if provision is there, otherwise allow some resting period, flexible upto recovery, if the employee admits in the hospital, visit them and so you are concern about his/her health and ask if he needs any help, if it is admissible, tell him speedy recovery of the person is very essential, meet the need all these are milestones in developing good HR. Be magnificent in your activities
- Recognize one's own feelings and sentiments—Administrator/Manager/Supervisor/Nurse educator has to understand the feelings, sentiments, values of colleagues or co workers, everyone will have their own sentiments, unless they are harmful to others, One should not criticize others, if anything one has to discuss think thrice, if it is necessary without hurting their inner feelings discuss on one on one basis
- Gentleness and Courtesy—If you want to give instructions for subordinates or juniors give gently smoothly without hurting inner feelings of the person, at the same time take precautions, work has to be done and mistakes has to be corrected. Be courteous, do not hurt the inner feelings. Be polite
- Generosity fetch high dividends—Be kind, open, broad, generous, show love and concern for others, help the person in need, with kindness, whenever the need arises
- Admit your mistake—Err is human, Admit your mistake, say sorry and then try to learn correct one
- Communication–Communicate the content clearly, openly, if doubt arises say sorry and explain again in detail. Avoid misunderstanding, try to understand what they are saying, if it is not clear ask twice and try to understand correct meaning
- Listen to others—Listening is both art and skill, Develop active listening skills, Listen completely, don't interrupt while they are talking, express joy and happiness when you heard positive information. Listen with your eyes, ears and with heart
- To work effectively as a member of the group and leader of the group—Keep trying, never put a stop, Don't leave the problem in between, try until you find a solution for the problem and reach the goal
- Elevate the general morale of the people—Build up loyalty, mutual sincerity, implement steps to improve morale of the group members. Ensure the goals and needs of the group members will be taken care
- Employee oriented leaders–Democratic leaders generally achieve better results than autocratic or task oriented leaders
- Accept change—In the world, nothing is static, everything is subjected for change, accept the change, flow along with the stream and not against the stream. Bring positive change within the mind and work with a hope
- Identify the hidden talents–Leader/administrator/supervisor has to identify the hidden talents/capabilities/strengths and weaknesses of the employees, encourage them to develop professional skills
- Maintain high level of ethics and morale—Leader has to be an exemplar/role model, has to maintain good ethics and positive morale, inculcate moral and ethical values to the group members. Give respect and take respect from group employees
- Administrator can not please everyone all the time, some times one has to take hard decisions to straighten up the things
- Social values—Give respect for the social values, encourage morality among the group members. Change is the law of nature, even though change everyone will not accept immediately, each one will take their own course of time, leader has to be persistent in bringing positive change among the employees
- Give self appraisal forms and do the performance appraisal of employees and get feed back from colleagues, subordinates and students. Have one on one meetings with each employee and advise for getting improvement. Encourage the fellow beings to improve further in their personal and professional skills
- Be judicious—Administrator has to equally delegate the work to all the group members. One should not be overloaded and one should not be under loaded. Delegation of the work should be equal based on the speciality administrator has to delegate the work to all group members and supervise their work
- Do not grudge or grumble at others. Think analytically and wisely while talking with your group members, maintain your good will
- Good to forget about bad issues which occurred, it is not good to recall every time and have the feeling of painful experiences, get stressed out, things which you can not change

- Do not reprimand in the presence of others—Call the person to administrator's office , have one on one meeting, discuss the problems and give suggestions, do not hurt the feelings by discussing in front of a group and his/her prestige will be hurted and the ego will be lowered
- Praise before criticism—Give appreciation first for the things accomplished first, then discuss the points where change is required
- Improve the group member's skills—Consider personality style and discuss the intrinsic factor first to improve the group member's skill
- Leadership style—Based on the situation, exhibit the leadership pattern like when the things are not proper use autocratic leadership and get the things straighten up, when all the group member's interest has to be considered and skills has to be encouraged be friendly and use democratic skills. Whenever necessary Lasizepiere skills has to be used. Encourage group members to enhance cohesion and improve coordination, professional skills
- Be detached—Love every one appreciate their goodness, but not get attached, be sensitive to the feelings of others, win the acceptance and approval, encourage creativity of the individuals.

Barriers in human relations

1. Human relation problems may develop because of the failure of people to share and understand messages
2. When a person uses a word has just one meaning
3. The particular meaning is what that person intends the word to mean
4. Bypassing is a barrier in communication because one single word or expression is complicated by several different meanings or several different words might have the same meaning
5. Employers and employees can cause communication problems by misusing language; two of the most serious
6. Problems that arise due to the misuse of language are:
   - Labeling or name—Calling to unfairly classify someone as a certain type of person. Typical labels given to people are:
     - Clown—A person who appears to do silly things
     - Troublemaker—A person who appears to be frequently involved in problems
     - Animal—a person lacking in manners.
   - Emotional confusion—Words that mean the same thing; some have pleasant sounds while others do not. Negative appeal, positive appeal death insurance, life insurance, garbage collector, sanitary engineer, stock salesperson, investment counselor
   - Avoid emotional confusion in human relations by using as many positive sounding words or titles as possible
   - Listening—When good listeners do not understand a message, they ask the speaker for a different explanation; good listeners must be alert; listening is much more than hearing—the process of listening requires an active mind.
   - Grapevine—The term dates back to the Civil War, when the United States sent secret messages by telegraph line strung through trees and bushes almost like a vine; today, the term "grapevine" includes all forms of unofficial communication, but messages by way of the grapevine are only about 80% reliable. Interpret data from various sources in formulating conclusions; demonstrate proficiency in medical terminology and skills related to the health care of an individual; and interpret knowledge and skills that are transferable among health science professions.
7. Use Cognitive Skills—By utilizing intellectual curiosity, engage in scholarly inquiry and dialogue, accept constructive criticism and revise personal views when valid evidence warrants
8. Reasoning—Consider arguments and conclusions of self and others, construct well-reasoned arguments to explain phenomena, validate conjectures, or support positions, gather evidence to support arguments, findings, or lines of reasoning, Support or modify claims based on the results of an inquiry
9. Problem solving—Analyze a situation to identify a problem to be solved, Develop and apply multiple strategies to solving a problem

10. Work habits—Work independently and collaboratively
    - Academic integrity—Attribute ideas and information to source materials and people, Evaluate sources for quality of content, validity, credibility, and relevance, Include the ideas of others and the complexities of the debate, issue, or problem
    - Understand and adhere to ethical codes of conduct—Reading across the curriculum, use effective pre-reading strategies, use a variety of strategies to understand the meanings of new words
    - Identify the intended purpose and audience of the text
    - Identify the key information and supporting details
    - Analyze textual information critically
    - Annotate, summarize, paraphrase, and outline texts when appropriate
    - Adapt reading strategies according to structure of texts—Connect reading to historical and current events and personal.

Human Relations in Health Care

In modern Health care Institutions, the Personnel department plays a vital role, it should be considered as integral part of the institution. Personnel manager is integral part of the education team, he/she held many responsibilities, sometimes acts as a link between the administrator and managerial authorities, establishes cordial relationship with all the personnel in the organization. All people work together cooperatively and productively. In order to develop good human relations in the working situation should possess sound knowledge of human behavior and basic needs are essential. They will be motivated and rewarded if they develop good human relations.

- Prepare the job responsibilities
- Fill the posts and vacancies as per statutory body's directions and orient them with the institutional policies and their duties
- Provide future security for all the employees in terms of health insurance and family benefits
- Maintain the sense of dignity, respect, trust with all the employees in the organization
- Develop and win the confidence of the present employees
- Foster an empathy, respect, genuineness
- Encourage constructive criticism and motivate them to utilize problem solvation techniques in dealing with the issues
- Authorities should make sincere efforts to implement the policies and work for employee's benefits
- Inform the group to work together, ability to share with the individuals, establish and maintain good working relationships
- Ability to share power, derive satisfaction
- Accomplish together work structure, goals, cohesion.

HEALTH BEHAVIOR

Behavior is the general term covering all the physical acts performed by individuals, e.g. physical acts—walking, interacting with others, writing, reading and preparing to learn. Behavior includes seeking or not seeking advice for health care and following or not following a prescribed medical regimen. Health Behavior is a complex behavior, motivated by stimuli in an individual's environment, motivation for health behavior is dynamic. Health behaviors expressed by individuals to protect, to maintain and to promote their health status. Lifestyle is closely associated with health behavior and factors influencing life style are: socioeconomic, educational and cultural. Every behavior or activity by an individual has an impact on health status. Health behaviors are distinguished from risk behaviors which are defined separately as behaviors associated with increased susceptibility to a specific cause of ill-health. Health behaviors and risk behaviors are often related in clusters in a more complex pattern of behaviors referred to as lifestyles. it includes not only observable, overt actions but also the mental events and feeling states that can be reported and measured. Health state must also be considered in the field of health behavior. This should be considered to encompass physical functions and the effects of illness, including the adequacy with which stress is addressed by coping strategies and phenomena such as addiction and treatment effects. Health state can affect all three elements of the triangle. "Sets of concepts and propositions that articulate relations among variables to explain and predict situations and results."

Definitions

"Any activity undertaken by an individual, regardless of actual or perceived health status, for the purpose of promoting, protecting and maintaining health, whether or not such behavior is objectively effective towards that end"

"Personal attributes such as beliefs, expectations, motives, values, perceptions and other cognitive elements; personality characteristics, including affective and emotional states, traits and overt behavior patterns, action and habits that relate to health maintenance, to health restoration, and to health improvement"—*Gochman, 1982 and 1997.*

"The actions of individuals, groups and organizations as well as their determinants, correlates and consequences, including social change, policy development and implementation, improved coping skills and enhanced quality of life"—*Parkerson and others, 1993.*

Types of Health Behavior

- Health-directed behavior
  Observable acts that are undertaken with a specific health outcome in mind, e.g. performing exercises, yoga, meditation etc. to have better health
- Health-related behavior
  Those actions that a person does that may have health implications but are not undertaken with a specific health objective in mind, e.g. parents are the first teachers in the child's life. They teach the child to cultivate specific behavior like Prayer, Hygienic Practices, Adequate Nutrition, Rest, Sleep, Recreation, Social interaction and establishing good inter personal relationships, Educating the child about Balance Mind, Coping Strategies, etc. to attain holistic health and desired behavior for the child direct or indirectly.
- Preventive Health Behavior
  Action taken when a person wants to avoid being ill or having a problem. Any activity undertaken by an individual for the purpose of preventing or detecting illness in an asymptomatic state. For example parents will immunize the child to protect against specific diseases.
- Illness behavior
  Any activity undertaken by an individual who perceives himself to be ill, to define the state of health, and to discover a suitable remedy. Action taken when a person recognises signs or symptoms that suggest a pending illness, e.g. a mother gives her child cough medicine to suppress child's cough, administers antibiotics as per doctor's advice to cure infections.
- Sick-role behavior
  Action taken once an individual has been diagnosed (either self or medical diagnosis).
  Any activity undertaken by an individual who considers himself to be ill, for the purpose of getting well. It includes receiving treatment from medical providers, generally involves a whole range of dependent behaviors and leads to some degree of exemption from one's usual responsibilities. For example, a mother decides that her child has Malaria when she observes the child is having fever with chills and takes him to the clinic for confirming diagnosis and obtains treatment, follows doctors' advise and implement necessary steps to control the Disease and its' manifestations. Parents strive for child's survival and for better health improvement.

Determinants of health behavior

- Psychological factors, e.g. Euphoria, joy, happiness—Healthybehavior, sick behavior, e.g. emotional behavior
- Cultural factors, e.g. customs, traditions, specific habits, values promotes healthy behavior
- Social factors, e.g. economic qualitative, productive, healthy life style
- Environmental factors, e.g. sanitation; proper disposal of waste products maintaining good
- Hygiene, e.g. physical and mental hygiene.

Cognitive theories of health behavior

Most models of behavioral change are based on an assumption of volitional, that is cognitively determined, behavior, e.g. the health belief model and its offshoots are based on the premise that attitudes and beliefs are the major determinants of health behavior and that any behavior in response to a health threat is based on two major types of cognition: the expectation that a specific action will lead to improve the health and the subjective value that is placed on improved health. Any divergence in behavior is thus related to the adequacy of cognition and how readily cognition is adapted to new experience. Cognitive theories have been used to investigate the roles of motivation, fear and misperception. In all, the basic premise is the same: preventive behavior is a function of the perception of threat and of the belief that the best course of action includes new behavior. With the recognition that context also plays a role, evolving theory includes cues to action and general orientation to health as subjective cultural values. Models of behavior have been developed from Rogers' concept that adoption of new behavior is a process and diffuses across society from individuals at various stages (diffusion of innovations). Models of individual behavior are based on the hypothesis of interactions between behavior and cognition, so that different types of cognition operate at different stages. For example, the trans theoretical model of stages of change proposes that an individual passes through a growing degree of readiness for change before initiating that change. Interventions based on stage models encourage identification of stage, and the cognitions associated with that stage are targeted. In stage theories, intention is considered to be the last step before a new behavior is practised. Cognitive models generally assume that self-efficacy (the confidence of having the means to enact change) is in operation, and the specific role of the context is added as an aspect of perception of social norms and barriers to action. health education is based on the assumption of a more direct line between knowledge and behavior.

Theories of the context of behavior

Environmental theories tend to go beyond individual volition and to varying degrees discount volition or other cognition. They are based on the premise that even if attitude mediates a person's responses to a context, it is the environment that influences behavioral choices. A general theory related to context is the *'ecological'* *approach*, in which multiple and reciprocal levels of influence are identified, including intrapersonal or individual factors (Biology, Psychology and Behavior), interpersonal factors, institutional or organizational factors, community factors and public policy factors. In this perspective, cognitive elements play a relatively small role in health behavior in relation to context, which is divided into several categories. **In structural models**, change in individual behavior is considered to be a result of changes in the organizational conditions within which the individuals live and work. By changing the structure, change is allowed to occur. The observed decrease in the incidence of stomach cancer has been attributed not to individuals deciding to change their eating patterns, but rather to the quality and variety of foods that have become available with modern refrigeration and food preservation techniques. Research into health-care systems is based on a structural model of behavior. In **grounded theory**, a social and structural model often used in work on sex differences in health, subjective experiences are examined qualitatively to determine the dominant social and structural processes that account for the greatest variation in behavior in a particular situation, and these become the focus for change. **Participatory models** are based on the premise that sustained change comes about through social change orchestrated by the community itself. Participatory studies address community programs that involve the collaboration of various sectors of society for change designated and desired by the community. **Advocacy** is a major strategy for social change. It is a systematic attempt to gain political and social support for changes related to health in the population. It does not involve promotion of individual solutions but support for changes in the social environment that legitimize or delegitimize certain behavior, creating the changes in social conditions that allow individuals to adopt healthy behavior.

Phases between knowledge and behavior (Fig. 15.6)

- In some cases, knowledge may be sufficient to elicit changes in behavior, but in other cases it may be low, where an individual requires to modify
- It should not be assumed that individuals are always knowledgeable about an appropriate health behavior, but it assumed that knowledge will guarantee changes in behavior
- Where knowledge is deemed important, this should be expressed in terms that are salient to the target audience

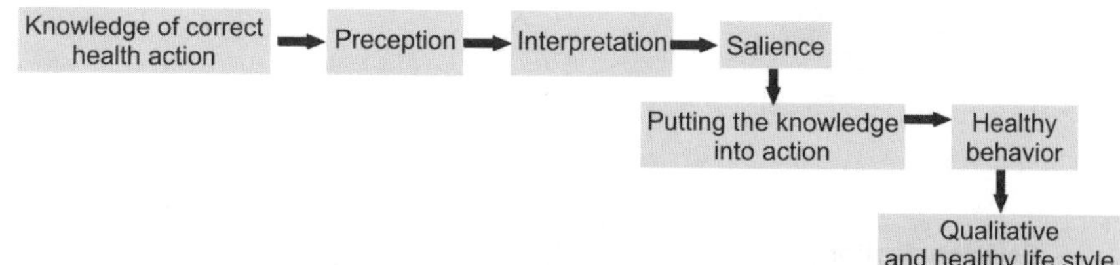

Fig. 15.6: Knowledge and health behavior

- The transfer of knowledge into action is dependent on a wide range of internal and external factors, including values, attitudes and beliefs
- For most individuals, the translation of knowledge into behavior requires the development of specific skills (enabling factors) which may include interpersonal skills.

Attitudes, values and behavior
- An individual's attitude to a specific action and their intention to adopt it is influenced by beliefs, motivation which comes from the person's values, attitudes and drives (instincts) and the influence from social norms
- A belief represents the information a person has about an object or action. It links the object to some attribute
- Values are acquired through socialization and are those emotionally charged beliefs which make up what a person thinks is important
- Attitudes are value-ladened social judgments which possess a strong evaluative component
- Attitudes have different components-cognitive (belief), emotional (feeling) and behavioral (predispositions to act)
- Values and attitudes help to explain the knowledge-action gap in many instances
- Most people are at ease when their knowledge is consistent with their attitude and values
- If discord arises, the facts are often interpreted so that contradiction between knowledge is removed
- There is no clear or linear progression from attitudes to behavior
- Often, attitude change precedes behavioral change, e.g. often assumed that changing attitudes to smoking will influence smokers to quit, yet a majority of smokers continue to smoke despite a negative attitude to smoking and aware of the effects associated with it
- But equally, behavior change may precede and influence attitudes – On the other hand, quitting smoking is often a stimulus for indifferent smokers to develop a negative attitude to smoking.

MODELS OF BEHAVIOR CHANGE

Cognitive dissonance model (Festinger-1957)
- The model holds that inconsistency is a painful or uncomfortable state
- Since dissonance is psychologically uncomfortable, it will motivate an individual to reduce dissonance to achieve consonance
- In addition, the individual will actively avoid situations and information that are likely to increase the dissonance
- The consequences of this are vital for anyone involved in the process of influence
- For example, if a respected role model with whom an individual identifies makes a statement or declaration with which the individual disagrees, consonance is achieved by either: (a) changing the belief or by (b) changing attitudes to the respected person.

Maslow's hierarchy of needs (Maslow-1968) (Fig. 15.7)
- Behavior is motivated by a hierarchy of human needs
- Explains why not everybody responds to the obviously beneficial and well-meaning interventions
- Health needs may be compromised for the sake of satisfaction of low-order needs.

1st segment: Base of Triangle—Physiological needs (Basic Needs-Essential for survival, e.g. Food, Water, Air, Sleep, Rest, Relaxation, Sex, Homeostasis, Excretion, Shelter/stay for living/Home, clothing/apparel)

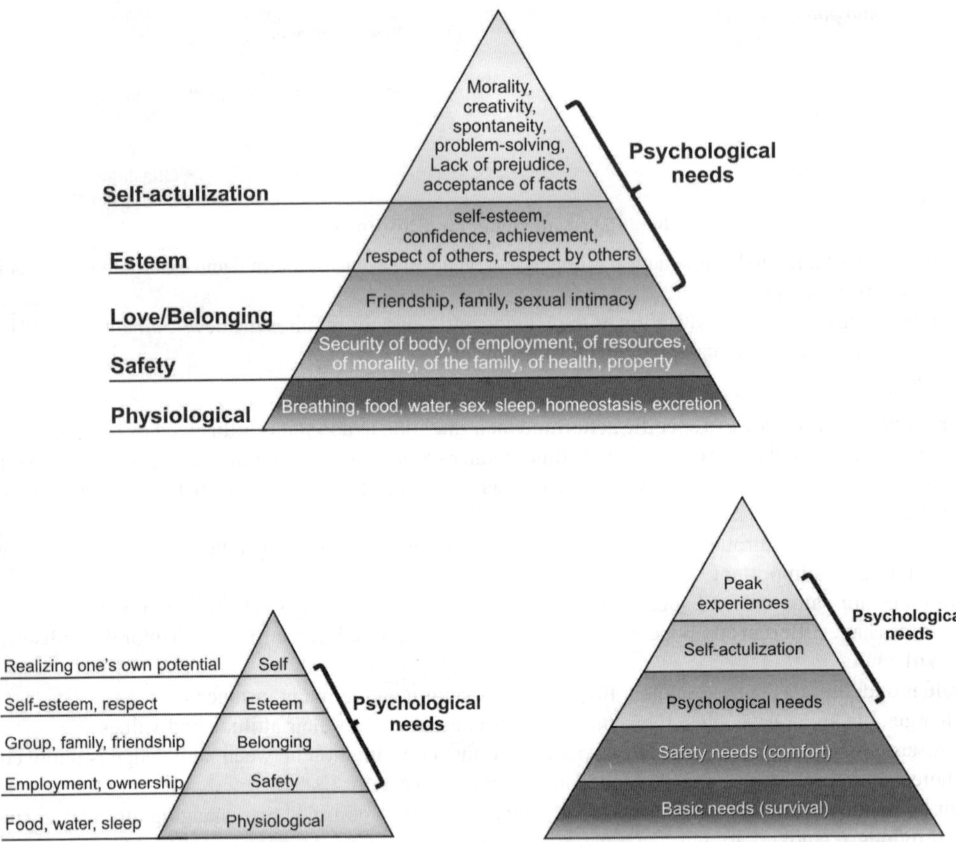

Fig. 15.7: Maslow's Hierarchy of needs

2nd segment: Safety/Comfort/Security Needs/Protective needs, e.g. Security of–Body, Employment, Resources, Morality, Family, Health, Wealth, Ownership, Property, Social Stability, free from the threat, free from pain, free from terror, praise, awards, decorations, gifts

3rd segment: Love and Belonging Needs, e.g. Family, Friends, Sexual intimacy, Sense of Connection

4th segment: Self Esteem Needs, e.g. Confidence, Achievement, Respect of others, Respect by others. The need to be a unique individual.

5th segment: Self Actualization Needs (Realization of one's own potential/the need and desire to act as they pleased according to their talents and interests), e.g. Morality, Creativity, Spontaneity, Problem – solving, Lack of Prejudice, Acceptance of facts, experience, purpose, Meaning and inner potential

6th segment: Peak experience highest achievements in one's own life.

The health belief model (Rosenstock and Becker - 1974) (Fig. 15.8)

Two major factors influence the likelihood that a person will adopt a recommended preventive health action

- First: They must feel personally threatened by disease, i.e. they must feel personally susceptible to a disease with serious or severe consequences
- Second: They must believe that the benefits of taking the preventive action outweigh the perceived barriers to (and/or cost of) preventive action seeks healthy behavior.

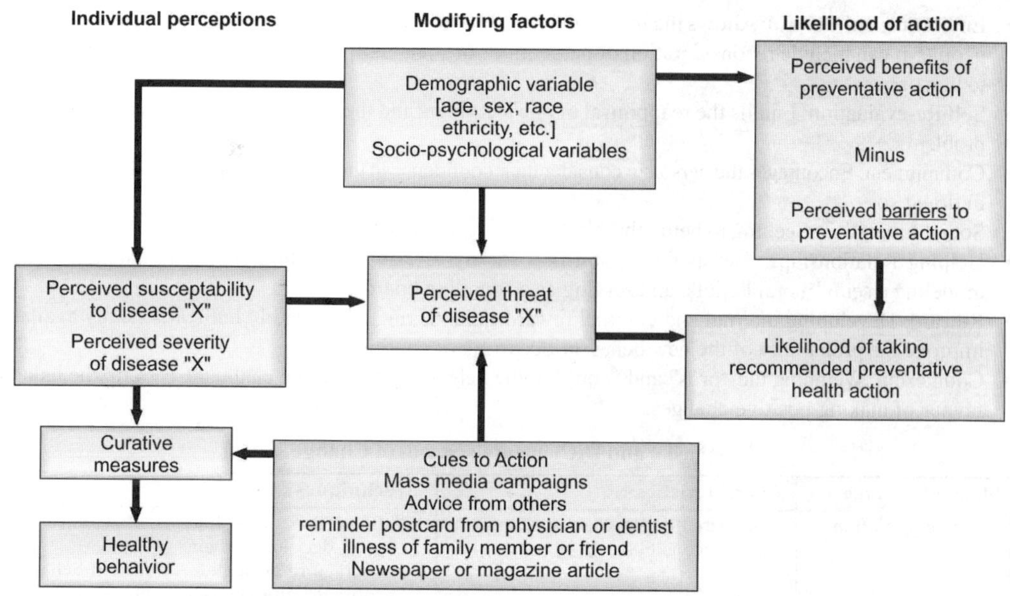

Fig. 15.8: Modified form of Health Belief model

Stages of change model (Prochaska and Diclemente-1984)

* The model identifies a number of stages which a person can go through during the process of behavior change
* It takes a holistic approach, integrating a range of factors such as the role of personal responsibility and choices and the impact of social and environmental forces that set very real limits on the individual potential for behavior change
* It provides a framework for a wide range of potential interventions by health promoters.

Stages of Change
* Pre-contemplation
* Contemplation
* Preparation
* Maintenance
* Action

Pre-contemplation: Has no intention to take action within the next 6 months.

Contemplation: Intends to take action within the next 6 months.

Preparation: Intends to take action within the next 30 days and has taken some behavioral steps in this direction.

Action: Has changed overt behavior for less than 6 months.

Maintenance: Has changed overt behavior for more than 6 months.

Termination: Overt behavior will never return and there is complete confidence that you can cope without tear of relapse.

Process of Change
* Any activity that you initiate to help modify your thinking, feeling or behavior

Major process of change

* Consciousness Raising: Involves providing information regarding the nature and risk of unsafe behaviors and the value and drawbacks of the safer behavioral alternatives.
* Dramatic Relief: Fosters the identification, experiencing, and expression of emotions related to the risk the safer alternatives in order to work toward adaptive

- Environmental Control: Allows the individual to reflect on the consequences of his or her behavior for other people. It can include reconsideration of perceptions of social norms and the opinions of people important to him or her.
- Self Re-evaluation: Entails the reappraisal of one's problem and the kind of person one is exposed for given problem
- Commitment: Encourages the person to consider their confidence in their ability to change and their commitment in doing so.
- Social Liberation: Seeking to help others with similar situations.
- Helping Relationships: Assists the person In a variety of ways, Including providing emotional support, modeling a set of moral beliefs, and serving as a sounding board.
- Reward: Developing internal and external rewards and making them readily but contingently available to improve the probability of the new behavior occurring or continuing.
- Countering: Weighing the "pros" and "cons" of the behavior change. The challenge is to tip the balance in favour of making positive changes.

Prochaska and DiClemente's Stages of Change Model

Stage of Change	Characteristics	Techniques
Pre-contemplation	Not currently considering change: "Ignorance is bliss"	Validate lack of readiness Clarify: decision is theirs Encourage re-evaluation of current behavior Encourage self-exploration, not action Explain and personalize the risk
Contemplation	Ambivalent about change: "Sitting on the fence" Not considering change within the next month	Validate lack of readiness Clarify: decision is theirs Encourage evaluation of pros and cons of behavior change Identify and promote new, positive outcome expectations

COLLECTIVE BARGAINING

Definitions

"A process between employers and employees to reach an agreement regarding the rights and duties of people at work".

"It will address equity issues from the point of view of employees—Issues such as a fair wage, working conditions and the equal distribution of wage increases to all".

"The Process whereby workers organize collectively and bargain with employers regarding the work place. In a broad sense, it is the coming together of workers to negotiate their employment".

"Collective action or simply acting as a group with a single voice, is one method by which to deal with problems".

"The practice of bargaining with reference to wages, work practice and other benefits by employees in a collective group with management".

"A labor contract between an employer and one or more unions. It consists of the process of negotiation between representatives of a union and employers, in respect of the terms and conditions of employment of employees, such as wages, hours of work, working conditions and grievance—Procedures and about the rights and responsibilities of trade unions, The parties often refer to the result of the negotiation as a collective bargaining agreement (CBA) or as a collective employment agreement (CEA)".

"A type of negotiation between organized workers or employees and their employer or employers—Usually to determine wages, hours, rules and working conditions".

"A recognized way of creating a system of industrial jurisprudence. It acts as a method of introducing civil rights in the industry, that is, the management should be conducted by rules rather than arbitrary decision making. It establishes rules which define and restrict the traditional authority exercised by the management".

"Voluntary negotiation between employers or employers' organizations and workers' organizations, with a view to the regulation of terms and conditions of employment by collective agreements" – ILO.

"The process or means and collective agreements to the possible result of bargaining. Collective bargaining may not always lead to a collective agreement."

"Collective bargaining allows both workers and managers to discuss specific terms that can , depending on national law: determine the rules that govern their relationship, determine wages, deal with other matters of mutual interest eg: hiring practices, lay offs, promotions, job functions, working conditions and hours, work safety, worker discipline, termination and benefit programs".

Aims

- Develops a sense of self respect and responsibility among the employees
- To reach a collective agreement which usually sets out issues such as employees pay, working hours, training, health and safety and rights to participate in workplace or company affairs
- During the bargaining process, employees are typically represented by a trade union. The union may negotiate with a single employer or may negotiate with a federation of businesses, depending on the country, to reach an industry wide agreement
- Permits workers to achieve a form of workplace democracy
- To reduce the conflictual issues it is more effective for employers and their employees to establish joint consultation mechanisms to achieve an understanding on how to increase the productivity 'cake'. In that event, in collective bargaining the areas of dispute would be narrowed and both parties would be likely to share a common view about the issues and even arrive at a basic agreement on them
- To ensure the rule of law in the workplace. Workers gain a voice to influence the establishment of rules that control a major aspect of their lives
- Collective bargaining includes not only negotiations between the employers and unions but also includes the process of resolving labor–management conflicts. Thus collective bargaining is, essentially, a recognized way of creating a system of introducing civil rights in the industry i.e., the management should be conducted by rules rather than arbitrary decision-making. It establishes rules which define and restrict the traditional authority exercised by the management.

Importance to employees

- It develops a sense of self-respect and responsibility among the employees
- It increases the strength of the workforce, thereby increasing their bargaining capacity as a group
- Increases the morale and productivity of employees
- Restricts management's freedom for arbitrary action against the employees. Unilateral actions by the employer are also discouraged
- It strengthens the Trade Unions movement
- Employees feel motivated as they can approach the management on various matters and bargain for higher benefits
- It helps in securing a prompt and fair settlement of grievances. It provides a flexible means for the adjustment of wages and employment conditions to economic and technological changes in the industry, as a result of which the chances for conflicts are reduced.

Importance to employers

- It becomes easier for the management to resolve issues at the bargaining level rather than taking up complaints of individual workers
- Collective bargaining tends to promote a sense of job security among employees and thereby tends to reduce the cost of labor turnover to management
- Collective bargaining opens up the channel of communication between the workers and the management and increases worker participation in decision-making
- Collective bargaining plays a vital role in settling and preventing industrial disputes.

Importance to society
- Collective bargaining leads to industrial peace in the country
- It results in establishment of a harmonious industrial climate which supports which helps the pace of a nation's efforts towards economic and social development since the obstacles to such a development can be reduced considerably
- The discrimination and exploitation of workers is constantly being checked
- It provides a method or the regulation of the conditions of employment of those who are directly concerned about them.

Pros
- Can lead to high-performance workplace where labor and management jointly engage in problem solving, addressing issues on an equal standing
- Provides legally based bilateral relationship
- Management's rights are clearly spelled out
- Employer's and employee's rights protected by binding collective bargaining agreement
- Multi-year contracts may provide budgetary predictability on salary and other compensation issues
- Unions may become strong allies in protecting higher education from the effects of an economic slowdown
- Promotes fairness and consistency in employment policies and personnel decisions within and across institutions
- Employees may choose whether they want union representation
- A strong labor management partnership may enable the workforce development needed for engaging the technology revolution
- Board of Regents maintains right to establish the labor-related activities that may take place on the work site, subject to labor's right to appeal to State Labor Relations Board (SLRB)
- Individual institutions may negotiate sub agreements on any issue, preserving institutional distinctions on matters subject to collective bargaining
- Board of Regents has the authority to assign titles and positions to bargaining units, subject to labor's right to appeal to SLRB
- Elections may take place at reasonable intervals (every 2 years)
- Employees are prohibited from striking and engaging in other similar work stoppages or slowdowns
- Lack of impasse procedures favors management
- Employees who are not members of unions are not required to pay service fees
- Employees may still discuss any matter with the employer
- The management rights section is extensive
- A broad range of employees are exempted
- An election is required before employees can choose to bargain collectively or not
- Protect patients from inadequate and unsafe care
- Ensure that nurses have fair pay, good benefits and safe/satisfactory working conditions
- Establish effective channels of communication with those who make decisions that impact nursing practice.
- Advance nurse's professional growth and development
- Participates in decision making
- Protects economic security
- Improves the quality of patient care
- Settlement through dialogue and consensus rather than through conflict and confrontation
- Collective bargaining agreements often institutionalize settlement through dialogue
- Collective bargaining is a form of participation, it involves a sharing of rule-making power between employers and unions in areas which in earlier times were regarded as management prerogatives, e.g. transfer, promotion, redundancy, discipline, modernization and production norms
- Collective bargaining agreements sometimes renounce or limit the settlement of disputes through trade union action. Such agreements have the effect of guaranteeing industrial peace for the duration of the agreements, either generally or more usually on matters covered by the agreement

- Collective bargaining is an essential feature in the concept of social partnership towards which labor relations should strive. Social partnership in this context may be described as a partnership between organised employer institutions and organised labor institutions designed to maintain non-confrontational processes in the settlement of disputes which may arise between employers and employees
- Collective bargaining has valuable by-products relevant to the relationship between the two parties. For instance, a long course of successful and bonafide dealings leads to the generation of trust. It contributes towards mutual understanding by establishing a continuing relationship. The process, once the relationship of trust and understanding has been established, creates an attitude of attacking problems together rather than each other in societies where there is a multiplicity of unions and shifting union loyalties
- Collective bargaining and consequent agreements tend to stabilize union membership. For instance, where there is a collective agreement employees are less likely to change union affiliations frequently. This is of value also to employers who are faced with constant changes in union membership and consequent inter-union rivalries resulting in more disputes in the workplace than otherwise collective bargaining usually has the effect of improving industrial relations. This improvement can be at different levels. The continuing dialogue tends to improve relations at the workplace level between workers and the union on the one hand and the employer on the other
- It also establishes a productive relationship between the union and the employers' organization where the latter is involved in the negotiation process.

Cons

- Management's authority and freedom are much more restricted by negotiated rules
- Creates significant potential for polarization between employees and managers
- Disproportionate effect of relatively few active employees on the many in the bargaining unit. This is particularly the case when collective bargaining involves a system-wide structure of elections
- Increases bureaucratization and requires longer time needed for decision making
- Increases participation by external entities (e.g. arbitrators, State Labor Relations Board) in higher education's decision-making
- Negotiation of system wide bargaining contracts will be cumbersome and time-consuming, requiring agreement among system wide managers before negotiations begin and restricting flexibility during negotiations
- The sub agreement process will be difficult to administer. There will be an increased burden on the Board of Regents to craft a flexible management plan to serve as the basis of the negotiation with the exclusive bargaining agent
- The votes of employees within a bargaining unit at a single large institution may dominate the decision whether that system wide bargaining unit will engage in collective bargaining
- Legislative approval may be required on certain matters that are now within the Board of Regents' authority, running counter to the spirit of autonomy
- A very strong system of shared governance will be restricted to a very limited number of areas
- Under the guise of inconsistency and unfairness, labor will attempt to negotiate away the different conditions of work and various economic benefits necessary to the unique requirements of an institution
- Protects the status quo, thereby inhibiting innovation and change. This is particularly the case when the change involves privatizations
- More difficult for employees at smaller campuses to have their voices heard
- Higher management costs associated with negotiating and administering the agreements
- Eliminates ability of management to make unilateral changes in wages, hours and other terms and conditions of employment
- Restricts management's ability to deal directly with individual employees
- Increased dependence on the private sector for certain services, particularly those requiring technological competence, may be compromised
- Contract administration is a very difficult process to manage and significantly changes the skill set required of managers and supervisors.

Collective Action Models

- Shared governance—is where nurses and managers work together to define their roles and expected outcomes. It holds everyone accountable for his or her role and expected outcomes. For example, Partnership, Equity, Accountability and Ownership
- Workplace advocacy—refers to the activities nurses undertake to address problems in their everyday workplace setting. Activities include forming committees to address problems, devising alternatives to achieve optimal care and inventing new ways to implement change
- Collective action—is simply acting as a group with a single voice. When a group acts with a single voice and brings ideas to management, it changes from collective action to collective bargaining. If the group cannot achieve its desires through informal collective bargaining with management, the group may decide to form a union
- Whistle blowing—is the act where an individual discloses information regarding a violation of a law, rule or regulation or a substantial and specific danger to public health or safety. A collective bargaining agent—is an agent who works with employees to formalize collective bargaining though unionization.

Theories

- Collective bargaining is a human right and thus deserving of legal protection. The *Universal Declaration of Human Rights* identifies the ability to organize trade unions as a fundamental human right and the *International Labor Organization's* Declaration on Fundamental Principles and Rights at Work defines the "freedom of association and the effective recognition of the right to collective bargaining" as an essential right of workers. The right to bargain collectively with an employer enhances the human dignity, liberty and autonomy of workers by giving them the opportunity to influence the establishment of workplace rules and thereby gain some control over a major aspect of their lives, namely their work
- *Monopoly Union Model* (*Dunlop*, 1944)—States that the monopoly union has the power to maximize the wage rate; the firm then chooses the level of employment
- The *Right-to-Manage Model*—Developed by the British school during the 1980s (*Nickell*) views the labor union and the firm bargaining over the wage rate
- The *efficient bargaining Model* (McDonald and *Solow*, 1981)—Sees the union and the firm bargaining over both wages and employment (or more realistically, hours of work).

Collective Bargaining Process/Collective Bargaining Agreement (CBA)

Collective bargaining includes negotiations between the two parties (Employee's & Employer's representatives). It consists of negotiations between an employer and a group of employees that determine the conditions of employment. Often employees are represented in the bargaining by "Union or other labor organization". The result of collective bargaining procedure is called Collective Bargaining Agreement (CBA). Collective agreements may be in the form of "Procedural agreements or Substantive agreements". Procedural agreements deal with the relationship between workers and management and the procedures to be adopted for resolving individual or group disputes. It include procedures in respect of individual grievances, disputes and discipline. Procedural agreements are put into the company rule book which provides information on the overall terms and conditions of employment and codes of behavior. A Substantive agreement deals with specific issues, e.g. Basic Pay, Overtime premiums, bonus arrangements, holiday entitlements and hours of work, etc. In many companies, agreements have a fixed time scale and a collective bargaining process will review the Procedural agreement when negotiations take place on pay and conditions of employment (Fig. 15.9).

Steps

1. Prepare—It involves composition of a Negotiation team, consists of representatives of both the parties with adequate knowledge and skills for negotiation. In this phase both the employer's representatives and the Union examine their own situation in order to develop the issues that they believe will be most important. The first thing to be done is to determine whether there is actually any reason to negotiate at all. A correct understanding of the main issues to be covered and intimate knowledge of operations, working conditions, production norms and other relevant conditions is required.

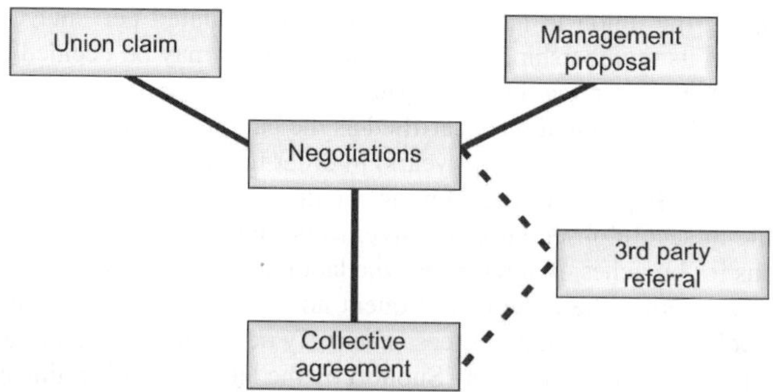

Fig. 15.9: The process of collective bargaining

2. Discuss—The parties decide the ground rules that will guide the negotiations. A process well begun is half done and this is no less true in case of collective bargaining. An environment of mutual trust and understanding is also created so that the collective bargaining agreement would be reached.
3. Propose—Involves initial opening statements and the possible options that exists to resolve them. It is brain storming, the exchange of messages takes place and the opinion of both parties is sought.
4. Bargain—Negotiations are becoming easy, if problem solving is adopted. This stage comprises time, that when " what ifs" and "Supposals" were set forth and drafting of agreements takes place.
5. Settlement—Once the parties are through with the bargaining process, a consensual agreement is reached upon wherein both the parties agree a common decision regarding the problem or the issue. This stage is describing as consisting of effective joint implementation of the agreement through shared visions, strategic planning and negotiated change.

Nature of Collective Bargaining
- It is a method used by trade unions to improve the terms and conditions of employment of their members
- It seeks to restore the unequal bargaining position between employer and employee. Where it leads to an agreement, it modifies, rather than replaces, the individual contract of employment, because it does not create the employer-employee relationship
- The process is bipartite, but in some developing countries the State plays a role in the form of a conciliator where disagreements occur or where collective bargaining impinges on government policy.

Conditions for Successful Collective Bargaining
- Pluralism and the Freedom of Association–A pluralistic outlook involves the acceptance within a political system of pressure groups (e.g. religious groups, unions, business associations, political parties) with specific interests with which a government has dialogue, with a view to effecting compromises by making concessions. Pluralism implies a process of bargaining between these groups and between one or more of them on the one hand and the government on the other. It is therefore recognizes these groups as the checks and balances which guarantee democracy. It is natural that in labor relations in a pluralist society, collective bargaining is recognized as a fundamental tool, through which stability is maintained, while the freedom of association because without the right of association the interest groups in a society would be unable to function effectively. Thus pluralism's theme is that, men associate together to further their common interests and desires; their associations exert pressure on each other and on the government; the concessions which follow help to bind society together; thereafter stability is maintained by further concessions and adjustments as new associations emerge and power shifts from one group to another. Therefore, no meaningful collective bargaining without the freedom of association accorded to both employers and workers
- Trade Union Recognition—The existence of the freedom of association does not necessarily mean that there would automatically be recognition of unions for bargaining purposes. Especially in systems where there is a multiplicity of trade unions, there should be some pre-determined objective criteria operative within the industrial relations system to decide when and how a union should be recognized for collective bargaining purposes. The accepted principle is to recognize the most representative union, but what criteria is used to decide it and by whom may differ from system to system. In some systems the issue would be

determined by requiring the union to have not less than a stipulated percentage of the workers in the enterprise or category in its membership. The representativeness may be decided by a referendum in the workplace or by an outside certifying authority (such as a labor department or an independent statutory body). There could be a condition that once certified as the bargaining agent, there cannot be a change of agent for a prescribed period (e.g. one or two years) in order to ensure the stability of the process.

- Observance of Agreements - Especially in developing countries where there is a multiplicity of unions, unions are sometimes unable to secure observance of agreements by their members. Where a labor law system provides for sanctions for breaches of agreements, the labor administration authorities may be reluctant to impose sanctions on workers. Where there is frequent non-observance of agreements or understandings reached through the collective bargaining process, the party not in default would lose faith in the process.
- Support of Labor Administration Authorities - Support by the labor administration authorities is necessary for successful collective bargaining. This implies that they will:
  - Provide the necessary climate for it. For instance, they should provide effective conciliation services in the event of a breakdown in the process, and even provide the necessary legal framework for it to operate in where necessary, e.g. provision for the registration of agreements
  - It will not support a party in breach of agreements concluded consequent to collective bargaining
  - As far as practicable, secure observance of collective bargaining agreements
  - Provide methods for the settlement of disputes arising out of collective bargaining if the parties themselves have not so provided
- Good Faith—Collective bargaining is workable only if the parties bargain in good faith. If not, there will be only the process of bargaining without a result viz., an agreement. Good faith is more likely where certain attitudes are shared among employers, workers and their organizations, e.g. a belief and faith in the value of compromise through dialogue, in the process of collective bargaining and in the productive nature of the relationship collective bargaining requires and develops. Strong organizations of workers and employers contribute to bargaining in good faith, because there would be some parity in the bargaining strength of the two parties
- Proper Internal Communication—Both the management and union should keep their managers and members respectively well-informed, as a lack of proper communication and information can lead to misunderstandings and even to strikes. Sometimes managers and supervisors who are ill-informed may inadvertently mislead workers who work under them about the current state of negotiations, the management's objectives and so on. In fact, it is necessary to involve managers in deciding on objectives and solutions and such participation is likely to ensure greater acceptance and therefore better implementation by them.

Levels of bargaining

Originally collective bargaining at the national or the industry level was viewed by employers as a means of reducing competition based on labor costs through standardized wage rates. Employers no longer view collective bargaining from this perspective. Instead, centralized and industry level negotiation is considered as depriving enterprises of the needed flexibility to compete on the basis of adjustments at the level of the enterprise in relation to pay, working hours and conditions, work organization, manpower utilization and so on. The efficiency gains are considerably greater and more easily realizable—When negotiations take place at the enterprise level. Therefore, the major thrust in all countries where the pattern hitherto was national or industry level bargaining, towards increased enterprise-level bargaining, has been by employers. Not all unions favor this trend; their power position can be automatically eroded by this trend, just as it is enhanced through centralized or industry level bargaining.

Steps in Organizing a Collective Bargaining Unit

- Assemble a group of nurses who support collective bargaining
- Arrange a meeting with a representative of the State Nurse's Association
- Assess the feasibility of an organizing campaign
- Conduct necessary research to develop a plan of action
- Establish an organizing committee and subcommittees
- Begin the process of obtaining union authorization cards
- Schedule an informal meeting for nurses eligible for the collective bargaining unit

- Keep the lines of communication open with nurses
- Seek voluntary recognition from the employer
- Move toward formal organization of the unit
- Seek certification by the National Labor Relations Board as the exclusive bargaining agent of the unit
- Initiate contract negotiations
- Manager's role during process—Unions may increase the cost for the hospital and limit the authority of its managers
- Manager's role during initiation of unionization—Know the law and make sure rights of the nurses as well as management are clearly understood, Act clearly within the law, no matter what the organization delegates to you as manager. Find out the reasons the nurses want collective action. Discuss and deal with the nurses and the problems directly and effectively. Distribute lists of disadvantages of unionization, such as paying dues distribute examples of unions that did not help with patient care issues
- Employees' role during process—Nurses desiring to choose a collective bargaining agent must be sure they know the laws that have been instituted and follow them carefully, Know your legal rights and the rights of the manager, Act clearly within the law at all times
- If a manager acts unlawfully, e.g. by firing an employee for organizing, report the employer's actions to the National Labor Relations Board
- Keep all nurses informed through regular meetings held close to the hospital
- Set meeting times conveniently around shift changes and assist with child care during meetings
- Striking
  - A collective bargaining agent cannot make the decision to strike
  - The decision to strike can be made only by a majority of union members
  - Most nursing collective bargaining agents put a no-strike clause in the contract
- Collective Bargaining Agents
  - Service Employees International Union
  - State Nurses' Council, The Trained Nurses Association of India
  - National Union of Hospital and Health Care Employees.

Organizational Behavior

In every field of Social Science, or even Physical Science has a philosophical foundation of basic concepts that guide its development. There are some certain philosophical concepts in organizational behavior also. Organizational behavior studies encompasses the study of organizations from multiple viewpoints, methods and levels of analysis. The study of "micro" organizational behavior refers to individual and *group dynamics* in an organizational setting and "macro" strategic management and organizational theory studies whole organizations and industries, how they adapt and the strategies, structures and contingencies that guide them. Understanding organizational behavior is a major factor for increased opportunity and success in the world. Gaining an awareness of an organizations culture is necessary for continued diverse growth. In order to attract the best talent to an organization, a culture of diversity and open communication is needed. Once an organization has the best talent it can find, the organization can improve efficiency and have more wide spread viewpoints to learn from. Care must be taken, to make sure the organizational culture is compatible with the strategic goals of an organization. Organizations must consider what employees want and what concerns they may have. Consistent responses such as recognition for work well done, job security, a balance between work and family life and competitive salary and benefits. There is a fundamental need for organizations and managers to know what their employees value, how they feel, and be accommodating so as to keep the organization on the leading edge of productivity, profitability and productivity.

Definitions

"The study of human behavior in organization. It uses scientific methods to test hypotheses. It is also a multi-disciplinary study, taking knowledge from Social and Behavioral sciences and applying it to real world situations"

—Schermerhorn, et al (2005)

"The systematic study and careful application of knowledge about how people—As individuals and as groups act within organizations"

"The study and application of knowledge about how people, individuals and groups act in organizations. It does this by taking a *system approach*. That is, it interprets people - organization relationships in terms of the whole person, whole group, whole organization, and whole social system. Its purpose is to build better relationships by achieving human objectives, organizational objectives, and social objectives"

"The array of ways humans behave in task-oriented groupings—Employers, military, churches, etc. Organizational behavior includes the study of motivation, leadership, interpersonal relations and performance"

"The study of what people do in an organization and how the behavior affects the performance of the organization is concerned with the employment status"

"The systematic study of how people, individual or group thinks, feels, behaves and acts within the organization as well as outside the organization and applying this"

"Values and beliefs that are shared among members of an organization that affects the way they interact and accomplish certain task"

"The study of the many factors that have an impact on how individuals and groups respond to and act in organizations and how organizations manage their environments"

" A concept or tool for businesses motivated to meet the needs of its employees while being aware of the impact each individual has on an organization's behavior"

"The systematic study and careful application of knowledge about how people act within organizations."

Models of Organizational behavior

- Autocratic—The basis of this model is power with a managerial orientation of authority. The employees in turn are oriented towards obedience and dependence on the boss. The employee need that is met is subsistence. The performance result is minimal. has its roots in the industrial revolution
- Custodial—The basis of this model is economic resources with a managerial orientation of money. The employees in turn are oriented towards security and benefits and dependence on the organization. The employee need i.e., met is security. The performance result is passive cooperation
- Supportive—The basis of this model is leadership with a managerial orientation of support. The employees in turn are oriented towards job performance and participation. The employee need i.e., met is status and recognition. The performance result is awakened drives
- Collegial—The basis of this model is partnership with a managerial orientation of teamwork. The employees in turn are oriented towards responsible behavior and self-discipline. The employee need that is met is self-actualization. The performance result is moderate enthusiasm.

  Although there are four separate models, almost no organization operates exclusively in one. There will usually be a predominate one, with one or more areas over-lapping in the other models.

  The three models (Custodial, Supportive and Collegial) begin to build on *McGregor's Theory Y*. They have each evolved over a period of time and there is no one best model. In addition, the collegial model should not be thought as the last or best model, but the beginning of a new model or paradigm.

Concepts

- A social system—is a complex set of human relationships interacting in many ways. Within an organization, the social system includes all the people in it and their relationships to each other and to the outside world. The behavior of one member can have an impact, either directly or indirectly, on the behavior of others. Also, the social system does not have boundaries—It exchanges goods, ideas, culture, etc. with the environment around it and status. Their behavior is influenced by their group's individual drives. Organization environment in a social system is dynamic. All parts of the system are interdependent.
- Culture—is the conventional behavior of a society that encompasses beliefs, customs, knowledge and practices. It influences human behavior, even though it seldom enters into their conscious thought. People depend on culture as it gives them stability, security, understanding and the ability to respond to a given situation. This is why people fear change. They fear the system will become unstable, their security will be lost, they will not understand the new process and they will not know how to respond to the new situations.

- Individualization—is when employees successfully exert influence on the social system by challenging the culture.

The quadrant shown shows (Fig. 15.10) how individualization affects different organizations (Schein, 1968):
- Quadrant A—Too little socialization and too little individualization creates isolation.
- Quadrant B—Too little socialization and too high individualization creates rebellion.
- Quadrant C—Too high socialization and too little individualization creates conformity.
- Quadrant D—While the match that organizations want to create is high socialization and high individualization for a creative environment.

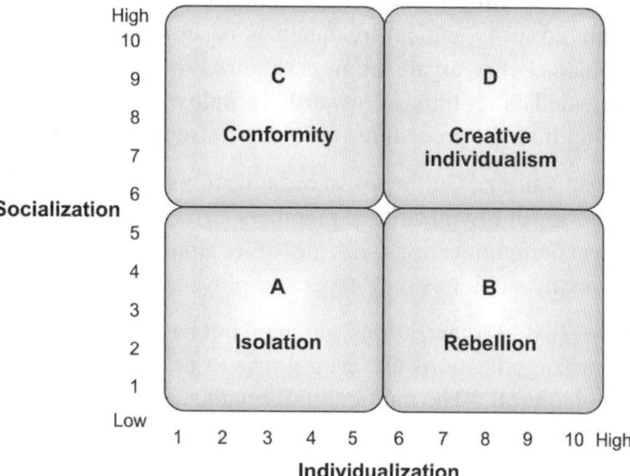

Fig. 15.10: Impact of indivisualization on an organization

This is what it takes to survive in a very competitive environment having people grow with the organization, but doing the right thing when others want to follow the easy path.

This can become quite a balancing act. Individualism favors individual rights, loosely knit social networks, self-respect, personal rewards and careers—It may become look out for Number One, Socialization or collectivism favors the group, harmony and asks "What is best for the organization?" Organizations need people to challenge, question and experiment while still maintaining the culture that binds them into a social system.

Individual differences—Every individual in the world is different from others. This idea is supported by Science. Each person is different from all others, probably in million ways, just as each persons' DNA profile is different. The idea of individual difference comes originally from Psychology. From the day of birth, each person is unique and individual experiences after birth tend to make people even more different.

Perception—Peoples' perceptions are also differ when they see an object. Two people can differently present a same object and this is occurring for their experiences. A person always organizes and interprets what he sees according to his lifetime of experience and accumulated value. Employees also see work differently for differ in their personalities, needs, demographics factors, past experiences and social surrounding.

A whole person—An employee's personal life is not detached from his working life, e.g. A women who attend the office at 8:30 AM is always anxious for her children's school time (if her children able to attend the school or not). As a result, its impact falls on her concentration that means her working life. For this reason, we cannot separate it. So manager should treat an employee as a whole person.

Motivated behavior—An employee has so many needs inside him. So, they want to fulfill those needs. That's why; they have to perform well in the organization. Some motivations are needed to enrich the quality of work. A path toward increased need fulfillment is the better way that enriches the quality of work.

Desire for involvement—Every employee is actively seeking opportunities at work to involve in decision-making problems. They hunger for the chance to share what they know and to learn from the experience. So, organization should provide them a chance to express their opinions, ideas and suggestion for decision-making problem. A meaningful involvement can bring mutual benefit for both parties.

Value of the person—An employee wants to be treated separately from other factor of production . They refuse to accept the old idea that they are simply treated as economic tools because they are best creation of almighty, God. For this reason, they want to be treated with carrying respect, dignity and other things from their employers and society.

Mutual interest—In order to develop the organization behavior mutually of interest organizations and people is necessary. Organizations need people and people in turn need organizations. People satisfy their needs through organization and organization accomplish their goal through people.

Ethics—In order to attract and retain valuable employees in an era in which good employees are constantly required away, ethical treatment is necessary. To succeed, organization must treat employees in an ethical fashion. Every organization is required to establish codes of ethics, publicized statements of ethical values, provided ethics training, rewarded employees for notable ethical behavior, publicized positive role models and set up internal procedures to handle misconduct.

Organizational Culture—An organizations culture stems from "the shared beliefs and values that influence the behavior of organizational members". Every organization has a different culture. The culture also encourages direct communications with any other employee no matter what level on the organization chart they are. Other company's cultures may expect employees to only do their job and not give input at all.

Diversity—Organizations which do not have a culture of encouraging diversity are at a decided disadvantage. Some organizations are even going to the extreme of trying to eliminate all subcultures and become truly multicultural. "The multicultural organization is a firm that values diversity but systematically works to block the transfer of societally based subcultures into the fabric of the organization".

Communication—Two types of organizational communication exist: formal and informal. Organizations of all sizes make use of both, whether directly or indirectly. Formal channels of communication generally follow the chain of command or organizational chart and are top down. Informal channels on the other hand tend to be more open and spontaneous. Gossip is also considered forms informal organizational communication. Many small companies rely more on informal communications channels. Small organizations by and large adhere less to formal command structures and all employees are generally more active in feedback and decision making.

Organizational Effectiveness and Efficiency—Organizational effectiveness measures how well an organization is in sync. Even with the best management, superior strategy and flawless execution an organization can be less successful than it could be. Organizations who understand employees as partners stand as much better chance of achieving high organizational effectiveness and efficiency. "Organizational effectiveness is about each individual doing everything they know how to do and doing it well. Smaller organizations should exhibit more organizational efficiency due to less bureaucratic management. This is not always the case as smaller organizations oftentimes have less clear strategic goals and incomplete systems. Smaller organizations tend to not have as many mature systems in place for employees. This creates inefficiency as several, and oftentimes conflicting, methods are created by employees and not management. These systems may also conflict with management's strategic plan.

Organizational Learning—In today's fast paced, global business environment, organizations need to adapt quickly to threats and opportunities. How an organization learns directly affects the speed and efficiency of an organization to handle opportunities and threats., "A Learning Organization" is one in which people at all levels, individually and collectively, are continually increasing their capacity to produce results they really care about" .

Motivation in organizations—"Motivation is the forces either internal or external to a person that arouse enthusiasm and resistance to pursue a certain course of action."Although motivation is a broad and complex concept, organizational scientists have agreed on its basic characteristics. Drawing from various social sciences, we define *motivation* as, "the set of processes that arouse, direct, and maintain human behavior toward attaining some goal".

Organization Development (OD)—The systematic application of behavioral science knowledge at various levels, such as group, inter-group, organization, etc. to bring about planned change. Its' objectives is a higher quality of work-life, productivity, adaptability and effectiveness. It accomplishes this by changing attitudes, behaviors, values, strategies, procedures and structures so that the organization can adapt to competitive actions, technological advances and the fast pace of change within the environment.

Characteristics of Organizational Behavior

Newstrom, Davis, 1993 described characteristics
- Humanistic Values: Positive beliefs about the potential of employees (McGregor's Theory)

- Systems Orientation: All parts of the organization, to include structure, technology, and people, must work together
- Experiential Learning: The learner's experiences in the training environment should be the kind of human problems they encounter at work. The training should not be all theory and lecture
- Problem-Solving: Problems are identified, data is gathered, corrective action is taken, progress is assessed and adjustments in the problem-solving-process are made as needed. This process is known as Action Research
- Contingency Orientation: Actions are selected and adapted to fit the need
- Change Agent: Stimulate, facilitate and coordinate change
- Levels of Interventions: Problems can occur at one or more level in the organization so the strategy will require one or more interventions.

Elements of organizational Behavior

The organization's base rests on management's Philosophy, values, vision and goals. This in turn drives the organizational culture which is composed of the formal organization, informal organization and the social environment. The culture determines the type of leadership, communication and group dynamics within the organization. The workers perceive this as the quality of work life which directs their degree of motivation. The final outcome are performance, individual satisfaction and personal growth and development. All these elements combine to build the model or framework that the organization operates.

Need /Aims

- If people are in organizations, most important asset then understanding how humans behave in organizations will improve productivity
- Understanding OB allows better worker relations, more realistic expectations and improves job satisfaction.

Theories

- **Incentive theory**—A concept of *human resources* or *management* theory. In the corporate sense, it states that firm owners should structure employee compensation in such a way that the employees' goals are aligned with owners' goals. As it applies to the operations of firms, it is more accurately called the *principal-agent problem.*
- **Classical organization theory**—Evolved during the first half of this century. It represents the merger of scientific management, bureaucratic theory and administrative theory.

  Frederick Taylor (1917) developed scientific management theory. His theory had four basic principles:
  - Find the one "best way" to perform each task.
  - Carefully match each worker to each task.
  - Closely supervise workers, and use reward and punishment as motivators.
  - The task of management is planning and control.

  Initially, Taylor was very successful at improving production. His methods involved getting the best equipment and people, and then carefully scrutinizing each component of the production process. By analyzing each task individually, Taylor was able to find the right combinations of factors that yielded large increases in production.
- **Taylor's scientific management theory**—Proved successful in the simple industrialized companies at the turn of the century, it has not faired well in modern companies. The philosophy of "production first, people second" has left a legacy of declining production and quality, dissatisfaction with work, loss of pride in workmanship and a near complete loss of organizational pride. Max Weber (1947) expanded on Taylor's theories and stressed the need to reduce diversity and ambiguity in organizations. The focus was on establishing clear lines of authority and control.
- **Weber's bureaucratic theory**—Emphasized the need for a hierarchical structure of power. It recognized the importance of division of labor and specialization. A formal set of rules was bound into the hierarchy structure to insure stability and uniformity. Weber also put forth the notion that organizational behavior is a network of human interactions, where all behavior could be understood by looking at cause and effect

- **Administrative theory** (i.e., principles of management)—Was formalized in the 1930's by Mooney and Reiley (1931). The emphasis was on establishing a universal set of management principles that could be applied to all organizations.
- **Classical management theory**—Was rigid and mechanistic. The shortcomings of classical organization theory quickly became apparent. Its major deficiency was that it attempted to explain people's motivation to work strictly as a function of economic reward
- **Neoclassical Organization theory**—The human relations movement evolved as a reaction to the tough, authoritarian structure of classical theory. It addressed many of the problems inherent in classical theory. activity, individual growth, and motivation. Neoclassical theory displayed genuine concern for human needs.
- **The Hawthorne experiment**—An organization might continually involve itself in the latest management fads to produce a continuous string of Hawthorne effects. "The result is usually a lot of wheel spinning and cynicism" (Pascale, 1990). Pascale believes that the Hawthorne effect is often misinterpreted. It is a "parable about researchers (and managers) manipulating and 'playing tricks' on employees." Erroneous conclusions are drawn because it represents a controlling and manipulative attitude toward workers
- **Writing in 1939, Barnard (1968)** proposed one of the first **Modern Theories of Organization** by organization as a system of consciously coordinated activities. He stressed in role of the executive in creating an atmosphere where there is coherence of values and purpose. Organizational success was linked to the ability of a leader to create a cohesive environment. He proposed that a manager's authority is derived from subordinates' acceptance, instead of the hierarchical power structure of the organization
- **Barnard's theory contains elements of both classical and neoclassical approaches**—Since there is no consensus among scholars, it might be most appropriate to think of Barnard as a **Transition Theorist.**
- Simon (1945) made an important contribution to the study of organizations when he proposed a model of **"limited Rationality"** to explain the Hawthorne experiments—The theory stated that workers could respond unpredictably to managerial attention. The most important aspect of Simon's work was the rigorous application of the scientific method. Reductionism, quantification and deductive logic were legitimized as the methods of studying organizations.
- **Contingency Theory**—Classical and neoclassical theorists viewed conflict as something to be avoided because it interfered with equilibrium. Contingency theorists view conflict as inescapable, but manageable. Chandler (1962) ideas was that organizations would act in a rational, sequential and linear manner to adapt to changes in the environment. Effectiveness was a function of management's ability to adapt to environmental changes.
- **Lawrence and Lorsch (1969)** studied how organizations adjusted to fit their environment. In highly volatile industries, they noted the importance of giving managers at all levels the authority to make decisions over their domain. Managers would be free to make decisions contingent on the current situation.
- **Systems Theory**—Proposed by Hungarian biologist Ludwig von Bertalanffy in 1928, although it has not been applied to organizations until recently (Kast and Rosenzweig, 1972; Scott, 1981). The foundation of systems theory is that all the components of an organization are interrelated and that changing one variable might impact many others. Organizations are viewed as open systems, continually interacting with their environment. They are in a state of dynamic equilibrium as they adapt to environmental changes.

  Senge (1990) describes systems as: understanding how our actions shape our reality. If I believe that my current state was created by somebody else or by forces outside my control, why should I hold a vision? The central premise behind holding a vision is that somehow I can shape my future, Systems thinking helps us see how our own actions have shaped our current reality, thereby giving us confidence that we can create a different reality in the future.
- **A central theme of systems theory**—is that nonlinear relationships might exist between variables. Small changes in one variable can cause huge changes in another and large changes in a variable might have only a nominal effect on another. The concept of nonlinearity adds enormous complexity to our understanding of organizations. In fact, one of the most salient argument against systems theory is that the complexity introduced by nonlinearity makes it difficult or impossible to fully understand the relationships between variables.

Organizational Structure

Organizations followed Weber's concept of bureaucratic structures. The increased complexity of multinational organizations created the necessity of a new structure that Drucker (1974) called "federal decentralization". In federal decentralization, a company is organized so that there are a number of independent units operating simultaneously. "Each unit has its own management which, in effect, runs its own autonomous business." This structure has resulted in large conglomerates which have diversified into many different fields in order to minimize risk. The project management organizational structure has been used effectively in highly dynamic and technological environments (French, Kast and Rosenzweig, 1985). The project manager becomes the focal point for information and activities related to a specific project. The goal is to provide effective integration of an organization's resources towards the completion of a specific project. Implementing a project management approach often involves dramatic changes in the relationships of authority and responsibility.

The matrix organizational structure evolved from the project management form (Kolodny, 1979). It represents a compromise between the traditional bureuacratic approach and the autonomous project management approach. A matrix organization has permanently established departments that provide integration for project management. The matrix form is superimposed on the hierarchical structure, resulting in dual authority and responsibilities. Permanent functionality departments allocate resources to be shared among departments and managers.

Systems theory views organizational structure as the "established pattern of relationships among the parts of the organization" (French, Kast and Rosenzweig, 1985), of particular importance are the patterns in relationships and duties. These include themes of 1) integration (the way activities are coordinated), 2) differentiation (the way tasks are divided), 3) the structure of the hierarchical relationships (authority systems) and 4) the formalized policies, procedures and controls that guide the organization (administrative systems).

The relationship between the environment and organizational structure is especially important. Organizations are open systems and depend on their environment for support. Generally, more complex environments lead to greater differentiation. The trend in organizations is currently away from stable (mechanistic) structures to more adaptive (organic) structures. The advantage is that organizations become more dynamic and flexible. The disadvantage is that integration and coordination of activities require more time and effort.

The relationship between an organization and its environment is characterized by a two-way flow of information and energy. Most organizations attempt to influence their environment. Advertising campaigns and lobbying efforts are two examples. Some theorists believe that "environments are largely invented by organizations themselves. Organizations select their environments from ranges of alternatives, then they subjectively perceive the environments they inhabit" (Starbuck, 1976). Strategic decisions regarding product lines and distribution channels contribute to the selection of the organizational structure and the environment. It is a commonly held tenant that people are less satisfied with their work in highly structured organizations. Older (i.e., larger) organizations have become more rigid in their ways and they are less able to adapt to change. Another popular theory is that in larger organizations, workers' jobs become more specialized. The lack of variety creates a less motivating environment. Other theories have proposed that excessive size creates crippling coordination problems (Filley and Aldag, 1980; Zald and Ash, 1966).

Organizational Birth and Growth

The first stage in organizational growth is "**entrepreneurial**", characterized by early innovation, niche formation and high creativity. The entrepreneur is convinced that their idea for a product or service is needed and wanted in the marketplace. The common characteristic of all entrepreneurs and new businesses is the desire to find a pattern of operation that will survive in the marketplace. Nearly all new businesses fail within the first five years. the entrepreneurial stage involves a series of trial and error endeavours. This is followed by a stage of "**collectivity**", where there is high cohesion and commitment among the members, organizational growth is characterized by a complete reversal in strategy. The next stage is one of "**formalization and control**", where the goals are stability and institutionalization. The last stage is one of "**elaboration**", characterized by domain expansion and decentralization. The striking feature of these life-cycle models is that they did not include any notion of organizational decline. They covered birth, growth, and maturity, but none included decline or death. The classic S-curve typifies these life-cycle models.

Land and Jarman (1992) have attempted to redefine the traditional S-curve that defines birth, growth, and maturity. The second phase in Where the next stage is the standardization of rules that define how the organizational system operates and interacts with the environment. The chaotic methods of the entrepreneur are replaced with structured patterns of operation. Internal processes are regulated and uniformity is sought. During this phase, growth actually occurs by limiting diversity. "Management procedures, processes and controls are geared to maintain order and predictability" (Land and Jarman, 1992)

Organizational growth does not continue indefinitely. An upper asymptopic limit can be imposed by a number of factors. Land and Jarman (1992) identify the most common reasons why organizations reach upper growth limits:

- Rapidly increasing a product proliferation and market divisions
- Internal competition for resources
- Increasing cost of manufacturing and sales
- Diminishing returns
- Declining share of the market
- Decreasing productivity gains
- Growing external pressures from regulators and influence groups
- Increasing impact of new technologies
- New and unexpected competitors.

"The organization must open up to permit what was never allowed in to become a part of the system, not only by doing things differently, but by doing different things" (Land and Jarman, 1992). The organization needs to continue its core business, while at the same time engaging in inventing new business. This bifurcation is necessary because the entrepreneurial environment (of inventing business) is incompatible with the controlling environment of the core business.

The goal is a continuing integration of the new inventions into the mainstream business, where a recreated organization emerges. The core business is changed by the inventions it assimilates, and the organization takes on a new form.

There are several factors that contribute to organizational growth (Child and Kieser, 1981). The most obvious is that growth is a by product of another successful strategy. A second factor is that growth is deliberately sought because it facilitates management goals, e.g. it provides increased potential for promotion, greater challenge, prestige and earning potential. A third factor is that growth makes an organization less vulnerable to environmental consequences. Larger organizations tend to be more stable and less likely to go out of business (Caves, 1970; Marris and Wood, 1971; Singh, 1971). Increased resources make diversification feasible, thereby adding to the security of the organization.

Child and Kieser (1981) suggest four distinct operational models for organizational growth.

1. Growth can occur within an organization's existing domain. This is often manifest as a striving for dominance within its field.
2. Growth can occur through diversification into new domains. Diversification is a common strategy for lowering overall risk and new domains often provide fertile new markets.
3. Technological advancements can stimulate growth by providing more effective methods of production.
4. Improved managerial techniques can facilitate an atmosphere that promotes growth.

    Organizational growth was an indicator of successful management.

Organizational Decline

Kenneth Boulding (1950) proposed a biological model of economics, characterized by birth, maturation, decline and death. He argued that in all organisms, there is an "inexorable and irreversible movement towards the equilibrium of death."

The 1980's ushered in a new era where organizational decline was apparent everywhere. Management strategies involved reducing employees, salary freezes and reductions, cutting administrative overhead and consolidating operations.

Decline is 'a decrease in profit or budget. Most theorists agree that decline negatively impacts individuals and the organization as a whole'. Cameron, Whetten and Kim (1987) argue that decline results in decreased morale, innovativeness, participation, leader influence and long-term planning. They associate decline with, conflict, secrecy, rigidity, centralization, formalization, scapegoating and conservatism.

Nystrom and Starbuck (1984) attribute organizational decline to over-confidence. According to this theory, a successful past can lure an organization to become over-confident in its ability to prosper. This leads to a attitude towards new innovations, quality and customer satisfaction.

Another theory is that large size promotes rigidity, which makes it cumbersome for an organization to respond to environmental changes (Whetten, 1987).

Bibeault (1982) proposed a four-stage model to describe the process of turning around an organization in decline. The key to the process was to replace the top personnel.
- Change in management
- Evaluation stage
- Implementing emergency actions and stabilization procedures
- A return to growth.

Zammuto and Cameron (1985) model was based on the idea that turn around could be accomplished by addressing five process domains.
- The defense domain involves strategies for protecting the organization from a hostile environment, e.g. an organization that forms a common-purpose coalition with other organizations
- The offense domain involves expanding on the activities that the organization already does well
- Creating new domains consists of diversification activities
- The consolidation domain involves reducing the scope of activities by cutting back to core products and services
- The substitution domain involves replacing one set of activities with another.

The most common response to organizational decline is retrenchment. Whetten (1987) identifies three sequential stages involved in the process.
- Identification: Management must be sensitive to problems when they first appear and be able to meet the problems head on.
- Communication: Management must communicate a clear message of the organization's situation and instill confidence in its ability to meet the crisis.
- It involves the implementation of a downsizing program.

Sutton (1983) surveyed managers to examine their beliefs regarding how employees would react to an organizational closing. It was found that managers had several inaccurate perceptions

The Learning Organization

Peter Senge (1990) defines learning as enhancing ones capacity to take action. So learning organizations are organizations that are continually enhancing their capacity to create.

Senge (1990) believes that new organizations can be built by adopting a set of disciplines, where a discipline is defined as a "particular theory, translated into a set of practices, which one spends one's life mastering." Thus, mastering a discipline becomes a life-long learning process.

According to Senge, there are five disciplines important to the learning organization.
1. "Building a shared vision". "Building" involves an ongoing process and "shared" implies that the vision is held in common by individuals.
2. "Personal mastery" demonstrates a commitment to the vision.
3. involves the idea of mental models, where we construct internal representations of reality. An important element of using mental models is the need to balance inquiry and advocacy.
4. Shared mental models are important for organizational learning.
5. A commitment to a systems approach.

Classical organization theory—Bureaucracy, Power and Control

Bureaucratic administration means fundamentally the exercise of control on the basis of knowledge (Weber, 1947). For the sociologist, power is principally exemplified within organizations by the process of control. Max Weber distinguished between authority and power by defining the latter as any relationship within which one person could impose his will, regardless of any resistance from the other, whereas authority existed when there was a belief in the legitimacy of that power.

Weber classified organizations according to the nature of that legitimacy
- Charismatic authority, based on the sacred or outstanding characteristic of the individual
- Traditional authority, essentially a respect for custom
- Rational legal authority, which was based on a code or set of rules

According to Weber rational legal authority is attained through the most efficient form of organization: bureaucracy. He argued that managers should not rule through arbitrary personal whim but by a formal system of rules. He listed the beliefs which underlie rational legal authority:
- A legal code can be established which can claim obedience from members of the organization
- The law is a system of abstract rules which are applied to particular cases; and administration looks after the interests of the organization within the limits of that law
- The person exercising authority also obeys this impersonal order
- Only through being a member does the member obey the law
- Obedience is due not to the person who holds the authority but to the impersonal order which has granted him this position.

Weber is usually described as having believed that bureaucracy is the most efficient form of organization. In fact, Weber believed bureaucracy to be the most formally rational form of organization. As such, Weber conceived of bureaucracy as being more effective than alternative forms. In his day administration was based on written documents. This tended to make the office (bureau) the focus of organization. He did not share the modern conception of a bureaucratic organization as being slow, rigid and inefficient. His primary concern was to establish ways of behaving which avoided the corruption, unfairness and nepotism characterizing most 19th century organizations. Based on his ideas concerning the legitimacy of power

Weber outlined the characteristics of bureaucracy in its purest form.
- A continuous organization of official functions bound by rules'
- Specialization: Each office has a defined sphere of competence, involving division of labor. The tasks of the organization are divided into distinct functions given to separate offices. These functions are clearly specified so that the staff know exactly what is expected of them. Job-holders are given the authority necessary to carry out their roles.
- A clearly defined hierarchy of offices: A firm system of supervision based on clear levels of authority. Each official knows whom to report to with specified rights of control and complaint procedures.
- Rules: A stable, comprehensive system of conduct which can be learned and may require technical qualifications to understand and administer.
- Impersonality: No hatred or passion with equality of treatment for all clients of the organization. Staff members are free of any external responsibilities and constraints. They are able to attend to their duties in a fair and objective way.
- Free selection of appointed officials: on the basis of professional qualifications, with proof shown by a diploma of degree gained through examinations. They are selected and appointed rather than elected so that there is no question of bias or favor.
- Full-time paid officials: Usually paid on the basis of hierarchical rank, the office being their sole or major concern. Officials are appointed on the basis of a contract. They have a monetary salary and usually pension rights. The salary is graded according to the position in the hierarchy. The officers can leave their posts and under certain circumstances employment can be terminated.
- Career officials: There is a career structure and a system of promotion based on seniority or merit based on the judgment of superiors.
- Private/public split: Separates business and private life. The official works in a detached fashion from the ownership of the organization. The finances and interests of the two should be kept firmly apart: the resources of the organization are quite distinct from those of the members as private individuals. Officials may appropriate neither posts nor the resources which go with them. A radical notion at a time when bribery was the norm and officials regularly took a cut of any fee or payment due to their office.
- There is a strict, systematic discipline and control of the official's work.

Despite being based on the idea of formal rationality, Weber's concepts were idealistic. He believed that bureaucratic control would lead to a number of social consequences.

- A tendency to a levelling of the social classes by allowing a wide range of recruits with technical competence to be taken by any organization
- Plutocracy, because of the time required to achieve the necessary technical training;
- Greater degree of social equality due to the dominance of the spirit of impersonality or objectivity.

QUESTIONS

- Attitude Change (5M, NTRUHS, July, 2008)
- Barriers of developing I.P.R with adolescents (5M, RGUHS, Feb, 2010)
- Define inter personal relationship, Explain the phases of IPR, Barriers of IPR (2+8+5=15M, NTRUHS, Nov. 2010)
- Discuss Human Relation in context of Nursing, explain methods of overcoming barriers in Interpersonal Relationships (8M + 8M, Rajasthan UHS, Feb, 2010)
- Discuss the barriers to interpersonal communication and the methods to overcome them in the context of dealing with patients and their families (10M, NIMS, May, 2008)
- Discuss the factors influencing healthy behaviour (10M, RGUHS, May, 2010 and 10M, NTRUHS, July, 2008)
- Discuss the importance of Human Relations (10M, Rajasthan UHS, March, 2010)
- Explain how will you establish effective interpersonal relations with patient, families and co-workers in context of nursing (10M, RGUHS, Sept, 2009)
- Explain Johari window and its use in improving IPR in Nursing Practice (5 + 5 M, Baba Farid UHS, 2008)
- Explain the methods of overcoming barriers in Interpersonal Relations in context of Nursing? (10M, Rajasthan UHS, March, 2010)
- Explain the strategies to develop effective human relations in the context of Nursing (10M, NIMS, May, 2008)
- Explain the term "Public relations", How would you establish and Maintain Public relations in the Community (15 M, RGUHS, May, 2010)
- Human Relations in Nursing (7.5 Baba Farid UHS, 2010 &5M, NIMS, Dec, 2009)
- Importance of Team Work in Nursing(5M, RGUHS, Aug, 2010)
- Interpersonal Model (5M, RGUHS, 1997; 5M, GULBU, 2001; 5M, NTRUHS, 2001)
- Interpersonal relationship with patients (15M, NTRUHS, June, 2009)
- Introspection (5M, NTRUHS, June, 2009)
- Johari Window (7.5M, Baba Farid UHS, Punjab, 2010; 5M, NIMS, May, 2010)
- Justify the importance of public relations in hospital administration (10M, RGUHS, Oct, 2009)
- Phases of Interpersonal Relationship (4M, NIMS, Dec, 2009 and 10M, Baba Farid UHS, 2010)
- Public relation in context of Nursing (5M, NTRUHS, Nov, 2010)
- Public relations (10M, RGUHS, May, 2006)
- Public relations in Nursing (5M, NIMS, April, 2008)
- Social behaviour (5M, Baba Farid UHS, 2009)
- Social behavior among nursing students—explain (5M, NTRUHS, June, 2010)
- What are the barriers of interpersonal relations and explain how to overcome such barriers? (5M, NTRUHS, June, 2010)
- What are the biological bases of Motivation, bring out its relation with Learning (15M, NTRUHS, July, 2008).

Bibliography

1. Abel WM, Freeze M. Evaluation of concept mapping in an associate degree Nursing program. Journal of Nursing Education 2006;45(9): 356-64.
2. Andrews PV, Schwarz J, Helme RD. Students can learn medicine with computers. Med J Aust 1992.
3. Angelo T. Classroom assessment and research: An update on uses, approaches and research findings, 1998.
4. Asgari Jirhandeh N, Haywood J. Computer awareness amongst medical students: a survey. Med Educ 1997;31:225-31.
5. 5. Au W Unequal by design: High-stakes testing and the standardization of inequality. Routledge: London 2008.
6. Azarmsa R. Educational computing: Principles and applications. Englewood Cliffs, NJ: Educational Technology Publications 1991.
7. Basavanthappa BT. Nursing Education. 1st Edition, Jaypee Brothers Medical Publishers (P) Ltd, New Delhi, India 2003;68-70,71-5.
8. Basavantappa BT. Communication and Education Technology for Nurses. Jaypee Brothers Medical Publishers (P) Ltd, New Delhi, 2010.
9. Basavanthappa BT: Nursing Administration. Jaypee Brothers Publishers (P) Ltd, New Delhi. 2003; 152-8.
10. Berkow R etal. The Merck Manual of Medical Information. Merck & Co., NJ, Whitehouse Station: 2001.
11. Berlo DK. The process of communication. Holt, Rinehart & Winston, New York. 1960, 24.
12. Berscheid E, Peplau LA The emerging science of relationships. 1983
13. Bettinghaus EP. Health promotion and the knowledge–attitude–behaviour continuum. 1986, Prev Med. 15:475–91.
14. Bhatia and Craig. Elements of psychology and mental hygiene for nurses in India. 2nd edition, university press private limited, hyd. 1998, 32-34.
15. Biggs JC. Teaching for Quality Learning at University. 2nd edition. Open University Press, Berkshire. 2003.
16. Bion WR. Experiences in Groups. Tavistock.1989.
17. Black, et al. Administrative Intervention: A Discipline Handbook for Effective School Administrators. Colorado. 1992.
18. Brandt RC et al. Flip charts: How to draw them and how to use them. Richmond, VA, 1986.
19. Brian Myers, et al. A publication of the Agricultural Education and Communication Department; 2009.
20. Brian Myers. Bridging the language barrier - School of Teaching and Learning. University of Florida, Gainesville, FL 32611, 2010.
21. Brodinsky Ben. Student Discipline: Problems and Solutions. American Association of School Administrators Critical Issues Report, California 1980.
22. Brookfield SD. The skillful teacher: On technique, trust, and responsiveness in the classroom. Jossey-Bass: San Francisco; 1990.
23. Brown E, Gibbs G, Glover C. Evaluation tools for assessing the impact of assessment regimes on student learning; 2003.
24. Brown, JS et al. Situated cognition and the culture of learning. Educational Researcher. 1989;32-42.
25. Bryan C, Clegg K. Innovative Assessment in Higher Education. Routledge; London. 2006.
26. Byrne D. Interpersonal attraction and attitude similarity. Journal of Abnormal and Social Psychology; 1961 62, 713–5.
27. CM Charles. Building Classroom Discipline Sixth Edition. © Allyn & Bacon.1999.
28. Campbell JK, Johnson C. Trend spotting: fashions in Medical Education. Br Med J 1999;318:1272-5.
29. Clayden GS, Wilson B. Computer-assisted learning in Medical Education. Med Educ 1988;456-7.
30. Craig SE, et al. Creating a performance management system. Training and Development Journal. 1986, April: 38-42; May: 74-79.

31. Close relationships. WH Freeman and Company:New York. 1–19.
32. Dale E. Audiovisual Methods in Teaching. 3rd ed Dryden Press:NY; 1969.
33. Davis RH, Alexander LT. Guides for the improvement of instruction in higher education Vol. 4. Effective uses of media. East Lansing, MI: Michigan State University, Instructional Media Center; 1977.
34. De Dombal FT, Hartley JR, Sleeman DA. A compuiter-assisted system for learning clinical diagnosis—Evaluation of a problem-oriented learning;1998.
35. Devitt P, Palmer E. Computers in Medical Education. Aust N Z J Surg 68:284-7.
36. Di Leonardi BC. Tips for Facilitating Learning: The Lecture Deserves Some Respect. The Journal of Continuing Education in Nursing; 2007;38(4), 154-1.
37. Diamond RM. Designing and improving courses and curricula in higher education: A systematic approach. Jossey-Bass, San Francisco 1989.
38. Diane Andrica. Nursing image: our public relations responsibility. Nursing Economics; 2010.
39. Diane M Billings and Judith A. Halstead. Teaching in Nursing A guide for faculty. 3rdEdition, Sunders, Elsevier. 2005, 189-193.
40. Duckworth, Kenneth. School Discipline Policy. A Problem of Balance. Eugene, Oregon: Center for Educational Policy and Management;1984.
41. Duke, Daniel L. School Organization, Leadership, and Student Behavior. In Strategies to Reduce Student Misbehavior. edited by Oliver C. Moles. Washington, DC; Office of Educational Research and Improvement, US Department of Education;1989.
42. Dyer, William. Team Building. 3rd Edition. Prentice Hall; 1994.
43. Einstein, WO, LeMere-Labonte J. Performance appraisal: dilemma or desire? Sam Advanced Management Journal;1989, 54 (2): 26-0.
44. Elizabeth A Franko. Microscopy for Public Health Nurses. Georgia Department of human resources. Division of Public Health;2007.
45. Elwood F Holton, Others. Toward development of a generalized instrument to measure Andragogy;2007.
46. Eugene D Gennaro. The Effectiveness of Using Previsit Instructional Materials on Learning for a Museum Field Trip Experience. Journal of Research in Science Teaching;1981;275–9.
47. Elizabeth Davies. A model for inservice education. The Australian Nurses Journal, Queensland.
48. Facts for life. UNICEF. 2002
49. Feenberg A. The Written World. Mindweave: Communication, Computers, and Distance Education. R. Mason and A. Kaye (Eds). Oxford. Pergamon Press; 1989, 22-9.
50. Fincham FD, Beach, SRH. Toward a positive relationship science. Journal of Family Theory & Review. 2010; 2:4 – 24.
51. Fonteyn M. Concept mapping an easy teaching strategy that contributes to understanding and may improve critical thinking. Nurse Educator; 2007, 46(5). 199-0.
52. Forsyth DR. Group Dynamics. 4th Edition. Belmont, CA: Thomson Wadsworth;2006.
53. Frame, John Christopher. Homeless at Harvard: Street Culture Relationships and a Theology of Relational Care (Thesis, Harvard University Divinity School).
54. Fraser RC. Clinical method. a general practice approach. 3rd edition.
55. Frels, Kelly, others. School Discipline Policies and Procedures: A Practical Guide, Alexandria, Virginia: National School Boards Association; 1990.
56. Freud, Sigmund. Group Psychology and the Analysis of the Ego. New York: Liveright Publishing company; 1922.
57. Gable S L, Reis HT. Capitalizing on Positive Events in an Interpersonal Context. Advances in Experimental Social Psychology; 2010; 42, 195-257.
58. Garrud P, others. Non-verbal communication: evaluation of a computer assisted learning package. Med Educ; 27:474 - 8.
59. Gaustad, Joan. Schools Respond to Gangs and Violence. OSSC Bulletin. Eugene, Oregon: Oregon School Study Council;1993.
60. Glanz K, Lewis, Others: Health Behavior and Health Education: Theory Research and Practice. San Francisco, CA. Jossey-Bass Publishers; 1997.

61. Graeff JA, others. Communication for Health and Behavior Change: A Developing Country Perspective". San Francisco, CA: Jossey-Bass Publishers; 1993.
62. Hase, Others. The Johari Window and the Dark Side of Organisations. Southern Cross University; 1999.
63. Health Metrics Network. WHO. Components of a strong Health Information system Mastering Human Relations. A Falikowski . Pearson Education; 2002.
64. Hildegard E. Peplau. Interpersonal Relations in Nursing, A conceptual frame of reference for Psychodynamic Nursing; 1999.
65. Hill C: Integrating clinical experiences into the concept mapping process. Nurse Educator; 2006; 31(1), 36-9.
66. Homans GC. Social Behavior- Its Elementary Forms. Rev. Ed. New York. Harcourt Brace Jovanovich; 1974.
67. HortonW, Horton K: E-learning tools and technologies: A consumer's guide for trainers, teachers, educators and instructional designers. Indianapolis: John Wiley & Sons; 2003.
68. Humanism in Nursing: contradictions and conflicts. J Adv Nurs; 1995 Nov;22(5): 1995, 979-4. England
69. Bonnie W Duldt-Battey. Humanism, Nursing, Communication, And Holistic Care Bellflower Drive Antioch, California
70. Houghton Mifflin Company. Stanford University: Active learning: Getting students to work and think in the classroom.Speaking of Teaching. Stanford University; 1993.
71. Importance of a Nursing Education|eHow.com; 2008.
72. Sriyan de Silva. International Labour Organisation Collective Bargaining Negotiations Act/Emp Publications; 1996.
73. Irby DM. Three exemplary models of case-based teaching; 1994.
74. Jones, John E. A model of group development. Journal of Research in Science Teaching. Annual Handbook for Group Facilitators. University Associates: La Jolla, CA; 1973, 275–279.
75. Joyce Margulies: Performance Appraisals, Archer North & Associatiates,1998.
76. Jung CG.. Two Essays on Analytical Psychology. Collected Works, Volume 7, Princeton, NJ: Princeton University Press; 1966.
77. Jung CG. Psychological Types, Collected Works. Volume 6, Princeton, NJ: Princeton University Press, 1971.
78. Moser K. Ten Tips for a Successful Field Trip Teaching K–8; 44–5.
79. Kathleen B.Amman Gaberson Adult Learning, Principles, applications for preceptor programs. AORN Journal. April 1987. Vol.45. No.4
80. Kelly, Anita E, McKillop, Kevin J: Consequences of Revealing Personal Secrets; 1996.
81. Khadra MH, Guinea AI, Hill DA: The acceptance of computer assisted learning by medical students. Aust N Z J Surg. 1995.
82. Kidd MR. What do medical students know about computers? 1993.
83. Kroeger L. Choose the visual-Aids medium carefully. Prentice Hall of fame, New Delhi; 1998, 129-135.
84. Kroeger L. using visual aids & Machinery, The complete Idiot's guide to successful business presentation, prentice Hall of fame, New Delhi; 1998, 239-247.
85. L. Cullen, L Whitaker: Making the Most of Field Trips; 2004,163:26. 54.
86. Laboratory equipments and articles. Indian Nursing Council. Combined council building, kotla road, temple lane, New Delhi - 110002.
87. Le Bon G: The Crowd: A Study of the Popular Mind. London: Ernest Benn Limited; 1896.
88. Learn Med: 2000,12:91-5.
89. Levinger G: Development and change. In H. H. Kelley, et al. (Eds), Close relationships. (315–9). New York: W. H. Freeman and Company; 1983.
90. Lewin K. Frontiers in group dynamics, Human Relations; 1947;1:5-1.
91. Luft J, Ingham H. The Johari window, a graphic model of interpersonal awareness. Proceedings of the western training laboratory in group development (Los Angeles: UCLA); 1955.
92. Luft, Joseph. Of Human Interaction, Palo Alto, CA:National Press; 1969.
93. Lynn Cohen. How to Run First-Rate Field Trips. Instructor-Intermediate; 1988, 85, (107) 6, .
94. Mangione S, Others: Comparison of computer-based learning and seminar teaching of pulmonary auscultation to first-year medical students. Acad Med; 1992;67:S63-65.

95. Maniaci MR, Reis HT. The Marriage of Positive Psychology and Relationship Science; 2010.
96. McKeachie WJ. Teaching tips: A guidebook for the beginning college teacher. 8th ed; 1986.
97. Lansing M Prescott. Microbiology, 6th Edition.
98. Tortora Gerard J. Microbiology An introduction. 2nd Edition.
99. Rajeshwar ReddyK. Microbiology and Parasitology. 3rd Edition.
100. MIT Human Resources, Creating an Effective Employee Performance Management System.
101. Monga ML. Management of Performance Appraisal. Bombay: Himalaya Publishing House; 1983.
102. Myers DG. Social psychology. New York: McGraw Hill. 1993; 116.
103. National Disaster Management guidelines, Psycho Social support and Mental Health services in Disasters., Dec 2009. National Disaster.
104. Neeraja KP. Essentials of Mental Health and Psychiatric Nursing. Vol.1, Jaypee brothers and Medical Publishers (P) Ltd. New Delhi; 2008, 304-9.
105. Neeraja K P. Text Book of Sociology for Nursing students. Jaypee brothers and Medical Publishers (P) Ltd. New Delhi; 2005, 100-5.
106. Neeraja KP. Text Book of Community Health Nursing–II. (MPHWM). State Institute of Vocational Education. Hyderabad; 2001, 322-2.
107. Newble D, Cannon R: A handbook for teach-ers in universities and colleges: A guide to improving teaching methods (4th ed.). New York, NY: Taylor & Francis Group; 2000.
108. Newby TJ, others. Instructional technology for teaching and learning: Designing instruction, integrating comput-ers, and using media. 2nd ed. Upper Saddle River, NJ: Prentice Hall Career & Technology. 1999.
109. Nursing and Midwifery Council. The Code of Professional Conduct: standards for conduct, performance and ethics. NMC, London; 2004.
110. Patricia Kelly-Heidenthal. Nursing Leadership & Management, PPS. Delmar Learning, a Thomson Learning company; 2003.
111. Oberg W. Make performance appraisal relevant. Harvard Business Review; 1972.
112. David S Walonick. Barnard C. Organizational Theory and Behaviour. The Functions of the Executive. Cambridge. Harvard University Press. 1968.
113. Park K. Park's Text book of Preventive and Social Medicine. 20th edition. M/s Banarsidas, Bhanot Publishers. Jabalpur; 2009.
114. Patten TH. A Manager's Guide to Performance Appraisal. London: Free Press; 1982.
115. Paulsen MF. Moderating Educational Computer Conferences. Computer-mediated communication and the on-line classroom in Distance Education. Cresskill, NJ: Hampton Press. 1995.
116. Peck MS. The Different Drum: Community-Making and Peace; 1987, 95-103.
117. Pettersson R. Visuals for information: Research and practice. Englewood Cliffs, NJ: Educational Technology Publications; 1989.
118. Polyakov A, Others. Clinicians and computers; friends or foes. Teach; 1989.
119. Power F Clark, Hart, Stuart N. The Way Forward to Constructive Child Discipline, in Hart, Stuart N (ed.), Eliminating Corporal Punishment: The Way Forward to Constructive Child Discipline. Paris: UNESCO Publishing; 2005.
120. Ojomo W Olusegun . Principles and Practice of Public Relations. National Open University of Nigeria. Victoria Island, Lagos.
121. Prochaska JO: Systems of Psychotherapy: a Transtheoretical Analysis. Pacific, CA:Brooks-Cole; 1979.
122. Prochaska JO, DiClemente CC: Transtheoretical therapy toward a more integrative model of change. Psychotherapy Theory, Research and Practice; 1982, 19(3), 276-7.
123. Prochaska JO, Norcross JC, DiClemente CC: Changing for Good. New York, NY: William Morrow. Psychological Bulletin; 1994, v120(3), 450.
124. Rao TV. Performance Appraisal Theory and Practice. New Delhi: Vikas Publishing House; 1985.
125. Margaret A Richardson. Recruitment Strategies Managing/Effecting The Recruitment Process Government of the Republic of Trinidad and Tobago.
126. Resolving Social Conflicts: Selected Papers on Group Dynamics. Harper & Row: New York; 1948.
127. Roan, Shari. Our secrets are spilling out all over, Los Angeles Times; 1996.

128. Rooda LA. Effects of mind mapping on student achievement in a Nursing research course. Nurse educator, 1994, 19[6], 25-27.

129. Ruchi Sachdeva: Barriers & Gateways In Communication.

130. Rumar S teaching learning Medie: The means to an end, Medical Education Principles & Practice, 2nd edition, 64-1.

131. S Martin, R Seevers: A Field Trip Planning Guide for Early Childhood Classes - Preventing School Failure. 47:4 2003, 177-180.

132. Saha TK & Bhatnnagar R. Audio-Visual Aids, workshop on lecture-A tool for Medical Teaching. Dept of Medical Education, AFMC, Pune; 2000.

133. Schermerhorn JR. Teaching material M.Sc. Psychology, Institute of Distance Education, University of Madras, Chennai; 2005.

134. Schuler, Randall S. Personnel and Human Resource Management. Third Edition; 1987.

135. Schutz W. A Three-Dimensional Theory of Interpersonal Behavior. New York: Holt, Rinehart & Winston; 1958.

136. Snyder CR, Lopez, Shane J. Positive psychology: the scientific and practical explorations of human strengths, Thousand Oaks, California: Sage Publications, 2007, 297–1.

137. Sujayalakshmi. Concept Mapping, Nursing Times. New Delhi. 2010.

138. Sujayalakshmi. Clickers in Nursing Education: Nursing Times. New Delhi. 2009.

139. Susskind JE. Power in the classroom: Enhancing students, self-efficacy and attitudes. Computers & Education; 2005, 45, 203-5.

140. The Council on Ethical and Judicial Affairs. Policy Compendium of the American Medical Association. Chicago: American Medical Association; 1999.

141. The Microscope – A practical guide by World Health Organization; 1999

142. The role of education in promoting creativity: potential barriers and enabling factors-Pasi Sahlberg-European Training Foundation at scribd.com

143. The Theory and Practice of Group Psychotherapy, third edition, Basic Books, hardback; 1985, ISBN 0-465-08447-8.

144. Thomas F Patterson: Refining Performance Appraisal; 1987.

145. Topping KJ. Trends in Peer Learning. Educational Psychology; 2005, 25 (6), 631-5.

146. Tuckman B. Developmental sequence in small groups. Psychological bulletin 63; 1965, 384-9.

147. US Department of the Interior, Performance Appraisal Handbook.

148. Vidushi Kanwar. Barriers To Communication, Presented at scribd.com.

149. Virginia 1 Rockwell. Better patient care through inservice education, AORN Journal, NY

150. WJ Krepel, CR Duvall. Field trips: A guide for planning and conducting educational experiences. Washington, D.C. National Education Association; 1981.

151. Weber, Max : The Theory of Social and Economic Organization. Translated by A. M. Henderson & Talcott Parsons, The Free Press; 1947.

152. White, Lois. Foundations of Nursing: Caring for the Whole Person. Albany, NY: Delmar Thomson Learning; 2001.

153. Wilma G van. An instrument for reviewing the effectiveness of HE & Health Promotion". "Patient Education and Counselling, Driel; 1996.

154. Wray etal. Fundamentals of Human Relations: Applications for Life and Work. Cincinnati, OH: Southwestern Publishing; 1996.

155. Yeolekar M. Teaching Learning Methodologies. The Art of Teaching Medical Students; 1998, 8-12.

156. RGUHS, B.Sc (N) syllabus. Revised ordinance governing B.Sc (N) (Basic) Degree course regulations and curricula. Bangaluru; 2006 and 2009.

157. NTRUHS, Hand book for students, B.Sc (N) course (4 YDC) vijayawada; 2007-08.

158. Diploma in General Nursing and Midwifery training programme syllabus; 2006.

WEBSITES

http://www.performance-appraisal.com/intro.htm

http://en.wikipedia.org/wiki/Interpersonal_relationship

http://novaonline.nvcc.edu/eli/spd110td/interper/relations/relations.html

http://www.pmhut.com/creating-an-effective-employee-performance-management-system. http://classes.aces.uiuc.edu/ACES100/Mind/c-m2.html

http://www-personal.umich.edu/~jmargeru/conceptmap/types.htm

http://www.joe.org/joe/1987winter/a5.html.

http://www.bnabooks.com/ababna/eeo/2004/eeo55.pdf.

http://www.strategic-human-resource.com/performance-appraisal-methods.html

http://www.definitionofwellness.com/dictionary/health-behavior.html

http://www.infosihat.gov.my/artikelHP/bahanrujukan/HEam/Health%20Behaviour.pdf

http://en.wikipedia.org/wiki/Objective_structured_clinical_examination

OSCE http://vig.pearsoned.co.uk/catalog/uploads/Bloomfield%20-%20Chapter%202.pdf

http://www.ukzn.ac.za/musiced/general_principles_of_education.htm

http://en.wikipedia.org/wiki/Compact_Cassette

http://en.wikipedia.org/wiki/VCR

http://en.wikipedia.org/wiki/Gramophone_record

http://en.wikipedia.org/wiki/Tape_recorder

http://www.ehow.com/about_5316664_importance-nursing-education.html#ixzz0zVHkjrdP

http://www.tutorvista.com/content/math/statistics-and-probability/graphical-representation/bar-graphs-animation.php

http://www.tutorvista.com/content/math/statistics-and-probability/graphical-representation/graphical-representationindex.php

http://www.usask.ca/education/coursework/mcvittiej/methods/fieldtrip.htmlHelathypeople.gov.

http://712educators.about.com/od/teacherresources/a/field_trips.htm

Newsletter on Teaching, 5(1), 1-4.

http://ctl.stanford.edu/Newsletter/active_learning.pdf.

Bob." How Paging and Intercoms work over the network http://www.imakenews.com/kin2/e_article000855106.cfm?x=b8v5FDQ,b25tl0b3,w

http://www.vocalist.org.uk/equipment_maintenance.html

How do I use a computer in medical and nursing education? |

http://www.answerbag.com/q_view/1867586

http://www.sci.brooklyn.cuny.edu/~marciano/detailExp.html

http://www.nald.ca/connect/v5i1/db/lesson1.htm

http://www.stutzfamily.com/mrstutz/eisgeneral/computerparts.html

http://www.businessdictionary.com/definition/career-ladder.html#ixzz18YysK4fJ

http://en.wikipedia.org/wiki/Career_ladder

http://en.wikipedia.org/wiki/Health_education

http://www.nursingcollegemalaysia.com/nursing-opportunities.html

http://www.unesco.org/education/educprog/ste/projects/health/planning.htm#Philosophies of health education

http://www.unesco.org/education/educprog/ste/projects/health/planning.htm#Philosophieof health education

http://www.indiannursingcouncil.org/contact-indian-nursing-council.asp

http://gsociology.icaap.org/ Free Resources for Methods in Program Evaluation

http://gsociology.icaap.org/methods

http://hubpages.com/hub/Types-of-Budgeting

http://www.ehow.com/about_4869424_what-different-types-budgeting.html

http://en.wikipedia.org/wiki/Cost-benefit_analysis

http://www.sjsu.edu/faculty/watkins/cba.htm

NIH (2004). Organizational Effectiveness and Efficiency. Retrieved October 10, 2007, from http://clinicalcenter.nih.gov/about/profile/profile_archives/2004/effectiveness.html

Karash, R. (2002). What is a "Learning Organization". Retrieved October 10, 2007, from http://world.std.com/~lo/en.wikipedia.org/wiki/Organizational_Behavior

http://www.dattnerconsulting.com/presentations/performanceappraisal.pdf

http://www.minurses.org/Labor/benefits.shtml

http://industrialrelations.naukrihub.com/process.html

http://industrialrelations.naukrihub.com/importance-of-collective-bargaining.html

http://en.wikipedia.org/wiki/Collective_bargaining

Positive Discipline: An Approach and a Definition. http://www.brainsarefun.com/Posdis.html.2005

Borgerson, Bruce. 2007." Sound & Video Contractor. 1. 18 Feb. <http://svconline.com/mag/avinstall_pa_sr/index.html>.

http://en.wikipedia.org/wiki/Public_address

http://findarticles.com/p/articles/mi_qa3689/is_199706/ai_n8762766/ Page 194 to 196

Index